Textbook of Stroke Medicine

Edited by

Michael Brainin MD FESO FAHA
Center of Clinical Neurosciences, Danube University, Krems, Austria

Wolf-Dieter Heiss MD
Max Planck Institute for Neurological Research, Cologne, Germany

Editorial Assistant

Susanne Heiss MD

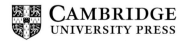

CAMBRIDGE
UNIVERSITY PRESS

CAMBRIDGE UNIVERSITY PRESS
Cambridge, New York, Melbourne, Madrid, Cape Town, Singapore,
São Paulo, Delhi

Cambridge University Press
The Edinburgh Building, Cambridge CB2 8RU, UK

Published in the United States of America by
Cambridge University Press, New York

www.cambridge.org
Information on this title: www.cambridge.org/9780521518260

First published 2010

Printed in the United Kingdom at the University Press, Cambridge

A catalogue record for this publication is available from the British Library

Library of Congress Cataloging-in-Publication Data

Textbook of stroke medicine / edited by Michael Brainin, Wolf-Dieter
Heiss; editorial assistant, Susanne Heiss.
    p. ; cm.
  Includes bibliographical references and index.
  ISBN 978-0-521-51826-0 (hardback)
1. Cerebrovascular disease. I. Brainin, M. (Michael) II. Heiss,
W.-D. (Wolf-Dieter), 1939– III. Heiss, Susanne. IV. Title.
  [DNLM: 1. Stroke. WL 355 T355 2010]
  RC388.5.T42 2010
  616.8′1–dc22
                                                          2009034872

ISBN 978-0-521-51826-0 Hardback

Contents

v

Preface

This book is designed to improve the teaching and learning of stroke medicine in postgraduate educational programs. It is targeted at "beginning specialists", either medical students with a deeper interest or medical doctors entering the field of specialized stroke care. Therefore the text contains what is considered essential for this readership but, in addition, goes into much greater depth, e.g. the coverage of less frequent causes of stroke, and describing the more technical facets and settings of modern stroke care.

The textbook leads the reader through the many causes of stroke, its typical manifestations, and the practical management of the stroke patient. We have tried to keep the clinical aspects to the fore, giving relative weight to those chapters that cover clinically important issues; however, the pathological, pathophysiological and anatomical background is included where necessary. The book benefits from the experience of many specialized authors, thereby providing expert coverage of the various topics by international authorities in the field. In places this leads to some differences of opinion in the approach to particular patients or conditions; as Editors we have tried not to interfere with the individual character of each chapter, leaving only duplicate presentations when they were handled from different topological or didactic aspects, e.g. on genetics or rarer forms of diseases.

The development of this textbook has been triggered by the "European Master in Stroke Medicine Programme" held at Danube University in Austria. This program has been fostered by the European Stroke Organisation and has been endorsed by the World Stroke Organization. This book has been shaped by the experiences of the lecturers – most of them also leading authors for our chapters – and the feedback of our students during several runs of this course. Thus, we hope to satisfy the needs of students and young doctors from many different countries, both within and outside Europe.

Finally, we would like to thank Dr Susanne Heiss for her expert editorial assistance and her diligent and expert help in summarizing the chapters' contents. Thanks also to Nick Dunton and his team at Cambridge University Press for their help and patience.

Michael Brainin
Wolf-Dieter Heiss

Contributors

Gregory W. Albers MD
Department of Neurology,
Stanford University Medical Center,
Stanford, CA, USA

Sylvan J. Albert MD
Department of Neurology and
Neurorehabilitation, Rehabilitation Centre,
Valens, Switzerland

Marta Altieri MD PhD
Department of Neurology,
"Sapienza" University,
Rome, Italy

Eitan Auriel MD
Department of Neurology,
Souraski Medical Center,
Tel-Aviv, Israel

Natan M. Bornstein MD
Department of Neurology,
Souraski Medical Center,
Tel-Aviv, Israel

Michael Brainin MD FESO FAHA
Center of Clinical Neurosciences,
Danube University,
Krems, Austria

Lara Caeiro PhD
Department of Neurosciences,
Hospital de Santa Maria and
Instituto de Medicina Molecular,
University of Lisbon, Lisbon, Portugal

Valeria Caso MD PhD
Stroke Unit, Department of Internal Medicine,
University of Perugia,
Perugia, Italy

László Csiba MD PhD DSc
Department of Neurology,
University Medical School,
Debrecen, Hungary

Hans-Christoph Diener MD PhD FAHA
Department of Neurology,
University of Essen,
Essen, Germany

Raoul Eckhardt MD
Department of Neurology,
Landesklinikum Donauregion Tulln,
Tulln, Austria

José M. Ferro MD PhD
Department of Neurosciences,
Hospital de Santa Maria and Instituto
de Medicina Molecular,
University of Lisbon,
Lisbon, Portugal

Jens Fiehler MD
Klinik und Poliklinik für Neuroradiologische
Diagnostik und Intervention,
Diagnostikzentrum Universitaetsklinikum
Eppendorf, Hamburg, Germany

Josef Finsterer MD PhD
Department of Neurology,
Hospital Rudolfsstiftung,
Vienna, Austria

Wolf-Dieter Heiss MD
Max Planck Institute for Neurological Research,
Cologne, Germany

Konstantin A. Hossmann MD PhD
Max Planck Institute for Neurological Research;
Klaus-Joachim-Zülch-Laboratories of the Max Planck
Society;

Faculty of Medicine of the University of Cologne,
Cologne, Germany

Achim J. Kaasch MD
Institute for Medical Microbiology,
Immunology and Hygiene,
University of Cologne,
Cologne, Germany

Markku Kaste MD PhD FAHA FESO
Department of Neurology,
Helsinki University Central Hospital,
University of Helsinki,
Helsinki, Finland

Jürg Kesselring MD
Department of Neurology and Neurorehabilitation,
Rehabilitation Centre,
Valens, Switzerland

Wilfried Lang MD
Neurologische Abteilung,
KH der Barmherzigen Brüder Wien,
Vienna, Austria

Kennedy R. Lees MD
Division of Cardiovascular and Medical Sciences,
University of Glasgow,
Western Infirmary, Glasgow, UK

Didier Leys MD PhD
Department of Neurology,
University Lille II,
CHU Hopital Roger Salengro,
Lille, France

Markku Mähönen
Department of Public Health,
University of Helsinki, Helsinki, Finland

Isabel P. Martins MD PhD
Department of Neurosciences,
Hospital de Santa Maria and Instituto
de Medicina Molecular,
University of Lisbon,
Lisbon, Portugal

Karl Matz MD
Center of Clinical Neurosciences,
Danube University, Krems, Austria

Patrik Michel MD
Neurology Service, Centre Hospitalier
Universitaire Vaudois,
University of Lausanne,
Lausanne, Switzerland

Bo Norrving MD PhD FESO
Department of Neurology,
University Hospital, Lund, Sweden

Richard O'Brien MBChB MRCP
Division of Cardiovascular and Medical Sciences,
University of Glasgow,
Western Infirmary,
Glasgow, UK

Céline Odier MD
Neurology Service, Centre Hospitalier
Universitaire Vaudois,
University of Lausanne,
Lausanne, Switzerland

Risto O. Roine MD PhD
Department of Neurology,
Turku University Hospital,
Turku, Finland

Jobst Rudolf MD
Department of Neurology,
General Hospital "Papageorgiou",
Thessaloniki, Greece

Cinzia Sarti
Department of Public Health,
University of Helsinki,
Helsinki, Finland,
Department of Chronic Disease Prevention,
National Institute of Health and Welfare,
Helsinki, Finland

Harald Seifert MD
Institute for Medical Immunology and Hygiene,
University of Cologne,
Cologne, Germany

Thorsten Steiner MD PhD MME
Department of Neurology,
University of Heidelberg,
Heidelberg, Germany

Claudia Stöllberger MD
Second Medical Department,
Hospital Rudolfsstiftung,
Vienna, Austria

Yvonne Teuschl PhD
Center of Clinical Neurosciences,
Danube University,
Krems, Austria

Jaakko Tuomilehto MD PhD
Department of Public Health,
University of Helsinki,
Helsinki, Finland;
South Ostrobothnia Central Hospital,
Seinäjoki, Finland

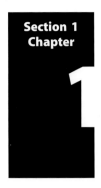

Section 1
Chapter

1

Etiology, pathophysiology and imaging

Neuropathology and pathophysiology of stroke

Konstantin A. Hossmann and Wolf-Dieter Heiss

The vascular origin of cerebrovascular disease

All cerebrovascular diseases (CVD) have their origin in the vessels supplying or draining the brain. Therefore, knowledge of pathological changes occurring in the vessels and in the blood is essential for understanding the pathophysiology of the various types of CVD and for the planning of efficient therapeutic strategies. Changes in the vessel wall lead to obstruction of blood flow, by interacting with blood constituents they may cause thrombosis and blockade of blood flow in this vessel. In addition to vascular stenosis or occlusion at the site of vascular changes, disruption of blood supply and consecutive infarcts can also be produced by emboli arising from vascular lesions situated proximally to otherwise healthy branches located more distal in the arterial tree or from a source located in the heart. At the site of occlusion, the opportunity exists for thrombus to develop in anterograde fashion throughout the length of the vessel, but this event seems to occur only rarely.

Changes in large arteries supplying the brain, including the aorta, are mainly caused by atherosclerosis. Middle-sized and intracerebral arteries can also be affected by acute or chronic vascular diseases of inflammatory origin due to subacute to chronic infections, e.g. tuberculosis and lues, or due to collagen disorders, e.g. giant cell arteriitis, granulomatous angiitis of the CNS, panarteritis nodosa, and even more rarely systemic lupus erythematosus, Takayasu's arteriitis, Wegener granulomatosis, rheumatoid arteriitis, Sjögren's syndrome, or Sneddon and Behcet's disease. In some diseases affecting the vessels of the brain the etiology and pathogenesis are still unclear, e.g. moyamoya disease and fibromuscular dysplasia, but these disorders are characterized by typical locations of the vascular changes. Some arteriopathies are hereditary, such as CADASIL (cerebral autosomal

dominant arteriopathy with subcortical infarcts and leukoencephalopathy), and in some such as cerebral amyloid angiopathy a degenerative cause has been suggested. All these vascular disorders can cause obstruction, and lead to thrombosis and embolizations. Small vessels of the brain are affected by hyalinosis and fibrosis; this "small-vessel disease" can cause lacunes and, if widespread, is the substrate for vascular cognitive impairment and vascular dementia.

Atherosclerosis is the most widespread disorder leading to death and serious morbidity including stroke. The basic pathological lesion is the atheromatous plaque, and the most commonly affected sites are the aorta, the coronary arteries, the carotid artery at its bifurcation, and the basilar artery. Arteriosclerosis, a more generic term describing hardening and thickening of the arteries, includes as an additional type Mönkeberg's sclerosis and is characterized by calcification in the tunica media and arteriolosclerosis with proliferative and hyaline changes affecting the arterioles. Atherosclerosis starts at a young age, and lesions accumulate and grow throughout life and become symptomatic and clinically evident when end organs are affected [1].

> Atherosclerosis: atheromatous plaques, most commonly in the aorta, the coronary arteries, the bifurcation of the carotid artery and the basilar artery.

The initial lesion of atherosclerosis has been attributed to the "fatty streaks" and the "intimal cell mass". Those changes occur in childhood and adolescence and do not necessarily correspond to the future sites of atherosclerotic plaques. Fatty streaks are focal areas of intracellular lipid collection in both macrophages and smooth muscle cells. Various concepts have been proposed to explain the progression of such precursor lesions to definite atherosclerosis [1, 2], the most remarkable of which is the response-to-injury

1

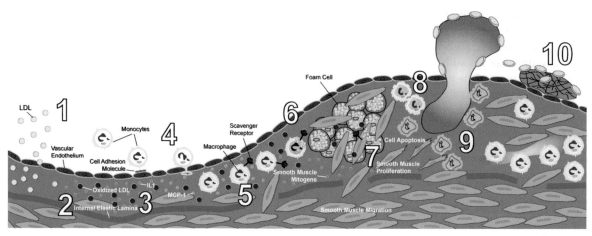

Figure 1.1. The stages of development of an atherosclerotic plaque. (1) LDL moves into the subendothelium and (2) is oxidized by macrophages and smooth muscle cells (SMC). (3) Release of growth factors and cytokines (4) attracts additional monocytes. (5) Macrophages and (6) foam cell accumulation and additional (7) SMC proliferation result in (8) growth of the plaque. (9) Fibrous cap degradation and plaque rupture (collagenases, elastases). (10) Thrombus formation. (Modified from Faxon et al. [5].)

hypothesis postulating a cellular and molecular response to various atherogenic stimuli in the form of an inflammatory repair process [3]. This inflammation develops concurrently with the accumulation of minimally oxidized low-density lipoproteins [4, 5], and stimulates vascular smooth muscle cells (VSMCs), endothelial cells and macrophages, and as a result foam cells aggregate with an accumulation of oxidized LDL. In the further stages of atherosclerotic plaque development VSMCs migrate, proliferate, and synthesize extracellular matrix components on the luminal side of the vessel wall, forming the fibrous cap of the atherosclerotic lesion [6]. In this complex process of growth, progression and finally rupture of an atherosclerotic plaque a large number of matrix modulators, inflammatory mediators, growth factors and vasoactive substances are involved. The complex interactions of these many factors are discussed in the specialist literature [4–6]. This fibrous cap covers the deep lipid core with a massive accumulation of extracellular lipids (*atheromatous plaque*) or fibroblasts and extracellular calcifications may contribute to a *fibrocalcific lesion*. Mediators from inflammatory cells at the thinnest portion of the cap surface of a *vulnerable plaque* – which is characterized by a larger lipid core and a thin fibrous cap – can lead to plaque disruption with formation of a thrombus or hematoma or even to total occlusion of the vessel. During the development of atherosclerosis the entire vessel can enlarge or constrict in size [7]. However, once the plaque enlarges to >40%

of the vessel area, the artery no longer enlarges, and the lumen narrows as the plaque grows. In vulnerable plaques thrombosis forming on the disrupted lesion further narrows the vessel lumen and can lead to occlusion or be the origin of emboli. Less commonly, plaques have reduced collagen and elastin with a thin and weakened arterial wall, resulting in aneurysm formation which when ruptured may be the source of intracerebral hemorrhage (Figure 1.1).

> Injury hypothesis of progression to atherosclerosis: fatty streaks (focal areas of intra-cellular lipid collection) → inflammatory repair process with stimulation of vascular smooth muscle cells → atheromatous plaque.

Thromboembolism

Immediately after plaque rupture or erosion, subendothelial collagen, the lipid core and procoagulants such as tissue factor and von Willebrand factor are exposed to circulating blood. Platelets rapidly adhere to the vessel wall through the platelet glycoproteins (GP) Ia/IIa and GP Ib/IX [8] with subsequent aggregation to this initial monolayer through linkage with fibrinogen and the exposed GP IIb/IIIa on activated platelets. As platelets are a source of nitrous oxide (NO), the resulting deficiency of bioactive NO, which is an effective vasodilator, contributes to the progression of thrombosis by augmenting platelet activation, enhancing VSMC proliferation and migration, and participating in neovascularization [9]. The activated platelets also release adenosine diphosphate (ADP) and thromboxane A2 with subsequent activation of the clotting cascade. The growing thrombus obstructs or even blocks the blood flow in the vessel. Athero-sclerotic thrombi are also the source of embolisms, which are the primary pathophysiological mechanisms of ischemic strokes, especially from carotid artery disease or of cardiac origin.

> Rupture or erosion of atheromatous plaques → adhesion of platelets → thrombus → obstruction of blood flow and source of emboli.

Small-vessel disease usually affects the arterioles and is associated with hypertension. It is caused by subendothelial accumulation of a pathological protein, the hyaline, formed from mucopolysaccharides and matrix proteins. It leads to narrowing of the lumen or even occlusion of these small vessels. Often it is associated with fibrosis, which affects not only arterioles, but also other small vessels and capillaries and venules. Lipohyalinosis also weakens the vessel wall, predisposing it to the formation of "miliary aneurysms". Small-vessel disease results in two pathological conditions: status lacunaris (lacunar state) and status cribrosus (state criblé). Status lacunaris is characterized by small irregularly shaped infarcts due to occlusion of small vessels; it is the pathological substrate of lacunar strokes and vascular cognitive impairment and dementia. In status cribrosus small round cavities develop around affected arteries due to disturbed supply of oxygen and metabolic substrate. These "criblures" together with miliary aneurysms are the sites of vessel rupture causing typical hypertonic intracerebral hemorrhages [10–13]. The etiology and pathophysiology of the various specific vascular disorders are discussed in specialist articles and handbooks [14].

> Small-vessel disease: subendothelial accumulation of hyaline in arterioles.

Types of acute cerebrovascular diseases

Numbers relating to the frequency of the different types of acute CVD are highly variable depending on the source of data. The most reliable numbers come from the in-hospital assessment of stroke in the Framingham study determining the frequency of complete stroke: 60% were caused by athero-thrombotic brain infarction, 25.1% by cerebral emboli, 5.4% by subarachnoid hemorrhage, 8.3% by intracerebral hemorrhage and 1.2% by undefined diseases. In addition, isolated transient ischemic attacks (TIAs) accounted for 14.8% of the total cerebrovascular events [15].

Ischemic strokes are caused by a critical reduction of regional cerebral blood flow and, if the critical blood flow reduction lasts beyond a critical duration, they are caused by atherothrombotic changes of the arteries supplying the brain or by emboli from sources in the heart, the aorta or the large arteries. The pathological substrate of ischemic stroke is ischemic infarction of brain tissue; the location, extension and shape of these infarcts depend on the size of the occluded vessel, the mechanism of arterial obstruction and the compensatory capacity of the vascular bed. Occlusion of arteries supplying defined brain territories by atherothrombosis or embolizations leads to *territorial infarcts* of variable size: they might be large – e.g. the whole territory supplied by the middle cerebral artery (MCA) – or small, if branches of large arteries are occluded or if compensatory collateral perfusion – e.g. via the circle of Willis or leptomeningeal anastomoses – is efficient in reducing the area of critically reduced flow [12, 13] (Figure 1.2). In a smaller number of cases *infarcts* can also develop *at the borderzones* between vascular territories, when several large arteries are stenotic and the perfusion in these "last meadows" cannot be maintained above the critical threshold during special exertion [16]. *Borderzone infarctions* are a subtype of the *low-flow* or hemodynamically induced *infarctions* which are the result of critically reduced cerebral perfusion pressure in far-downstream brain arteries that leads to a reduced cerebral blood flow and oxygen supply in certain vulnerable brain areas. Borderzone infarcts are located in cortical areas between the territories of major cerebral arteries; the more common low-flow infarctions affect subcortical structures within a vascular bed but with marginal irrigation [17]. *Lacunar infarcts* reflect disease of the vessels penetrating the brain to supply the capsule, the basal ganglia, thalamus and paramedian regions of the brain stem [18]. Most often they are caused by lipohyalinosis of deep arteries (small-vessel disease); less frequent causes are stenosis of the MCA stem and microembolization to penetrant arterial territories. Pathologically these

3

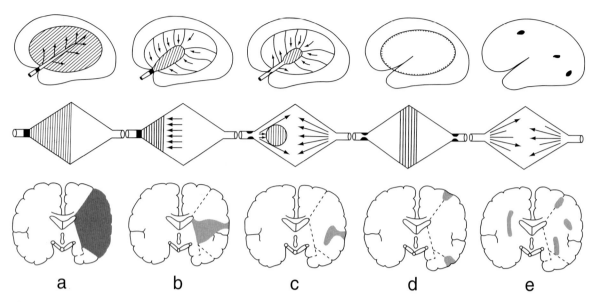

Figure 1.2. Various types and sizes of infarcts due to different hemodynamic patterns. (a) Total territorial infarct due to defective collateral supply. (b) Core infarct, meningeal anastomosis supply peripheral zones. (c) Territorial infarct in center of supply area, due to branch occlusion. (d) Borderzone infarction in watershed areas due to stenotic lesions in arteries supplying neighboring areas. (e) Lacunar infarctions due to small-vessel disease. (Modified from Zülch [13].)

lacunes are defined as small cystic trabeculated scars about 5 mm in diameter, but they are more often observed on magnetic resonance images, where they are accepted as lacunes up to 1.5 cm diameter. The classic lacunar syndromes include pure motor, pure sensory, and sensorimotor syndromes, sometimes ataxic hemiparesis, clumsy hand, dysarthria and hemichorea/hemiballism, but higher cerebral functions are not involved.

> Territorial infarcts are caused by an occlusion of arteries supplying defined brain territories by athero-thrombosis or embolizations.
> Borderzone infarcts develop at the borderzone between vascular territories and are the result of a critically reduced cerebral perfusion pressure (low flow infarctions).
> Lacunar infarcts are mainly caused by small-vessel disease.

Hemorrhagic infarctions, i.e. "red infarcts" in contrast to the usual "pale infarcts", are defined as ischemic infarcts in which varying amounts of blood cells are found within the necrotic tissue. The amount can range from a few petechial bleeds in the gray matter of cortex and basal ganglia to large hemorrhages involving the cortical and deep hemispheric regions. Hemorrhagic transformation frequently appears

during the second and third phase of infarct evolution, when macrophages appear and new blood vessels are formed in tissue consisting of neuronal ghosts and proliferating astrocytes. However, the only significant difference between "pale" and "red infarcts" is the intensity and extension of the hemorrhagic component, since in at least two-thirds of all infarcts petechial hemorrhages are microscopically detectable. Macroscopically red infarcts contain multifocal bleedings which are more or less confluent and predominate in cerebral cortex and basal ganglia which are richer in capillaries than the white matter [19]. If the hemorrhages become confluent intrainfarct hematomas might develop, and extensive edema may contribute to mass effects and lead to malignant infarction. The frequency of hemorrhagic infarctions (HIs) in anatomic studies ranged from 18 to 42% [20], with a high incidence (up to 85% of HIs) in cardioembolic stroke [21].

Mechanisms for hemorrhagic transformation are manifold and vary with regard to the intensity of bleeding. Petechial bleeding results from diapedesis rather than vascular rupture. In severe ischemic tissue vascular permeability is increased and endothelial tight junctions are ruptured. When blood circulation is spontaneously or therapeutically restored, blood can leak out of these damaged vessels. This can also happen with fragmentation and distal migration of an

Textbook of Stroke Medicine

embolus (usually of cardiac origin) in the damaged vascular bed, explaining delayed clinical worsening in some cases. For the hemorrhagic transformation the collateral circulation might also have an impact: in some instances reperfusion via pial networks may develop with the diminution of peri-ischemic edema at borderzones of cortical infarcts. Risk of hemorrhage is significantly increased in large infarcts, with mass effect supporting the importance of edema for tissue damage and the deleterious effect of late reperfusion when edema resolves. In some instances also the rupture of the vascular wall secondary to ischemia-induced endothelial necrosis might cause an intrainfarct hematoma. Vascular rupture can explain very early hemorrhagic infarcts and early intrainfarct hematoma (between 6 and 18 hours after stroke), whereas hemorrhagic transformation usually develops within 48 hours to 2 weeks.

> Hemorrhagic infarctions (HI) are defined as ische-mic infarcts in which varying amounts of blood cells are found within the necrotic tissue. They are caused by leakage from damaged vessels, due to increased vascular permeability in ischemic tissue or vascular rupture secondary to ischemia.

Intracerebral hemorrhage (ICH) occurs as a result of bleeding from an arterial source directly into the brain parenchyma and accounts for 5–15% of all strokes [22, 23]. Hypertension is the leading risk factor, but in addition old age and race, and also cigarette smoking, alcohol consumption and high serum cholesterol levels, have been identified. In a number of instances ICH occurs in the absence of hypertension, usually in atypical locations. The causes include small vascular malformations, vasculitis, brain tumors and sympathomimetic drugs (e.g. cocaine). ICH may also be caused by cerebral amyloid angiopathy and rarely damage is elicited by acute changes in blood pressure, e.g. due to exposure to cold. The occurrence of ICH is also influenced by the increasing use of antithrombotic and throm-bolytic treatment of ischemic diseases of the brain, heart and other organs [24, 25].

Spontaneous ICH occurs predominantly in the deep portions of the cerebral hemispheres ("typical ICH"). Its most common location is the putamen (35–50% of cases). The subcortical white matter is the second most frequent location (approx. 30%). Hemorrhages in the thalamus are found in 10–15%, in the pons in 5–12% and in the cerebellum in 7%

[26]. Most ICHs originate from the rupture of small, deep arteries with diameters of 50 to 200 μm, which are affected by lipohyalinosis due to chronic hypertension. These small-vessel changes lead to weakening of the vessel wall and miliary micro-aneurysm and consecutive small local bleedings, which might be followed by secondary ruptures of the enlarging hematoma in a cascade or avalanche fashion [27]. After active bleeding starts it can continue for a number of hours with enlargement of hematoma, which is frequently associated with clinical deterioration [28].

Putaminal hemorrhages originate from a lateral branch of the striate arteries at the posterior angle, resulting in an ovoid mass pushing the insular cortex laterally and displacing or involving the internal capsule. From this initial putaminal-claustral location a large hematoma may extend to the internal capsule and lateral ventricle, into the corona radiata and into the temporal white matter. Putaminal ICHs were considered the typical hypertensive hemorrhages.

Caudate hemorrhage, a less common form of bleeding from distal branches of lateral striate arteries, occurs in the head of the caudate nucleus. This bleeding soon connects to the ventricle and usually involves the anterior limb of the internal capsule.

Thalamic hemorrhages can involve most of this nucleus and extend into the third ventricle medially and the posterior limb of the internal capsule laterally. The hematoma my press on or even extend into the midbrain. Larger hematomas often reach the corona radiata and the parietal white matter.

Lobar (white matter) hemorrhages originate at the cortico-subcortical junction between gray and white matter and spread along the fiber bundles most commonly in the parietal and occipital lobes. The hematomas are close to the cortical surface and usually not in direct contact with deep hemisphere structures or the ventricular system. As atypical ICHs they are not necessarily correlated with hypertension.

Cerebellar hemorrhages usually originate in the area of the dentate nucleus from rupture of distal branches of the superior cerebellar artery and extend into the hemispheric white matter and into the fourth ventricle. The pontine tegmentum is often compressed. A variant, the midline hematoma, originates from the cerebellar vermis, always communicates with the fourth ventricle and frequently extends bilaterally into the pontine tegmentum.

Pontine hemorrhages from bleeding of small para-median basilar perforating branches cause medially placed hematomas involving the basis of the pons. A unilateral variety results from rupture of distal long circumferential branches of the basilar artery. These hematomas usually communicate with the fourth ventricle and extend laterally and ventrally into the pons.

The frequency of recurrent of ICHs in hypertensive patients is rather low (6%) [29]. The recurrence rate is higher with poor control of hypertension and also in hemorrhages due to other causes. In some instances multiple simultaneous ICHs may occur, but also in these cases the cause is other than hypertension.

In ICHs, the local accumulation of blood destroys the parenchyma, displaces nervous structures and dissects the tissue. At the bleeding sites fibrin globes are formed around collections of platelets. After hours or days extracellular edema develops at the periphery of the hematoma. After 4 to 10 days the red blood cells begin to lyse, granulocytes and thereafter microglial cells arrive and foamy macrophages are formed, which ingest debris and hemosiderin. Finally, the astrocytes at the periphery of the hematoma proliferate and turn into gemistocytes with eosinophilic cytoplasm. When the hematoma is removed, the astrocytes are replaced by glial fibrils. After that period – extending to months – the residue of the hematoma is a flat cavity with a reddish lining resulting from hemosiderin-laden macrophages [26].

> Intracerebral hemorrhage (ICH) occurs as a result of bleeding from an arterial source directly into the brain parenchyma, predominantly in the deep portions of the cerebral hemispheres (typical ICH). Hypertension is the leading risk factor, and the most common location is the putamen.

Cerebral venous thrombosis

Thrombi of the cerebral veins and sinuses can develop from many causes and because of predisposing conditions. Cerebral venous thrombosis (CVT) is often multifactorial, when various risk factors and causes contribute to the development of this disorder [30]. The incidence of septic CVT has been reduced to less than 10% of cases, but septic cavernous sinus thrombosis is still a severe, however rare, problem. Aseptic CVT occurs during puerperium and less frequently during pregnancy, but may also be related to use of oral contraceptives. Among the non-infection causes of CVT are congenital thrombophilia,

particularly prothrombin gene and factor V Leiden mutations, and prothrombin mutation, as well as antithrombin, protein C and protein S deficiencies must be considered. Other conditions with risk for CVT are malignancies, inflammatory diseases and systemic lupus erythematodes. However, in 20–35% of CVT the etiology remains unknown.

The fresh venous thrombus is rich in red blood cells and fibrin and poor in platelets. Later on, it is replaced by fibrous tissue, occasionally with recanalization. The most common location of CVT is the superior sagittal sinus and the tributary veins.

Whereas some thromboses, particularly of the lateral sinus, may have no pathological consequences for the brain tissue, occlusion of cerebral veins usually leads to a venous infarct. These infarcts are located in the cortex and adjacent white matter and often are hemorrhagic. Thrombosis of the superior sagittal sinus might lead only to brain edema, but usually causes bilateral hemorrhagic infarcts in both hemispheres. These venous infarcts are different from arterial infarcts: cytotoxic edema is absent or mild, vasogenic edema is prominent, and hemorrhagic transformation or bleeding is usual. Despite this hemorrhagic component heparin is the treatment of choice.

> Cerebral venous thrombosis can lead to a venous infarct. Venous infarcts are different from arterial infarcts: cytotoxic edema is absent or mild, vasogenic edema is prominent, and hemorrhagic transformation or bleeding is usual.

Cellular pathology of ischemic stroke

Acute occlusion of a major brain artery causes a stereotyped sequel of morphological alterations which evolve over a protracted period and which depend on the topography, severity and duration of ischemia [31, 32]. The most sensitive brain cells are neurons, followed – in this order – by oligodendrocytes, astrocytes and vascular cells. The most vulnerable brain regions are hippocampal subfield CA_1, neocortical layers 3, 5 and 6, the outer segment of striate nucleus, and the Purkinje and basket cell layers of cerebellar cortex. If blood flow decreases below the threshold of energy metabolism, the primary pathology is necrosis of all cell elements, resulting in ischemic brain infarct. If ischemia is not severe enough to cause primary energy failure, or if it is of so short duration that energy metabolism recovers after reperfusion, a delayed type of cell death may evolve which exhibits the morphological characteristics of necrosis, apoptosis or a combination of both. In the following, primary and delayed cell death will be described separately.

Cellular pathology of ischemic stroke
Primary ischemic cell death

In the core of the territory of an occluded brain artery the earliest sign of cellular injury is neuronal swelling or shrinkage, the cytoplasm exhibiting microvacuolation (MV), which ultrastructurally has been associated with mitochondrial swelling [33]. These changes are potentially reversible if blood flow is restored before mitochondrial membranes begin to rupture. One to two hours after the onset of ischemia, neurons undergo irreversible necrotic changes (red neuron or

ischemic cell change (ICC)), characterized by condensed acidophilic cytoplasm, formation of triangular nuclear pyknosis and direct contact with swollen astrocytes. Electronmicroscopically mitochondria exhibit flocculent densities which represent denaturated mitochondrial proteins. After 2–4 hours, ischemic cell change with incrustations appears, which has been associated with formaldehyde pigments deposited after fixation in the perikaryon. Ischemic cell change must be distinguished from artifactual dark neurons which stain with all (acid or base) dyes and are not surrounded by swollen astrocytes (Figure 1.3).

With ongoing ischemia, neurons gradually lose their stainability with hematoxylin; they become mildly eosinophilic and, within 4 days, transform into ghost cells with a hardly detectable pale outline. Interestingly, neurons with ischemic cell change are mainly

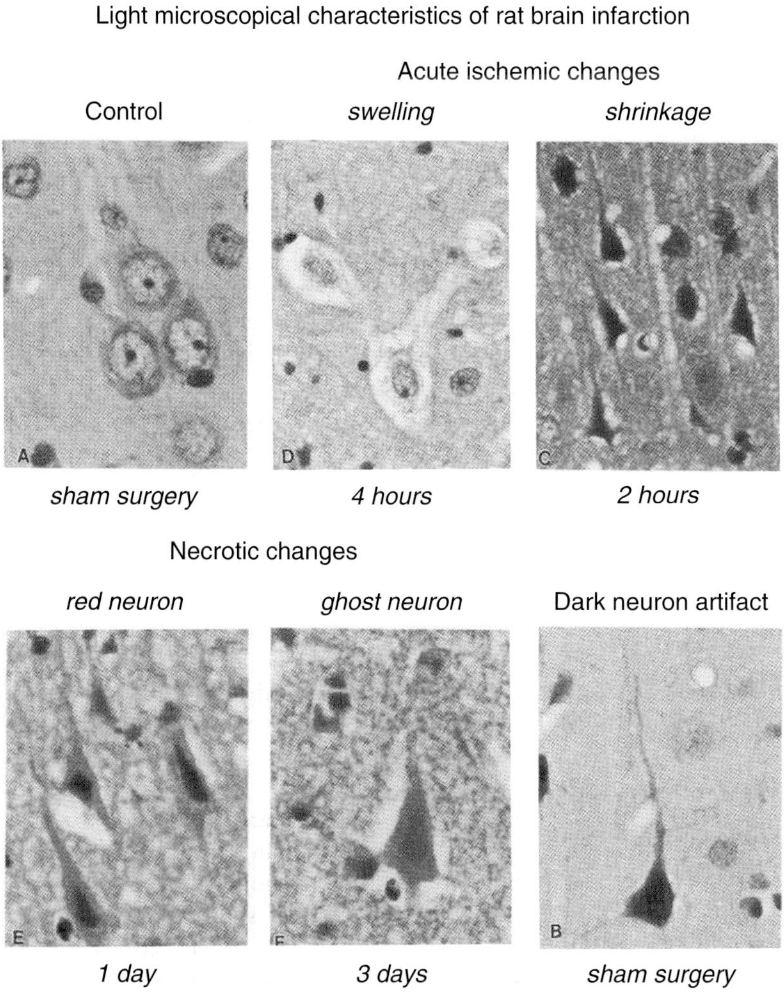

Light microscopical characteristics of rat brain infarction

Acute ischemic changes

Control — sham surgery

swelling — 4 hours

shrinkage — 2 hours

Necrotic changes

red neuron — 1 day

ghost neuron — 3 days

Dark neuron artifact — sham surgery

Figure 1.3. Light-microscopical evolution of neuronal changes after experimental middle cerebral occlusion. (Modified from Garcia et al. [94].)

Inflammation and cavitation of ischemic infarction

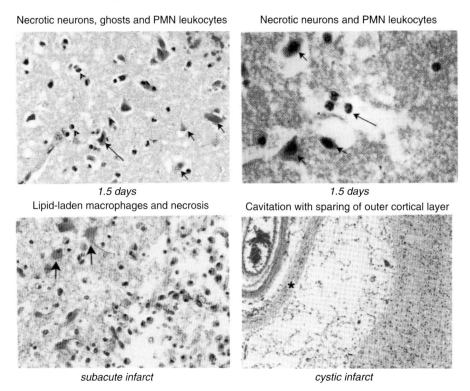

Figure 1.4. Transformation of acute ischemic alterations into cystic infarct. Note pronounced inflammatory reaction prior to tissue cavitation. (Modified from Petito [32].)

located in the periphery and ghost cells in the center of the ischemic territory, which suggests that manifestation of ischemic cell change requires some residual or restored blood flow, whereas ghost cells may evolve in the absence of flow [32].

Primary ischemic cell death induced by focal ischemia is associated with reactive and secondary changes. The most notable alteration during the initial 1–2 hours is perivascular and perineuronal astrocytic swelling; after 4–6 hours the blood–brain barrier breaks down, resulting in the formation of vasogenic edema; after 1–2 days inflammatory cells accumulate throughout the ischemic infarct, and within 1.5 to 3 months cystic transformation of the necrotic tissue occurs together with the development of a peri-infarct astroglial scar.

Delayed neuronal death

The prototype of delayed cell death is the slowly progressing injury of pyramidal neurons in the CA_1 sector of the hippocampus after a brief episode of global ischemia [34]. In focal ischemia delayed neuronal death may occur in the periphery of cortical infarcts or in regions which have been reperfused before ischemic energy failure becomes irreversible. Cell death is also observed in distant brain regions, notably in the substantia nigra and thalamus.

The morphological appearance of neurons during the interval between ischemia and cell death exhibits a continuum that ranges from necrosis to apoptosis with all possible combinations of cytoplasmic and nuclear morphology that are characteristic of the two types of cell death [35]. In its pure form, necrosis combines karyorrhexis with massive swelling of endoplasmic reticulum and mitochondria, whereas in apoptosis mitochondria remain intact and nuclear fragmentation with condensation of nuclear chromatin gives way to the development of apoptotic bodies (Figure 1.4). A frequently used histochemical method for the visualization of apoptosis is terminal deoxyribonucleotidyl transferase (TdT)-mediated biotin-16-dUTP nick-end labeling (TUNEL assay), which detects DNA strand breaks. However, as this method may also stain necrotic neurons, a clear differentiation is not possible [36].

A consistent ultrastructural finding in neurons undergoing delayed cell death is disaggregation of ribosomes, which reflects the inhibition of protein synthesis at the initiation step of translation [37]. Light-microscopically, this change is equivalent to tigrolysis, visible in Nissl-stained material. Disturbances of protein synthesis and the associated endoplasmic reticulum stress are also responsible for cytosolic protein aggregation and the formation of stress granules [38]. In the hippocampus, stacks of accumulated endoplasmic reticulum may become visible but in other areas this is not a prominent finding.

> Severe ischemia induces primary cell death due to necrosis of all cell elements.
> Not so severe or short-term ischemia induces delayed cell death with necrosis, apoptosis or a combination of both.

Pathophysiology of stroke
Animal models of focal ischemia

According to the Framingham study, 65% of strokes that result from vascular occlusion present lesions in the territory of the middle cerebral artery, 2% in the anterior and 9% in the posterior cerebral artery territories; the rest are located in brainstem or cerebellum, or in watershed or multiple regions. In experimental stroke research, this situation is reflected by the preferential use of middle cerebral artery occlusion models.

Transorbital middle cerebral artery occlusion: this model was introduced in the seventies for the production of stroke in monkeys [39], and later modified for use in cats, dogs, rabbits and even rats. The procedure is technically demanding and requires microsurgical skills. The advantage of this approach is the possibility of exposing the middle cerebral artery at its origin from the internal carotid artery without retracting parts of the brain. Vascular occlusion can thus be performed without the risk of brain trauma. On the other hand, removal of the eyeball is invasive and may evoke functional disturbances which should not be ignored. Surgery may also cause generalized vasospasm which may interfere with the collateral circulation and, hence, induce variations in infarct size. The procedure therefore requires extensive training before reproducible results can be expected.

The occlusion of the middle cerebral artery at its origin interrupts blood flow to the total vascular territory, including the basal ganglia which are supplied by the lenticulo-striate arteries. These MCA branches are end-arteries which, in contrast to the cortical branches, do not form collaterals with the adjacent vascular territories. As a consequence, the basal ganglia are consistently part of the infarct core whereas the cerebral cortex exhibits a gradient of blood flow which decreases from the peripheral towards the central parts of the vascular territory. Depending on the steepness of this gradient, a cortical core region with the lowest flow values in the lower temporal cortex is surrounded by a variably sized penumbra which may extend up to the para-sagittal cortex.

Transcranial occlusion of the middle cerebral artery: post- or retro-orbital transcranial approaches for middle cerebral artery occlusion are mainly used in rats and mice because in these species the main stem of the artery appears on the cortical surface rather close to its origin from the internal carotid artery [40]. In contrast to transorbital middle cerebral artery occlusion, transcranial models do not produce ischemic injury in the basal ganglia because the lenticulo-striate branches originate proximal to the occlusion site. Infarcts, therefore, are mainly located in the temporo-parietal cortex with a gradient of declining flow values from the peripheral to the central parts of the vascular territory.

Filament occlusion of the middle cerebral artery: the currently most widely used procedure for middle cerebral artery occlusion in rats and mice is the intraluminal filament occlusion technique, first described by Koizumi et al. [41]. A nylon suture with an acryl-thickened tip is inserted into the common carotid artery and orthogradely advanced, until the tip is located at the origin of the middle cerebral artery. Modifications of the original technique include different thread types for isolated or combined vascular occlusion, adjustments of the tip size to the weight of the animal, poly-L-lysine coating of the tip to prevent incomplete middle cerebral artery occlusion, or the use of guide-sheaths to allow remote manipulation of the thread for occlusion during polygraphic or magnetic resonance recordings.

The placement of the suture at the origin of the middle cerebral artery obstructs blood supply to the whole MCA-supplied territory, including the basal ganglia. It may also reduce blood flow in the anterior and posterior cerebral arteries, particularly when the common carotid artery is ligated to facilitate the insertion of the thread. As this minimizes collateral blood supply from these territories, infarcts are very large and produce massive ischemic brain edema with a high mortality when experiments last for more than a few hours. For this reason, threads are frequently withdrawn 1–2 hours following insertion. The resulting reperfusion salvages the peripheral parts of the MCA territory, and infarcts become smaller [42]. However, the pathophysiology of transient MCA occlusion differs basically from that of the clinically more relevant permanent occlusion models, and neither the mechanisms of infarct evolution nor the pharmacological responsiveness of the resulting lesions are comparable.

Transient filament occlusion is also an inappropriate model for the investigation of spontaneous or thrombolysis-induced reperfusion. Withdrawal of the intraluminal thread induces instantaneous reperfusion whereas spontaneous or thrombolysis-induced recanalization results in slowly progressing recirculation. As post-ischemic recovery is greatly influenced by the dynamics of reperfusion, outcome and pharmacological responsiveness of transient filament occlusion is distinct from most clinical situations of reversible ischemia where the onset of ischemia is much less abrupt.

Clot embolism of middle cerebral artery: middle cerebral artery embolism with autologous blood clots is a clinically highly relevant but also inherently variable stroke model which requires careful preparation and placement of standardized clots to induce reproducible brain infarcts [43]. The most reliable procedure for clot preparation is thrombin-induced clotting, which results in cylindrical clots that can be dissected into segments of equal length. Selection of either fibrin-rich (white) or fibrin-poor (red) segments influences the speed of spontaneous reperfusion and results in different outcomes. Clots can also be produced *in situ* by microinjection of thrombin [44] or photochemically by UV illumination of the middle cerebral artery following injection of rose Bengal [45].

The main application of clot embolism is for the investigation of experimental thrombolysis. The drug most widely used is human recombinant tissue plasminogen activator (rt-PA) but the dose required in animals is much higher than in humans, which must be remembered when possible side effects such as t-PA toxicity are investigated. The hemodynamic effect, in contrast, is similar despite the higher dose and adequately reproduces the slowly progressing recanalization observed under clinical conditions.

> Various procedures for artery occlusion models, mostly middle cerebral artery occlusion models, were developed to study focal ischemia in animals.

Regulation of blood flow

In the intact brain, cerebral blood flow is tightly coupled to the metabolic requirements of tissue (metabolic regulation) but the flow rate remains essentially constant despite alterations in blood pressure (autoregulation). An important requirement for metabolic regulation is the CO_2 reactivity of cerebral vessels, which can be tested by the application of carbonic anhydrase inhibitors or CO_2 ventilation. Under physiological conditions, blood flow doubles when CO_2 rises by about 30 mmHg and is reduced by approximately 35% when CO_2 falls to 25 mmHg. The vascular response to CO_2 depends mainly on changes in extracellular pH, but it is also modulated by other factors such as prostanoids, nitric oxide and neurogenic influences.

Autoregulation of cerebral blood flow is the remarkable capacity of the vascular system to adjust its resistance in such a way that blood flow is kept constant over a wide range of cerebral perfusion pressures (80–150 mmHg). The range of autoregulation is shifted to the right, i.e. to higher values, in patients with hypertension and to the left during hypercarbia. The myogenic theory of autoregulation suggests that changes in vessel diameter are caused by the direct effect of blood pressure variations on the myogenic tone of vessel walls. Other influences are mediated by metabolic and neurogenic factors but these may be secondary and are not of great significance.

Metabolic regulation: cerebral blood flow is coupled to metabolic requirements of tissue by a vascular response to CO_2.

Autoregulation: cerebral blood flow is kept constant over a wide range of cerebral perfusion pressures.

Disturbances of flow regulation

Focal cerebral ischemia is associated with tissue acidosis which leads to vasorelaxation and, in consequence, to a severe disturbance of the regulation of blood flow [46]. In the center of the ischemic territory, CO_2 reactivity is abolished or even reversed, i.e. blood flow may decrease with increasing arterial pCO_2. This paradoxical "steal" effect has been attributed to the rerouting of blood to adjacent non-ischemic brain regions in which CO_2 reactivity remains intact.

Stroke also impairs autoregulation but the disturbance is more severe with decreasing than with increasing blood pressure. This is explained by the fact that a decrease of local brain perfusion pressure cannot be compensated by further reduction of vascular resistance whereas an increase may shift the local perfusion pressure into the autoregulatory range and cause vasoconstriction. An alternative explanation is "false autoregulation" due to brain edema which causes an increase in local tissue pressure that precludes a rise of the actual tissue perfusion pressure. Failure of cerebral autoregulation can be demonstrated in such instances by dehydrating the brain in order to reduce brain edema.

After transient ischemia, vasorelaxation persists for some time, which explains the phenomenon of post-ischemic hyperemia or luxury perfusion. During luxury perfusion, oxygen supply exceeds the oxygen requirements of the tissue, as reflected by the appearance of red venous blood. With the cessation of tissue acidosis, vascular tone returns, and blood flow declines to or below normal. Subsequently, autoregulation, but not CO_2 reactivity, may recover, resulting in failure of metabolic regulation. This is one of the reasons why primary post-ischemic recovery may be followed by delayed post-ischemic hypoxia and secondary metabolic failure [47].

Disturbances of flow regulation through ischemia: tissue acidosis leads to vasorelaxation, CO_2 reactivity is abolished or even reversed and autoregulation is impaired.

Anastomotic steal phenomena

The connection of ischemic and non-ischemic vascular territories by anastomotic channels may divert blood from one brain region to another, depending on the magnitude and direction of the blood pressure gradients across the anastomotic connections (for review see Toole and McGraw [48]). Inverse steal has also been referred to as the Robin Hood syndrome in analogy to the legendary hero who took from the rich and gave to the poor.

Steals are not limited to a particular vascular territory and may affect both the extra- and intracerebral circulation. Examples of extracerebral steals are the subclavian, the occipital-vertebral and the ophthalmic steal syndrome. Intracerebral steals occur across collateral pathways of the brain, notably the circle of Willis and Heubner's network of pial anastomoses. The pathophysiological importance of steal has been disputed but as it depends on the individual hemodynamic situation it may explain unintended effects when flow is manipulated by alterations of arterial pCO_2 or vasoactive drugs. Most authors, therefore, do not recommend such manipulations for the treatment of stroke.

"Steal": decrease in flow in a region because blood is diverted from one brain region to another by anastomotic channels; "inverse steal" if that results in an improvement in flow.

The concept of ischemic penumbra
Energy requirements of brain tissue

The energy demand of the nervous tissue is very high and therefore sufficient blood supply to the brain must be maintained consistently. A normal adult male's brain containing approx. 130 billion neurons (21.5 billion in the neocortex) [49] comprises only 2% of total body mass, yet consumes at rest approximately 20% of the body's total basal oxygen consumption supplied by 16% of the cardiac blood output. The brain's oxygen consumption is almost entirely for the oxidative metabolism of glucose, which in normal physiological conditions is the almost exclusive substrate for the brain's energy metabolism [50] (Table 1.1). It must be kept in mind that the glucose metabolized in neuronal cell bodies is mainly to support cellular vegetative and house-keeping functions, e.g. axonal transport, biosynthesis of nucleic acids, proteins, lipids, as well as other energy-consuming processes not related directly to action potentials. Therefore the rate of glucose consumption of neuronal cell bodies is essentially unaffected by neuronal functional activation. Increases in glucose consumption (and regional blood flow) evoked by functional activation are confined to synapse-rich regions, i.e. neuropil which contains axonal terminals, dendritic processes, and also the astrocytic processes that envelop the synapses. The magnitudes of these increases are linearly related to the frequency of action potentials in the afferent pathways, and increases in the projection zones occur regardless of whether the pathway is excitatory or inhibitory. Energy metabolism by functional activation is due mostly to stimulation of the Na^+K^+-ATPase

activity to restore the ionic gradients across the cell membrane and the membrane potentials that were degraded by the spike activity and is rather high compared to the demand of neuronal cell bodies [51] (Figure 1.5).

In excitatory glutamanergic neurons, which account for 80% of the neurons in the mammalian cortex, glucose utilization during activation is mediated by astrocytes which by anaerobic glycolysis provide lactate to the neurons where lactate is further oxidatively phosphorylated [52]. Overall, 87% of the total energy consumed is required by signaling, mainly action potential propagation and postsynaptic ion fluxes, and only 13% is expended in maintaining membrane resting potential [53] (Figure 1.5).

The mechanisms by which neurotransmitters other than glutamate influence blood flow and energy metabolism in the brain are still not understood [54].

A normal adult male's brain comprises only 2% of total body mass, yet consumes at rest approximately 20% of the body's total basal oxygen consumption. Glucose is the almost exclusive substrate for the brain's energy metabolism; 87% of the total energy consumed is required by signaling, mainly action potential propagation and postsynaptic ion fluxes.

Table 1.1. Cerebral blood flow, oxygen utilization and metabolic rates of glucose in man (approximate values).

	Cortex	White matter	Global
CBF (ml/100 g/min)	65	21	47
CMRO$_2$ (mol/100 g/min)	230	80	160
CMRGlc (mol/100 g/min)	40	20	32

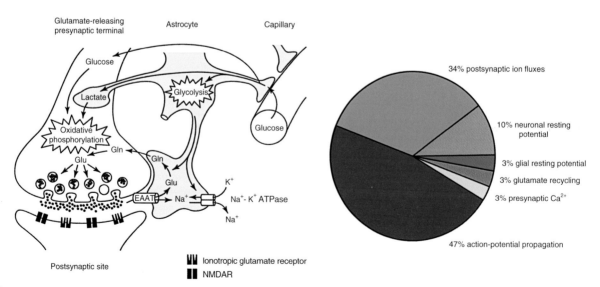

Figure 1.5. (a) Schematic representation of the mechanism for glutamate-induced glycolysis in astrocytes during physiological activation [95]. (b) Distribution of energy expenditure in rat cortex at a mean spike rate of 4 Hz: most energy is required for activity, only 13% is used for maintenance of resting potential for both neurons and glial cells [53, 96].

Flow thresholds for preservation of function and morphological integrity

The different energy requirements for maintenance of membrane function and for propagation of information (signals) lead to different thresholds of energy consumption and consequently blood flow required for preservation of neuronal function and morphological integrity. The range of perfusion between those limits – a blood flow level below which neuronal function is impaired and a lower threshold below which irreversible membrane failure and morphological damage occur – was called the "ischemic penumbra" [55]; it is characterized by the potential for functional recovery without morphological damage, provided that local blood flow can be re-established at a sufficient level and within a certain time window [56, 57].

The functional threshold was demonstrated in ischemic monkeys gradually developing a neurological deficit progressing from mild paresis at 22 ml/100 g/min to complete paralysis at 8 ml/100 g/min. Concurrently the electrocorticogram and the evolved potentials (EPs) were abolished at 15–20 ml/100 g/min, and the spontaneous activity of cortical neurons disappeared at approximately 18 ml/100 g/min. The large variability of the functional thresholds of individual neurons (6–22 ml/100 g/min) indicates selective vulnerability even within small cortical sectors. This explains the gradual development of neurological deficits, which might additionally be related to altered single-cell activity with grouped or regular discharges at flow levels above the threshold. Spontaneous neuronal activity as well as EPs were restored when blood flow was re-established above the critical values.

Whereas neuronal function is impaired immediately when flow drops below the threshold, the development of irreversible morphological damage is time-dependent. It starts at low flow values (below 10 ml/100 g/min) after short duration of ischemia with leakage of K^+ out of cell bodies, indicating loss of membrane function and leading to anoxic depolarization. In larger ischemic areas this final step is indicated by depolarization of the cortical DC potential. The interaction of severity and duration of ischemia in the development of irreversible cell damage was studied by simultaneous recordings of cortical neuronal activity and local blood flow. Based on recordings from a considerable number of neurons during and after ischemia of varying degree and duration it was possible to construct a discriminant curve representing the worst possible constellation of residual blood flow and duration of ischemia still permitting neuronal recovery (Figure 1.6). These results broaden the concept of the ischemic penumbra: the potential for recovery (or irreversible damage) is determined not only by the level of residual flow but also by the duration of the flow disturbance. Each level of decreased flow can, on average, be tolerated for a defined period; flow between 17 and 20 ml/100 g/min can be tolerated for prolonged but yet undefined periods. As a rule used in many experimental models, flow rates of 12 ml/100 g/min lasting for 2–3 hours lead to large infarcts, but individual cells may become necrotic after shorter periods and at higher levels of residual flow. However, in some instances critical, but not detrimental, flow disturbance may trigger dynamic processes, leading to delayed neuronal death in vulnerable brain regions [58].

> The ischemic penumbra is the range of perfusion between the flow threshold for preservation of function and the flow threshold for morphological integrity. It is characterized by the potential for functional recovery without morphological damage.

Imaging of penumbra

Based on the threshold concept of brain ischemia, the penumbra can be localized on quantitative flow images using established flow thresholds. A more direct approach is the imaging of threshold-dependent biochemical disturbances and demarcating the mismatch between disturbances which occur only in the infarct core and others which also affect the penumbra [59] (Figure 1.7). Under experimental conditions the most reliable way to localize the infarct core is the loss of ATP on bioluminescent images of tissue ATP content. A biochemical marker of core plus penumbra is tissue acidosis or the inhibition of protein synthesis. The penumbra is the difference between the respective lesion areas. The reliability of this approach is supported by the precise co-localization of gene transcripts that are selectively expressed in the penumbra, such as the stress protein hsp70 or the documentation of the gradual disappearance of the penumbra with increasing ischemia time [60] (Figure 1.7).

13

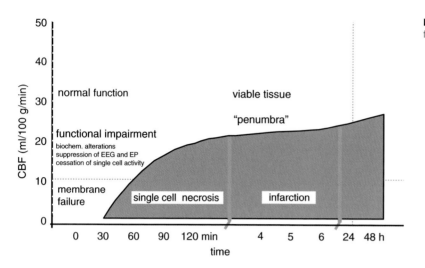

Figure 1.6. Diagram of cerebral blood flow (CBF) threshold.

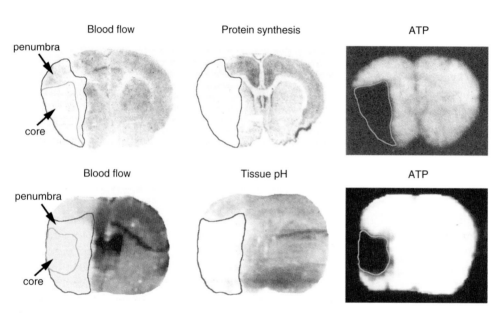

Figure 1.7. Biochemical imaging of infarct core and penumbra after experimental middle cerebral artery occlusion. The core is identified by ATP depletion and the penumbra by the mismatch between the suppression of protein synthesis and ATP depletion (top) or by the mismatch between tissue acidosis and ATP (bottom) (Hossmann and Mies [59]).

Non-invasive imaging of the penumbra is possible using positron emission tomography (PET) or magnetic resonance imaging (NMR). Widely used PET parameters are the increase in oxygen extraction or the mismatch between reduced blood flow and the preservation of vitality markers, such as flumazenil binding to central benzodiazepine receptors [61]. An alternative PET approach is the use of hypoxia markers such as 18F-nitromidazol (F-MISO), which is trapped in viable hypoxic but not in normoxic or necrotic tissue [62].

The best-established NMR approach for penumbra imaging is the calculation of mismatch maps between the signal intensities of perfusion (PWI) and diffusion-weighted images (DWI), but its reliability has been questioned [63]. An alternative method is quantitative mapping of the apparent diffusion coefficient (ADC) of water, which reveals a robust correlation with the biochemically characterized penumbra for ADC values between 90% and 77% of control [64]. Recently MR stroke imaging has been performed by combining PWI, DWI and pH-weighted imaging (pHWI), where the mismatch between DWI and pHW detects the penumbra, and that between PWI and pHWI the area of benign oligemia [65].

Finally, new developments in non-invasive molecular imaging are of increasing interest for stroke research [66]. These methods make use of contrast probes that trace gene transcription or of intracellular conjugates that reflect the metabolic status and/or bind to stroke markers. The number of molecules that can be identified by these methods rapidly expands and greatly facilitates the regional analysis of stroke injury.

> Non-invasive imaging of the penumbra is possible using positron emission tomography (PET) or magnetic resonance imaging (NMR).

Progression of ischemic injury

With the advent of non-invasive imaging evidence has been provided that brain infarcts grow. This growth is not due to the progression of ischemia because the activation of collateral blood supply and spontaneous thrombolysis tend to improve blood flow over time. Infarct progression can be differentiated into three phases. During the acute phase tissue injury is the direct consequence of the ischemia-induced energy failure and the resulting terminal depolarization of cell membranes. At flow values below the threshold of energy metabolism this injury is established within a few minutes after the onset of ischemia. During the subsequent subacute phase, the infarct core expands into the peri-infarct penumbra until, after 4–6 hours, core and penumbra merge. The reasons for this expansion are peri-infarct spreading depressions and a multitude of cell biological disturbances, collectively referred to as molecular cell injury. Finally, a delayed phase of injury evolves which may last for several days or even weeks. During this phase secondary phenomena such as vasogenic edema, inflammation and possibly programmed cell death may contribute to a further progression of injury.

The largest increment of infarct volume occurs during the subacute phase in which the infarct core expands into the penumbra. Using multiparametric imaging techniques for the differentiation between core and penumbra, evidence could be provided that 1 hour after occlusion of the middle cerebral artery the penumbra is still approximately of the same size

as the infarct core [60]. However, after 3 hours more than 50% and between 6 and 8 hours almost all of the penumbra has disappeared and is now part of the irreversibly damaged infarct core. In the following, the most important mediators of infarct progression will be discussed.

> Brain infarcts grow in three phases:
>
> - acute phase, within a few minutes after the onset of ischemia; terminal depolarization of cell membranes;
> - subacute phase, within 4–6 hours; molecular cell injury, the infarct core expands into the peri-infarct penumbra;
> - delayed phase, several days to weeks; vasogenic edema, inflammation and possibly programmed cell death.

Peri-infarct spreading depression

A functional disturbance contributing to the growth of the infarct core into the penumbra zone is the generation of peri-infarct spreading depression-like depolarizations. These depolarizations are initiated at the border of the infarct core and spread over the entire ipsilateral hemisphere. During spreading depression the metabolic rate of the tissue markedly increases in response to the greatly enhanced energy demands of the activated ion-exchange pumps. In the healthy brain the associated increase of glucose and oxygen demands is coupled to a parallel increase of blood flow but in the peri-infarct penumbra this flow response is suppressed or even reversed [67]. As a result, a misrelationship arises between the increased metabolic workload and the low oxygen supply, leading to transient episodes of hypoxia and the stepwise increase in lactate during the passage of each depolarization.

The pathogenic importance of peri-infarct depolarizations for the progression of ischemic injury is supported by the linear relationship between the number of depolarizations and infarct volume. Correlation analysis of this relationship suggests that during the initial 3 hours of vascular occlusion each depolarization increases the infarct volume by more than 20%. This is probably one of the reasons that glutamate antagonists reduce the volume of brain infarcts because these drugs are potent inhibitors of spreading depression.

15

Peri-infarct spreading depressions are depolarizations initiated at the border of the infarct core and may contribute to progression of ischemic injury.

Molecular mechanisms of injury progression (Figure 1.8)

In the border zone of permanent focal ischemia or in the ischemic territory after transient vascular occlusion, cellular disturbances may evolve that cannot be explained by a lasting impairment of blood flow or energy metabolism. These disturbances are referred to as molecular injury, where the term "molecular" does not anticipate any particular injury pathway (Figure 1.8). The molecular injury cascades (Figure 1.8) are interconnected in complex ways, which makes it difficult to predict their relative

pathogenic importance in different ischemia models. In particular, molecular injury induced by transient focal ischemia is not equivalent to the alterations that occur in the core or the penumbra of permanent ischemia. Therefore, the relative contribution of the following injury mechanisms differs in different types of ischemia.

Acidotoxicity: during ischemia oxygen depletion and the associated activation of anaerobic glycolysis cause an accumulation of lactic acid which, depending on the severity of ischemia, blood glucose levels and the degree of ATP hydrolysis, results in a decline of intracellular pH to levels between 6.5 and below 6.0. As the severity of acidosis correlates with the severity of ischemic injury, it has been postulated that acidosis is neurotoxic. Recently, evidence has been provided that ASICs (acid-sensing ion channels) are glutamate-independent vehicles of calcium flux, and

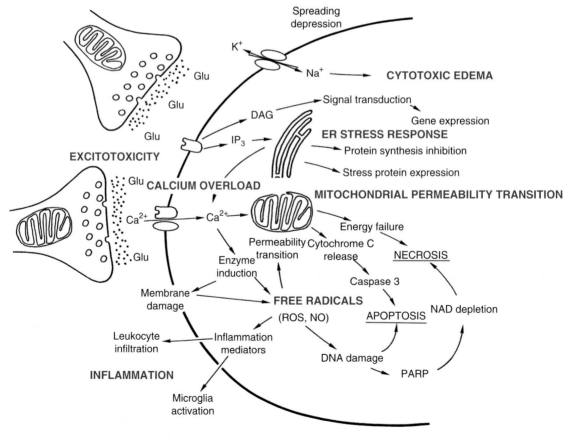

Figure 1.8. Schematic representation of molecular injury pathways leading to mitochondrial failure and the endoplasmic reticulum stress response. Injury pathways can be blocked at numerous sites, providing multiple approaches for the amelioration of both necrotic and apoptotic tissue injury.

that blockade of ASICs attenuates stroke injury. This suggests that acidosis may induce calcium toxicity, and that this effect is the actual mechanism of acidotoxicity [68].

Excitotoxicity: shortly after the onset of ischemia, excitatory and inhibitory neurotransmitters are released, resulting in the activation of their specific receptors. Among these neurotransmitters, particular attention has been attributed to glutamate, which at high concentrations is known to produce excitotoxicity [69]. The activation of ionotropic glutamate receptors results in the inflow of calcium from the extracellular into the intracellular compartment, leading to mitochondrial calcium overload and the activation of calcium-dependent catabolic enzymes. The activation of metabotropic glutamate receptors induces the IP$_3$-dependent signal transduction pathway, leading inter alia to the stress response of endoplasmic reticulum, and by induction of immediate-early genes (IEG) to adaptive genomic expressions. At high concentration, glutamate results in primary neuronal necrosis. However, following pharmacological inhibition of ionotropic glutamate receptors, an apoptotic injury mechanism evolves that may prevail under certain pathophysiological conditions. The importance of excitotoxicity for ischemic cell injury has been debated, but this does not invalidate the beneficial effect of glutamate antagonists for the treatment of focal ischemia. An explanation for this discrepancy is the above-described pathogenic role of peri-infarct depolarizations in infarct expansion. As glutamate antagonists inhibit the spread of these depolarizations, the resulting injury is also reduced.

Calcium toxicity: in the intact cell, highly efficient calcium transport systems ensure the maintenance of a steep calcium concentration gradient of approximately 1:10 000 between the extra- and the intracellular compartment on the one hand, and between the cytosol and the endoplasmic reticulum (ER) on the other. During ischemia anoxic depolarization in combination with the activation of ionotropic glutamate and acid-sensing ion channels causes a sharp rise of cytosolic calcium [70]. At the onset of ischemia this rise is further enhanced by activation of metabotropic glutamate receptors which mediate the release of calcium from endoplasmic reticulum (ER), and after recovery from ischemia by activation of transient receptor potential (TRP) channels which perpetuate intracellular calcium overload despite the restoration

of ion gradients (Ca^{2+} paradox) [71]. The changes in intracellular calcium activity are highly pathogenic: prolonged elevation of cytosolic calcium causes mitochondrial dysfunction and induces catabolic changes, notably by activation of Ca^{2+}-dependent effector proteins and enzymes such as endonucleases, phospholipases, protein kinases and proteases that damage DNA, lipids and proteins. The release of calcium from the ER evokes an ER stress response, which mediates a great number of ER-dependent secondary disturbances, notably inhibition of protein synthesis. Calcium-dependent pathological events are therefore complex and contribute to a multitude of secondary molecular injury pathways.

Free radicals: in brain regions with low or intermittent blood perfusion, reactive oxygen species (ROS) are formed which produce peroxidative injury of plasma membranes and intracellular organelles [72]. The reaction with nitric oxide leads to the formation of peroxynitrate, which also causes violent biochemical reactions. Secondary consequences of free radical reactions are the release of biologically active free fatty acids such as arachidonic acid, the induction of endoplasmic reticulum stress, the induction of mitochondrial disturbances and fragmentation of DNA. The latter may induce apoptosis and thus enhance molecular injury pathways related to mitochondrial dysfunction. The therapeutic benefit of free radical scavengers, however, is limited, as recently documented by the therapeutic failure of the free-radical-trapping agent NXY-059 [73].

Nitric oxide toxicity: nitric oxide (NO) is a product of NO synthase (NOS) acting on argenin. There are at least three isoforms of NOS: eNOS is constitutively expressed in endothelial cells, nNOS in neurons and the inducible isoform iNOS mainly in macrophages. Pathophysiologically, NO has two opposing effects [74]. In endothelial cells the generation of NO leads to vascular dilatation, an improvement of blood flow and the alleviation of hypoxic injury, whereas in neurons it contributes to glutamate excitotoxicity and – by formation of peroxynitrate – to free-radical-induced injury. The net effect of NO thus depends on the individual pathophysiological situation and is difficult to predict.

Zinc toxicity: zinc is an essential catalytic and structural element of numerous proteins and a secondary messenger which is released from excitatory synapses during neuronal activation. Cytosolic zinc

17

overload may promote mitochondrial dysfunction and generation of reactive oxygen species (ROS), activate signal transduction pathways such as protein kinase C or enhance glutamate toxicity by inhibiting $GABA_A$ channels and blocking excitatory amino acid transporters. However, zinc may also exhibit neuroprotective properties, indicating that cells may possess a specific zinc set-point by which too little or too much zinc can promote ischemic injury [75].

Inhibition of protein synthesis: a robust molecular marker for the progression of ischemic injury is inhibition of protein synthesis, which persists throughout the interval from the onset of ischemia until the manifestation of cell death [37]. It is initiated by the ischemia-induced release of calcium stores from the endoplasmic reticulum (ER), which results in ER stress and various cell biological abnormalities such as misfolding of proteins, expression of stress proteins and a global inhibition of the protein-synthesizing machinery [76]. The latter is due to the activation of protein kinase R (PKR), which causes phosphorylation and inactivation of the alpha subunit of eukaryotic initiation factor eIF_2. This again leads to selective inhibition of polypeptidepol chain initiation, disaggregation of ribosomes and inhibition of protein synthesis at the level of translation.

Other consequences of ER stress are ubiquination and trapping of proteins which are crucial for cellular function, and SUMOylation (i.e. conjugation with the small ubiquitin-like modifier, SUMO), which causes suppression of most transcription factors. The former is presumably the reason for the irreversibility of translation arrest because protein aggregates include components of the translation complex [77]. Obviously, persistent inhibition of protein synthesis is incompatible with cell survival but, as the interval between onset of ischemia and cell death greatly varies, other factors are also involved.

Mitochondrial disturbances: the concurrence of an increased cytosolic calcium activity with the generation of reactive oxygen species leads to the increase in permeability of the inner mitochondrial membrane (mitochondrial permeability transition, MPT), which has been associated with the formation of a permeability transition pore (PTP). The PTP is thought to consist of a voltage-dependent anion channel (VADC), the adenine nucleotide translocator (ANT), cyclophilin D and other molecules. The increase in permeability of the inner mitochondrial membrane has two pathophysiologically important consequences. The breakdown of the electrochemical gradient interferes with mitochondrial respiration and, in consequence, with aerobic energy production. Furthermore, the equilibration of mitochondrial ion gradients causes swelling of the mitochondrial matrix, which eventually will cause disruption of the outer mitochondrial membrane and the release of pro-apoptotic mitochondrial proteins (see below). Ischemia-induced mitochondrial disturbances thus contribute to delayed cell death both by impairment of the energy state and by the activation of apoptotic injury pathways [78].

A large number of biochemical substrates, molecules and mechanisms are involved in the progression of ischemic damage.

Inflammation

Brain infarcts evoke a strong inflammatory response which is thought to contribute to the progression of ischemic brain injury. Gene expressions related to this response have, therefore, been extensively investigated in the search for possible pharmacological targets (for review see Rothwell and Luheshi [79]). The inflammatory response of the ischemic tissue has been associated, inter alia, with the generation of free radicals in reperfused or critically hypoperfused brain tissue. The prostaglandin-synthesizing enzyme cyclooxygenase-2 (COX-2) and NF-kappa B, a transcription factor that responds to oxidative stress, are strongly upregulated and may be neurotoxic, as suggested by the beneficial effect of COX-2 inhibitors. Infarct reduction was also observed after genetic or pharmacological inhibition of matrix metalloproteinase (MMP)-9, but this effect has been disputed.

A key player in the intracellular response to cytokines is the JAK (janus kinase)/STAT (signal transducer and activator of transcription) pathway, which induces alterations in the pattern of gene transcription. These changes are associated with either cell death or survival and suggest that inflammation may be both neurotoxic and neuroprotective [80]. Inflammatory reactions and the associated free-radical-mediated processes are, therefore, important modulators of ischemic injury but the influence on the final outcome is difficult to predict.

Inflammatory reactions are important modulators of ischemic injury.

Brain edema

Ischemic brain edema can be differentiated into two pathophysiologically different types: an early cytotoxic type, followed after some delay by a late vasogenic type of edema. The cytotoxic type of edema is threshold-dependent. It is initiated at flow values of approx. 30% of control when stimulation of anaerobic metabolism causes an increase of brain tissue osmolality and, hence, an osmotically obliged cell swelling. At flow values below 20% of control, anoxic depolarization and equilibration of ion gradients across the cell membranes further enhance intracellular osmolality and the associated cell swelling. The intracellular uptake of sodium is also associated with a coupled movement of water that is independent of an osmotic gradient and which is referred to as "anomalous osmosis".

In the absence of blood flow, cell swelling occurs at the expense of the extracellular fluid volume, leading to the shrinkage of the extracellular compartment, but not to a change in the net water content. The shift of fluid is reflected by a decrease in the apparent diffusion coefficient of water, which is the reason for the increase in signal intensity in diffusion-weighted MR imaging [64]. However, if some residual blood flow persists, water is taken up from the blood, and the net tissue water content increases. After MCA occlusion this increase starts within a few minutes after the onset of ischemia and causes a gradual increase in brain volume.

With the evolution of tissue necrosis and the degradation of basal lamina, the blood–brain barrier breaks down [81], and after 4–6 hours serum proteins begin to leak from the blood into the brain. This disturbance initiates a vasogenic type of edema which further enhances the water content of the tissue. Vasogenic edema reaches its peak at 1–2 days after the onset of ischemia and may cause an increase of tissue water by more than 100%. If brain infarcts are large, the volume increase of the edematous brain tissue may be so pronounced that transtentorial herniation results in compression of the midbrain. Under clinical conditions, this "malignant" form of brain infarction is by far the most dangerous complication of stroke and an indication for decompressive craniectomy [82].

Vasogenic edema, in contrast to the early cytotoxic type of edema, is isoosmotic and accumulates mainly in the extracellular compartment. This reverses the narrowing of the extracellular space and explains the "pseudonormalization" of the signal intensity observed in diffusion-weighted MR imaging [83]. However, as the total tissue water content is increased at this time, the high signal intensity in T_2-weighted images clearly differentiates this situation from a "real" recovery to normal.

The formation of cytotoxic and, to a lesser extent, also vasogenic edema requires the passage of water through aquaporin channels located in the plasma membrane [84]. Inhibition of aquaporin water conductance may, therefore, reduce the severity of ischemic brain edema. Similarly, the inhibition of sodium transport across sodium channels has been suggested to reduce edema formation. However, as the driving force for the generation of edema is the gradient of osmotic and ionic concentration differences built up during ischemia, aquaporin channels may modulate the speed of edema generation but not the final extent of tissue water accumulation. Their pathophysiological importance is, therefore, limited.

> Early cytotoxic edema is caused by osmotically induced cell swelling; the later vasogenic edema is isoosmotic, caused by breakdown of the blood–brain barrier, and accumulates in the extracellular compartment.

Apoptosis

Apoptosis is an evolutionarily conserved form of programmed cell death that in multicellular organisms matches cell proliferation to preserve tissue homeostasis. It is an active process that requires intact energy metabolism and protein synthesis, and it is initiated essentially by two pathways: an extrinsic death receptor-dependent route, and an intrinsic pathway which depends on the mitochondrial release of pro-apoptotic molecules such as apoptosis inducing factor (AIF) and cytochrome c. Both pathways involve a series of enzymatic reactions and converge in the activation of caspase 3, a cystine protease which contributes to the execution of cell death. An endstage of this process is the ordered disassembly of the genome, resulting in a laddered pattern of oligonucleosomal fragments as detected by electrophoresis or terminal deoxyribonucleotidyl transferase (TdT)-mediated biotin-16-dUTP nick-end labeling (TUNEL).

19

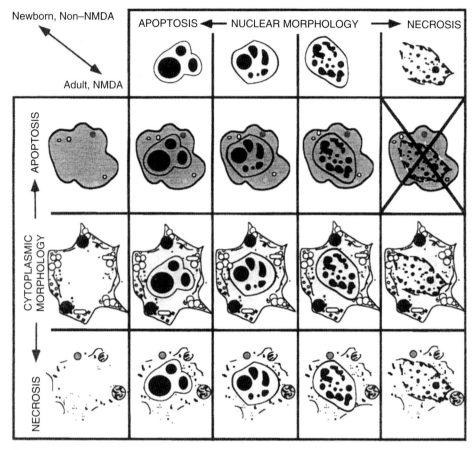

Figure 1.9. The concept of the apoptosis–necrosis continuum of neuronal cell death. The matrix shows possible combinations between nuclear and cytoplasmic morphologies near or at the terminal stages of degeneration [35].

Although apoptosis is mainly involved in physiological cell death, it is widely assumed to contribute to the pathogenesis of diseases, including cerebral ischemia [85]. In the context of stroke this is difficult to understand because in areas with primary cell death the obvious cause is energy failure, and in regions with delayed injury protein synthesis is irreversibly suppressed (Figure 1.9). However, ischemia induces a multitude of biochemical reactions that are reminiscent of apoptosis, such as the expression of p53, JNK, c-jun, p38, cycline-dependent kinase 5 or caspase 3, all of which correlate to some degree with the severity of injury. Conversely, inhibition of these reactions by gene manipulation or pharmacological interventions reduces the volume of brain infarcts. It has, therefore, been suggested that ischemic cell death is a hybrid of necrosis and apoptosis, appearing on a continuum with the two forms of cell death at its poles [86] (Figure 1.9).

Apoptosis, an active form of programmed cell death, may contribute to a certain extent to ischemic cell death.

Ischemic pre- and postconditioning

The molecular signaling cascades initiated by brain ischemia are not solely destructive but may also exert a neuroprotective effect. In fact, most of the above-described injury pathways including ischemia itself induce a transient state of increased ischemic tolerance, provided the initial injury remains subliminal for tissue destruction. This effect is called "ischemic preconditioning" and can be differentiated into three phases: during the induction phase molecular sensors which respond to the preconditioning stimulus are activated by transcription factors; the transduction phase results in the amplification of the signal; and during the effector phase proteins with a protective impact are switched on [87]. The increase in ischemia tolerance appears 2–3 days after the preconditioning stimulus, and it slowly disappears after 1 week.

An important preconditioning pathway is the up-regulation of the hypoxia-inducible factor 1 (HIF-1) in astrocytes. HIF-1 is a transcription factor that inter alia induces the expression of erythropoietin (EPO), which binds to the neuronal EPO receptor and which exhibits potent neuroprotective effects. Another putative mechanism is the endoplasmic reticulum stress response. Depletion of ER calcium stores causes accumulation of unfolded proteins in the ER lumen and induces the activation of two highly conserved stress responses, the ER overload response (EOR) and the unfolded protein response (UPR). EOR triggers activation of the transcription factor NF-kappa B, and UPR causes a suppression of the initiation of protein synthesis. As the latter contributes to delayed ischemic injury (see above) its reduction may have a neuroprotective effect.

Recently, evidence has been provided that ischemic injury can also be alleviated by repeated mechanical interruptions of blood reperfusion after a period of transient focal ischemia [88]. This phenomenon, termed "ischemic postconditioning", has been associated with the phosphorylation of several prosurvival protein kinases, such as extracellular signal-regulated kinase (ERK), p38 mitogen-activated protein kinase (MAPK) and Akt. The possibility of influencing ischemic injury after the primary impact is challenging but it remains to be shown for which kind of clinical situation this finding is of practical relevance.

> Short episodes of ischemia can improve the tolerance of brain tissue for subsequent blood flow disturbance.

Regeneration of ischemic injury

Brain infarcts produced by focal ischemia are seemingly irresolvable, in agreement with Cajal's classic statement that in the adult brain "everything may die, nothing may be regenerated". This dogma was reversed by the discovery of three permanently neurogenic regions, i.e. the subventricular zone (SVZ), the subgranular zone (SGZ) and the posterior perireticular (PPr) area, which provide lifelong supply of newly generated neurons to the hippocampus and olfactory bulb. After stroke, neurogenesis increases in these areas, and some of the newly formed cells migrate to the infarct penumbra, differentiate into glia and mature neurons, and survive for at least several weeks [89]. Neurogenesis may also occur within cerebral cortex, but this finding is debated.

Ischemia-induced neurogenesis is enhanced by growth factors, nitric oxide, inflammation, and various hormones and neurotransmitters, notably estradiol and dopamine, but it is repressed by activation of the NMDA subtype of glutamate receptors. The functional consequences of spontaneous or drug-enhanced neurogenesis are modest but optimism is increasing for targeted interventions. Similarly, considerable expectations are placed on the transplantation of neural progenitor cells, particularly in combination with growth factors and/or strategies that permit recruitment of transplanted cells to the site of injury. However, major breakthroughs have not yet been achieved, and further research is necessary to explore the actual potentials of stroke regenerative medicine.

> Several brain regions may provide lifelong supply of newly generated neurons.

Translation of experimental concepts to clinical stroke

Experimental research has advanced our knowledge about brain physiology and the pathophysiology of brain disorders, but the transfer of this knowledge into clinical application is difficult and often lags behind. One of the reasons is the differences between the brains of experimental animals and man with respect to evolutionary state (non-gyrencephalic vs. gyrencephalic), anatomy (amount of gray vs. white matter), relative size, cellular density, blood supply and metabolism (see Table 1.1); additionally, experimental models in animals cannot be easily compared to complex human diseases often affecting multimorbid patients. The other problem arises from the investigative procedures, which cannot be equally applied in animals and patients. This is especially true when pathophysiological changes obtained by invasive procedures in animals, e.g. by analysis of tissue samples, by autoradiography or by histology, should be related to the course of a disease, but cannot be assessed repeatedly and regionally. To facilitate the transfer of knowledge from experimental neuroscience to clinical neurology it is necessary to develop methods which can be equally applied in patients and animal models, and which are not invasive and can be performed repeatedly without affecting or harming the object. To this task of transferring experimental results into clinical application, functional imaging modalities are successfully applied.

Positron emission tomography (PET) is still the only method allowing quantitative determination of various physiological variables in the brain and was applied extensively for studies in patients with acute, subacute or chronic stages of ischemic stroke (review in Heiss [61]). The introduction of scanners with high resolution (2.5 to 5 mm for human, 1 mm for animal application) made PET a tool for studying animal models and to compare repeat examinations of various variables from experiments to the course of disease in humans. The regional decrease of cerebral blood flow (CBF) can be directly observed in PET as in other studies (SPECT, PW-MRI, PCT). However, even in early PET studies [90] preserved glucose consumption was observed in regions with decreased flow in the first hours after the ictus. In the 1980s, PET with oxygen-15 tracers became the gold standard for the evaluation of pathophysiological changes in early ischemic stroke [91]. The quantitative measurement of CBF, $CMRO_2$, OEF and CBV permitted the independent assessment of perfusion and energy metabolism, and demonstrated the uncoupling of these usually closely related variables. These studies provided data on flow and metabolic variables predicting final infarction on late CTs (rCBF less than 12 ml/(100 g min), $CMRO_2$ less than 65 µmol/ (100 g min)). Relatively preserved $CMRO_2$ indicated maintained neuronal function in regions with severely reduced CBF; this pattern was coined "misery perfusion" and served as a definition for the penumbra, which is characterized by increased oxygen extraction fraction (up to more than 80% from the normal 40–50%). Late CT or MRI often showed these regions as morphologically intact.

Sequential PET studies of CBF, $CMRO_2$ and CMRGlc before and repeatedly up to 24 hours after MCA occlusion in cats could demonstrate the development and growth of irreversible ischemic damage. Immediately after MCA occlusion CBF within the supplied territory dropped, but $CMRO_2$ was less diminished and was preserved at an intermediate level. As a consequence, OEF was increased, indicating misery perfusion, i.e. penumbra tissue. With time,

OEF was decreased, a process which started in the center and developed centrifugally to the borderline of the ischemic territory, indicating the conversion into irreversible damage and the growth of the MCA infarct. In experiments with transient MCA occlusion it could be demonstrated that an infarct did not develop when reperfusion was initiated to tissue with increased OEF. Comparable to patients with early thrombolysis, reperfusion could salvage ischemic tissue in the condition of "penumbra" (Figure 1.10). Similar results were obtained in ischemia models of baboons.

In conclusion, PET permits the definition of various tissue compartments within an ischemic territory: irreversible damage by decreased flow and oxygen consumption below critical thresholds; misery perfusion, i.e. penumbra, by decreased flow, but preserved oxygen utilization above a critical threshold, expressed by increased OEF; luxury perfusion by flow increased above the metabolic demand; anaerobic glycolysis by a change in the ratio between glucose metabolism and oxygen utilization. However, PET has severe disadvantages limiting its routine application in patients with stroke: it is a complex methodology, requires multi-tracer application, and quantitative analysis necessitates arterial blood sampling.

> Positron emission tomography (PET) is the only quantitative method to reliably identify irreversible tissue damage and penumbra.

Prediction of irreversible tissue damage

The prediction of the portion of irreversibly damaged tissue within the ischemic area early after the stroke is of utmost importance for the efficiency of treatment. Meticulous analyses of CBF and $CMRO_2$ data indicated that $CMRO_2$ below 65 µmol/(100 g min) predicted finally infarcted tissue, but also large portions with flow and oxygen utilization in the penumbra range were included in the final cortical–subcortical infarcts. Determination of oxygen utilization additionally requires arterial blood sampling, which limits clinical applicability. These facts stress the need for a marker of neuronal integrity that can identify irreversibly damaged tissue irrespective of the time elapsed since the vascular attack and irrespective of the variations in blood flow over time.

Central benzodiazepine receptor (BZR) ligands can be used as markers of neuronal integrity as they

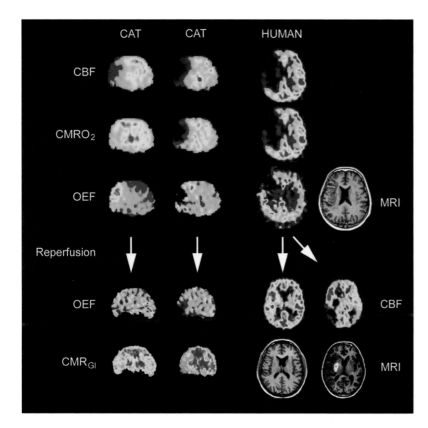

Figure 1.10. Sequential PET images of CBF, CMRO₂ and OEF of·permanent MCA occlusion in a cat compared to images of a patient 12 hours after stroke: in the cat, the progressive decrease of CMRO₂ and the reduction of OEF predicts final infarction, in the patient the area with preserved OEF is finally not infarcted (outside area indicated on late MRI). If reperfusion occurs before OEF is reduced, tissue can be salvaged (left cat and left patient in lower part of figure). If reperfusion is achieved after this therapeutic window, tissue cannot be salvaged (right cat, right patient).

bind to the GABA receptors abundant in cerebral cortex that are sensitive to ischemic damage. After successful testing in the cat MCA occlusion model, cortical binding of flumazenil (FMZ) was investigated in patients with acute ischemic stroke [92]. In all patients, defects in FMZ binding were closely related to areas with severely depressed oxygen consumption and predicted the size of the final infarcts, whereas preserved FMZ binding indicated intact cortex. Additionally, FMZ distribution within 2 min after tracer injection was highly correlated with CBF measured by $H_2^{15}O$ and therefore can be used as a relative flow tracer yielding reliable perfusion images. PET with FMZ therefore can be used as non-invasive procedure to image irreversible damage and critically reduced perfusion (i.e. penumbra) in early ischemic stroke. This method yields more reliable results than the determination of mismatch by PW-DW-MRI, where changes in the diffusion signal overestimate the volume of final infarct, and changes in kinetics of Gd distribution do not permit a reliable estimation of critically decreased blood flow [93].

Chapter Summary

Atherosclerosis is the most widespread disorder leading to death and serious morbidity including stroke. It develops over years from initial fatty streaks to atheromatous plaques with the potential for plaque disruption and formation of thrombus, from which emboli might originate. Lipohyalinosis affects small vessels, leading to lacunar stroke. The vascular lesions and emboli from the heart cause territorial infarcts, whereas borderzone infarcts are due to low perfusion in the last meadows. Ischemic infarcts may be converted into hemorrhagic infarctions by leakage of vessels, whereas intracerebral hemorrhages (5–15% of all strokes) result from rupture of arteries typically in deep portions of the hemispheres. Venous infarcts usually result from thrombosis of sinuses or veins and are often accompanied by edema, hemorrhagic transformation and bleeding.

Primary ischemic cell death is the result of severe ischemia; early signs are potentially reversible swelling or shrinkage; irreversible necrotic neurons have condensed acidophilic cytoplasm and pyknotic nuclei. Delayed neuronal death can occur after moderate or short-term ischemia; it goes along with nuclear fragmentation and development of apoptotic bodies.

The pathophysiology of ischemic cell damage was studied in a large number of animal models, which usually reflect only certain aspects of ischemia and cannot give a complete picture of ischemic stroke in man. From these experimental models principles of regulation of cerebral blood flow and flow thresholds for maintenance of function and morphology were deduced. As the energy requirement of the brain is very high, decreases of blood supply lead to potentially reversible disturbance of function and, if the shortage persists for certain periods, to irreversible morphological damage. Tissue perfused in the range between these two thresholds was called the penumbra, a concept which has great importance for treatment.

The ischemia-induced energy failure triggers a complex cascade of electrophysiological disturbances, biochemical changes and molecular mechanisms, which lead to progressive cell death and growth of infarction. The progression of ischemic injury is further boosted by inflammatory reactions and the development of early cytotoxic and later vasogenic brain edema. The translation of these experimental concepts into clinical application and management of stroke patients, however, is difficult. It can be achieved in some instances by special functional imaging techniques, e.g. positron emission tomography.

References

1. Rajamani K, Fisher M, Fisher M. Atherosclerosis – pathogenesis and pathophysiology. In: Ginsberg MD, Bogousslavsky J, eds. *Cerebrovascular Disease: Pathophysiology, Diagnosis and Management*, Vol. 2. London: Blackwell Science; 1998:308–18.

2. Willeit J, Kiechl S. Biology of arterial atheroma. *Cerebrovasc Dis (Basel)* 2000;**10** Suppl 5:1–8.

3. Ross R. Atherosclerosis—an inflammatory disease. *N Engl J Med* 1999; **340**:115–26.

4. Aikawa M, Libby P. The vulnerable atherosclerotic plaque: pathogenesis and therapeutic approach. *Cardiovasc Pathol* 2004; **13**:125–38.

5. Faxon DP, Fuster V, Libby P, Beckman JA, Hiatt WR, Thompson RW, et al. Atherosclerotic Vascular Disease Conference: Writing Group III: pathophysiology. *Circulation* 2004; **109**:2617–25.

6. Dzau VJ, Braun-Dullaeus RC, Sedding DG. Vascular proliferation and atherosclerosis: new perspectives and therapeutic strategies. *Nature Med* 2002; **8**:1249–56.

7. Glagov S, Weisenberg E, Zarins CK, Stankunavicius R, Kolettis GJ. Compensatory enlargement of human atherosclerotic coronary arteries. *N Engl J Med* 1987; **316**:1371–5.

8. Rauch U, Osende JI, Fuster V, Badimon JJ, Fayad Z, Chesebro JH. Thrombus formation on atherosclerotic plaques: pathogenesis and clinical consequences. *Ann Intern Med* 2001; **134**:224–38.

9. Loscalzo J. Nitric oxide insufficiency, platelet activation, and arterial thrombosis. *Circ Res* 2001; **88**:756–62.

10. Fisher CM. Cerebral miliary aneurysms in hypertension. *Am J Pathol* 1972; **66**:313–30.

11. Rossrussell RW. Observations on intracerebral aneurysms. *Brain* 1963; **86**:425–42.

12. Zülch K-J. Über die Entstehung und Lokalisation der Hirninfarkte. *Zentralbl Neurochir* 1961; **21**:158–78.

13. Zülch K-J. *The Cerebral Infarct. Pathology, Pathogenesis, and Computed Tomography*. Berlin: Springer-Verlag; 1985.

14. Mohr JP, Choi DW, Grotta JC, Weir B, Wolf PA. *Stroke – Pathophysiology, Diagnosis, and Management*. 4th ed. Philadelphia: Churchill Livingstone; 2004.

15. Wolf PA. Epidemiology of stroke. In: Mohr JP, Choi DW, Grotta JC, Weir B, Wolf PA, eds. *Stroke – Pathophysiology, Diagnosis, and Management*. Philadelphia: Churchill Livingstone; 2004: 13–34.

16. Stochdorph O. Der Mythos der letzten Wiese. *Zentralbl Allg Pathol Path Anat* 1977; **121**:554.

17. Ringelstein EB, Zunker P. Low-flow infarction. In: Ginsberg MD, Bogousslavsky J, eds. *Cerebrovascular Disease: Pathophysiology, Diagnosis, and Management*, Vol. 2. London: Blackwell Science; 1998: 1075–89.

18. Fisher CM. Lacunes: small, deep cerebral infarcts. *Neurology* 1965; **15**:774–84.

19. Beghi E, Bogliun G, Cavaletti G, Sanguineti I, Tagliabue M, Agostoni F, et al. Hemorrhagic infarction: risk factors, clinical and tomographic features, and outcome. A case-control study. *Acta Neurol Scand* 1989; **80**:226–31.

20. Lodder J, Krijne-Kubat B, Broekman J. Cerebral hemorrhagic infarction at autopsy: cardiac embolic cause and the relationship to the cause of death. *Stroke* 1986; **17**:626–9.

21. Fisher M, Adams RD. Observations on brain embolism with special reference to the mechanism of hemorrhagic infarction. *J Neuropathol Exp Neurol* 1951; **10**:92–4.

22. Mohr JP, Caplan LR, Melski JW, Goldstein RJ, Duncan GW, Kistler JP, et al. The Harvard Cooperative Stroke

Registry: A prospective registry. *Neurology* 1978; **28**:754–62.

23. Sacco RL, Wolf PA, Bharucha NE, Meeks SL, Kannel WB, Charette LJ, et al. Subarachnoid and intracerebral hemorrhage: natural history, prognosis, and precursive factors in the Framingham Study. *Neurology* 1984; **34**:847–54.

24. Feldman E. *Intracerebral Hemorrhage*. Armonk, NY: Futura; 1994.

25. Schütz H. *Spontane intrazerebrale Hämatome. Pathophysiologie, Klinik und Therapie*. Berlin: Springer-Verlag; 1988.

26. Kase CS, Mohr JP, Caplan LR. Intracerebral Hemorrhage. In: Mohr JP, Choi DW, Grotta JC, Weir B, Wolf PA, eds. *Stroke – Pathophysiology, Diagnosis, and Management*. Philadelphia: Churchill Livingstone; 2004: 327–76.

27. Fisher CM. Pathological observations in hypertensive cerebral hemorrhage. *J Neuropathol Exp Neurol* 1971; **30**:536–50.

28. Brott T, Broderick J, Kothari R, Barsan W, Tomsick T, Sauerbeck L, et al. Early hemorrhage growth in patients with intracerebral hemorrhage. *Stroke* 1997; **28**:1–5.

29. Gonzalez-Duarte A, Cantu C, Ruiz-Sandoval JL, Barinagarrementeria F. Recurrent primary cerebral hemorrhage: frequency, mechanisms, and prognosis. *Stroke* 1998; **29**:1802–5.

30. Bousser MG, Barnett HJM. Cerebral venous thrombosis. In: Mohr JP, Choi DW, Grotta JC, Weir B, Wolf PA, eds. *Stroke – Pathophysiology, Diagnosis, and Management*, 4th ed. Philadelphia: Churchill Livingstone; 2004: 301–25.

31. Auer RN, Benveniste H (eds). *Hypoxia and Related Conditions*. London: Arnold; 1997: 283–98.

32. Petito CK (ed). *The Neuropathology of Focal Brain Ischemia*. Basel: ISN Neuropath Press; 2005: 215–21.

33. Brown AW, Brierley JB. Anoxic-ischaemic cell change in rat brain. Light microscopic and fine-structural observations. *J Neurol Sci* 1972; **16**:59–84.

34. Kirino T, Sano K. Selective vulnerability in the gerbil hippocampus following transient ischemia. *Acta Neuropathol* 1984; **62**:201–8.

35. Martin LJ. The apoptosis-necrosis cell death continuum in CNS development, injury and disease: contributions and mechanisms. In: Lo EH, Marwah J, eds. *Neuroprotection*. Scotsdale, AZ: Prominent Press; 2001: 378–412.

36. Charriaut-Marlangue C, Benari Y. A cautionary note on the use of the TUNEL stain to determine apoptosis. *NeuroReport* 1995; **7**:61–4.

37. Hossmann K-A. Disturbances of cerebral protein synthesis and ischemic cell death. *Prog Brain Res* 1993; **96**:161–77.

38. DeGracia DJ, Rafols JA, Morley SJ, Kayali F. Immunohistochemical mapping of total and phosphorylated eukaryotic initiation factor 4G in rat hippocampus following global brain ischemia and reperfusion. *Neuroscience* 2006; **139**:1235–48.

39. Hudgins WR, Garcia JH. Transorbital approach to the middle cerebral artery of the squirrel monkey: a technique for experimental cerebral infarction applicable to ultrastructural studies. *Stroke* 1970; **1**:107–11.

40. Tamura A, Graham DI, McCulloch J, Teasdale GM. Focal cerebral ischaemia in the rat: 1. Description of technique and early neuropathological consequences following middle cerebral artery occlusion. *J Cereb Blood Flow Metab* 1981; **1**:53–60.

41. Koizumi J, Yoshida Y, Nakazawa T, Ooneda G. Experimental studies of ischemic brain edema. 1. A new experimental model of cerebral embolism in rats in which recirculation can be introduced in the ischemic area. *Jpn J Stroke* 1986; **8**:1–8.

42. Rogers DC, Campbell CA, Stretton JL, Mackay KB. Correlation between motor impairment and infarct volume after permanent and transient middle cerebral artery occlusion in the rat. *Stroke* 1997; **28**:2060–5.

43. DiNapoli VA, Rosen CL, Nagamine T, Crocco T. Selective MCA occlusion: A precise embolic stroke model. *J Neurosci Methods* 2006; **154**:233–8.

44. Orset C, Macrez R, Young AR, Panthou D, Angles-Cano E, Maubert E, et al. Mouse model of in situ thromboembolic stroke and reperfusion. *Stroke* 2007; **38**:2771–8.

45. Chen F, Suzuki Y, Nagai N, Jin LX, Yu J, Wang HJ, et al. Rodent stroke induced by photochemical occlusion of proximal middle cerebral artery: evolution monitored with MR imaging and histopathology. *Eur J Radiol* 2007; **63**:68–75.

46. Symon L. Regional vascular reactivity in the middle cerebral arterial distribution. An experimental study in baboons. *J Neurosurg* 1970; **33**:532–41.

47. Hata R, Maeda K, Hermann D, Mies G, Hossmann K-A. Evolution of brain infarction after transient focal cerebral ischemia in mice. *J Cereb Blood Flow Metab* 2000; **20**:937–46.

48. Toole JF, McGraw CP. The steal syndromes. *Annu Rev Med* 1975; **26**:321–9.

49. Pakkenberg B, Gundersen HJ. Neocortical neuron number in humans: effect of sex and age. *J Comp Neurol* 1997; **384**:312–20.

25

50. Clarke DD, Sokoloff L. Circulation and energy metabolism of the brain. In: Siegel G, Agranoff B, Albers RW, Fisher S, eds. *Basic Neurochemistry: Molecular, Cellular, and Medical Aspects*, 6th ed. Philadelphia: Lippincott-Raven; 1999: 637–69.

51. Sokoloff L. Energetics of functional activation in neural tissues. *Neurochem Res* 1999; **24**:321–9.

52. Magistretti PJ, Pellerin L. Astrocytes couple synaptic activity to glucose utilization in the brain. *News Physiol Sci* 1999; **14**:177–82.

53. Laughlin SB, Attwell D. The metabolic cost of neural information: from fly eye to mammalian cortex. In: Frackowiak RSJ, Magistretti PJ, Shulman RG, Altman JS, Adams M, eds. *Neuroenergetics: Relevance for Functional Brain Imaging*. Strasbourg: HFSP Workshop XI, 2001; 54–64.

54. Frackowiak RSJ, Magistretti PJ, Shulman RG, Altman JS, Adams M (eds). *Neuroenergetics: Relevance for Functional Brain Imaging*. Strasbourg: HFSP Workshop XI, 2001.

55. Astrup J, Siesjö BK, Symon L. Thresholds in cerebral ischemia – the ischemic penumbra. *Stroke* 1981; **12**:723–5.

56. Heiss WD. Experimental evidence of ischemic thresholds and functional recovery. *Stroke* 1992; **23**:1668–72.

57. Hossmann KA. Viability thresholds and the penumbra of focal ischemia. *Ann Neurol* 1994; **36**:557–65.

58. Kirino T. Delayed neuronal death in the gerbil hippocampus following ischemia. *Brain Res* 1982; **239**:57–69.

59. Hossmann K-A, Mies G (eds). *Multimodal Mapping of the Ischemic Penumbra in Animal Models*. New York: Marcel Dekker; 2007: 77–92.

60. Hata R, Maeda K, Hermann D, Mies G, Hossmann K-A. Dynamics of regional brain metabolism and gene expression after middle cerebral artery occlusion in mice. *J Cereb Blood Flow Metab* 2000; **20**:306–15.

61. Heiss WD. Ischemic penumbra: evidence from functional imaging in man [Review]. *J Cereb Blood Flow Metab* 2000; **20**:1276–93.

62. Takasawa M, Beech JS, Fryer TD, Hong YT, Hughes JL, Igase K, et al. Imaging of brain hypoxia in permanent and temporary middle cerebral artery occlusion in the rat using F-18-fluoromisonidazole and positron emission tomography: a pilot study. *J Cereb Blood Flow Metab* 2007; **27**:679–89.

63. Kane I, Sandercock P, Wardlaw J. Magnetic resonance perfusion diffusion mismatch and thrombolysis in acute ischaemic stroke: a systematic review of the evidence to date. *J Neurol Neurosurg Psychiatry* 2007; **78**:485–90.

64. Hoehn-Berlage M, Norris DG, Kohno K, Mies G, Leibfritz D, Hossmann K-A. Evolution of regional changes in apparent diffusion coefficient during focal ischemia of rat brain: the relationship of quantitative diffusion NMR imaging to reduction in cerebral blood flow and metabolic disturbances. *J Cereb Blood Flow Metab* 1995; **15**:1002–11.

65. Sun PZ, Zhou JY, Sun WY, Huang J, van Zijl PCM. Detection of the ischemic penumbra using pH-weighted MRI. *J Cereb Blood Flow Metab* 2007; **27**:1129–36.

66. Heckl S. Future contrast agents for molecular imaging in stroke. *Curr Med Chem* 2007; **14**:1713–28.

67. Strong AJ, Anderson PJ, Watts HR, Virley DJ, Lloyd A, Irving EA, et al. Peri-infarct depolarizations lead to loss of perfusion in ischaemic gyrencephalic cerebral cortex. *Brain* 2007; **130**:995–1008.

68. Simon R, Xiong Z. Acidotoxicity in brain ischaemia. *Biochem Soc Trans* 2006; **34**:1356–61.

69. Choi DW. Excitotoxic cell-death. *J Neurobiol* 1992; **23**:1261–76.

70. Siesjö BK. Calcium, excitotoxins, and brain damage. *News Physiol Sci* 1990; **5**:120–5.

71. MacDonald JF, Xiong ZG, Jackson MF. Paradox of Ca^{2+} signaling, cell death and stroke. *Trends Neurosci* 2006; **29**:75–81.

72. Chan PH. Role of oxidants in ischemic brain damage. *Stroke* 1996; **27**:1124–9.

73. Shuaib A, Lees K, Lyden P, Grotta J, Davalos A, Davis S, et al. NXY-059 for the treatment of acute ischemic stroke. *N Engl J Med* 2007; **357**:562.

74. Dalkara T, Moskowitz MA. The complex role of nitric oxide in the pathophysiology of focal cerebral ischemia. *Brain Pathol* 1994; **4**:49–57.

75. Sensi SL, Jeng JM. Rethinking the excitotoxic ionic milieu: the emerging role of $Zn2^+$ in ischemic neuronal injury. *Curr Mol Med* 2004; **4**:87–111.

76. Paschen W. Dependence of vital cell function on endoplasmic reticulum calcium levels: implications for the mechanisms underlying neuronal cell injury in different pathological states [Review]. *Cell Calcium* 2001; **29**:1–11.

77. DeGracia DJ, Hu BR. Irreversible translation arrest in the reperfused brain. *J Cereb Blood Flow Metab* 2007; **27**:875–93.

78. Norenberg MD, Rao KVR. The mitochondrial permeability transition in neurologic disease. *Neurochem Int* 2007; **50**:983–97.

79. Rothwell NJ, Luheshi GN. Interleukin I in the brain: biology, pathology and therapeutic target [Review]. *Trends Neurosci* 2000; **23**:618–25.

80. Planas AM, Gorina R, Chamorro A. Signalling pathways mediating inflammatory responses in brain ischaemia. *Biochem Soc Trans* 2006; **34**:1267–70.

81. Wang CX, Shuaib A. Critical role of microvasculature basal lamina in ischemic brain injury. *Prog Neurobiol* 2007; **83**:140–8.

82. Walz B, Zimmermann C, Bottger S, Haberl RL. Prognosis of patients after hemicraniectomy in malignant middle cerebral artery infarction. *J Neurol* 2002; **249**:1183–90.

83. Lansberg MG, Thijs VN, O'Brien MW, Ali JO, de Crespigny AJ, Tong DC, et al. Evolution of apparent diffusion coefficient, diffusion-weighted, and T2-weighted signal intensity of acute stroke. *Am J Neuroradiol* 2001; **22**:637–44.

84. Badaut T, Lasbennes T, Magistretti PJ, Regli L. Aquaporins in brain: distribution, physiology, and pathophysiology. *J Cereb Blood Flow Metab* 2002; **22**:367–78.

85. Johnson EM, Greenlund LJS, Akins PT, Hsu CY. Neuronal apoptosis: current understanding of molecular mechanisms and potential role in ischemic brain injury. *J Neurotrauma* 1995; **12**:843–52.

86. MacManus JP, Buchan AM. Apoptosis after experimental stroke: Fact or fashion? [Review]. *J Neurotrauma* 2000; **17**:899–914.

87. Dirnagl U, Simon RP, Hallenbeck JM. Ischemic tolerance and endogenous neuroprotection. *Trends Neurosci* 2003; **26**:248–54.

88. Zhao H, Sapolsky RM, Steinberg GK. Interrupting reperfusion as a stroke therapy: ischemic postconditioning reduces infarct size after focal ischemia in rats. *J Cereb Blood Flow Metab* 2006; **26**:1114–21.

89. Wiltrout C, Lang B, Yan YP, Dempsey RJ, Vemuganti R. Repairing brain after stroke: a review on post-ischemic neurogenesis. *Neurochem Int* 2007; **50**:1028–41.

90. Kuhl DE, Phelps ME, Kowell AP, Metter EJ, Selin C, Winter J. Effects of stroke on local cerebral metabolism and perfusion: Mapping by emission computed tomography of 18 FDG and 13 NH 3. *Ann Neurol* 1980; **8**:47–60.

91. Baron JC, Frackowiak RS, Herholz K, Jones T, Lammertsma AA, Mazoyer B, et al. Use of PET methods for measurement of cerebral energy metabolism and hemodynamics in cerebrovascular disease. *J Cereb Blood Flow Metab* 1989; **9**:723–42.

92. Heiss WD, Grond M, Thiel A, Ghaemi M, Sobesky J, Rudolf J, et al. Permanent cortical damage detected by flumazenil positron emission tomography in acute stroke. *Stroke* 1998; **29**:454–61.

93. Sobesky J, Weber OZ, Lehnhardt FG, Hesselmann V, Neveling M, Jacobs A, et al. Does the mismatch match the penumbra? Magnetic resonance imaging and positron emission tomography in early ischemic stroke. *Stroke* 2005; **36**:980–5.

94. Garcia JH, Liu KF, Ho KL. Neuronal necrosis after middle cerebral artery occlusion in Wistar rats progresses at different time intervals in the caudoputamen and the cortex. *Stroke* 1995; **26**:636–42.

95. Magistretti PJ. Coupling synaptic activity to glucose metabolism. In: Frackowiak RSJ, Magistretti PJ, Shulman RG, Altman JS, Adams M, eds. *Neuroenergetics: Relevance for Functional Brain Imaging*. Strasbourg: HFSP Workshop XI, 2001: 133–42.

96. Attwell D, Laughlin SB. An energy budget for signaling in the grey matter of the brain. *J Cereb Blood Flow Metab* 2001; **21**:1133–45.

Common causes of ischemic stroke

Bo Norrving

Introduction

This chapter focuses on the major causes of ischemic stroke. Common and less common stroke syndromes are described in Chapters 8 and 9.

Ischemic stroke is not a single disease but a heterogeneous condition with several very different pathophysiological mechanisms. Identification of the underlying cause is important for several reasons. It helps to group patients into specific subtypes for the study of different aspects of prognosis, which may be used for planning and information purposes. It also helps for selecting patients for some specific therapies, which are among the most effective secondary preventive measures currently available. Identification of the mechanism of ischemic stroke should therefore be part of the routine diagnostic workup in clinical practice.

Cerebral infarction is generally caused by one of three pathogenic mechanisms:

- large artery atherosclerosis in extracranial and large intracranial arteries
- embolism from the heart
- intracranial small-vessel disease (lacunar infarcts).

These three types account for about 75% of all ischemic strokes (Figure 2.1). In about 20% of patients no clear cause of ischemic stroke can be identified despite appropriate investigations; this is labeled cryptogenic stroke. About 5% of all ischemic strokes result from more uncommon causes. These frequencies relate to ischemic stroke aggregating all age groups: in younger patients with stroke the pathogenic spectrum is much different, with arterial dissection as the most common single cause in patients <45 years of age (Chapter 9, Less common stroke syndromes).

As described in Chapter 8 (Common stroke syndromes), there are several classification schemes for ischemic stroke based on the underlying pathophysiology. The most widely used is the Trial of Organon

in Acute Stroke (TOAST) classification, which divides ischemic stroke into atherothrombotic, cardio-embolic, small-vessel occlusion, other determined cause, and undetermined cause [1]. The latter category comprises both truly cryptogenic strokes, ischemic strokes that are "undetermined" because of incomplete investigation, and strokes that are "undetermined" because multiple possible causes coexist in the same patient. In a further development of the TOAST classification the "undetermined cause" category has been subdivided, and definitions of subtypes have been further refined, taking more recent advances in diagnostic tools into account [2]. A computerized algorithm of this classification has been developed [3], and further defines categories into evident, probable, and possible based on the level of diagnostic support (Table 2.1). Although these classification schemes were developed for use in clinical trials, they also form a useful framework for identifying causes of stroke in clinical practice.

> The TOAST classification divides ischemic stroke into atherothrombotic, cardioembolic, small-vessel occlusion, other determined cause, and undetermined cause.

Large artery atherosclerosis

Atherosclerosis of the major vessels supplying the brain is an important mechanism in ischemic stroke. Although the common occurrence of atherosclerosis in the region of the carotid bifurcation was observed early in the twentieth century, and the mechanism of distal embolization in causing strokes was proposed, it was widely assumed that most cerebral ischemic strokes were caused by in situ middle cerebral artery (MCA) thrombosis. The full implications of extracranial atherosclerosis for ischemic stroke were not recognized until the mid-twentieth century with the advent of the diagnostic techniques of

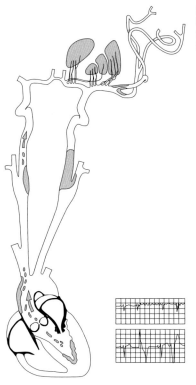

Figure 2.1.
Graphic illustration of the major causes of ischemic stroke.

Table 2.1. Causative Classification System for Ischemic Stroke (CCS) [3].

Large artery atherosclerosis	Evident – probable – possible
Cardio-aortic embolism	Evident – probable – possible
Small artery occlusion	Evident – probable – possible
Other causes	Evident – probable – possible
Undetermined causes	
unknown – cryptogenic embolism	
unknown – other cryptogenic	
unknown – incomplete evaluation	
unclassified	

commonly present also in patients with other stroke subtypes.

Large-vessel disease may cause ischemia through embolism or reduction of blood flow.

catheter angiography and later ultrasound, the links with clinical syndromes, and the therapeutic implications of carotid surgery for carotid bifurcation disease.

Large-vessel disease may cause ischemia through embolism (artery-to-artery embolism) or reduction of blood flow (hemodynamic causes). Emboli from large-vessel disease are usually platelet aggregates or thrombus formed on atherosclerotic plaques. Atherosclerotic debris and cholesterol crystals may also contribute. In many patients carotid or vertebral artery occlusion occurs without symptoms because good collateral supply is provided through the circle of Willis, the external carotid artery and cortical pial anastomoses.

Patients with stroke often have generalized atherosclerosis in other vascular beds. About one-quarter of patients with TIA or stroke have a history of a symptomatic coronary event, and an additional 25–50% have asymptomatic coronary plaques, stenoses or silent myocardial infarcts [4, 5]. Although coronary heart disease is somewhat more prevalent in patients with large atherosclerosis of the cervical arteries, it is

Prevalence of large atherosclerosis: extra- and intracranial

Symptomatic atherosclerosis is most common at the bifurcation of the common carotid artery into the external and internal carotid arteries. Other common extracranial sites are the aortic arch, the proximal subclavian arteries, and the vertebral artery origins (Figure 2.2). Severe carotid stenosis (50–99%) is present in 10–15% of patients with anterior circulation ischemic strokes, with proportions increasing with age. The proportions are similar in patients with TIAs. Intracranial atherosclerosis, in Caucasian populations less common than extracranial, most often affects the carotid siphon, the intracranial vertebral arteries as they penetrate the dura, and the basilar artery. Severe atherosclerosis in the proximal MCA is rarer; in Caucasians MCA occlusion is usually the result of embolism from the heart or a proximal arterial site. Overall, large artery atherosclerosis is estimated to account for about 30% of all ischemic strokes.

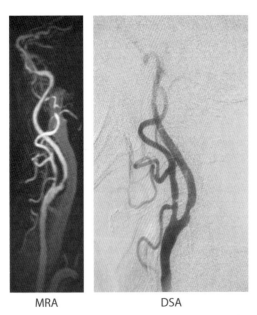

MRA   DSA

Figure 2.2. An extracranial carotid stenosis (degree of stenosis 67%) as visualized by MR angiography (left) and digital subtraction angiography (right). (Courtesy Dr Mats Cronqvist.)

However, the pattern of atherosclerosis is widely different in other populations. Intracranial atherosclerosis appears to be much more common in the Asian and African-American population (Figure 2.3). Intracranial large artery disease has long been a relatively neglected disorder because of a research focus on the more accessible extracranial carotid artery occlusive disease lesions. However, intracranial large artery disease appears to be the most common stroke subtype worldwide [6]. In Chinese and Japanese populations intracranial atherosclerosis accounts for up to half of all strokes, and in Korean studies up to a quarter. The underlying causes of racial differences in the distribution of extracranial and intracranial occlusive disease are not fully understood: they are presumably related to differences in risk-factor patterns but findings from different regions do not show a consistent pattern.

Large artery atherosclerosis in the aortic arch

The link between atherosclerosis of the aortic arch and ischemic stroke was not clearly recognized until the early 1990s when autopsy studies revealed a high prevalence of such lesions in particular in patients with cryptogenic strokes [7]. At that time examination of the aortic arch was not part of the routine echocardiographic examination. Protruding aortic atheromas (>4–5 mm) have been found to be 3–9 times more common in stroke patients than in healthy controls. Later studies have established that aortic arch atheroma is clearly associated with ischemic stroke, possibly both by serving as a source of emboli and by being a marker of generalized large artery atherosclerosis including cerebral vessels. In stroke patients thick or complex aortic atheromas are associated with advanced age, carotid stenosis, coronary heart disease, atrial fibrillation, diabetes and smoking. For the long-term prognosis, the characteristics of thickness over 4–5 mm, ulceration, non-calcified plaque and presence of mobile components are associated with a 1.6–4.3 times increased risk of recurrent stroke.

> Protruding aortic atheromas are frequently found in stroke patients.

Mechanisms of cerebral ischemia resulting from extracranial and intracranial large artery atherosclerosis

Artery-to-artery embolism is considered the most common mechanism of TIA and ischemic stroke due to large artery atherosclerosis. Thrombosis at the site of an atherosclerotic lesion is due to interplay between the vessel wall lesion, blood cells and plasma factors. Severe stenosis alters blood flow characteristics, and turbulence replaces laminar flow when the degree of stenosis exceeds about 70%. Platelets are activated when exposed to abnormal or denuded endothelium in the region of an atheromatous plaque. Plaque hemorrhage may contribute to thrombus formation, similar to the mechanisms in coronary artery disease. Plaque instability appears to be a dynamic phenomenon [8], and may explain the observation that the risk of recurrent ischemic events is highest early after a TIA and is much lower from 1–3 months and onwards [9, 10]. Plaque instability is characterized by a thin fibrous cap, large lipid core, reduced smooth muscle content, and a high macrophage density. Complicating thrombosis occurs mainly when the thrombogenic center of the plaque is exposed to flowing blood.

Reduction of blood flow in the carotid artery is not affected until the degree of stenosis approaches

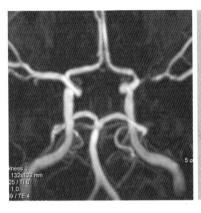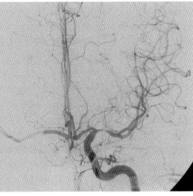

Figure 2.3. Stenosis of the middle cerebral artery visualized by MR angiography (left) and digital subtraction angiography (right). (Courtesy Dr Mats Cronqvist.)

70%, corresponding to a luminal diameter of less than 1.5 mm. However, the degree of carotid stenosis correlates poorly with intracranial hemodynamic alterations because of the variability of the collateral circulation. Embolic and hemodynamic causes of ischemic stroke and TIA are not mutually exclusive mechanisms. Ultrasound studies with transcranial Doppler have documented the frequent occurrence of microembolic signals not associated with apparent clinical symptoms in patients with symptomatic ischemic vascular disease of the brain. Hemodynamically compromised brain regions appear to have a diminished capacity for wash-out or clearance of small emboli which are more likely to cause infarcts in low-flow areas [11].

> Blood flow in the carotid artery is reduced if stenosis is more than 70%.

Clinical features of large artery atherosclerosis

Large artery atherosclerosis is a prototype of stroke mechanism that may cause almost any clinical stroke syndrome. Furthermore, some degree of atherosclerosis in brain-supplying arteries is present in most patients with ischemic stroke, raising the issue of determining the likely cause if multiple potential causes are identified. The clinical spectrum of large artery atherosclerosis ranges from asymptomatic arterial disease, TIA affecting the eye or the brain, and ischemic stroke of any severity in the anterior and posterior circulation. Less common clinical syndromes due to large artery atherosclerosis, e.g. those due to hemodynamic causes, are detailed in Chapter 9.

Cardioembolic stroke

Cardioembolic stroke accounts for 25–35% of all ischemic strokes, making cardiac disease the most common major cause of stroke overall – a practical point often forgotten. Non-valvular atrial fibrillation is the commonest cause of cardioembolic stroke. The heart is of particular importance in ischemic stroke for other reasons also: cardiac disorders (in particular coronary heart disease) frequently co-exist in patients with stroke and are important long-term prognostic determinants. Whereas recurrent stroke is the most common vascular event during the first few years after a first stroke, with time an increasing proportion of new vascular events are due to coronary heart disease.

> Cardiac disease is the most common cause of stroke overall.

Proportion of all strokes due to cardioembolic stroke

The proportion of strokes associated with cardioembolic strokes increases sharply with age, mainly because of the epidemiological characteristics in the population of atrial fibrillation, the single most common major cardioembolic source.

In some cases of cardioembolic stroke the association may be coincidental. This is certainly true for several of the minor cardioembolic sources (see below), for which findings from case-control studies show divergent results. As technology advances further more cardiac conditions that may constitute potential causes of stroke are detected. It is also true for atrial fibrillation, which is associated with several other stroke risk factors, and is very common in the general population. However, the finding that anti-coagulant therapy reduces the risk of ischemic stroke by about 60% in patients with atrial fibrillation suggests that the majority of strokes associated with atrial fibrillation are the result of cardiac embolism. A recent autopsy study of patients with stroke dying within 30 days showed that 70% of patients with a diagnosis of cardioembolic stroke in this study (based on cardiac conditions that may produce emboli in the heart or through the heart) were found to have intra-cardiac thrombi, which were of similar composition to persistent emboli detected in the major intracerebral arteries [12].

Cardioembolic sources: major and minor

There are several cardiac disorders that may consti-tute a source of embolus, but not all sources pose equal threats. They are commonly divided by origin in the heart (atrial, valvular, ventricular) and potential for embolism (high risk versus low or uncertain risk, or major versus minor) (Table 2.2). The clinically most important cardioembolic sources are non-rheumatic atrial fibrillation (AF), infective endocard-itis, prosthetic heart valve, recent myocardial infarc-tion, dilated cardiomyopathy, intracardiac tumors and rheumatic mitral valve stenosis.

Atrial fibrillation

Non-valvular atrial fibrillation (AF) is by far the commonest major cardioembolic source, and an arrhythmia of considerable importance for ischemic stroke due to its prevalence in the population and the substantial increase in stroke risk. In the general population 5–6% of persons >65 years and 12% of persons >75 years have AF. Fifty-six percent of people with AF are over 75 years of age. Epidemi-ological studies have shown that non-valvular atrial fibrillation is associated with at least a five-fold increased risk of stroke. However, the individual risk of embolism in AF varies 20-fold among atrial fib-rillation patients, depending on age and other asso-ciated risk factors. To predict the future risk for embolism in AF risk stratification schemes have been developed. Of the many schemes available, CHADS2 score is best validated; this score takes congestive heart failure (1 point), hypertension (1 point), age (1 point), diabetes (1 point) and prior stroke and TIA (2 points) into account; 1 point

Table 2.2. Cardioembolic sources and risk of embolism. (Modified from Ferro [21].)

High risk	Low/uncertain risk
I Atrial	
Atrial fibrillation	Patent foramen ovale
Sustained atrial flutter	Atrial septal aneurysm
Sick sinus syndrome	Atrial auto-contrast
Left atrial/atrial appendage thrombus	
Left atrial myxoma	
II Valvular	
Mitral stenosis	Mitral annulus calcification
Prosthetic valve	Mitral valve prolapse
Infective endocarditis	Fibroelastoma
Non-infective endocarditis	Giant Lambl's excrescences
III Ventricular	
Left ventricular thrombus	Akinetic/dyskinetic ventricular wall segment
Left ventricular myxoma	Subaortic hypertrophic cardiomyopathy
Recent anterior myocardial infarct	Congestive heart failure
Dilated cardiomyopathy	

corresponds to 1.4% annual stroke risk [13]. CHADS2 and other scores mainly refer to the pri-mary prevention setting. Patients in whom cerebral embolism has occurred generally fall into the cat-egories of very high risk.

> Atrial fibrillation carries at least a five-fold increased risk of stroke.

The proportion of ischemic strokes associated with AF increases with age, and in the highest age group >80 years about 40% of all strokes occur in patients with this arrhythmia [14]. The mean age of patients with stroke associated with AF is 79 years in European stroke registries, about 4 years higher than the average age of stroke in general. The importance of AF for ischemic stroke is likely to increase even further in the future because the prevalence of AF in the population is increasing (because persons with AF tend to live longer, and a larger proportion of people are reaching a higher age).

Paroxysmal atrial fibrillation carries a risk for embolism similar to the average risk for chronic AF, which is of importance for therapeutic purposes. Paroxysmal AF after ischemic stroke appears to be undetected in a substantial proportion of patients. By subsequent use of Holter monitoring and other monitoring techniques new AF is detected in at least 5% of all patients with ischemic stroke who are initially in sinus rhythm [15].

Prosthetic heart valves

Mechanical prosthetic heart valves are well recognized for their propensity to produce thrombosis and embolism, whereas tissue prostheses appear to have a much lower risk. Long-term anticoagulant therapy is standard practice for patients with mechanical prosthetic heart valves, but despite therapy embolism occurs at a rate of about 2% per year. Any type of prosthetic valve may be complicated by infective endocarditis, which should be considered in patients who experience embolic events.

Endocarditis

Infectious and non-infectious endocarditis is covered in Chapter 9 (Less common stroke syndromes).

Recent anterior myocardial infarct

Ischemic stroke may occur in close temporal proximity (hours, days, weeks) to an acute myocardial infarct, suggesting a cause-and-effect relationship due to embolism. Left ventricular mural thrombi have been diagnosed by echocardiography in up to 20% of patients with large anterior infarcts, but the frequency has not been well determined in the current era of much more active antithrombotic drug treatments and endovascular procedures in the acute phase of coronary heart disease. Studies have reported a frequency of about 5% for ischemic stroke during the first few weeks after myocardial infarction. After this period the stroke risk appears to be much lower, and is probably related to the presence of shared risk factors for coronary heart disease and ischemic stroke in the vast majority of these patients.

Five percent of ischemic strokes are related to a myocardial infarct.

Dilated cardiomyopathy

Dilated cardiomyopathies are a well-recognized cause of embolism, which may be due to the formation of intracardiac thrombus from severe ventricular dysfunction, atrial fibrillation or endocarditis. In contrast, hypertrophic cardiomyopathies appear not to be associated with an increased risk of stroke per se.

Patent foramen ovale (PFO) and atrial septal aneurysm

Patent foramen ovale (PFO) has been linked to ischemic stroke mainly in young adults, in whom frequencies for this cardiac finding of up to 40% are detected, about twice the rate in the general population [16, 17]. PFO is more commonly observed in patients with cryptogenic stroke than in those with a known cause, and this association appears to hold also for elderly patients [18]. PFO may cause stroke through paradoxical embolism, which requires the coexistence of thrombosis in lower limb, pelvic or visceral veins or pulmonary embolism, a cardiac right-to-left shunt, or cough or other Valsalva maneuver immediately preceding stroke onset. However, the exact mechanism by which PFO may cause stroke is still not clear, and evidence mainly comes indirectly from statistical associations. Concurrent venous thrombosis or pulmonary embolism is rarely detected even in patients with a high suspicion of paradoxical embolism. Besides paradoxical embolism PFO may be linked to stroke through causing a propensity for supraventricular arrhythmias, and through thrombus from a coexisting ASA. The long-term risk of recurrent stroke from PFO has not been precisely determined; it appears that mainly the coexistence of PFO and ASA is associated with a clearly increased risk of recurrence. PFO has also been linked to migraine (which increases the risk of stroke in young adults), but recent studies have not confirmed this association [19].

Patent foramen ovale may cause strokes through paradoxical embolism.

Mitral valve prolapse

Early studies proposed mitral valve prolapse to be the major cause of unexplained stroke in particular in young persons. However, revised diagnostic criteria and subsequent observational and case–control studies have questioned the overall role of mitral valve prolapse as a cardioembolic source.

Clinical and neuroimaging features of cardioembolic ischemic strokes

Although cardioembolism may cause almost any clinical stroke syndrome, some features are statistically linked to this cause and are therefore characteristic (Table 2.3). However, it should be borne in mind that the positive predictive value of clinical features suggesting cardioembolism is very modest, at only about 50% [20, 21]. Conversely, some clinical and neuroimaging syndromes, such as a lacunar syndrome found on dw-MRI to be due to a single small infarct, are very unlikely to be due to cardioembolism.

Traditionally it was thought that cardioembolic strokes almost always had a sudden onset of symptoms that were maximal from the beginning, but this doctrine has not stood the test of time. Exceptions with gradual and stuttering progressive courses are not rare, and may be due to distal migration of an embolus or early recurrence of embolism in the same vascular territory [22]. Strokes due to cardioembolism are usually more severe than average, probably because emboli from the heart tend to be larger than emboli from arterial sources. However, cardioembolism may well cause TIAs, and the proportion of cardioembolic strokes preceded by TIA is similar to findings in other stroke subtypes.

> Strokes due to cardioembolism are usually more severe than those from other causes.

The risk of early hemorrhagic transformation (multifocal or in the form of secondary hematoma) is about twice as high in cardiac embolism compared to other stroke subtypes [23]. Hemorrhagic transformation has been thought to be due to leakage of blood through a vessel wall with ischemic-induced increased permeability, but the process is likely to be much more complex. In patients with cardioembolism predictive factors of hemorrhagic transformation are decreased level of consciousness, high stroke severity, proximal occlusion, extensive early infarct signs in the MCA territory and delayed recanalization [24].

Some patients with a major cerebral hemispheric stroke syndrome due to distal internal carotid artery or proximal middle cerebral artery occlusion may have rapid spontaneous improvement of neurological deficits, a phenomenon that has been labeled "spectacular shrinking deficit" [25]. This clinical syndrome is usually, but not exclusively, caused by

Table 2.3. Features suggestive of cardioembolic stroke.

Sudden onset of maximal deficit

Decreased level of consciousness

Rapid regression of initially massive symptoms ("spectacular shrinking deficit")

Supratentorial stroke syndromes of isolated motor or sensory dysphasia, or visual field defects

Infratentorial ischemic stroke involving the cerebellum (PICA or SCA territories), top-of-the basilar

Hemorrhagic transformation

Neuroimaging finding of acute infarcts involving multiple vascular territories in the brain, or multiple levels of the posterior circulation

cardioembolism. The rapid improvement is due to distal propagation, fragmentation and subsequent spontaneous lysis of the embolus.

Emboli from the heart may occlude the internal artery in the neck, but more commonly they occlude one of the main intracranial vessels. In the anterior circulation cardioembolism and artery-to-artery embolism are the two major causes of full MCA infarcts due to proximal MCA occlusion as well as partial (pial territorial) MCA infarcts due to more distal occlusions. Large artery disease tends to be somewhat more common for anterior MCA infarcts, whereas cardioembolism is more common in posterior MCA lesions. Cardioembolism is also a recognized cause of the restricted cortical MCA syndrome of acute ischemic distal arm paresis, which may mimic peripheral radial or ulnar nerve lesion [26].

In the posterior circulation cardioembolism is no less frequent and tends to occur at characteristic "embolic" sites, common for embolism from cardiac and arterial sources (Figure 2.4). Cardioembolism is the cause of about a quarter of all lateral medullary infarcts, and about three-quarters of cerebellar infarcts in the PICA and SCA territories, and distal basilar artery occlusions. Basilar artery occlusion presenting with sudden onset of severe brainstem symptoms is often due to cardioembolism [27].

Studies with dw-MRI in patients with acute ischemic stroke have demonstrated that acute ischemic abnormalities involving multiple territories are much more common than previously thought; about 40% of

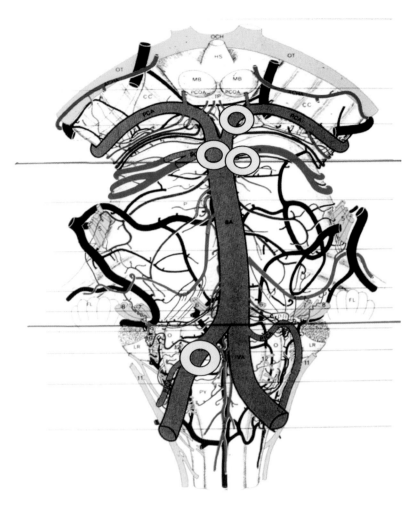

Figure 2.4. Main emboli recipient sites in the posterior circulation. (From Caplan LR, *Posterior Circulation Disease. Clinical Findings, Diagnosis and Management.* Cambridge MA: Blackwell Science 1996).

all patients have scattered lesions in one vascular territory or multiple lesions in multiple vascular territories. As should be logically plausible, these ischemic lesion patterns have been associated with embolism from cardiac or large artery sources [28].

Small-vessel disease

Infarcts due to small-vessel disease of the brain were first recognized by French neurologists and neuropathologists in the nineteenth century, who also coined the term "lacune" from the autopsy finding of a small cavitation. However, the importance of lacunar infarcts as one of the main ischemic stroke subtypes was not clearly recognized until the investigations of C. Miller Fisher in the 1960s, who on the basis of careful clinico-pathological observations laid the foundation for our pathological understanding of lacunar infarction.

Lacunar infarcts are small (<15 mm diameter) subcortical infarcts that result from occlusion of a single penetrating artery (Figure 2.5). Lacunar infarcts are usually located in the basal ganglia, thalamus, internal capsule, corona radiate and the brainstem. The arterial pathology is characterized by intracranial atherosclerosis (in situ atheroma either at the mouth or along the length of the penetrating vessel) and segmental arterial disorganization or lipohyalinosis secondary to the effects of hypertension. However, the detailed microvascular characteristics of lacunar infarcts are based on quite few observations, partly due to the difficulties in obtaining adequate and timely autopsy specimens. In the current era of better blood-pressure control lipohyalinosis appears to have become rarer [29].

Lacunar infarcts result from occlusion of single penetrating arteries.

35

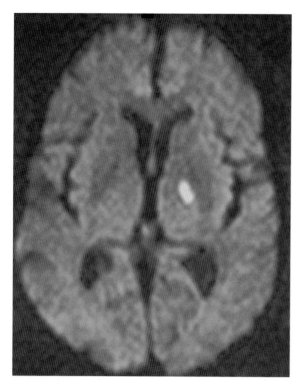

Figure 2.5. Diffusion-weighted MRI of a lacunar infarct in the internal capsule. (Courtesy Professor Stig Holtås.)

Prevalence and risk factors

In most series lacunar infarcts are thought to account for about one-quarter of all ischemic strokes, a proportion similar to cardioembolic stroke and infarcts due to large-vessel atherosclerosis. Patients with lacunar infarcts are on average a few years younger than patients with ischemic stroke in general. This is likely to be indirectly linked to the fact that cardioembolic sources become more prevalent with age and consequently patients with cardiac embolism tend to be older.

Lacunar infarcts are formed on a risk-factor profile that comprises age, gender, hypertension, diabetes, smoking, previous TIA and possibly ischemic heart disease. In particular, hypertension was initially thought to be a prerequisite for the development of small-vessel occlusion. However, later studies have demonstrated that the vascular risk-factor profile is not specific for lacunar infarction, but is largely similar to other stroke types [30]. Lacunar infarcts are also part of the clinical spectrum of cerebral autosomal dominant arteriopathy with subcortical infarcts and leukencephalopathy (CADASIL), a genetic disease affecting the small arteries of the brain (see Chapter 9).

Clinical features

Lacunar infarcts cause stroke, i.e. give rise to acute stroke symptoms, when they occur at strategic sites where descending and ascending long tracts are concentrated in their course subcortically or in the brainstem.

Classic lacunar syndromes

When symptomatic, lacunar infarcts are associated with clinical "lacunar" syndromes, five of which are well recognized: pure motor hemiparesis, pure sensory stroke, sensorimotor stroke, dysarthria–clumsy hand syndrome, and ataxic hemiparesis. Face, arm and leg involvement are characteristic of the first three syndromes. The most important clinical feature is the absence of cognitive symptoms or signs and visual field defects. Preceding TIAs occur in about 25% of all cases, usually only shortly before the infarct occurs. Sometimes patients present with a burst of dramatic TIAs with dense hemiparesis for 5–15 minutes alternating with normal function – the "capsular warning syndrome". About half of these patients go on to develop a lacunar infarct within the first 1–2 days, despite routine antiplatelet and even heparin therapies. Initial progression of the neurological deficit is observed in up to 40% of all cases, making lacunar infarct the most common subtype of progressive stroke. The exact mechanisms of the progression are unclear [31].

The classic lacunar syndromes are further detailed in Chapter 8.

Other clinical presentations of lacunar infarcts

Several other rarer clinical syndromes may also be caused by occlusion of single penetrating arteries, but the clinicopathological evidence for this is more limited. Descriptions include movement disorders such as chorea, dystonia, hemibalismus and asterixis. Brainstem syndromes (such as internuclear ophthalmoplegia, horizontal gaze palsy, Bendikt's syndrome, Claude's syndrome, pure motor hemiplegia plus sixth nerve palsies) and isolated cranial nerve palsies (most often third nerve palsies) may be caused by a microinfarct in the brainstem (visualized only by MRI), presumably most often due to occlusion of a small penetrating artery, though the mechanism is likely to vary. Occlusion of a branch artery at its origin by disease of the parent vessel (basilar branch occlusion) appears to occur more commonly in the posterior circulation than in the anterior circulation, where the mechanism is more often in situ disease in penetrating vessels. The old doctrine that isolated vascular cranial nerve syndromes were usually caused by affection of vasa vasorum to the peripheral nerve outside the brainstem is probably incorrect [32].

Silent lacunar infarcts

Lacunar infarcts cause clinical symptoms when they affect the long motor and sensory tracts in the subcortical areas, linked to their clinical presentation. However, MRI studies of the general population have disclosed that most lacunar infarcts do not produce acute stroke symptoms but are clinically unrecognized or "silent". Silent brain infarcts (95% of which are "lacunar") are at least five times as common as symptomatic ones, and have been shown to increase the risk of vascular events (including stroke), cognitive decline and dementia [33].

> Silent lacunar infarcts are five times more frequent than symptomatic ones.

Specificity of the clinical lacunar syndromes

Studies have shown that the majority of patients with lacunar syndromes have dw-MRI findings suggestive of lacunar infarcts, i.e. that the imaged ischemic abnormality is compatible with the territory of a single perforating artery. In the acute stage the diameter should be less than 15 mm, but may extend up to 20 mm in some cases. The infarct size shrinks by at least half from the acute to the chronic stage, and most late lacunar infarcts are less than 5 mm in diameter. However, with dw-MRI in no less than one-third of patients lesion patterns of multiple ischemic areas in the cortex or subcortex are seen, suggesting embolism as the underlying cause [34, 35]. Because multiple small embolic infarcts are present in a proportion of all patients presenting with a lacunar syndrome, carotid artery ultrasound, ECG and cardiac monitoring to detect atrial fibrillation should also be part of clinical routine in such patients.

Multiple overlapping causes of ischemic stroke

In some patients multiple overlapping causes of ischemic stroke are identified. In such cases, whether these findings are purely coincidental or represent the cause of the infarct is not clear. For example, patients with clinical and neuroimaging features that are compatible with lacunar infarction may have associated findings of large artery atherosclerosis or a cardioembolic source (most commonly atrial fibrillation). In one study, 4% of all stroke patients had small artery disease coexisting with large artery disease or a cardiac embolic source [36]. The cause of stroke in such patients is difficult to establish on an individual basis, but large artery or cardiac causes of stroke are not always coincidental. A causative rather than coincidental role of an ipsilateral carotid stenosis (70–99%) is indirectly suggested by a pooled analysis of individual patient data from randomized controlled trials of carotid surgery, which showed that surgery was also beneficial in a subgroup of patients with a lacunar infarct as defined by CT criteria [37].

Cryptogenic ischemic stroke

Patients experiencing a TIA/stroke frequently have no determined etiology after standard diagnostic evaluation. Previous reports show that 20–25% of stroke survivors are classified as cryptogenic stroke, but it is a matter of debate which strokes should be labeled cryptogenic – what level of evidence is needed for accepting a finding or risk factor as the "cause"? Such debate has surrounded PFO, which can be an incidental finding or possibly an underlying mechanism: methods for distinguishing incidental PFOs from pathogenic ones in cryptogenic stroke patients and for identifying patients at high risk of recurrence would be clinically most useful but are currently not available.

Many, if not most, of such 'cryptogenic' strokes may stem from unrecognized cardiac embolism in younger patients, and from subclinical aortic and large artery atherothrombotic embolism in older individuals. However, the identification of a potential underlying cause also relates to how far the diagnostic evaluations are pursued. Intermittent fibrillation was detected by long-term rhythm monitoring in 23% of such patients in a recent study [38].

Chapter Summary

> The Trial of Organon in Acute Stroke (TOAST) classification divides ischemic stroke into
> - atherothrombotic (30% of ischemic strokes, mostly emboli from the bifurcation of the carotid artery)

- cardioembolic (25–35% of ischemic strokes, mostly due to atrial fibrillation)
- small-vessel occlusion (25% of ischemic strokes, leading to lacunar infarcts)
- other determined cause
- and undetermined cause.

Sometimes, overlapping causes can be identified. Large artery atherosclerosis is estimated to account for about 30% of all ischemic strokes. Large-vessel disease may cause ischemia through embolism (artery-to-artery embolism) or reduction of blood flow (hemodynamic causes) or both (hemodynamically compromised brain regions appear to have a diminished capacity for wash-out or clearance of small emboli). The clinical spectrum of large artery atherosclerosis ranges from asymptomatic arterial disease, TIA affecting the eye or the brain, and ischemic stroke of any severity in the anterior and posterior circulation.

Cardioembolic stroke accounts for 25–35% of all ischemic strokes. The clinically most important cardioembolic sources are non-rheumatic atrial fibrillation (AF), infective endocarditis, prosthetic heart valve, recent myocardial infarction, dilated cardiomyopathy, intracardiac tumors and rheumatic mitral valve stenosis. Strokes due to cardioembolism are usually more severe than average.

In most series lacunar infarcts are thought to account for about one-quarter of all ischemic strokes. Lacunar infarcts are small (<15 mm diameter) subcortical infarcts that result from occlusion of a single penetrating artery. Lacunar infarcts are formed on a risk-factor profile that comprises age, gender, hypertension, diabetes, smoking, previous TIA and possibly ischemic heart disease. The most important clinical feature is the absence of cognitive symptoms or signs and visual field defects.

References

1. Adams HP, Bendixen BH, Kappelle LJ, et al. Classification of subtype of acute ischemic stroke. Definitions for use in a multicenter clinical trial. *Stroke* 1993; **24**:35–41.

2. Ay H, Furie KL, Singhal A, Smith WS, Sorensen AG, Koroshettz WJ. An evidence-based causative classification system for acute ischemic stroke. *Ann Neurol* 2005; **58**:688–97.

3. Ay H, Benner T, Arsava EM, Furie KL, Jensen MB, et al. A computerized algorithm for etiologic classification of ischemic stroke: the Causative Classification of Stroke System. *Stroke* 2007; **38**:2979–84.

4. Adams RJ, Chimowitz MI, Alpert JS, et al. Coronary risk evaluation in patients with transient ischemic attack and ischemic stroke: a scientific statement for healthcare professionals from the Stroke Council and the Council on Clinical Cardiology of the American Heart Association/American Stroke Association. *Stroke* 2003; **34**:2310–22.

5. Gongora-Rivera F, Labreuche J, Jaramillo A, et al. Autopsy prevalence of coronary atherosclerosis in patients with fatal stroke. *Stroke* 2007; **38**:1203–10.

6. Gorelick PB, Ka Sing Wong, Hee-Joon Bae, Pandey DK. Large artery intracranial occlusive disease. A large worldwide burden but a relatively neglected frontier. *Stroke* 2008; **39**:2396–99.

7. Amarenco P, Cohen A, Tzuorio C, et al. Atherosclerotic disease of the aortic arch and the risk of ischemic stroke. *N Engl J Med* 1994; **331**:1474–9.

8. Rothwell PM. Atherothrombosis and ischaemic stroke. *BMJ* 2007; **334**:379–80.

9. Giles MF, Rothwell PM. Risk of stroke early after transient ischaemic attack: a systematic review and meta-analysis. *Lancet Neurology* 2007; **6**:1063–72.

10. Wu CM, McLaughlin K, Lorenzetti DL, Hill MD, Manns BJ, Ghali WA. Early risk of stroke after transient ischemic attack. A systematic review and meta-analysis. *Arch Intern Med* 2007; **167**:2417–22.

11. Caplan LR, Wong KS, Gao S, Hennerici MH. Is hypoperfusion an important cause of strokes? If so, how? *Cerebrovasc Dis* 2006; **21**(3):145–53.

12. Ogata J, Yutani C, Otsubo R, Yamanishi H, Naritomi H, Yamaguchi T, et al. Heart and vessel pathology underlying brain infarction in 142 stroke patients. *Ann Neurol* 2008; **63**:770–81.

13. Gage BF, van Walraven C, Pearce L, Hart RG, Koudstaal PJ, Boode BS, et al. Selecting patients with atrial fibrillation for anticoagulation: stroke risk stratification in patients taking aspirin. *Circulation* 2004; **110**:2287–92.

14. Marini C, De Santis F, Sacco S, et al. Contribution of atrial fibrillation to incidence and outcome of ischemic stroke: results from a population-based study. *Stroke* 2005; **36**:1115–19.

15. Liao J, Khalid Z, Scallan C, Morillo C, O'Donnell M. Noninvasive cardiac monitoring for detecting paroxysmal atrial fibrillation or flutter after acute ischemic stroke: a systematic review. *Stroke* 2007; **38**:2935–40.

16. Mas JL, Arquizan C, Lamy C, Zuber M, Cabanes I, Derumeaux G, et al. Recurrent cerebrovascular events associated with patent foramen ovale, atrial septal aneurysm, or both. *N Engl J Med* 2001; **345**:1740–6.

17. Lamy C, Giannesini C, Zuber M, Arquizan C, Meder JF, Trystram D, et al. Clinical and imaging findings in cryptogenetic stroke patients with and without patent foramen ovale: the PFO-ASA Study. *Stroke* 2002; **33**:706–11.

18. Handke M, Harloff A, Olschewski M, Hetzel A, Geibel A. Patent foramen ovale and cryptogenic stroke in older patients. *N Engl J Med* 2007; **357**:2262–8.

19. Rundek T, Elkind MS, Di Tullio MR, Carrera E, Jin Z, Sacco RL, et al. Patent foramen ovale and migraine: a cross-sectional study from the Northern Manhattan Study (NOMAS). *Circulation* 2008; **118**:1419–24.

20. Palacio S, Hart RG. Neurologic manifestations of cardiogenic embolism: an update. *Neurol Clin* 2002; **20**:179–93.

21. Ferro JM. Cardioembolic stroke: an update. *Lancet Neurology* 2003; **2**:177–88.

22. Kang DW, Latour LL, Chalela JA, Dambrosia J, Warach S. Early ischemic lesion recurrence within a week after acute ischemic stroke. *Ann Neurol* 2003; **54**:66–74.

23. Paciaroni M, Agnelli G, Corea F, Ageno W, Alberti A, et al. Early hemorrhagic transformation of brain infarction: rate, predictive factors, and influence on clinical outcome: results of a prospective multicenter study. *Stroke* 2008; **39**:2249–56.

24. Molina CA, Montaner J, Abilleira S, et al. Timing of spontaneous recanalization and risk of hemorrhagic transformation in acute cardioembolic stroke. *Stroke* 2001; **32**:1079–84.

25. Minematsu K, Yamaguchi T, Omae T. Spectacular shrinking deficit: rapid recovery from a major hemispheric syndrome by migration of an embolus. *Neurology* 1992; **42**:17–62.

26. Gass A, et al. A diffusion-weighted MRI study of acute ischemic distal arm paresis. *Neurology* 2001; **57**:1589–94.

27. Caplan LR. *Posterior Circulation Disease. Clinical Findings, Diagnosis and Management.* Cambridge MA: Blackwell Science; 1996.

28. Kang DW, Chalela JA, Ezzeddine MA, et al. Association of ischaemic lesion patterns on early diffusion-weighted imaging with TOAST stroke subtypes. *Arch Neurol* 2003; **60**:1730–4.

29. Lammie GA, Brannan F, Slattery J, Warlow C. Nonhypertensive cerebral small-vessel disease: an autopsy study. *Stroke* 1997; **28**:2222–9.

30. Jackson C, Sudlow C. Are lacunar strokes really different? A systematic review of differences in risk factor profiles beween lacuna and nonlacunar infarcts. *Stroke* 2005; **36**:891–901.

31. Steinke W and Ley SC. Lacunar stroke is the major cause of progressive motor deficits. *Stroke* 2002; **33**:1510–16.

32. Thömke F, Gutmann L, Stoeter P, Hopf HC. Cerebrovascular brainstem diseases with isolated cranial nerve palsies. *Cerebrovasc Dis* 2002; **13**:147–55.

33. Vermeer S, Longstreth Jr WT, Koudstaal PJ. Silent brain infarcts: a systematic review. *Lancet Neurology* 2007; **6**:611–19.

34. Wessels T, Rottger C, Jauss M, Kaps M, Traupe H, Stolz E. Identification of embolic stroke patterns by diffusion-weighted MRI in clinically defined lacunar stroke syndromes. *Stroke* 2005; **36**:757–61.

35. Caso V, Budak K, Georgiadis D, Schuknecht B, Baumgartner RW. Clinical significance of detection of multiple acute brain infarcts on diffusion weighted magnetic resonance imaging. *J Neurol Neurosurg Psychiatry* 2005; **76**:514–18.

36. Moncayo J, Devuyst G, Van Melle G, Bogousslavsky J. Coexisting causes of ischemic stroke. *Arch Neurol* 2000; **57**:1139–44.

37. Rothwell PM, Eliaziw M, Gutnikov SA, et al. Analysis of pooled data from the randomized trials of endarterectomy for symptomatic carotid stenosis. *Lancet* 2003; **361**:107–16.

38. Tayal AH, Tian M, Kelly KM, Jones SC, Wright DG, et al. Atrial fibrillation detected by mobile cardiac outpatient telemetry in cryptogenic TIA or stroke. *Neurology* 2008; **71**:1696–701.

Neuroradiology

PART A: IMAGING OF ACUTE ISCHEMIC AND HEMORRHAGIC STROKE: CT, PERFUSION CT, CT ANGIOGRAPHY

Patrik Michel

Non-contrast CT (NCCT)

NCCT can be performed in less than a minute with a helical CT scanner, and is considered sufficient to select patients for intravenous thrombolysis with iv-RTP within 4.5 hours, or endovascular treatment within 6 hours. It is a highly accurate method for identifying acute intracerebral hemorrhage and sub-arachnoid hemorrhage, but quite insensitive for detecting acute ischemia. The approximate sensitivity of CT and perfusion CT (PCT) in different ischemic stroke subtypes is depicted in Figure 3.1. Focal hypoattenuation (hypodensity) is very specific and predictive for irreversible ischemia, whereas early edema without hypoattenuation indicates low perfusion pressure with increased MCV and therefore represents potentially salvageable tissue [1]. The "fogging effect" relates to the potential disappearance of hypoattenuation from approximately day 7 for up to 2 months after the acute stroke. It may result in false-negative NCCT in the subacute stage of ischemic stroke.

Prognosis in thrombolysed and non-thrombolysed patients is worse if there are clear early ischemic signs on NCCT [2, 3]. However, patients benefit from early intravenous and intra-arterial thrombolysis despite early ischemic signs [3, 4].

> Non-contrast CT (NCCT) is highly accurate for identifying acute intracerebral hemorrhage and sub-arachnoid hemorrhage, but quite insensitive for detecting acute ischemia.

Perfusion CT (PCT)

PCT with iodinated contrast may be used in two ways:
- as a slow-infusion/whole-brain technique
- as dynamic perfusion CT with first-pass bolus-tracking methodology.

The latter is preferable as it is quantitative and allows accurate identification of the ischemic penumbra [5].

In a patient with suspected acute ischemic stroke, a non-contrast baseline cerebral CT is immediately followed by PCT. Then, a CTA of the head and neck, and a contrast-enhanced CT of the brain are performed, with a total of about 15 minutes from the start to the end of the examination. If the patient fulfils criteria for intravenous thrombolysis based on the NCCT, treatment may be started in the scanner while the patient is undergoing PCT and CTA. Similarly, image acquisition and processing usually overlap.

PCT examinations usually consist of two 40-second series separated by 5 minutes. For each series, CT scanning is initiated 7 seconds after injection of 50 ml of isoosmolar iodinated contrast material into an antecubital vein using a power injector. Multidetector-array technology currently allows the acquisition of data from four adjacent 5–10 mm sections for each series. The lowest of these eight cerebral CT sections usually cuts through the midbrain and hippocampi; the other slices cover most of the supratentorial brain.

The perfusion CT data are analyzed according to the central volume principle to create parametric maps of regional cerebral blood volume (rCBV), mean transit time (MTT), and regional cerebral blood flow (rCBF). The rCBV map is calculated from a quantitative estimation of the partial size averaging effect, which is completely absent in a reference pixel at the center of the large superior sagittal venous sinus. The

MTT maps result from a deconvolution of the parenchymal time–concentration curves by a reference arterial curve. Finally, the rCBF values can be calculated from the rCBV and MTT values for each pixel using the following equation: rCBF = rCBV/MTT. The maps can then be displayed graphically (Figure 3.2A–C).

Total ischemic area (penumbra and infarct) is defined as cerebral pixels with a greater than 145% prolongation of MTT compared with the corresponding region in the contralateral cerebral hemisphere [6]. Within this selected area, 2.0 ml/100 g represents the rCBV threshold: pixels belong to the infarct core if the rCBV value is inferior to the threshold, and to the penumbra if the rCBV value is superior to the threshold. Salvageable penumbra is displayed in green, and

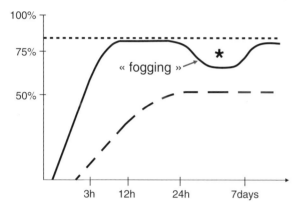

Figure 3.1. Approximate likelihood of detecting ischemic stroke on non-contrast CT (NCCT) in territorial (continuous line) and lacunar (dashed line) infarcts. * indicates the fogging effect observed in the subacute phase on NCCT. The dotted line indicates approximate sensitivity of perfusion CT in non-lacunar supratentorial strokes. PCT data are from the ASTRAL registry.

tissue with low likelihood of survival (infarct core) is displayed in red (Figure 3.2D).

Raw maps of PCT images may be interpreted in a non-quantitative way by comparing the different parameters given in Table 3.1.

MTT is the most sensitive measure for decreased blood flow but overestimates ischemia. rCBF is more specific in identifying salvageable tissue, and rCBV is the most specific parameter for irreversibly damaged tissue [7, 8], also in white matter [9]. Threshold maps separate reversible from irreversible ischemia [10, 11] and result in high inter-observer agreement [11].

The 64-slice CT scanners allowing for eight or more brain slices have increased the detection rate for acute ischemic stroke [12], which is now similar to that of DWI [13]. PCT has an overall sensitivity of about 75% for ischemic stroke, above 85% for non-lacunar supratentorial infarcts (Figure 3.1), and a high specificity for ischemia [7, 11 14]. PCT also predicts mass effect in the MCA territory [15].

Comparison of PCT with PET in healthy controls shows that quantitative measures of blood flow are accurate [16], but this comparison still needs to be performed in acute stroke patients.

PCT also shows brain perfusion alterations in about 25% of patients with TIAs, which is sometimes still present after the resolution of the patients' symptoms [17]. Focal hyperperfusion in relationship with epileptic seizures has been described, and focal hypoperfusion is rare [18]. During the aura of migrainous patients, occasional poorly delimited hemispheric hypoperfusion contralateral to the aura symptoms is found [19].

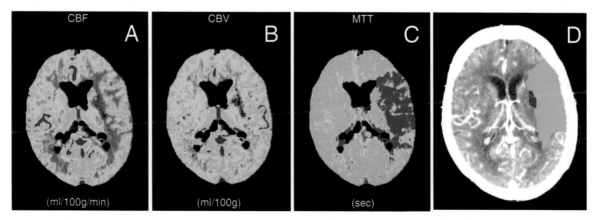

Figure 3.2. A 77-year-old patient, found on awakening with aphasia and right hemiparesis, NIHSS = 20. Perfusion CT maps depicting (A) regional cerebral blood flow, (B) regional cerebral blood volume, (C) mean transit time, and (D) core infarct maps according to a threshold model (Wintermark, *Ann Neurol* 2002 [10]). In (D), green: reversible ischemia (penumbra), and red: low likelihood of survival (infarct).

Overall, in the absence of an abnormality on PCT in a patient with stroke symptoms, one might suspect a posterior fossa stroke, a lacunar stroke, small cortical stroke [12] or a stroke-imitating condition (migraine, Todd's paralysis, venous thrombosis, encephalitis, conversion syndrome). Acute recanalization treatments might be inappropriate in some of these patients.

Baseline PCT volumes correlate with stroke severity in the acute stage, and do so better in left-sided infarctions [20]. As compared to standard imaging [3], acute advanced functional imaging performs better in predicting the clinical status and outcome [21].

PCT predictors of treatment response are not yet established. In a series of 75 patients [22], the best predictors for dependency (mRS > 2) at 3 months were patient age and the total ischemia volume on PCT. The presence or absence of a large-vessel occlusion before thrombolysis was not a significant predictor of outcome in this group [21]. This suggests that i.v. thrombolysis may be particularly effective if an initial large-vessel occlusion is present. It has been shown that thrombolysis saves salvageable tissue as identified by PCT [23].

> Perfusion CT (PCT) has an overall sensitivity of about 75% for ischemic stroke, above 85% for non-lacunar supratentorial infarcts, and a high specificity for ischemia.

CT angiography

Cerebral and cervical CT angiography is performed using intravenous administration of 50 ml of iodinated contrast material at a rate of 3 ml per second, and an acquisition delay of about 15 seconds. Data acquisition is performed from the origin of the aortic arch branch vessels to the circle of Willis and reconstructed as maximum-intensity projections (MIP) (Figure 3.3E) and three-dimensional reconstructions (Figure 3.3B).

Table 3.1. Alterations of MTT, rCBV and rCBF in case of ischemia (comparison with contralateral homologous region).

	MTT	rCBF	rCBV
Healthy parenchyma	=	=	=
Penumbra	↑↑	↓	= or ↑
Infarct	↑↑↑	↓↓	↓

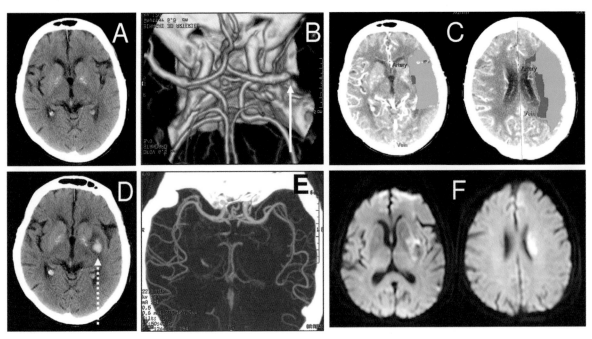

Figure 3.3. Same patient as in Figure 3.2. **Upper row**: imaging at 12 hours after going to bed: (A) plain CT, (B) CT angiography with occlusion of the middle cerebral artery (white arrow), and (C) perfusion CT with threshold maps. The patient was then given intravenous thrombolysis with rTPA at 13 hours after going to bed and 2.5 hours after awaking (approved study protocol with informed consent from family). **Lower row**: (D) plain CT at 24 hours with a small left basal ganglion bleed (dotted arrow). (E) CT angiography with repermeabilization, and (F) diffusion-weighted MRI at 5 days, showing a small, partially hemorrhagic lesion.

CTA has been shown to identify the site of arterial occlusion in acute ischemic stroke patients, with similar accuracy compared to DSA and MRA [24]. Clot burden scores and collateral circulation [25] can be assessed. A few pilot studies have considered its predictive value [10, 21], but its value for predicting treatment response remains insufficiently known [26].

> CT angiography (CTA) has been shown to identify the site of arterial occlusion in acute ischemic stroke patients.

Comparison of MR- and CT-based acute stroke imaging

Both CT- and MR-based perfusion and arterial imaging are feasible in the emergency setting. With regard to information about brain perfusion, PCT appears at least equivalent to MRI [13, 27–30]. Significant correlation has been demonstrated between PCT-CBV and DWI, between PCT-MTT and PWI-TTP, and between CTA source images and DWI [28, 29]. If threshold models are used, the PCT core correlates well with DWI and PCT total ischemia with PWI-MTT [10, 13].

The linear relationship between contrast concentration and signal intensity is an important advantage of CT perfusion imaging over gadolinium-based MR perfusion imaging, allowing a more quantitative estimation of cerebral blood flow [31].

Both CTA and MRA detect significant stenosis and vascular malformations quite reliably [24, 32]. Whereas CTA better identifies arterial calcifications, MRA is probably more specific in diagnosing cervical artery dissections [33].

Valid criticisms of MR imaging include its cost, limited availability, more difficult patient monitoring, pace-maker incompatibility, and the longer time required for scanning [34]. Exposure to radiation prohibits frequent use of PCT and CTA. Iodinated contrast can occasionally be associated with allergy, hyperthyroidism, or renal failure, although this seems to occur rarely [35]. These drawbacks are counterbalanced by the availability of CT in most emergency rooms, its easy accessibility, and the easy monitoring of patients. Patients with known severe renal failure (creatinine clearance <30 ml/min.) should probably receive neither iodinated contrast agents nor gadolinium [36].

> PCT appears to be at least equivalent to MRI for information about brain perfusion.

CT and intracranial hemorrhage

Hyperintensity in acute intracranial hemorrhage (ICH) is present on NCCT from its onset in virtually all patients. Intraparenchymal calcifications or melanin-containing metastases may sometimes give false-positive results. Adding CTA is debated, but is probably useful in patients with higher risk of vascular malformations underlying the ICH, such as patients with ICH outside the perforator (deep) localizations, without hypertension, and of younger age. One main advantage of adding iodinated contrast in ICH is that contrast extravasation ("leakage") is an independent predictor of hematoma growth and poorer clinical outcome. It may constitute a target for aggressive antihypertensive or hemostatic therapy. Various radiological methods, including PCT [37], indicate that there is no ischemia around the hematoma but rather point to edema formation.

> Intracranial hemorrhage (ICH) can be diagnosed with NCCT. Adding CTA can be useful in patients with higher risk of vascular malformations.

PART B: IMAGING OF ACUTE ISCHEMIC AND HEMORRHAGIC STROKE: MRI AND MR ANGIOGRAPHY

Jens Fiehler

Practical aspects of acute stroke MRI

Magnetic resonance imaging (MRI) can be used as the sole modality for the emergency imaging of patients with suspected acute stroke, whether ischemic or hemorrhagic. Multiparametric stroke imaging combining diffusion and perfusion-weighted MRI (DWI and PWI), MR angiography (MRA) and conventional MR sequences such as fluid-attenuated inversion recovery (FLAIR) is increasingly utilized as the primary imaging modality in major stroke centers. Short acquisition times reduce motion artifacts and enable the study of acute stroke patients with moderate cooperation. Fast image reconstruction makes the results of MRA or PWI available within a few minutes. The advantage of a multiparametric MRI approach lies in the characterization of the lesion extension and of the stroke mechanism, thus providing a pathophysiological basis for rational decision-making. In a recent prospective study it has been shown that MRI is more effective than plain CT for detection of acute ischemia, and can detect acute and chronic hemorrhage; it should be the preferred test for accurate diagnosis of patients with suspected acute stroke [38].

> Multiparametric MRI (using a combination of diffusion- and perfusion-weighted MRI (DWI and PWI)), MR angiography (MRA) and conventional MR sequences such as fluid-attenuated inversion recovery (FLAIR) can provide a characterization of the extension of the lesion and of the underlying mechanism in acute stroke.

Diffusion-weighted imaging (DWI)

DWI is based on the additional signal intensity increase caused by slow-moving spins between two diffusion-sensitizing magnetic field gradients. DWI signal intensity in acute stroke reveals a typical sequel of an early decrease (minutes to <1 hour; cell depolarization and cytotoxic edema) when T2w imaging may still be normal, and "pseudonormalization" after 1–10 days (increased extracellular water content = vasogenic edema) followed by a further rise above normal ranges (cell lysis and necrosis).

Magnetic resonance angiography (MRA)

In contrast to PWI, MRA directly reveals the location of the vessel occlusion. The size of the thrombus – related to the site of vessel occlusion in MRA – is an important determinant of vessel recanalization rates and cannot be derived from diffusion or perfusion-weighted imaging alone. Most patients with more proximal occlusions on MRA reveal a considerable lesion growth and a poor outcome [39]. Without MRA available signal intensity changes within vessels ("vessel signs") in conventional MRI sequences can be helpful in diagnosing the site of vessel occlusion. However, the hypointense vessel sign in T2*-weighted MRI and the hyperintense vessel sign in FLAIR do not independently predict recanalization, ICH, or clinical outcome [40].

Perfusion-weighted imaging (PWI) and the mismatch concept

PWI maps are derived from the signal intensity change caused by the passage of contrast agent through the capillary bed and reflect several aspects of cerebral perfusion such as cerebral blood volume and flow and the mean transit time. Both the volume and the severity of the initial perfusion deficit are associated with the growth of the initial DWI lesion at follow-up imaging.

The penumbra in acute stroke patients has been defined as brain tissue with loss of electrical activity and potential recovery after timely recanalization of the occluded artery. It is widely accepted that extension of the lesion in acute stroke as delimited in perfusion-weighted MRI (PWI) beyond the corresponding lesion boundary in diffusion-weighted imaging (DWI) is indicative of the penumbra [41, 42]. This PWI > DWI mismatch has been used, validated and refined in several studies [42–44]. Especially for stroke patients treated 3–6 hours after onset, such baseline MRI findings can identify subgroups that are likely to benefit from reperfusion therapies and can potentially identify subgroups that are unlikely to benefit or may be harmed [45, 46]. However, the PWI > DWI mismatch concept has also been challenged [47, 48] on the grounds that the PWI lesion cannot discriminate reliably between benign oligemia and true penumbra, and because of noted overestimation of the extent of infarction seen at follow-up [49, 50]. A likely factor in these shortcomings is that the same degree of perfusion impairment might have a different impact on the tissue depending on patient age, the anatomic location and time from stroke onset.

Susceptibility-weighted imaging and intracerebral hemorrhage

Measurement of transverse relaxation times that characterize the signal loss caused by local susceptibilities (T2') is sensitive to changes of the local concentration of deoxy-Hb in brain tissue as a direct indicator of an increased oxygen extraction fraction in the presence of a perfusion deficit, and T2' lesions exceeding the dimensions of the corresponding ADC lesion were a more specific predictor of infarct growth than the traditional PWI > DWI mismatch [51]. Another way to improve diagnostic accuracy is the use of multivariate prediction models that integrate all available imaging parameters into one prediction model [52]. In the future such information might be most beneficial in patients where the decision whether or not to treat with thrombolysis is difficult, for example in a patient arriving after >3 h or with known elevated risk of bleeding complications.

For the evaluation of intracranial hemorrhage (ICH) clinicians have traditionally relied on CT, in fear of missing or misdiagnosing an ICH by utilizing MRI only. Recent studies suggest that this is not the case, and that MRI in fact may be superior [53], especially for the detection of small chronic hemorrhages, the cerebral microbleeds (CMBs). CMBs in the brain parenchyma diagnosed in T2*-weighted MRI should be interpreted in the light of the patient's history as well as the location, number, and distribution of the lesions and associated imaging findings. Current data do not support the hypothesis that CMBs are associated with a higher risk of a clinically relevant intracerebral hemorrhage after anticoagulation/antiaggregation therapy or after thrombolytic therapy in stroke patients, and thus do not support the general exclusion of patients from therapy based on the presence of CMBs [54, 55]. Subdural hematomas (SDHs) and subarachnoid hemorrhages (SAHs) can be identified reliably by using appropriate MRI techniques. In the hyperacute setting SDHs are best demonstrated on FLAIR sequences. Since FLAIR imaging nulls the effect of cerebrospinal fluid, SDHs are best appreciated on this sequence. On DWI SDHs appear hyperintense and on T2*-weighted images they tend to be hypointense. The presence of mixed signal intensity within the SDH may indicate the presence of blood with different ages and MRI may emerge as a tool in selecting the therapeutic approach to SDHs [56]. The best imaging sequences for MRI-based SAH detection are FLAIR and proton density-weighted images [57].

Chapter Summary

Imaging of acute ischemic and hemorrhagic stroke: CT

Non-contrast CT (NCCT) is highly accurate for identifying acute intracerebral hemorrhage and subarachnoid hemorrhage, but quite insensitive for detecting acute ischemia. Focal hypoattenuation (hypodensity) is very specific and predictive for irreversible ischemia. NCCT is considered sufficient to select patients for intravenous thrombolysis with iv-RTP within 4.5 hours or endovascular treatment within 6 hours.

Perfusion CT (PCT) has an overall sensitivity of about 75% for ischemic stroke, above 85% for non-lacunar supratentorial infarcts, and a high specificity for ischemia.

Mean transit time (MTT) is the most sensitive measure for decreased blood flow but overestimates ischemia. Regional blood flow (rCBF) is more specific in identifying salvageable tissue, and regional cerebral blood volume (rCBV) is the most specific parameter for irreversibly damaged tissue. Threshold maps separate reversible from irreversible ischemia. With regard to information about brain perfusion, PCT appears at least equivalent to MRI.

CT angiography (CTA) has been shown to identify the site of arterial occlusion in acute ischemic stroke patients, with similar accuracy compared to DSA and MRA. Hyperintensity in acute intracranial hemorrhage (ICH) is present on NCCT from its onset in virtually all patients. Adding CTA is probably useful in patients with higher risk of vascular malformations underlying the ICH.

Imaging of acute ischemic and hemorrhagic stroke: MRI

The advantage of a multiparametric MRI approach lies in the characterization of the lesion extension and of the stroke mechanism, thus providing a pathophysiological basis for rational decision-making. **Diffusion-weighted imaging (DWI)** reveals a typical early decrease of signal intensity in acute stroke when T2w imaging may still be normal. **Magnetic resonance angiography (MRA)** directly reveals the location of the vessel occlusion. **Perfusion-weighted imaging (PWI)** reflects several aspects of cerebral perfusion such as cerebral blood volume and flow and the mean transit time. A mismatch of DWI and PWI in the extension of the ischemic lesion is indicative of the penumbra (this concept has also been challenged, though). Cerebral microbleeds, subdural hematomas and subarachnoid hemorrhages can be identified reliably by using appropriate MRI techniques (fluid attenuated inversion recovery (FLAIR) and proton density-weighted images).

References

1. Na DG, Kim EY, Ryoo JW, et al. CT sign of brain swelling without concomitant parenchymal hypoattenuation: comparison with diffusion- and perfusion-weighted MR imaging. *Radiology* 2005; **235**(3):992–48.

2. Hill MD, von Kummer R, Levine S, et al. ASPECT overview of NINDS, ECASS, and ATLANTIS. TAST Symposium, Whistler, Canada; 2004.

3. Hill MD, Rowley HA, Adler F, et al. Selection of acute ischemic stroke patients for intra-arterial thrombolysis with pro-urokinase by using ASPECTS. *Stroke* 2003; **34**(8):1925–31.

4. Demchuk AM, Hill MD, Barber PA, Silver B, Patel SC, Levine SR. Importance of early ischemic computed tomography changes using ASPECTS in NINDS rtPA Stroke Study. *Stroke* 2005; **36**(10):2110–15.

5. Latchaw RE, Yonas H, Hunter GJ, et al. Guidelines and recommendations for perfusion imaging in cerebral ischemia: A scientific statement for healthcare professionals by the writing group on perfusion imaging, from the Council on Cardiovascular Radiology of the American Heart Association. *Stroke* 2003; **34**(4):1084–104.

6. Wintermark M, Flanders AE, Velthuis B, et al. Perfusion-CT assessment of infarct core and penumbra: receiver operating characteristic curve analysis in 130 patients suspected of acute hemispheric stroke. *Stroke* 2006; **37**(4):979–85.

7. Koenig M, Kraus M, Theek C, Klotz E, Gehlen W, Heuser L. Quantitative assessment of the ischemic brain by means of perfusion-related parameters derived from perfusion CT. *Stroke* 2001; **32**(2):431–7.

8. Eastwood JD, Lev MH, Azhari T, et al. CT perfusion scanning with deconvolution analysis: pilot study in patients with acute middle cerebral artery stroke. *Radiology* 2002; **222**(1):227–36.

9. Murphy BD, Fox AJ, Lee DH, et al. White matter thresholds for ischemic penumbra and infarct core in patients with acute stroke: CT perfusion study. *Radiology* 2008; **247**(3):818–25.

10. Wintermark M, Reichhart M, Thiran JP, et al. Prognostic accuracy of cerebral blood flow measurement by perfusion computed tomography, at the time of emergency room admission, in acute stroke patients. *Ann Neurol* 2002; **51**(4):417–32.

11. Wintermark M, Fischbein NJ, Smith WS, Ko NU, Quist M, Dillon WP. Accuracy of dynamic perfusion CT with deconvolution in detecting acute hemispheric stroke. *Am J Neuroradiol* 2005; **26**(1):104–12.

12. Youn SW, Kim JH, Weon YC, Kim SH, Han MK, Bae HJ. Perfusion CT of the brain using 40-mm-wide detector and toggling table technique for initial imaging of acute stroke. *Am J Roentgenol* 2008; **191**(3):W120–6.

13. Schaefer PW, Barak ER, Kamalian S, et al. Quantitative assessment of core/penumbra mismatch in acute stroke. CT and MR perfusion imaging are strongly correlated when sufficient brain volume is imaged. *Stroke* 2008; **39**:epublish August 21.

14. Wintermark M, Fischbein NJ, Smith WS, Ko NU, Quist M, Dillon WP. Accuracy of dynamic perfusion CT with deconvolution in detecting acute hemispheric stroke. *Am J Neuroradiol* 2005; **26**(1):104–12.

15. Dittrich R, Kloska SP, Fischer T, et al. Accuracy of perfusion-CT in predicting malignant middle cerebral artery brain infarction. *J Neurol* 2008; **255**(6):896–902.

16. Kudo K, Terae S, Katoh C, et al. Quantitative cerebral blood flow measurement with dynamic perfusion CT using the vascular-pixel elimination method: comparison with H2(15)O positron emission tomography. *Am J Neuroradiol* 2003; **24**(3):419–26.

17. Michel P, Reichhart M, Wintermark M, Maeder P, Bogousslavsky R. Perfusion-CT in transient ischemic attacks (abstract). *Stroke* 2005; **36**:484.

18. Bezerra DC, Michel P, Reichhart M, Wintermark M, Meuli R, Bogousslavsky J. Perfusion-CT guided acute thrombolysis in patients with seizures at stroke onset (abstract). *Stroke* 2005; **36**:484.

19. Gonzalez-Delgado M, Michel P, Reichhart M, Wintermark M, Maeder P, Bogousslavsky J. The significance of focal hypoperfusion during migraine with aura. *Stroke* 2005; **36**:444.

20. Furtado AD, Smith WS, Koroshetz W, et al. Perfusion CT imaging follows clinical severity in left hemispheric strokes. *Eur Neurol* 2008; **60**(5):244–52.

21. Nabavi DG, Kloska SP, Nam EM, et al. MOSAIC: Multimodal Stroke Assessment Using Computed Tomography: novel diagnostic approach for the prediction of infarction size and clinical outcome. *Stroke* 2002; **33**(12):2819–26.

22. Reichhart MD, Bezerrra DC, Wintermark M, et al. Predictive value of penumbra and vascular occlusion state in stroke patients treated with iv rt-PA within 3 hours. *Neurology* 2005; **64**:A263.

23. Silvennoinen HM, Hamberg LM, Lindsberg PJ, Valanne L, Hunter GJ. CT perfusion identifies increased salvage of tissue in patients receiving intravenous recombinant tissue plasminogen activator within 3 hours of stroke onset. *Am J Neuroradiol* 2008; **29**(6):1118–23.

24. Knauth M, von KR, Jansen O, Hahnel S, Dorfler A, Sartor K. Potential of CT angiography in acute ischemic stroke. *Am J Neuroradiol* 1997; **18**(6):1001–10.

25. Tan JC, Dillon WP, Liu S, Adler F, Smith WS, Wintermark M. Systematic comparison of perfusion-CT and CT-angiography in acute stroke patients. *Ann Neurol* 2007; **61**(6):533–43.

26. Jovin TG, Yonas H, Gebel JM, et al. The cortical ischemic core and not the consistently present penumbra is a determinant of clinical outcome in acute middle cerebral artery occlusion. *Stroke* 2003; **34**(10):2426–33.

27. Wintermark M, Reichhart M, Cuisenaire O, et al. Comparison of admission perfusion computed tomography and qualitative diffusion- and perfusion-weighted magnetic resonance imaging in acute stroke patients. *Stroke* 2002; **33**(8):2025–31.

28. Schramm P, Schellinger PD, Fiebach JB, et al. Comparison of CT and CT angiography source images with diffusion-weighted imaging in patients with acute stroke within 6 hours after onset. *Stroke* 2002; **33**(10):2426–32.

29. Eastwood JD, Lev MH, Wintermark M, et al. Correlation of early dynamic CT perfusion imaging with whole-brain MR diffusion and perfusion imaging in acute hemispheric stroke. *Am J Neuroradiol* 2003; **24**(9):1869–75.

30. Wintermark M, Meuli R, Browaeys P, et al. Comparison of CT perfusion and angiography and MRI in selecting stroke patients for acute treatment. *Neurology* 2007; **68**(9):694–7.

31. Wintermark M, Maeder P, Thiran JP, Schnyder P, Meuli R. Quantitative assessment of regional cerebral blood flows by perfusion CT studies at low injection rates: a critical review of the underlying theoretical models. [Review] [81 refs]. *Eur Radiol* 2001; **11**(7):1220–30.

32. Liu Y, Karonen JO, Vanninen RL, et al. Acute ischemic stroke: predictive value of 2D phase-contrast MR angiography–serial study with combined diffusion and perfusion MR imaging. *Radiology* 2004; **231**(2): 517–27.

33. Schievink WI. Spontaneous dissection of the carotid and vertebral arteries. *N Engl J Med* 2001; **344**(12):898–906.

34. Lev MH, Koroshetz WJ, Schwamm LH, Gonzalez RG. CT or MRI for imaging patients with acute stroke: visualization of "tissue at risk"? *Stroke* 2002; **33**(12):2736–7.

35. Dittrich R, Akdeniz S, Kloska SP, et al. Low rate of contrast-induced nephropathy after CT perfusion and CT angiography in acute stroke patients. *J Neurol* 2007; **254**(11):1491–7.

36. Thomsen HS. ESUR guideline: gadolinium-based contrast media and nephrogenic systemic fibrosis. *Eur Radiol* 2007; **17**(10):2692–6.

37. Fainardi E, Borrelli M, Saletti A, et al. CT perfusion mapping of hemodynamic disturbances associated to acute spontaneous intracerebral hemorrhage. *Neuroradiology* 2008; **50**:729–40.

38. Chalela JA, Kidwell CS, Nentwich LM, Luby M, Butman JA, Demchuk AM, et al. Magnetic resonance imaging and computed tomography in emergency assessment of patients with suspected acute stroke: a prospective comparison. *Lancet* 2007; **369**:293–8.

39. Fiehler J, Knudsen K, Thomalla G, Goebell E, Rosenkranz M, Weiller C, et al. Vascular occlusion sites determine differences in lesion growth from early apparent diffusion coefficient lesion to final infarct. *Am J Neuroradiol* 2005; **26**:1056–61.

40. Schellinger PD, Chalela JA, Kang DW, Latour LL, Warach S. Diagnostic and prognostic value of early MR imaging vessel signs in hyperacute stroke patients imaged <3 hours and treated with recombinant tissue plasminogen activator. *Am J Neuroradiol* 2005; **26**:618–24.

41. Rovira A, Orellana P, Alvarez-Sabin J, Arenillas JF, Aymerich X, Grive E, et al. Hyperacute ischemic stroke: middle cerebral artery susceptibility sign at echo-planar gradient-echo MR imaging. *Radiology* 2004; **232**:466–73.

42. Thomalla G, Schwark C, Sobesky J, Bluhmki E, Fiebach JB, Fiehler J, et al. Outcome and symptomatic bleeding complications of intravenous thrombolysis within 6 hours in MRI-selected stroke patients: comparison of a German multicenter study with the pooled data of ATLANTIS, ECASS, and NINDS tPA trials. *Stroke* 2006; **37**:852–8.

43. Hacke W, Albers G, Al-Rawi Y, Bogousslavsky J, Davalos A, Eliasziw M, et al. The Desmoteplase in Acute Ischemic Stroke Trial (DIAS): a phase II MRI-based 9-hour window acute stroke thrombolysis trial with intravenous desmoteplase. *Stroke* 2005; **36**:66–73.

44. Butcher K, Parsons M, Allport L, Lee SB, Barber PA, Tress B, et al. Rapid assessment of perfusion-diffusion mismatch. *Stroke* 2008; **39**:75–81.

45. Albers GW, Thijs VN, Wechsler L, Kemp S, Schlaug G, Skalabrin E, et al. Magnetic resonance imaging profiles predict clinical response to early reperfusion: the diffusion and perfusion imaging evaluation for understanding stroke evolution (DEFUSE) study. *Ann Neurol* 2006; **60**:508–17.

46. Davis SM, Donnan GA, Parsons MW, Levi C, Butcher KS, Peeters A, et al. Effects of alteplase beyond 3 h after stroke in the Echoplanar Imaging Thrombolytic Evaluation Trial (EPITHET): a placebo-controlled randomised trial. *Lancet Neurol* 2008; **7**:299–309.

47. Kidwell CS, Alger JR, Saver JL. Beyond mismatch: evolving paradigms in imaging the ischemic penumbra with multimodal magnetic resonance imaging. *Stroke* 2003; **34**:2729–2735.

48. Fiehler J, Knudsen K, Kucinski T, Kidwell CS, Alger JR, Thomalla G, et al. Predictors of apparent diffusion coefficient normalization in stroke patients. *Stroke* 2004; **35**:514–19.

49. Grandin CB, Duprez TP, Smith AM, Oppenheim C, Peeters A, Robert AR, et al. Which MR-derived perfusion parameters are the best predictors of infarct

growth in hyperacute stroke? Comparative study between relative and quantitative measurements. *Radiology* 2002; **223**:361–70.

50. Kucinski T, Naumann D, Knab R, Schoder V, Wegener S, Fiehler J, et al. Tissue at risk is overestimated in perfusion-weighted imaging: MR imaging in acute stroke patients without vessel recanalization. *Am J Neuroradiol* 2005; **26**:815–19.

51. Siemonsen S, Fitting T, Thomalla G, Horn P, Finsterbusch J, Summers P, et al. T2' imaging predicts infarct growth beyond the acute diffusion-weighted imaging lesion in acute stroke. *Radiology* 2008; **248**:979–986.

52. Wu O, Christensen S, Hjort N, Dijkhuizen RM, Kucinski T, Fiehler J, et al. Characterizing physiological heterogeneity of infarction risk in acute human ischaemic stroke using MRI. *Brain* 2006; **129**:2384–93.

53. Kidwell CS, Chalela JA, Saver JL, Starkman S, Hill MD, Demchuk AM, et al. Comparison of MRI and CT for detection of acute intracerebral hemorrhage. *JAMA* 2004; **292**:1823–30.

54. Fiehler J. Cerebral microbleeds: old leaks and new haemorrhages. *Int J Stroke* 2006; **1**:122–30.

55. Fiehler J, Albers GW, Boulanger JM, Derex L, Gass A, Hjort N, et al. Bleeding risk analysis in stroke imaging before thromboLysis (BRASIL): pooled analysis of T2*-weighted magnetic resonance imaging data from 570 patients. *Stroke* 2007; **38**:2738–44.

56. Tanikawa M, Mase M, Yamada K, Yamashita N, Matsumoto T, Banno T, et al. Surgical treatment of chronic subdural hematoma based on intrahematomal membrane structure on MRI. *Acta Neurochir (Wien)* 2001; **143**:613–18; discussion 618–19.

57. Wiesmann M, Mayer TE, Yousry I, Medele R, Hamann GF, Bruckmann H. Detection of hyperacute subarachnoid hemorrhage of the brain by using magnetic resonance imaging. *J Neurosurg* 2002; **96**:684–9.

PART C: FUNCTIONAL IMAGING IN ACUTE STROKE, RECOVERY AND REHABILITATION

Wolf-Dieter Heiss

Role of functional imaging in stroke patients

The functional deficit after a focal brain lesion is determined by the localization and the extent of the tissue damage; recovery depends on the adaptive plasticity of the undamaged brain, especially the cerebral cortex, and of the non-affected elements of the functional network. Since destroyed tissue usually cannot be replaced in the adult human brain, improvement or recovery of neurological deficits can be achieved only by reactivation of functionally disturbed but morphologically preserved areas or by recruitment of alternative pathways within the functional network. This activation of alternative pathways may be accompanied by the development of different strategies to deal with the new functional-anatomical situation at the behavioral level. Additionally, the sprouting of fibers from surviving neurons and the formation of new synapses could play a role in long-term recovery. These compensatory mechanisms are expressed in altered patterns of blood flow or metabolism at rest and during activation within the functional network involved in a special task, and therefore functional imaging tools can be applied successfully for studying physiological correlates of plasticity and recovery noninvasively after localized brain damage. The observed patterns depend on the site, the extent, and also the type and the dynamics of the development of the lesion; they change over time and thereby are related to the course and the recovery of a deficit. The visualization of disturbed interaction in functional networks and of their reorganization in the recovery after focal brain damage is the domain of functional imaging modalities such as PET and functional magnetic resonance imaging (fMRI).

For the analysis of the relationship between disturbed function and altered brain activity studies can be designed in several ways: measurement at rest, comparing location and extent to deficit and outcome (eventually with follow-up); measurement during activation tasks, comparing changes in activation patterns to functional performance; and measurement at rest and during activation tasks early and later in the course of disease (e.g. after stroke) to demonstrate recruiting and compensatory mechanisms in the functional network responsible for complete or partial recovery of disturbed functions. Only a few studies have been performed applying this last and most complete design together with extensive testing for the evaluation of the quality of performance finally achieved.

A large amount of data has been collected over the past years with functional imaging of changes in activation patterns related to recovery of disturbed function after stroke [1–6].

> The visualization of disturbed interaction in functional networks and of their reorganization in the recovery after focal brain damage is the domain of functional imaging modalities such as PET and functional magnetic resonance imaging (fMRI).

The principle of functional and activation studies using positron emission tomography (PET)

The energy demand of the brain is very high and relies almost entirely on the oxidative metabolism of glucose (see Chapter 1). Mapping of neuronal activity in the brain can be primarily achieved by quantitation of the regional cerebral metabolic rate for glucose (rCMRGlc), as introduced for autoradiographic experimental studies by Sokoloff et al. [7] and adapted for positron emission tomography (PET) in humans by Reivich et al. [8]. The cerebral metabolic rate for glucose (CMRGlc) can be quantified with PET using 2-[^{18}F]fluoro-2-deoxyglucose (FDG) and a modification of the three-compartment model equation developed for autoradiography by Sokoloff et al. [7]. Like glucose, FDG is transported across the blood–brain barrier and into brain cells, where it is phosphorylated by hexokinase. However, FDG-6-phosphate cannot be metabolized to its respective fructose-6-phosphate analog, and does not diffuse out of the cells in significant amounts. The distribution of the radioactivity accumulated in the brain remains quite stable between 30 and 50 minutes after intravenous tracer injection, thus permitting multiple intercalated scans. Using (i) the local radioactivity concentration measured with PET during this steady-state period, (ii) the concentration–time course of tracer in arterial plasma, (iii) plasma glucose concentration, and (iv) a lumped constant correcting for the differing behavior in brain of FDG and glucose, CMRGlc can be computed pixel by pixel according to an optimized operational equation [9]. The resulting pseudocolor-coded images reflect all effects on cerebral glucose metabolism. Because of its robustness with regard to procedure and model assumptions, the FDG method has been employed in many PET studies.

Almost all commonly applied methods for the quantitative imaging of CBF are based on the principle of diffusible tracer exchange. Using ^{15}O-labeled water administered either directly by intravenous bolus injection or by the inhalation of ^{15}O-labeled carbon dioxide, which is converted into water by carbonic anhydrase in the lungs, CBF can be estimated from steady-state distribution or from the radioactivity concentration–time curves in arterial plasma and brain. Typical measuring times range between 40 seconds and 2 minutes, and, because of the short biological half-life of the radiotracers, repeat studies can be performed [10, 11].

Various PET methods have been developed for determining the cerebral metabolic rate for oxygen (CMRO$_2$), using continuous [11] or single-breath inhalation [12] of air containing trace amounts of ^{15}O-labeled molecular oxygen. All require the concurrent estimation or paired measurement of CBF in order to convert the measured oxygen extraction fractions (OEFs) into images of CMRO$_2$ as given by the product of arterial oxygen concentration, local OEF and local CBF. Because ^{15}O has a short half-life (123 seconds), an on-site cyclotron is necessary; this and other methodological complexities limit the use of CMRO$_2$ as a measure of brain function. Application of this method for detection of penumbra tissue is described in Chapter 1.

Functional activation studies as they are used now rely primarily on the hemodynamic response, assuming a close association between energy metabolism and blood flow. Whereas it is well documented that increases in blood flow and glucose consumption are closely coupled during neuronal activation, the increase in oxygen consumption is considerably delayed, leading to a decreased oxygen extraction fraction (OEF) during activation [13]. PET detects and, if required, can quantify changes in CBF and CMRGlc accompanying different activation states of brain tissue. The regional values of CBF or CMRGlc represent the brain activity due to a specific state, task or stimulus in comparison to the resting condition, and color-coded maps can be analyzed or correlated to morphological images. Due to the radioactivity of the necessary tracers, activation studies with PET are limited to a maximum of 12 doses of ^{15}O labeled tracers, e.g. 12 flow scans, or two doses of ^{18}F-labeled tracers, e.g. two metabolic scans. Especially for studies of glucose consumption, the time to metabolic equilibrium (20–40 min) must be taken into consideration, as well as the time interval between measurements required for isotope decay (HT for ^{18}F 108 min, for ^{15}O 2 min).

PET used to quantify the regional concentration of these tracers relies on the labeling of the compounds with short-lived cyclotron-produced radioisotopes (e.g. ^{15}O, ^{11}C, ^{13}N, ^{18}F) which are characterized by a unique decay scheme. A positron, i.e. a positively charged particle of the mass of an electron, is emitted from a labeled probe molecule. Following emission from the atomic nucleus, the positron takes a path marked by multiple collisions with ambient electrons. Approximately 1–3 mm from its origin, it has lost so much energy that it combines with an electron, resulting in the annihilation of the two oppositely charged particles by the emission at an angle of $180° \pm 0.5°$ of two 511 keV (kilo electron volt) photons that are recorded as coincident events, using pairs of uncollimated (convergent) detectors facing each other. Therefore, the origin of the photons can be localized directly to the straight line between these coincidence detectors. State-of-the-art PET scanners are equipped with thousands of detectors arranged in up to 24 rings, simultaneously scanning 47 slices of <5 mm thickness. Pseudocolor-coded tomographic images of the radioactivity distribution are then reconstructed from the many projected coincidence counts by a computer, using CT-like algorithms and reliable scatter and attenuation corrections. Typical in-plane resolution (full width at half-maximum) is <5 mm; 3D data accumulation and reconstruction permits imaging of the brain in any selected plane or view.

> In PET, radioactive tracers can be used to detect and quantify changes in cerebral blood flow (CBF) and cerebral metabolic rate of glucose (CMRGlc). Color-coded maps of different activation states of brain tissue can be analyzed or coregistered to morphological images.

Functional magnetic resonance imaging (fMRI)

fMRI measures signals that depend on the differential magnetic properties of oxygenated and deoxygenated hemoglobin, termed the blood-oxygen-level-dependent (BOLD) signal, which gives an estimate of changes in oxygen availability [14]. This means that mainly the amount of deoxyhemoglobin in small blood vessels is recorded, which depends on the flow of well-oxygenated arterial blood (CBF), on the outflow of O_2 to the tissue (CMRO$_2$) and on the cerebral blood volume (CBV) [15]. The magnitude of these changes in signal intensity relative to the resting conditions is color-coded to produce fMRI images that map changes in brain function, which can be superimposed on the anatomical image. This results in a spatial resolution of fMRI of 1–3 mm with a temporal resolution of approx. 10 sec. As fMRI does not involve ionizing radiation and thus is also used without limitation in healthy subjects, and allows more rapid signal acquisition and more flexible experimental set-ups, it has become the dominant technique for functional imaging. There are some advantages of PET, however – physiologically specific measures, better quantitation, better signal-to-noise ratio, fewer artifacts, actual activated and reference values – which support its continued use especially in complex clinical situations and in combination with special stimulating techniques, such as transcranial magnetic stimulation (TMS).

> Functional MRI (fMRI) detects changes in brain function by measuring differences in magnetic properties of hemoglobin depending on the blood oxygen level.

Motor and somatosensory deficits

Motor function may be impaired by damage to a widely distributed network, involving multiple cortical representations and complex fiber tracts. The degree of motor impairment and the potential for recovery depends on the site of the lesion, the association of lesions in cortical areas and in fiber tracts and the involvement of deep gray structures, e.g. the basal ganglia, thalamus and brainstem. The patterns of altered metabolism and blood flow and the patterns of activation after stimuli or during motor tasks are manifold and reflect the site and extent of the lesion, but they are also dependent on the paradigm of stimulus or task. With severe motor impairment, patients cannot carry out complex or even simple motor tasks, and the activation paradigm must be restricted to passive movement or imagination of motor performance. The diverging experimental conditions make the interpretation and comparison of different studies extremely difficult, and might help explain the lack of a clear concept of "neuronal plasticity" applicable to recovery from motor stroke

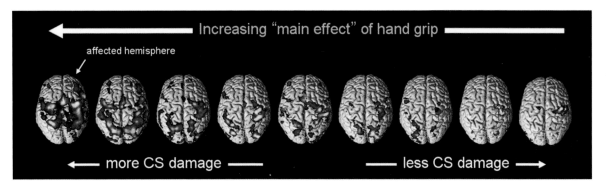

Figure 3.4. Brain activity for hand grip compared to rest for individual subjects with corticospinal damage. These fMRI studies demonstrate that increasing corticospinal damage leads to a shift in the pattern of activation from the primary to the secondary motor system. (Modified from Ward [5].)

(reviews in [2, 5, 6, 16–18]). A recent review concluded that "motor recovery after stroke depends on a variety of mechanisms including perilesional motor reorganization, use of motor pathways in subcortical structures, use of collateral pathways in the ipsilateral hemisphere, or use of collateral pathways in the contralateral hemisphere, or possibly the development of entirely new motor networks" [2]. In most fMRI or PET studies involving active or passive movements, a widespread network of neurons was activated in both hemispheres. The areas included frontal and parietal cortices, and sometimes the basal ganglia and cerebellum. In particular, (ipsilateral) premotor cortex, supplementary motor area (SMA), anterior parts of the insula/frontal operculum, and bilateral inferior parietal cortices are often activated (Figure 3.4). These results suggest that sensorimotor functions are represented in extended, variable, probably parallel processing, bilateral networks [19]. Whereas changes in both the damaged and the undamaged hemisphere can be observed, ipsilateral activation of motor cortex is consistently found to be stronger for movement of the paretic fingers after recovery from stroke, whereas movements of the unaffected hand (as in normal subjects) were accompanied mainly by activation of the contralateral cerebral cortex. In addition to stronger intensity, the spatial extent of activation in motor cortex was enlarged, and activation on the ipsilateral side was also seen in premotor and insular cortex. These results indicate that recruitment of ipsilateral cortices plays a role in recovery.

Task-oriented arm training increased activation bilaterally in the inferior parietal area, in premotor areas and in the contralateral sensorimotor cortex, suggesting an improved functional brain reorganization in the bilateral sensory and motor systems [20]. Similar results were obtained by fMRI, by which an evolution of the activation in the sensorimotor cortex from early contralesional activity to late ipsilateral activity was found [21], suggesting a dynamic bihemispheric reorganization of motor networks during recovery from hemiparesis. It was also shown that the over-activation observed a few weeks after a stroke diminishes over time, suggesting compensatory mechanisms appearing even late in the course (Figure 3.5) [22]. Ipsilateral cortical recruitment seems to be a compensatory cortical process related to the lesion of the contralateral primary motor cortex; this process of compensatory recruitment will persist if the primary motor cortex is permanently damaged. Newly learned movements after focal cortical injury are represented over larger cortical territories, an effect which is dependent on the intensity of rehabilitative training. It is of importance that the unaffected hemisphere actually inhibits the generation of a voluntary movement by the paretic hand [23]. This effect of transcallosal inhibition can be reduced by repetitive transcranial magnetic stimulation (rTMS) [24]. Recovery from infarction is also accompanied by substantial changes in the activity of the proprioceptive systems of the paretic and non-paretic limb, reflecting an interhemispheric shift of attention to proprioceptive stimuli associated with recovery [25].

During recovery from hemiparesis, a dynamic bihemispheric reorganization of motor networks takes place. fMRI and PET studies can display the compensatory cortical processes and show the importance of transcallosal inhibition.

7 weeks 31 weeks

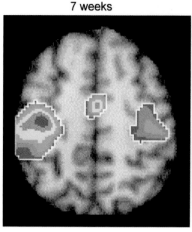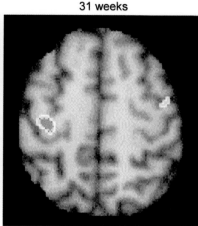

Figure 3.5. Overactivation in the primary and secondary motor area in five patients compared with normal controls 7 and 31 weeks after left capsular stroke during right thumb-index tapping. Decrease of initial bilateral overactivation to activation restricted to the primary sensorimotor cortex in the affected and primary motor cortex in the unaffected hemisphere. Left hemisphere is shown on the left of the standard MRI templates. (From Calautti C. et al. *Stroke* 2001, 32:2534–42.)

Post-stroke aphasia

Studies of glucose metabolism in aphasia after stroke have shown metabolic disturbances in the ipsilateral hemisphere caused by the lesion and contralateral hemisphere caused by functional deactivation (diaschisis) (review in [26]). In right-handed individuals with language dominance in the left hemisphere, the left temporo-parietal region, in particular the angular gyrus, supramarginal gyrus and lateral and transverse superior temporal gyrus are the most frequently and consistently impaired, and the degree of impairment is related to the severity of aphasia. In patients with aphasia attributable to purely subcortical strokes deactivation of temporo-parietal cortex is regularly found, which is probably responsible for the aphasic symptoms. The functional disturbance as measured by rCMRGlc in speech-relevant brain regions early after stroke is predictive of the eventual outcome of aphasia, where not only functional deactivation (diaschisis) but also neuronal loss may contribute to metabolic and perfusional changes in the neighborhood of the infarct. Therefore, metabolism in the hemisphere outside the infarct was significantly less in patients with a poor outcome of post-stroke aphasia than in those with good language recovery, indicating significant cell loss caused by the ischemic episode outside the ischemic core. In addition, the functionality of the network was reduced in patients with an eventual poor outcome; during task performance, patients with an eventual good recovery predominantly activated structures in the ipsilateral hemisphere. Although the brain recruits right-hemispheric regions for speech-processing when the left-hemispheric centers are impaired [27], outcome studies reveal that this strategy is significantly less effective than repair of the speech-relevant network in adults. That the quality of recovery is mainly dependent on undamaged portions of the language network in the left hemisphere and to a lesser extent on homologous right hemisphere areas [28] can be deduced from an activation study in the course after post-stroke aphasia [29]. Repeating words activated blood flow in 10 normal controls by more than 10% relative to resting condition in both upper temporal gyri, by 5–10% in planum temporale and Heschl gyrus of both sides and in the lower part of the central gyrus of the left side, and by less than 5% in the left Broca area. This test procedure was applied to 23 aphasic patients grouped according to the site of the MRI/CT lesion. Activation PET studies were performed in the subacute stage approximately 2 weeks after the stroke and repeated 6 weeks later. On matched MRIs regions of interest were defined in 14 identified structures of the bilateral language-related network. The three groups of aphasic patients showed different patterns of activation in the acute and chronic phase, and their improvement was different: whereas subcortical and frontal infarcts improved considerably in several tests, temporal infarcts showed only little improvement. These differences in improvement of speech deficits were reflected in different patterns of activation in the course after stroke (Figure 3.6): the subcortical and frontal groups improved substantially and activated the right inferior frontal gyrus and the right superior temporal gyrus (STG) at baseline and regained regional left

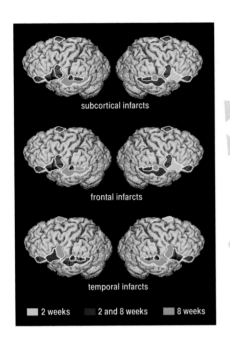

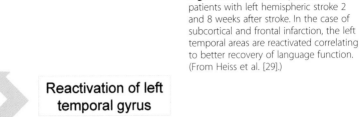

Figure 3.6. Activation patterns in patients with left hemispheric stroke 2 and 8 weeks after stroke. In the case of subcortical and frontal infarction, the left temporal areas are reactivated correlating to better recovery of language function. (From Heiss et al. [29].)

STG activation at follow-up. The temporal group improved only in word comprehension; it activated the left Broca area and supplementary motor areas at baseline and the precentral gyrus bilaterally as well as the right STG at follow-up, but could not reactivate the left STG. These results were confirmed in comparable studies [30–32]. In a randomized controlled study piracetam, which improved performance in a large multi-center trial [33] and was identified as effective in a Cochrane Review [34], improved performance in aphasia tests for spontaneous speech, which was reflected in increased activation in the left temporal gyrus, the triangular part of the left inferior frontal gyrus and the left posterior temporal gyrus [35].

> Studies of glucose metabolism in aphasia after stroke have shown metabolic disturbances in the ipsilateral hemisphere caused by the lesion and contralateral hemisphere caused by functional deactivation (diaschisis).

Combination of repetitive transcranial magnetic stimulation (rTMS) with activated imaging

rTMS is a non-invasive procedure to create electric currents in discrete brain areas which, depending on frequency, intensity and duration, can lead to transient increases and decreases in excitability of the affected cortex. Low frequencies of rTMS (below 5 Hz) can suppress excitability of the cortex, while higher-frequency stimulation (5–20 Hz) leads to an increase in cortical excitability [36]. Increases in relative cerebral blood volume in contralateral homologous language regions during overt propositional speech fMRI in chronic, non-fluent aphasia patients indicated over-activation of right language homologues. This right hemisphere over-activation may represent a maladaptive strategy and can be interpreted as a result of decreased transcallosal inhibition due to damage of the specialized and lateralized speech areas. TMS studies with blockade of this contralateral over-activation by series of 1 Hz rTMS [37] have reported improved picture-naming ability in chronic non-fluent aphasia patients. Collateral ipsilateral as well as transcallosal contralateral inhibition can be demonstrated by simultaneous rTMS and PET activation studies [38]: at rest, rTMS decreased blood flow ipsilaterally and contralaterally. During verb generation, rCBF was decreased during rTMS ipsilaterally under the coil, but increased ipsilaterally outside the coil and in the contralateral homologous area (Figure 3.7). The effect of rTMS was accompanied by a prolongation of reaction time latencies to verbal stimuli.

The role of activation in the right hemisphere for residual language performance can be investigated by combining rTMS with functional imaging, e.g. PET.

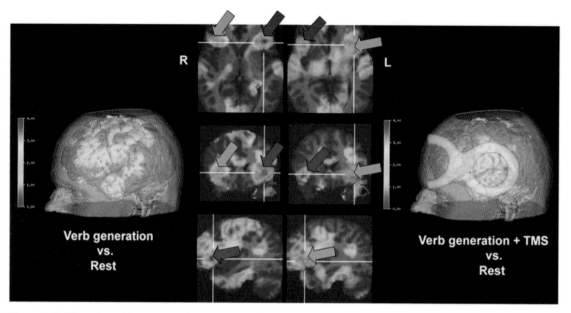

Figure 3.7. Effect of repetitive transcranial magnetic stimulation on activation pattern by verb generation. The coil position is shown in the 3D rendering. Image (A) shows inferior frontal gyrus activation during simple verb generation. Image (B) clearly shows the decreased activation on the left (blue arrow) and increased activity on the right side (yellow arrow) during rTMS interference. (Modified from Thiel et al. [38].)

In patients in whom verb generation activated predominantly the right inferior frontal gyrus, this response could be blocked by rTMS over this region. These patients had lower performance in verbal fluency tasks than patients with effects of rTMS only over the left IFG, suggesting a less effective compensatory potential of right-sided network areas. These results indicate a potential for rTMS in the treatment of post-stroke aphasia.

The activation studies in the course of recovery of post-stroke aphasia suggest various mechanisms for the compensation of the lesion within the functional network. Despite differences among the activation and stimulation paradigms and the heterogeneity of patients included in different imaging studies [39], a hierarchy for effective recovery might be deduced:

- Best, even complete, recovery can only be achieved by restoration of the original activation pattern after small brain damage outside primary centers.
- If primary functional centers are damaged, reduction of collateral inhibition leads to activation of areas around the lesion (intrahemispheric compensation).
- If the ipsilateral network is severely damaged, reduction of transcallosal inhibition causes

activation of contralateral homotopic areas, which is usually not as efficient as intrahemispheric compensation. In some patients with slowly developing brain damage the language function can be completely shifted to the right hemisphere.

In most instances the disinhibition of homotopic areas contralateral to the lesion impairs the capacity for recovery – a mechanism which might be counteracted by rTMS of these contralateral active areas. This approach might open a new therapeutic strategy for post-stroke aphasia.

The role of activation in the right hemisphere for residual language performance can be investigated by combining rTMS with functional imaging, e.g. PET. Counteraction by rTMS of contralateral active areas might open a new therapeutic strategy for post-stroke aphasia.

Chapter Summary

The visualization of disturbed interaction in functional networks and of their reorganization in the recovery after focal brain damage is the domain of functional imaging modalities such as PET and fMRI.

PET: Mapping of neuronal activity in the brain can be primarily achieved by quantitation of the regional **cerebral metabolic rate for glucose** (CMRGlc). Quantitative imaging of **cerebral blood flow** (CBF) is based on the principle of diffusible tracer exchange, using ^{15}O-labeled water.

PET detects and, if required, can quantify changes in CBF and CMRGlc accompanying different activation states of brain tissue. The regional values of CBF or CMRGlc represent the brain activity due to a specific state, task or stimulus in comparison with the resting condition, and color-coded maps can be analyzed or correlated to morphological images.

fMRI measures signals that depend on the differential magnetic properties of oxygenated and deoxygenated hemoglobin, termed the blood-oxygen-level-dependent (BOLD) signal, which gives an estimate of changes in oxygen availability. The amount of deoxyhemoglobin in small blood vessels depends on the flow of well-oxygenated arterial blood (CBF), on the outflow of O_2 to the tissue ($CMRO_2$) and on the cerebral blood volume (CBV). fMRI images map changes in brain function and can be superimposed on the anatomical image.

Motor and somatosensory deficits

In most fMRI or PET studies involving active or passive movements, a widespread network of neurons was activated in both hemispheres. During recovery from hemiparesis, a dynamic bihemispheric reorganization of motor networks takes place. Ipsilateral cortical recruitment seems to be a compensatory cortical process related to the lesion of the contralateral primary motor cortex. The unaffected hemisphere actually inhibits the generation of a voluntary movement by the paretic hand. This effect of transcallosal inhibition can be reduced by repetitive transcranial magnetic stimulation (rTMS).

Post-stroke aphasia

Studies of glucose metabolism in aphasia after stroke have shown metabolic disturbances in the ipsilateral hemisphere caused by the lesion and contralateral hemisphere caused by functional deactivation (diaschisis). Patients with an eventual good recovery predominantly activated structures in the ipsilateral hemisphere.

Combination of repetitive transcranial magnetic stimulation (rTMS) with activated imaging

Activation studies in the course of recovery of post-stroke aphasia suggest various mechanisms for the compensation of the lesion within the functional network: restoration of the original activation pattern, activation of areas around the lesion (intrahemispheric compensation) and reduction of transcallosal inhibition causing activation of contralateral homotopic areas. rTMS is a non-invasive procedure to create electric currents in discrete brain areas which, depending on frequency, intensity and duration, can lead to transient increases (with higher frequencies) and decreases (with lower frequencies) in excitability of the affected cortex. The role of activation in the right hemisphere for residual language performance can be investigated by combining rTMS with functional imaging, e.g. PET. Counteraction by rTMS of contralateral active areas might open a new therapeutic strategy for post-stroke aphasia.

References

1. Rijntjes M, Weiller C. Recovery of motor and language abilities after stroke: the contribution of functional imaging. *Prog Neurobiol* 2002; **66**:10922.

2. Thirumala P, Hier DB, Patel P. Motor recovery after stroke: lessons from functional brain imaging. *Neurol Res* 2002; **24**:453–8.

3. Weiller C. Imaging recovery from stroke. *Exp Brain Res* 1998; **123**:13–17.

4. Herholz K, Heiss WD. Functional imaging correlates of recovery after stroke in humans. *J Cereb Blood Flow Metab* 2000; **20**:1619–31.

5. Ward NS. Future perspectives in functional neuroimaging in stroke recovery. *Europa medicophysica* 2007; **43**:285–94.

6. Cramer SC. Repairing the human brain after stroke: I. Mechanisms of spontaneous recovery. *Ann Neurol* 2008; **63**:272–87.

7. Sokoloff L, Reivich M, Kennedy C, Des Rosiers MH, Patlak CS, Pettigrew KD, et al. The (14 C)-deoxyglucose method for the measurement of local cerebral glucose utilization: theory, procedure, and normal values in the conscious and anesthetized albino rat. *J Neurochem* 1977; **28**:897–916.

8. Reivich M, Kuhl D, Wolf A, Greenberg J, Phelps M, Ido T, et al. The (18 F)-fluorodeoxyglucose method for the measurement of local cerebral glucose utilization in man. *Circ Res* 1979; **44**:127–37.

9. Wienhard K, Pawlik G, Herholz K, Wagner R, Heiss WD. Estimation of local cerebral glucose utilization by positron emission tomography of [18F]2-fluoro-2-deoxy-D-glucose: a critical appraisal of optimization procedures. *J Cereb Blood Flow Metab* 1985; **5**:115–125.

10. Herscovitch P, Martin WRW, Raichle ME. The autoradiographic measurement of regional cerebral blood flow (CBF) with positron emission tomography: validation studies. *J Nucl Med* 1983; **24**:P62–3.

11. Frackowiak RSJ, Lenzi GL, Jones T, Heather JD. Quantitative measurement of regional cerebral blood flow and oxygen metabolism in man using 15 O and positron emission tomography: theory, procedure, and normal values. *J Comput Assist Tomogr* 1980; **4**:727–36.

12. Mintun MA, Raichle ME, Martin WRW, Herscovitch P. Brain oxygen utilization measured with O-15 radiotracers and positron emission tomography. *J Nucl Med* 1984; **25**:177–87.

13. Mintun MA, Lundstrom BN, Snyder AZ, Vlassenko AG, Shulman GL, Raichle ME. Blood flow and oxygen delivery to human brain during functional activity: theoretical modeling and experimental data. *Proc Natl Acad Sci USA* 2001; **98**:6859–64.

14. Ogawa S, Lee TM, Kay AR, Tank DW. Brain magnetic resonance imaging with contrast dependent on blood oxygenation. *Proc Natl Acad Sci USA* 1990; **87**:9868–72.

15. Turner R, Howseman A, Rees G, Josephs O. Functional imaging with magnetic resonance. In: Frackowiak RSJ, Friston KJ, Frith CD, Dolan RJ, Mazziotta JC, eds. *Human Brain Function*. San Diego: Academic Press; 1997: 467–86.

16. Weiller C. Recovery from motor stroke: human positron emission tomography studies. *Cerebrovasc Dis* 1995; **5**:282–91.

17. Heiss WD, Thiel A, Winhuisen L, Mühlberger B, Kessler J, Herholz K. Functional imaging in the assessment of capability for recovery after stroke. *J Rehab Med* 2003; **41**:27–33.

18. Liepert J, Weiller C. Recovery and plasticity imaging in stroke patients. In: Hennerici MG, ed. *Imaging in Stroke*. London: Remedica Group; 2003: 173–98.

19. Rizzolatti G, Luppino G, Matelli M. The organization of the cortical motor system: new concepts. *Electroencephalogr Clin Neurophysiol* 1998; **106**:283–96.

20. Nelles G, Jentzen W, Jueptner M, Müller S, Diener HC. Arm training induced brain plasticity in stroke studied with serial positron emission tomography. *Neuroimage* 2001; **13**:1146–54.

21. Marshall RS, Perera GM, Lazar RM, Krakauer JW, Constantine RC, DeLaPaz RL. Evolution of cortical activation during recovery from corticospinal tract infarction. *Stroke* 2000; **31**:656–61.

22. Calautti C, Leroy F, Guincestre JY, Baron JC. Dynamics of motor network overactivation after striatocapsular stroke: a longitudinal PET study using a fixed-performance paradigm. *Stroke* 2001; **32**:2534–42.

23. Murase N, Duque J, Mazzocchio R, Cohen LG. Influence of interhemispheric interactions on motor function in chronic stroke. *Ann Neurol* 2004; **55**:400–9.

24. Shimizu T, Hosaki A, Hino T, Sato M, Komori T, Hirai S, et al. Motor cortical disinhibition in the unaffected hemisphere after unilateral cortical stroke. *Brain* 2002; **125**:1896–1907.

25. Thiel A, Aleksic B, Klein J, Rudolf J, Heiss WD. Changes in proprioceptive systems activity during recovery from post-stroke hemiparesis. *J Rehabil Med* 2007; **39**:520–5.

26. Heiss WD, Thiel A, Kessler J, Herholz K. Disturbance and recovery of language function: correlates in PET activation studies. *Neuroimage* 2003; **20** Suppl 1:S42–9.

27. Raboyeau G, De Boissezon X, Marie N, Balduyck S, Puel M, Bezy C, et al. Right hemisphere activation in recovery from aphasia: lesion effect or function recruitment? *Neurology* 2008; **70**:290–8.

28. Rosen HJ, Petersen SE, Linenweber MR, Snyder AZ, White DA, Chapman L, et al. Neural correlates of recovery from aphasia after damage to left inferior frontal cortex. *Neurology* 2000; **55**: 1883–94.

29. Heiss WD, Kessler J, Thiel A, Ghaemi M, Karbe H. Differential capacity of left and right hemispheric areas for compensation of poststroke aphasia. *Ann Neurol* 1999; **45**:430–438.

30. Cao Y, Vikingstad EM, George KP, Johnson AF, Welch KMA. Cortical language activation in stroke patients recovering from aphasia with functional MRI. *Stroke* 1999; **30**:2331–40.

31. Warburton E, Price CJ, Swinburn K, Wise RJS. Mechanisms of recovery from aphasia: evidence from positron emission tomography studies. *J Neurol Neurosurg Psychiatry* 1999; **66**:155–61.

32. Saur D, Lange R, Baumgaertner A, Schraknepper V, Willmes K, Rijntjes M, et al. Dynamics of language reorganization after stroke. *Brain* 2006; **129**:1371–84.

33. Orgogozo JM. Piracetam in the treatment of acute stroke. *CNS Drugs* 1998; **9**:41–9.

34. Greener J, Enderby P, Whurr R. *Speech and language therapy for aphasia following stroke (Cochrane Review)*. Oxford: The Cochrane Library; 2001: 3.

35. Kessler J, Thiel A, Karbe H, Heiss WD. Piracetam improves activated blood flow and facilitates rehabilitation of poststroke aphasic patients. *Stroke* 2000; **31**:2112–16.

36. Kobayashi M, Pascual-Leone A. Transcranial magnetic stimulation in neurology. *Lancet Neurology* 2003; **2**:145–56.

37. Naeser MA, Martin PI, Nicholas M, Baker EH, Seekins H, Kobayashi M, et al. Improved picture naming in chronic aphasia after TMS to part of right Broca's area: an open-protocol study. *Brain Lang* 2005; **93**:95–105.

38. Thiel A, Schumacher B, Wienhard K, Gairing S, Kracht LW, Wagner R, et al. Direct demonstration of transcallosal disinhibition in language networks. *J Cereb Blood Flow Metab* 2006; **26**:1122–7.

39. Zahn R, Schwarz M, Huber W. Functional activation studies of word processing in the recovery from aphasia. *J Physiol Paris* 2006; **99**:370–85.

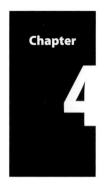

Ultrasound in acute ischemic stroke

László Csiba

Introduction

The results of non-invasive tests (e.g. ultrasound) can be highly variable, often providing ambiguous results. Although other parameters can be reviewed, calculation of overall accuracy, sensitivity and specificity as well as positive and negative predictive values are useful to the clinician who is managing the patient.

To calculate these statistics, ultrasound results must be compared to the established gold standards, usually angiography, surgery or autopsy findings. The simplest statistic compares the outcome of each test as either positive or negative. A true-positive result indicates that both tests are positive. A true-negative result indicates that both tests are negative. A false-positive result means that the gold standard is negative, indicating the absence of disease, while the non-invasive study is positive, indicating the presence of disease. A false-negative result occurs when the non-invasive test indicates the absence of disease but the gold standard is positive. True-positive and true-negative results can be used to calculate sensitivity and specificity. Sensitivity is the ability of a test to correctly diagnose disease. It can be calculated by dividing the number of true-positive tests by the total number of positive results obtained by the gold standard.

Specificity is the ability to diagnose the absence of disease and is calculated by dividing the true negative by the total number of negative results obtained by the gold standard. The positive predictive value (PPV) or likelihood means that disease is present and negative predictive values (NPV) means that disease is not present. Overall accuracy can be calculated by dividing the number of true negatives and true positives by the total number of tests performed. These results are not very specific and can be highly variable, based on the incidence of disease in the patient population. Because the patient population referred to the ultrasound lab is

diverse, high levels of sensitivity and specificity help to make the diagnosis optimal.

$$\text{Sensitivity } (\%) = \frac{\text{true positives}}{\text{true positives} + \text{false negatives}} \times 100$$

$$\text{Specificity } (\%) = \frac{\text{true negatives}}{\text{true negatives} + \text{false positives}} \times 100$$

$$\text{Positive predictive value } (\%)$$
$$= \frac{\text{true positives}}{\text{true positives} + \text{false positives}} \times 100$$

$$\text{Negative predictive value } (\%)$$
$$= \frac{\text{true negatives}}{\text{true negatives} + \text{false negatives}} \times 100$$

Extracranial ultrasound in acute stroke

The most important diagnostic question in ultrasonography is which extra- and intracranial vessel(s) is/are stenotic or occluded and can it/they be responsible for the clinical symptoms. Note that clinically silent stenotic processes might also influence the cerebral circulation.

Because of the interactions between extra- and intracranial hemodynamics, both extracranial and intracranial ultrasound techniques should be performed in acute stroke. Similarly, clinically silent stenoses should be detected by careful investigation of anterior, posterior or ipsi- and contralateral vasculature.

Doppler ultrasonography is the primary non-invasive test for evaluating carotid stenosis.

Carotid ultrasonography consists of two steps, imaging and spectral analysis. Images are produced with the brightness-mode (B-mode) technique and sometimes color flow information is superimposed on the grayscale image. By convention, the color of the pulsating artery is red. The echogenicity of an object on the image determines its brightness. An object that rebounds very little of the pulse is hypoechoic. An object that reflects much of the signal, such as calcified plaque, is hyperechoic. Plaques with irregular surface and/or heterogeneous echogenicity are more likely to embolize. Soft plaques present a higher embolic risk than hard plaques. The sonographic characteristics of symptomatic and asymptomatic carotid plaques are different. Symptomatic plaques are more likely to be hypoechoic and highly stenotic while asymptomatic plaques are hyperechoic and moderately stenotic. Evaluation of the surface of the plaque has not been demonstrated to be a satisfactory index of plaque instability.

The degree of stenosis is better measured on the basis of the waveform and spectral analysis of the CCA and its major branches, especially the ICA. Spectral (velocity) analysis is essential to identify stenosis or occlusion. An important general rule for ultrasound is the greater the degree of stenosis, the higher the velocity. Power Doppler provides color imaging that is independent of direction or velocity of flow and gives an angiographic-like picture of an artery.

Blood flow can be laminar, disturbed or turbulent. When no stenosis is present, blood flow is laminar. Flow of blood is even, with the fastest flow in the middle and the slowest at the edges of the vessel. When a small degree of stenosis is present, the blood flow becomes disturbed and loses its laminar quality. Even in normal conditions, such flow can be seen around the carotid bulb. With even greater stenosis, the flow can become turbulent [1].

In normal hemodynamics, as vessel length increases so does resistance. With increasing radius, the resistance decreases significantly.

As vessel diameter (and area) decreases, blood velocity increases to maintain volume flow.

The extracranial ultrasound procedure starts with the CCA, internal carotid artery (ICA) and external carotid artery (ECA); at least two or three spectral analyses of each vessel should be obtained. Color imaging and power Doppler may be used but may not necessarily provide additional information.

Note the carotid bifurcation, look for plaques, attempt to characterize the nature of the plaque, and color may be used at this point to identify flow within the artery and potential areas of high velocity.

CCA can be identified by pulsatile walls, smaller caliber than the jugular vein and systolic peak and diastolic endpoints in between those of external and internal carotid arteries on spectral analysis. ECA has a smaller caliber, while ICA is often posterolateral to ECA and ECA may have a superior thyroid artery branch coming off. ECA has virtually no diastolic flow (i.e. high-resistance vessel) on spectral analysis. ECA shows positive "temporal tap" (i.e. undulations in waveform with tapping of the temporal artery). Perform spectral analysis and find the highest velocity or frequency. After assessment of the anterior circulation, the sonographer should assess the vertebral circulation. Usually, the C4–C6 segment is accessible. Vertebral arteries can be identified with a probe parallel to the carotid: angle the probe laterally and inferiorly. The vertebral body processes appear as hypoechoic transverse bars. The vertebral artery runs perpendicular to vertebral processes.

Use of color flow Doppler enables the more rapid identification of vessels (especially the vertebral artery) and often helps identify the area of highest velocity, reduces scan time and may help in diagnosis of arterial occlusion [1].

> Doppler ultrasonography is the primary noninvasive test for evaluating carotid stenosis.
> Symptomatic and asymptomatic carotid plaques and the degree of stenosis can be analyzed with ultrasonography by examining the echogenicity of the structures and the velocity of the blood flow.

Degree of stenosis

Some sonographers characterize the degree of stenosis based on diameter or area reduction but estimation of stenosis solely based on this criterion is not reliable. Commonly used methods:

- peak systolic velocities (PSV) and end diastolic velocities
- ratios ICA/CCA maximal systolic flow velocity within the ICA stenosis
- maximal systolic flow velocity within the non-affected CCA
- ICA/ICA
- maximal systolic flow velocity within the ICA stenosis
- maximal systolic flow velocity of the nonaffected ICA.

The stroke risk depends on more than the degree of carotid artery narrowing (cardiac diseases, age, sex, hypertension, smoking and plaque structure). Most

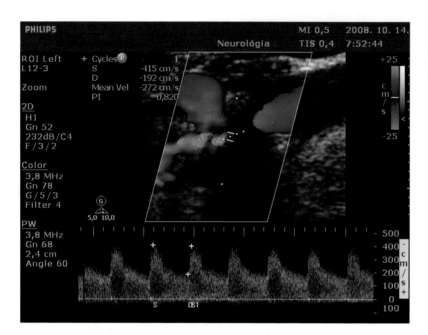

Figure 4.1. Duplex color-Doppler ultrasound. More than 300 cm/s systolic velocity could be measured in the stenotic area depicted by the color mode. (Courtesy of L. Oláh.)

studies consider carotid stenosis of 60% or greater to be clinically important. In a case of a suspected stenosis not only the intrastenotic but also the flow from vessel segments proximal and distal to a stenosis have to be analyzed. If normal flow signals are present before and behind the suspected lesion significant stenosis can be excluded. The stenosis ranges vary from laboratory to laboratory. When possible, laboratories should perform their own correlations with angiographic measurements for quality control. A consensus statement of the Society of Radiologists in Ultrasound recommended the following criteria for estimating stenosis [2]:

- Normal: ICA PSV <125 cm/s, no plaque or intimal thickening.
- <50% stenosis: ICA PSV <125 cm/s and plaque or intimal thickening.
- 50–69% stenosis: ICA PSV is 125–230 cm/s and plaque is visible.
- >70% stenosis to near occlusion: ICA PSV >230 cm/s and visible plaque and lumen narrowing.
- Near occlusion: a markedly narrowed lumen on c-Doppler ultrasound.
- Total occlusion: no detectable patent lumen is seen on grayscale ultrasound, and no flow is seen on spectral, power and color Doppler ultrasound.

With stenosis over 90% (near occlusion), velocities may actually drop as mechanisms that maintain

flow fail. Ratios may be particularly helpful in situations in which cardiovascular factors (e.g. poor ejection fraction) limit the increase in velocity [1].

> <50% stenoses ICA/CCA: <2.0.
>
> 50 − 69% stenoses ICA/CCA: 2.0−4.0.
>
> ≥70% stenoses ICA/CCA: >4.0.

Doppler ultrasonography associated with stenosis might result in false positive/negative results:

- Ipsilateral CCA-to-ICA flow ratios may not be valid in the setting of contralateral ICA occlusion.
- CCA waveforms may have a high-resistance configuration in ipsilateral ICA lesions.
- ICA waveforms may have a high-resistance configuration in ipsilateral distal ICA lesions.
- ICA waveforms may be dampened in ipsilateral CCA lesions.
- Long-segment ICA stenosis may not have high end-diastolic velocity.
- Velocities supersede imaging in grading stenosis.
- Imaging can be used to downgrade stenosis in the setting of turbulence caused by kinking [3].

A severe carotid stenosis is shown in Figure 4.1.

Most studies consider carotid stenosis of 60% or greater to be clinically important. This equals a peak systolic velocity over 125 cm/s. With stenosis over 90% (near occlusion), velocities may actually drop as mechanisms that maintain flow fail.

Ratios (maximal systolic flow velocity within the ICA stenosis/maximal systolic flow velocity within the non-affected CCA) may be particularly helpful in situations in which cardiovascular factors (e.g. poor ejection fraction) limit the increase in velocity.

IMT measurement

In the Cardiovascular Health Study, increases in the intimal-medial thickness (IMT) of the carotid artery were associated with an increased risk of myocardial infarction and stroke in older adults without a history of cardiovascular disease [4]. CCA IMT greater than 0.87 mm and ICA IMT greater than 0.90 mm were associated with a progressively increased risk of cardiovascular events. For each 0.20 mm increase in CCA IMT, the risk increased by approximately 27%. For each 0.55 mm increase in ICA IMT, the risk increased approximately 30%.

The following method is suggested by the American Society of Echocardiography and the Society for Vascular Medicine for measuring IMT: (1) use end-diastolic images for IMT measurements; (2) categorization of plaque presence and IMT; (3) avoid use of a single upper limit of normal for IMT because the measure varies with age, sex and race; and (4) incorporate lumen measurement, particularly when serial measurements are performed, to account for changes in distending pressure.

Treatment with lipid-lowering drugs has been shown to decrease the intimal thickness of the carotid artery. Decrease in the thickness of the intima of the CCA has been correlated directly with successful treatment with drugs that lower serum low-density lipoprotein levels.

With ultrasound, the intimal-medial thickness of the carotid artery can be measured. Increases in the intimal-medial thickness (IMT) of the carotid artery are associated with an increased risk of myocardial infarction and stroke.

ICA stenosis and occlusion

Mild stenoses (<50%) can be estimated by measurement of area and/or diameter in the cross-sectional and longitudinal image using the B- and color-mode of the ultrasound system. Area measurements in high-grade stenosis are difficult. Diagnosis of severe stenosis is based on hemodynamic parameters (measured by pre-, intra- and poststenotic Doppler spectrum analysis).

Investigation of flow direction in the ophthalmic artery is a simple, bedside, ancillary method in suspected ICA stenosis or occlusion (equally severe upper and lower extremity paresis). In a case of hemodynamically significant ICA stenosis or occlusion (proximal to the origin of the ophthalmic artery) a reversed (extra → intracranial) flow could be detected in the ophthalmic artery.

Occlusion results in a complete absence of color-flow signal in ICA, and the diagnosis can be confirmed by ultrasound contrast agents.

Using duplex ultrasound a proximal ICA occlusion (proximal to the origin of the ophthalmic artery, no color-mode signal and no Doppler flow) can be distinguished from the ICA occlusion distal to the ophthalmic origin (ICA has low flow velocities and a higher pulsatility but preserved diastolic velocity).

Extracranial vertebral and subclavian arteries

The origin of the vertebral artery (VA) is one of the most common locations of atherosclerotic stenosis, but is difficult to investigate, especially its origin. Raised flow velocities and spectral broadening can be seen in over 50% of stenoses. A distal extracranial VA occlusion may cause a stump signal or a high pulsatile flow signal with almost absent end-diastolic flow component.

A high grade of subclavian stenosis (>50%) results in increased flow velocities and a turbulent flow. In high-grade subclavian stenosis an alternating flow, or even a retrograde flow, can be detected within the ipsilateral VA. The levels of evidence of the European Federation of Neurological Societies are shown in Table 4.1 [5].

Ultrasound diagnosis of intracranial stenosis and occlusion

Intracranial disease corresponds to approximately 8–10% of acute ischemic stroke, depending on gender and race. Diagnosis is frequently reached through

Table 4.1. Highlights of the guidelines of the European Federation of Neurological Societies [5].

Domains	Class and level
Ultrasonography is the non-invasive screening technique indicated for the study of vessels involved in causing symptoms of carotid stenosis	class IV, GCPP
Transcranial Doppler (TCD) is useful for screening for intracranial stenosis and occlusion in patients with cerebrovascular disease	class II, level B
Transcranial Doppler is very useful for monitoring arterial reperfusion after thrombolysis of acute MCA occlusions	class II, level B
Clinical studies have suggested that continuous TCD monitoring in patients with acute MCA occlusion treated with intravenous thrombolysis may improve both early recanalization and clinical outcome	class II, level A
The presence of embolic signals with carotid stenosis predicts early recurrent stroke risk	class II, level A
Even in asymptomatic patients, TCD is the only imaging technique that allows detection of circulating emboli	class II, level A
Asymptomatic embolization is common in acute stroke, particularly in patients with carotid artery disease. In this group the presence of embolic signals has been shown to predict the combined stroke and transient ischemic attack (TIA) risk and more recently the risk of stroke alone	class II, level A

arteriography. TCD is an ancillary diagnosis tool with good sensitivity and specificity.

Transcranial color-coded duplex sonography (TCCD) combines the imaging of intracranial vessels and parenchymal structures. To penetrate the skull, TCCD uses low frequencies (1.75–3.5 MHz), which limit the spatial resolution. The duplex mode of TCCD enables sampling of vessels and Doppler measurements of angle-corrected blood-flow velocities.

General characteristics of the investigation [6–10]:

- About 15% of patients cannot be examined by TCCD, because of the insufficient acoustic window. Identification rates decline with advancing age.
- The mean velocity analysis is not enough to identify intracranial vessel abnormalities. It must be combined with other parameters such as asymmetry, segmental elevations, spectral analysis and knowledge of extracranial circulation.
- Either flow velocities (frequency-based TCCD) or the integrated power of the reflected signal (power TCCD) can be coded. The power TCCD does not display information on the flow direction.
- Flow velocities are determined by spectral Doppler sonography using the color Doppler image as a guide to the correct positioning of the Doppler sample volume.
- The angle correction should only be applied to velocity measurements when the sample volume

can be located in a straight vessel segment of at least 2 cm length.
- Flow velocities in the arterial as well as in the venous system are higher in women than in men, and decrease with age, whereas the pulsatility index increases.
- Intracranial stenosis: local increase in the peak systolic flow velocities, post-stenotic flow disturbances with low frequency and high-intensity Doppler signals.
- The intracranial vessel is occluded if the color signal is absent in one segment, while other vessels and parenchymal structures can be correctly visualized.
- The accuracy of ultrasound for detecting intracranial stenosis is summarized in Table 4.2.
- The use of Levovist increases the sensitivity and specificity and only 4% of examinations are inconclusive because of insufficient bone windows.
- After application of echo-contrast enhancing agents (ECE) the diagnostic confidence of TCCD for intracranial vessel occlusion is similar to that of magnetic resonance angiography.
- In an acute stroke study the ability of duplex ultrasound to diagnose main stem arterial occlusions within the anterior circulation was between 50% and 60% of studied vessels in unenhanced TCCS but reached 80–90% after intravenous contrast administration.

Table 4.2. Highlights of the American Academy of Neurology recommendations [7].

		Sensitivity (%)	Specificity (%)
Intracranial steno-occlusive disease	• Anterior circulation	70–90	90–95
	• Posterior circulation occlusion	50–80	80–96
	• MCA	85–95	90–98
	• ICA, VA, BA	55–81	96
	TCD is probably useful (**Type B, Class II–III**) for the evaluation of occlusive lesions of intracranial arteries in the basal cisterns (especially the ICA siphon and MCA).		
	The relative value of TCD compared with MR angiography or CT angiography remains to be determined (**Type U**).		
	Data are insufficient to recommend replacement of conventional angiography with TCD (**Type U**).		
Cerebral thrombolysis	• Complete occlusion	50	100
	• Partial occlusion	100	76
	• Recanalization	91	93
	TCD is probably useful for monitoring thrombolysis of acute MCA occlusions (**Type B, Class II–III**). More data are needed to assess the frequency of monitoring for clot dissolution and enhanced recanalization and to influence therapy (**Type U**).		
Cerebral microemboli detection	TCD monitoring is probably useful for the detection of cerebral microembolic signals in a variety of cardiovascular/cerebrovascular disorders/procedures (**Type B, Class II–IV**). Data do not support the use of this TCD technique for diagnosis or monitoring response to antithrombotic therapy in ischemic cerebrovascular disease (**Type U**).		
TCCS	TCCS is possibly useful (**Type C, Class III**) for the evaluation and monitoring of space-occupying ischemic MCA infarctions. More data are needed to show if it has value vs. CT and MRI scanning and if its use affects clinical outcomes (**Type U**).		
Contrast-enhanced TCCS	(CE)-TCCS may provide information in patients with ischemic cerebrovascular disease and aneurysmal SAH (**Type B, Class II-IV**).		
	Its clinical utility vs. CT scanning, conventional angiography, or non-imaging TCD is unclear (**Type U**).		

Type A: established as useful/predictive or not useful/predictive for the given condition in the specified population.
Type B: probably useful/predictive or not useful/predictive for the given condition in the specified population.
Type C: possibly useful/predictive or not useful/predictive for the given condition in the specified population.
Type U: data inadequate or conflicting; given current knowledge, test/predictor unproven.
Class I: evidence provided by prospective study in broad spectrum of persons with suspected condition, using a "gold standard" to define cases, where test is applied in blinded evaluation, and enabling assessment of appropriate tests of diagnostic accuracy.
Class II: evidence provided by prospective study in narrow spectrum of persons with suspected condition or well-designed retrospective study of broad spectrum of persons with suspected condition (by "gold standard") compared to broad spectrum of controls where test is applied in blinded evaluation and enabling assessment of appropriate tests of diagnostic accuracy.
Class III: evidence provided by retrospective study where either persons with established condition or controls are of narrow spectrum, and where test is applied in blinded evaluation.
Class IV: any design where test is not applied in blinded fashion OR evidence provided by expert opinion or descriptive case series.

Table 4.3. Ultrasound grading of intracranial stenosis. Modified from Baumgartner et al. [8] and Valdueza et al. [9].

Stenosis	≥50%	50–80%	≥80%
Middle cerebral artery	≥155 cm/s	≥220	distal M1/M2-MCA post-stenotic fp A1-ACA and/or P1/P2-PCA↑
Anterior cerebral artery	≥120	≥155	A2-ACA post-stenotic fp ipsilateral M1-MCA and/or contralat. A1↑
Posterior cerebral artery	≥100	≥145	distal PCA post-stenotic fp ipsilateral M1-MCA↑
Basilar artery	≥100	≥140	distal BA/PCA post-stenotic fp VA/proximal BA pre-stenotic fp
Vertebral artery	≥ 90	≥120	distal VA/BA post-stenotic fp VA extracranial pre-stenotic fp

Fp: flow pattern, ↑ increased velocity as collateral sign.

- The diagnostic strength of eTCCD can be the highly specific identification of a normal intracranial arterial status. Therefore, if an experienced sonographer detects no abnormalities by using eTCCD in a patient with sufficient bone windows, no more imaging is needed.
- A correctly performed TCD investigation also provides valuable information about the vascular status of the ICA. The presence of collaterals and delayed flow acceleration on TCD usually indicates a hemodynamically significant lesion (>80% ICA stenosis or occlusion).
- The investigation should start on the presumably non-affected side (road map → clinical symptoms).
- The sonographer looks for a focal velocity rise in a circumscribed vessel segment, and differences between the affected and non-affected sides, extending more than 30 cm/s.
- If a pathological finding is present, the proximal and distal vessel segments should also be evaluated.
- Occlusions are characterized by missing color and Doppler flow signals at the site of the occlusion or reduced flow signals in vessel segments proximal to the occlusion.

MCA stenosis

Stenoses of the M1-MCA can be graded according to flow velocity, turbulence and asymmetry into mild, moderate and high-grade stenoses and all detectable MCA segments should be insonated [7–9].

MCA occlusion

Depending on the location of the occlusion, the Doppler spectrum may be completely absent or reduced. If there is a proximal M1-MCA occlusion no flow signal is seen. In occlusions of the middle part of the MCA, a small orthograde flow with increased pulsatility may be present. In distal M1-MCA occlusion a reduced flow velocity is present with variable pulsatility depending on the presence of a temporal branch.

Distal MCA occlusion, e.g. of a relevant M2-MCA branch or more than one M2 branch, will result in a reduced flow with low velocities and a marked bilateral asymmetry.

ACA stenosis and occlusion

Clinical symptoms (contralateral lower leg paresis) can suggest ACA stenosis or occlusion. Altered velocity, the presence of turbulence or missing ACA and ipsilateral increased MCA flow velocities can help the diagnosis of ACA stenosis and occlusion [9].

Stenosis and occlusion in posterior circulation

Again the typical clinical symptoms of vertebrobasilar insufficiency should orient the sonographer. Alteration of flow velocities and turbulence, at least 30 cm/s flow velocity difference between the right and left sides, may also be useful. A proximal PCA occlusion can be diagnosed by absent flow signal. Vertebral stenoses can be diagnosed by flow velocity, profile disturbances, and pre- and post-stenotic flow patterns. Velocity values for mild and severe stenosis are given in Table 4.3. Flow signals in VA occlusion strongly depend on the site of the occlusion, mainly on their relation to the origin of the PICA (proximal or distal). Occlusions distal to the PICA origin will result in mild to moderate flow alterations of the extracranial VA, mainly depending on its diameter and its former relevance in the posterior circulation [9].

Basilar artery stenosis and occlusion

Transforaminal and transtemporal insonation allows the investigation of the total length of the basilar artery. The most distal segment of the basilar artery may be better insonated transtemporally, but the visualization of the distal part of the basilar artery appears to be difficult even using echo-enhancing agents.

Occlusions are difficult to assess and diagnostic certainty depends on the site of the occlusion. A proximal BA occlusion will always result in pre-stenotic flow alterations of both extracranial vertebral arteries [9]. Therefore, apparently normal VA and proximal BA velocities are not sufficient to exclude top of the basilar occlusion.

However, as this cannot exclude the presence of, for example, a fragmented thrombus, ultrasound should always be used together with other diagnostic tools such as CTA, MRA, or DSA in presumed BA pathology.

The highlights of the recommendation of the American Academy of Neurology [7] summarize the accuracy of TCD in intracranial steno-occlusive disorders (Table 4.2).

> With transcranial color-coded duplex sonography (TCCD), using low frequencies to penetrate the skull, most intracranial stenoses and occlusions can be detected by combining velocity analysis with other parameters. With the use of echo-contrast enhancing agents (ECE), the sensitivity and specificity can be increased and the diagnostic confidence of eTCCD for intracranial vessel occlusion can reach that of magnetic resonance angiography.

Fast-track neurovascular ultrasound examination

Recently, a practical algorithm has been published for urgent bedside neurovascular ultrasound examination with carotid/vertebral duplex and transcranial Doppler in patients with acute stroke [11, 12].

Using such a protocol, urgent TCD studies can be completed and interpreted quickly at the bedside. The expanded fast-track protocol for combined carotid and transcranial ultrasound testing in acute cerebral ischemia is shown in Table 4.4. Below, we highlight the most important details of the algorithm [11, 12].

The choice of fast-track insonation steps is determined by the clinical localization of ischemic arterial territory. For example, if patients present with middle cerebral artery symptoms, the insonation begins with the non-affected side. This is followed by locating the MCA on the affected side, with insonation starting at the mid-M1-MCA depth range, usually 50–58 mm. The waveforms and systolic flow acceleration are compared to the non-affected side. If a normal MCA flow is found, the distal MCA segments are insonated (range 40–50 mm); this is followed by proximal MCA and ICA bifurcation assessment (range 60–70 mm) [11, 12]. The non-invasive vascular ultrasound evaluation (NVUE) in patients with acute ischemic stroke has a high yield and accuracy in diagnosing lesions amenable to interventional treatment (LAIT). The ultrasound screening criteria for LAIT are shown in Table 4.5.

TCD has the highest sensitivity (>90%) for acute arterial obstructions located in the proximal MCA and ICAs. TCD has modest sensitivity (55–60%) for posterior circulation lesions if performed without transcranial color-coded duplex imaging or contrast enhancement (Table 4.2). However, with a completely normal spectral TCD, there is less than 5% chance that an urgent angiogram will show any acute obstruction [12].

While TCD demonstration of an arterial occlusion helps to determine the ischemic nature of acute focal neurological deficits, a normal TCD result would support a lacunar mechanism.

In summary, bedside ultrasound in acute stroke may identify thrombus presence, determine thrombus location(s), assess collateral supply, find the worst residual flow signal, and monitor recanalization and reocclusion.

> Recently, a practical algorithm has been published for urgent bedside neurovascular ultrasound examination with carotid/vertebral duplex and transcranial Doppler in patients with acute stroke.

Emboli monitoring and acute stroke

TCD identifies microembolic signs (MES) in intracranial circulation. The ultrasound distinguishes signal characteristics through embolic materials – solid or gaseous – from erythrocyte flow velocity. Microembolic signals appear as signals of high intensity and short duration within the Doppler spectrum as a result of their different acoustic properties compared to the circulating blood. MES have been proven

Table 4.4. Fast-track neurovascular ultrasound examination (Chernyshev et al. [11]).

Use portable devices with bright display overcoming room light. Stand behind patient headrest. Start with TCD because acute occlusion responsible for the neurological deficit is likely to be located intracranially. Extracranial carotid/vertebral duplex may reveal an additional lesion often responsible for intracranial flow disturbance. Fast-track insonation steps follow clinical localization of patient symptoms.

A. Clinical diagnosis of cerebral ischemia in the anterior circulation

STEP 1: Transcranial Doppler
1. If time permits, begin insonation on the non-affected side to establish the temporal window, normal MCA waveform (M1 depth 45–65 mm, M2 30–45 mm) and velocity for comparison with the affected side.
2. If short on time, start on the affected side: first assess MCA at 50 mm. If no signals detected, increase the depth to 62 mm. If an anterograde flow signal is found, reduce the depth to trace the MCA stem or identify the worst residual flow signal. Search for possible flow diversion to the ACA, PCA, or M2 MCA.
   Evaluate and compare waveform shapes and systolic flow acceleration.
3. Continue on the affected side (transorbital window). Check flow direction and pulsatility in the OA at depths 40–50 mm followed by ICA siphon at depths 55–65 mm.
4. If time permits or in patients with pure motor or sensory deficits, evaluate BA (depth 80–100 mm) and terminal VA (40–80 mm).

STEP 2: Carotid/vertebral duplex
1. Start on the affected side in transverse B-mode planes followed by color or power-mode sweep from proximal to distal carotid segments. Identify CCA and its bifurcation on B-mode and flow-carrying lumens.
2. Document if ICA (or CCA) has a lesion on B-mode and corresponding disturbances on flow images. In patients with concomitant chest pain, evaluate CCA as close to the origin as possible.
3. Perform angle-corrected spectral velocity measurements in the mid-to-distal CCA, ICA and external carotid artery.
4. If time permits or in patients with pure motor or sensory deficits, examine cervical portion of the vertebral arteries (longitudinal B-mode, color or power mode, spectral Doppler) on the affected side.
5. If time permits, perform transverse and longitudinal scanning of the arteries on the non-affected side.

B. Clinical diagnosis of cerebral ischemia in the posterior circulation

STEP 1: Transcranial Doppler
1. Start suboccipital insonation at 75 mm (VA junction) and identify BA flow at 80–100 mm.
2. If abnormal signals present at 75–100 mm, find the terminal VA (40–80 mm) on the non-affected side for comparison and evaluate the terminal VA on the affected side at similar depths.
3. Continue with transtemporal examination to identify PCA (55–75 mm) and possible collateral flow through the posterior communicating artery (check both sides).
4. If time permits, evaluate both MCAs and ACAs (60–75 mm) for possible compensatory velocity increase as an indirect sign of basilar artery obstruction.

STEP 2: Vertebral/carotid duplex ultrasound
1. Start on the affected side by locating CCA using longitudinal B-mode plane, and turn transducer downward to visualize shadows from transverse processes of midcervical vertebrae.
2. Apply color or power modes and spectral Doppler to identify flow in intratransverse VA segments.
3. Follow VA course to its origin and obtain Doppler spectra. Perform similar examination on other side.
4. If time permits, perform bilateral duplex examination of the CCA, ICA and external carotid artery as described above.

to represent solid or gaseous particles within the blood flow. They occur at random within the cardiac cycle and they can be acoustically identified by a characteristic "chirp" sound. Detection of MES can identify patients with stroke or TIA likely to be due to embolism. Potential applications of MES detection include determining the pathophysiology of cerebral ischemia, identifying patients at increased risk for stroke who may benefit from surgical and pharmacological intervention, assessing the effectiveness of novel antiplatelet therapies and perioperative monitoring to prevent intra- and postoperative stroke.

Table 4.5. Ultrasound screening criteria for lesions amenable for intervention (Chernyshev et al. [11]).

Lesion location	TCD criteria (at least one present)	CD criteria
M1/M2 MCA	*Primary:*	
	TIBI grades 0–4 (absent, minimal, blunted, dampened, or stenotic) at depths <45 mm (M2) and 45–65 mm (M1)	Extracranial findings may be normal or may show decreased ICA velocity on the side of the lesion
	Secondary:	
	Flow diversion to ACA, PCA, or M2	
	Increased resistance in ipsilateral TICA	
	Embolic, signals in MCA	
	Turbulence, disturbed flow at stenosis	
	Nonharmonic and harmonic covibrations (bruit or pure musical tones)	
TICA	*Primary:*	
	TIBI grades 0–4 at 60–70 mm	Decreased ICA velocity unilateral to lesion or normal extracranial findings
	Increased velocities suggest anterior cross-filling or collateral flow in posterior communicating artery	
	Secondary:	
	Embolic signals in unilateral MCA	
	Blunted unilateral MCA, MFV > 20 cm/s	
Proximal ICA	*Primary:*	
	Increased flow velocities suggest anterior cross-filling through ACommA or collateral flow through PcommA	B-mode evidence of a lesion in ICA ± CCA; Flow imaging evidence of no flow or residual lumen
	Reversed OA	
	Delayed systolic flow acceleration in or blunted ipsilateral MCA, MFV > 20 cm/s	
	Secondary:	ICA > 50% stenosis
		PSV > 125 cm/s
		EDV > 40 cm/s
		ICA/CCA PSV ratio > 2
	Embolic signals in unilateral MCA	ICA near-occlusion or occlusion
	Normal OA direction due to retrograde filling of siphon	Blunted, minimal, reverberating, or absent spectral Doppler waveforms in ICA
Tandem ICA/MCA stenosis/occlusion	*Primary:*	
	TIBI grades 0–4 and:	B-mode evidence of a lesion in ICA ± CCA; or: Flow imaging evidence of residual lumen or no flow

Table 4.5. (*cont.*)

Lesion location	TCD criteria (at least one present)	CD criteria
	Increased velocities in contralateral ACA, MCA, or unilateral PComma or:	
	Reversed unilateral DA	
		ICA > 50% stenosis
		PSV > 125 cm/s
		EDV > 40 cm/s
		ICA/CCA PSV ratio > 2
	Secondary:	
	Delayed systolic flow acceleration in proximal MCA or TICA	ICA near-occlusion or occlusion
	Embolic signals in proximal MCA or TICA	Blunted, minimal, reverberating, or absent spectral Doppler waveforms in ICA
Basilar artery	*Primary:*	
	TIBI flow grades 0–4 at 73–100 mm	Extracranial findings may be normal or showing decreased VA velocities or VA occlusion
	Secondary:	
	Flow velocity increase in terminal VA and branches, MCAs, or PCommAs	
	High resistance flow signals in VA(s)	
	Reversed flow direction in distal basilar artery (85 mm)	
Vertebral artery	*Primary (intracranial VA occlusion):*	
	TIBI flow grades 0–4 at 40–75 mm	Extracranial findings may be normal (intracranial VA lesion) or showing decreased VA velocities or VA occlusion
	Primary (extracranial VA occlusion)	
	Absent, minimal, or reversed high resistance flow signals in unilateral terminal VA	
	Secondary:	
	Embolic signals increased velocities or low pulsatility in contralateral VA	

TICA – terminal internal carotid artery; TIBI – thrombolysis in brain infarction; AComma – anterior communicating artery; PCommA – posterior communicating artery; CD – cervical duplex. Reproduced with permission from Chernyshev et al. [11].

The methodology includes simultaneous monitoring of both MCAs for at least 30 minutes, with fixed transducers in order to reduce movement artifacts. With two possible embolic sources – cardiogenic and carotid plaque – the identification of MES contributes higher diagnosis accuracy and support for therapy decision-making. MES detection, in addition, acts as a predictor for new cerebral ischemic event recurrence [13–16].

At present, monitoring of microembolisms is useful for patients with non-defined AIS, and which is of probable cardio- or carotid-embolic etiology.

Simultaneous monitoring for MES in different vessels may help identify the active embolic source (cardiac? carotid?). Simultaneous monitoring above (i.e. MCA) and below (i.e. common carotid artery) an internal carotid artery (ICA) stenosis is another possible way of differentiating between artery-to-artery and cardiogenic embolism.

The frequency of MES in acute stroke shows a wide range between 10% and 70%, probably due to different therapies, different criteria for MES detection, or different elapsed times after stroke. Some investigators used single registration, others serial measurements. The incidence of MES is maximal in the first week after stroke. The occurrence of MES showed more prevalence in completed stroke than in patients with TIA, and in symptomatic than asymptomatic hemispheres and a discrete subcortical or cortical pattern of infarction on computed tomography (CT) compared with a hemodynamic or small-vessel pattern.

Some authors have demonstrated that MES occur predominantly in patients with large-vessel territory stroke patterns and cases of artery-to-artery or cardiogenic embolism with persisting deficit. In contrast, MES are only occasionally detected in patients with small-vessel infarctions.

In addition, TCD monitoring may help to discriminate between different potential sources of embolism (i.e. artery-to-artery or cardioembolic strokes). Different types of emboli (i.e. cardiac or carotid) have different acoustic properties and ultrasonic characteristics, based on composition and size, which could permit differentiation.

MES detection by TCD in CEA candidates may allow identification of a particularly high-risk group of patients who merit an early intervention or, if this is not possible, more aggressive antithrombotic therapy. The Clopidogrel and Aspirin for Reduction of Emboli in Symptomatic Carotid Stenosis Study (CARESS) also revealed that the combination of clopidogrel and aspirin was associated with a marked reduction in MES, compared with aspirin alone (e.g. clopidogrel + aspirin versus aspirin) [17].

A recent meta-analysis confirmed the usefulness of microembolic signs (MES) detection by transcranial Doppler sonography. MES are a frequent finding in varying sources of arterial brain embolism and MES detection is useful for risk stratification in patients with carotid stenosis [18].

> TCD identifies MES in intracranial circulation. Detection of MES can identify patients with stroke or TIA likely to be due to embolism, acts as a predictor for new cerebral ischemic event recurrence and can influence therapy decision-making.

Diagnostic brain perfusion imaging in stroke patients

The availability of new ultrasound contrast agents (UCAs) and the development of contrast-specific imaging modalities have established the application of ultrasound in stroke patients for visualization of brain perfusion deficits. The UCAs consist of microbubbles composed of a gas that is associated with various types of shells for stabilization. Because of their small size, they can pass through the microcirculation. There are interactions between ultrasound and microbubbles: at low ultrasound energies UCA microbubbles produce resonance, emitting ultrasound waves at multiples of the insonated fundamental frequency.

The new microbubbles (e.g. SonoVue) generate a nonlinear response at low acoustic power without destruction, thus being particularly suitable for real-time imaging. Harmonic imaging differentiates echoes from microbubbles from those coming from tissue. The insonated tissue responds at the fundamental frequency, while resonating microbubbles cause scattering of multiples of the fundamental frequency – the harmonic frequencies.

Real-time visualization of middle cerebral artery infarction

Perfusion harmonic imaging after SonoVue bolus injection can be used in patients with acute stroke. In the early phase of acute ischemic stroke, bolus imaging after SonoVue injection is useful for analyzing cerebral perfusion deficits at the patient's bedside. The ultrasound imaging data correlate well with the definite area of infarction and outcome after ischemic stroke. Ultrasound perfusion imaging with SonoVue has allowed measurements not only in ischemic stroke but also in intracerebral hemorrhages, due to a characteristic reduction of contrast reaching the lesion.

In spite of continuous effort, perfusion imaging in acute stroke is still in the experimental phase [19–22].

New ultrasound contrast agents (UCAs) that can pass through the microcirculation and the development of contrast-specific imaging modalities make it possible to use ultrasound for the visualization of brain perfusion deficits.

Prognostic value of ultrasound in acute stroke

During recent years, ultrasound has become an important non-invasive imaging technique for bedside monitoring of acute stroke therapy and prognosis. By providing valuable information on temporal patterns of recanalization, ultrasound monitoring may assist in the selection of patients for additional pharmacological or interventional treatment. Ultrasound also has an important prognostic role in acute stroke. A prospective, multicenter, randomized study confirmed that a normal MCA finding is predictive of a good functional outcome in more than two-thirds of subjects. After adjustment for age, neurological deficit on admission, CT scan results, and preexisting risk factors, ultrasound findings remained the only independent predictor of outcomes [23].

The analysis of flow signal changes during thrombolysis acquired by TCD further confirmed the prognostic value of transcranial ultrasound. Acute arterial occlusion is a dynamic process since thrombus can propagate and break up, thereby changing the degree of arterial obstruction and affecting the correlation between TCD and angiography.

A complete occlusion should not produce any detectable flow signals. However, in reality, some residual flow around the thrombus is often present. The Thrombolysis in Brain Ischemia (TIBI) flow-grading system was developed to evaluate residual flow non-invasively and monitor thrombus dissolution in real time [24]:

- Grade 0: absent flow.
- Grade 1: minimal flow.
- Grade 2: blunted flow.
- Grade 3: dampened flow.
- Grade 4: stenotic flow.
- Grade 5: normal flow.

(TIBI 0 and 1 refer to proximal occlusion, TIBI 2 and 3 to distal occlusion and TIBI 4 to recanalization.)

Applying these criteria in acute stroke the TIBI classification correlates with initial stroke severity, clinical recovery and mortality in patients treated with recombinant tissue plasminogen activator (rt-PA). The grading system can be used also to analyze recanalization patterns.

The waveform changes ($0 \rightarrow 5$) correlate well with clinical improvement and a rapid arterial recanalization is associated with better short-term improvement, whereas slow flow improvement and dampened flow signals are less favorable prognostic signs [24].

Even incomplete or minimal recanalization determined 24 h after stroke onset results in more favorable outcome compared with persistent occlusion [25].

Reperfusion is important for prognosis. Both partial and full early reperfusion led to a lesser extent of neurological deficits irrespective of whether this occurred early or in the 6- to 24-hour interval.

Progressive deterioration after stroke due to cerebral edema, thrombus propagation, or hemodynamic impairment is closely linked to extra- and intracranial occlusive disease. Transcranial color-coded duplex is also useful for the evaluation of combined i.v.–intra-arterial (i.a.) thrombolysis. Patients receiving combined i.v.–i.a. thrombolysis show greater improvement in flow signal and higher incidence of complete MCA recanalization compared with those receiving i.v. thrombolysis, especially when the MCA was occluded or had only minimal flow [26].

Patients with distal middle cerebral artery occlusion are twice as likely to have a good long-term outcome as patients with proximal middle cerebral occlusion. Patients with no detectable residual flow signals as well as those with terminal internal carotid artery occlusions are least likely to respond early or long term. The distal MCA occlusions are more likely to recanalize with i.v. rt-PA therapy; terminal ICA occlusions were the least likely to recanalize or have clinical recovery with i.v. rt-PA compared with other occlusion locations [27].

Alexandrov et al. [28] described the patterns of the speed of clot dissolution during continuous TCD monitoring: sudden recanalization (abrupt normalization of flow velocity in a few seconds), stepwise recanalization as a progressive improvement in flow velocity lasting less than 30 min, and slow recanalization as a progressive improvement in flow velocity lasting more than 30 min. Sudden recanalization reflects rapid and complete restoration of flow, while stepwise and slow recanalization indicate proximal clot fragmentation, downstream embolization and continued clot migration. Sudden recanalization was associated with a higher degree of neurological improvement and better long-term outcome than stepwise or slow recanalization.

A tandem internal carotid artery/middle cerebral artery occlusion independently predicted a poor response to thrombolysis in patients with a proximal MCA clot, but not in those with a distal MCA clot [29].

> Ultrasound has an important prognostic role in acute stroke and can be used to monitor thrombus dissolution during thrombolysis.

Ultrasound accelerated thrombolysis and microbubbles

Transcranial Doppler can be used not only for diagnostic and prognostic purposes, but also for therapy. The ultrasound enhances the enzymatic thrombolysis, increasing the transport of t-PA into the thrombus and improving the binding affinity, and provides a unique opportunity to detect the recanalization during and after t-PA administration.

Continuous monitoring with 2 MHz TCD in combination with standard i.v. t-PA therapy results in significantly higher recanalization rate or dramatic recovery than i.v. t-PA therapy without TCD monitoring. In the CLOTBUST trial, 126 patients were randomly assigned to receive continuous TCD monitoring or placebo in addition to intravenous t-PA. Complete recanalization or dramatic clinical recovery within 2 h after the administration of a TPA bolus occurred in 49% of the target group as compared to 30% in the control group ($P = 0.03$). Only 4.8% of patients developed symptomatic intracerebral hemorrhage. These results showed the positive effects of 2 MHz continuous TCD monitoring in acute stroke, with no increase in the rate of intracerebral hemorrhage [30].

Recently, combining t-PA, ultrasound and gaseous microbubbles showed signs of further enhancing arterial recanalization. Although these microbubbles, previously known as diagnostic microbubbles or gaseous microspheres, were originally designed to improve conventional ultrasound images, facilitation of thrombolysis is now emerging as a new treatment application for this technology. Newer-generation bubbles use specific phospholipid molecules that, when exposed to mechanical agitation, arrange themselves in nanobubbles with a consistent 1–2 μm (or even less) diameter. When injected intravenously, nanobubbles carry gas

through the circulation. As the bubbles approach and permeate through the thrombus, they can be detected and activated by the ultrasound energy. Upon encountering an ultrasound pressure wave, the phospholipid shell breaks up and releases gas. The result is bubble-induced cavitation with fluid jets that erode the thrombus surface. In the presence of t-PA, this erosion increases the surface area for thrombolytic action and accelerates lysis of clots [12]. Recent studies evaluated the effects of administration of microbubbles on the initial MCA recanalization during systemic thrombolysis and continuous 2 MHz pulsed-wave TCD monitoring. The complete recanalization rate was significantly higher in the t-PA+ultrasound+microbubbles group (55%) than in the t-PA/ultrasound (41%) and t-PA (24%) groups [31] with no increase in sICH after systemic thrombolysis.

Although recent observations support the usefulness of ultrasound in facilitating thrombolysis, ultrasound-alone treatment should not be substituted for t-PA treatment.

> Arterial recanalization can be enhanced by combining t-PA with ultrasound, and even further with gaseous microbubbles, which increase the surface area for the thrombolytic action of t-PA.

Vasomotor reactivity

Vasomotor reactivity describes the ability of the cerebral circulation to respond to vasomotor stimuli; the changes in cerebral blood flow (velocity in TCD studies) in response to such stimuli can be studied by TCD. CO_2 is a widely used agent to measure cerebral vasomotor reactivity. Another widely used agent is i.v. acetazolamide (0.15 mg/kg).

CO_2 results in vasodilatation and increased cerebral blood flow velocity. Measuring vasomotor reactivity requires standard experimental conditions. Markus et al. [32] described a simple measurement of the MCA velocity in response to 30 s breath-holding and termed it the breath-holding index (BHI):

$$BHI = \frac{MFV_{end} - MFV_{baseline}}{MFV_{baseline}} \times \frac{100}{seconds\ of\ breath\ holding}$$

(MFV: mean flow velocity).

Others [33] evaluated BHI in different studies and showed that impaired vasomotor reactivity can help to identify patients at higher risk of stroke. Decreased vasomotor reactivity suggests failure of collateral flow to adapt to the stenosis. Various studies using different provocative measures for assessing cerebral vasomotor reactivity have demonstrated a remarkable ipsilateral event rate of approx. 30% risk of stroke over 2 years.

> The changes in cerebral blood flow in response to vasomotor stimuli can be studied by TCD.

Right-to-left shunt detection

Right-to-left shunts, particularly a patent foramen ovale (PFO), are common in the general population, with a prevalence of 10–35% in various echocardiography and autopsy studies for PFO. The prevalence is even higher in cryptogenic stroke or TIA and especially in younger patients without an apparent etiology. Contrast-enhanced TCD can be used for detecting the high-intensity transient signals (HITS) passing through the MCA, thus indicating the presence of a right-to-left shunt. The results of contrast-enhanced TCD have been compared with those of contrast-transesophageal echo and found to have a sensitivity and specificity of 68–100% and 67–100%, respectively [34]. Another study with TCD and TEE proved the strength of TCD in PFO detection and right-to-left (RLS) quantification [35].

In conclusion, TCD has an established clinical value in the diagnostic workup of stroke patients. TCD is also an evolving ultrasound method with increasing therapeutic potential.

> Contrast-enhanced TCD can also be used to identify patients with a patent foramen ovale.

Chapter Summary

> Doppler ultrasonography is the primary non-invasive test for evaluating carotid stenosis.
>
> The sonographic characteristics of symptomatic and asymptomatic carotid plaques are different: symptomatic plaques are more likely to be hypoechoic and highly stenotic, while asymptomatic plaques are hyperechoic and moderately stenotic. The degree of stenosis is better measured on the basis of the waveform and spectral analysis. When no stenosis is present, blood flow is laminar. With greater stenosis, the flow becomes turbulent. An

important general rule for ultrasound is the greater the degree of stenosis, the higher the velocity.

Most studies consider carotid stenosis of 60% or greater to be clinically important.

Commonly used methods to estimate stenosis with ultrasonography are:
- Peak systolic velocities:
  - Normal: ICA PSV <125 cm/s, no plaque or intimal thickening.
  - <50% stenosis: ICA PSV <125 cm/s and plaque or intimal thickening.
  - 50–69% stenosis: ICA PSV is 125–230 cm/s and plaque is visible.
  - >70% stenosis to near occlusion: ICA PSV >230 cm/s and visible lumen narrowing.
  - Near occlusion: a markedly narrowed lumen on c-Doppler ultrasound.
  - Total occlusion: no detectable patent lumen is seen on grayscale ultrasound, and no flow is seen on spectral, power and color Doppler ultrasound.
- Ratios of the maximal systolic flow velocity within the ICA stenosis divided by the maximal systolic flow velocity within the non-affected CCA:
  - <50% stenoses ICA/CCA: <2.0.
  - 50–69% stenoses ICA/CCA: 2.0–4.0.
  - ≥70% stenoses ICA/CCA: >4.0.

Ratios may be particularly helpful in situations in which cardiovascular factors (e.g. poor ejection fraction) limit the increase in velocity.

With ultrasound, the intimal-medial thickness of the carotid artery can be measured. Increases in the intimal-medial thickness (IMT) of the carotid artery are associated with an increased risk of myocardial infarction and stroke.

In case of hemodynamically significant ICA stenosis or occlusion (proximal to the origin of the ophthalmic artery) a reversed (extra → intracranial) flow can be detected in the ophthalmic artery. Occlusion results in a complete absence of color-flow signal in ICA, and the diagnosis can be confirmed by ultrasound contrast agents.

Intracranial stenosis and occlusion corresponds to approximately 8–10% of acute ischemic stroke. Transcranial color-coded duplex sonography (TCCD) combines the imaging of intracranial vessels and parenchymal structures. To penetrate the skull, TCCD uses low frequencies (1.75–3.5 MHz), which limit the spatial resolution. Some patients cannot be examined because of an insufficient acoustic window. The duplex mode of TCCD enables sampling of vessels and Doppler measurements of angle-corrected blood-flow velocities. Mean velocity analysis is not enough to identify intracranial vessel abnormalities. It must be combined with other parameters such as asymmetry, segmental elevations, spectral analysis and knowledge of extracranial circulation. The use of echo-contrast enhancing agents (ECE) increases the sensitivity and specificity and with ECE the diagnostic confidence of TCCD for intracranial vessel occlusion is similar to that of magnetic resonance angiography.

Recently, a practical algorithm has been published for urgent bedside neurovascular ultrasound examination with carotid/vertebral duplex and transcranial Doppler in patients with acute stroke. TCD has the highest sensitivity (>90%) for acute arterial obstructions located in the proximal MCA and ICAs. TCD has modest sensitivity (55–60%) for posterior circulation lesions if performed without transcranial color-coded duplex imaging or contrast enhancement. With a completely normal spectral TCD, there is less than 5% chance that an urgent angiogram will show any acute obstruction.

TCD identifies microembolic signs (MES) in the intracranial circulation. Detection of MES can identify patients with stroke or TIA likely to be due to embolism and, in addition, acts as a predictor for new cerebral ischemic event recurrence. TCD monitoring may help to discriminate between different potential sources of embolism (i.e. artery-to-artery or cardioembolic strokes). Different types of emboli (i.e. cardiac or carotid) have different acoustic properties and ultrasonic characteristics, based on composition and size, which could permit differentiation. MES detection by TCD in CEA candidates may allow identification of a particularly high-risk group of patients who merit an early intervention or, if this is not possible, more aggressive antithrombotic therapy.

New ultrasound contrast agents (UCAs) that can pass through the microcirculation and the development of contrast-specific imaging modalities make it possible to use ultrasound for the visualization of brain perfusion deficits. But perfusion imaging in acute stroke is still in the experimental phase.

Ultrasound has an important prognostic role in acute stroke and can be used to monitor thrombus dissolution during thrombolysis. The waveform changes correlate well with clinical improvement and a rapid arterial recanalization is associated with better short-term improvement, whereas slow flow improvement and dampened flow signals are less favorable prognostic signs.

Transcranial Doppler can be used not only for diagnostic and prognostic purposes, but also for therapy. The ultrasound enhances enzymatic thrombolysis, increasing the transport of t-PA into the thrombus and improving the binding affinity, and provides a unique opportunity to detect recanalization during and after t-PA administration. Arterial recanalization can be further enhanced by combining t-PA, ultrasound and gaseous microbubbles. Newer-generation bubbles permeate through the thrombus and erode the thrombus surface, which increases the surface area for the thrombolytic action of t-PA.

The changes in cerebral blood flow in response to vasomotor stimuli can be studied by TCD. Decreased vasomotor reactivity suggests failure of collateral flow to adapt to a stenosis and can help identify patients at higher risk of stroke.

Contrast-enhanced TCD can also be used to identify patients with a patent foramen ovale.

References

1. Silver B. http://emedicine.medscape.com/article/1155193-overview. Updated: 15 Dec 2008.

2. Grant EG, Benson CB, Moneta GL, et al. Carotid artery stenosis: grayscale and Doppler ultrasound diagnosis – Society of Radiologists in Ultrasound consensus conference. *Ultrasound Q* 2003; **19**(4):190–8.

3. Nadalo LA, Walters MC. Carotid artery, stenosis: imaging http://emedicine.medscape.com/article/417524-imaging.

4. Cao JJ, Thach C, Manolio TA, Psaty BM, Kuller LH, Chaves PH, et al. C-reactive protein, carotid intima-media thickness, and incidence of ischemic stroke in the elderly: the Cardiovascular Health Study. *Circulation* 2003; **108**(2):166–70.

5. Masdeu JC, Irimiaa P, Asenbaumb S, Bogousslavsky J, Brainin M, Chabriate H, et al. EFNS guideline on neuroimaging in acute stroke. Report of an EFNS task force. *Eur J Neurol* 2006; **13**:1271–83.

6. Zipper SG, Stolz E. Clinical application of transcranial colour-coded duplex sonography-a review. *Eur J Neurol* 2002; **9**:1–8.

7. Sloan MA, Alexandrov AV, Tegeler CH, Spencer MP, Caplan LR, Feldman E, et al. Assessment transcranial Doppler ultrasonography report of the therapeutics and technology assessment subcommittee of the American Academy of Neurology. *Neurology* 2004; **62**:1468–81.

8. Baumgartner RW. Transcranial color-coded duplex sonography. *J Neurol* 1999; **246**(8):637–47.

9. Valdueza JM, Schreiber SJ, Roehl JE, Klingebiel R. *Neurosonology and Neuroimaging of Stroke*. Stuttgart: Thieme; 2008.

10. Gerriets T, Goertler M, Stolz E, Postert T, Sliwka U, Schlachetzki F, et al. Feasibility and validity of transcranial duplex sonography in patients with acute stroke. *J Neurol Neurosurg Psychiatry* 2002; **73**:17–20.

11. Chernyshev OY, Garami Z, Calleja S, Song J, Campbell MS, Noser EA, et al. Yield and accuracy of urgent combined carotid-transcranial ultrasound testing in acute cerebral ischemia. *Stroke* 2005; **36**:32–7.

12. Sharma VK, Venketasubramanian N, Khurana DK, Tsivgoulis G, Alexandrov AV. Role of transcranial Doppler ultrasonography in acute stroke. *Ann Indian Acad Neurol* 2008; **11**:39–51.

13. Azarpazhooh MR, Chambers BR. Clinical application of transcranial Doppler monitoring for embolic signals. *J Clin Neurosci* 2006; **13**(8):799–810.

14. Segura T, Serena J, Castellanos M, Teruel J, Vilar C, Dávalos A. Embolism in acute middle cerebral artery stenosis. *Neurology* 2001; **56**:497–501.

15. Tegos TJ, Sabetai MM, Nicolaides AN, Robless P, Kalodiki E, Elatrozy TS, et al. Correlates of embolic events detected by means of transcranial Doppler in patients with carotid atheroma. *J Vasc Surg* 2001; **33**:131–8.

16. Del Sette M, Angeli S, Stara I, Finocchi C, Gandolfo C. Microembolic signals with serial transcranial Doppler monitoring in acute focal ischemic deficit. A local phenomenon? *Stroke* 1997; **28**:1311–13.

17. Markus HS, Droste DW, Kaps M, Larrue V, Lees KR, Siebler M, et al. Dual antiplatelet therapy with clopidogrel and aspirin in symptomatic carotid stenosis evaluated using doppler embolic signal detection: the Clopidogrel and Aspirin for Reduction of Emboli in Symptomatic Carotid Stenosis (CARESS) trial. *Circulation* 2005; **111**:2233–40.

18. Ritter MA, Dittrich R, Thoenissen N, Ringelstein EB, Nabavi DG. Prevalence and prognostic impact of microembolic signals in arterial sources of embolism. A systematic review of the literature. *J Neurol* 2008; **255**(7):953–61.

19. Della Martina A, Meyer-Wiethe K, Allemann E, Seidel G. Ultrasound contrast agents for brain perfusion imaging and ischemic stroke therapy. *J Neuroimaging* 2005; **15**:217–32.

20. Seidel G, Meyer-Wiethe K. Acute stroke: perfusion imaging. *Front Neurol Neurosci* 2006; **21**:127–39.

21. Meairs S. Contrast-enhanced ultrasound perfusion imaging in acute stroke patients. *Eur Neurol* 2008; **59**(suppl 1):17–26.

22. Seidel G, Meyer-Wiethe K, Berdien G, Hollstein D, Toth D, Aach T. Ultrasound perfusion imaging in acute middle cerebral artery infarction predicts outcome. *Stroke* 2004; **35**:1107–11.

23. Allendoerfer J, Goertler M, Reutern GM. Prognostic relevance of ultra-early doppler sonography in acute ischaemic stroke: a prospective multicentre study. *Lancet Neurol* 2006; **5**:835–40.

24. Demchuk AM, Burgin WS, Christou I, Felberg RA, Barber PA, Hill MD, et al. Thrombolysis in brain ischemia (TIBI) transcranial Doppler flow grades predict clinical severity, early recovery, and mortality in patients treated with intravenous tissue plasminogen activator. *Stroke* 2001; **32**:89–93.

25. Baracchini C, Manara R, Ermani M, Meneghetti G. The quest for early predictors of stroke evolution: can TCD be a guiding light? *Stroke* 2000; **31**:2942–7.

26. Perren F, Loulidi J, Graves R, Yilmaz H, Rüfenacht D, Landis T, et al. Combined IV–intraarterial thrombolysis: a color-coded duplex pilot study. *Neurology* 2006; **67**:324–26.

27. Saqqur M, Uchino K, Demchuk AM, Molina CA, Garami Z, Calleja S, et al. Site of arterial occlusion identified by transcranial doppler predicts the response to intravenous thrombolysis for stroke. *Stroke* 2007; **38**(3):948–54.

28. Alexandrov AV, Burgin SW, Demchuk AM, El-Mitwalli A, Grotta JC. Speed of intracranial clot lysis with intravenous tissue plasminogen activator therapy: sonographic classification and short-term improvement. *Circulation* 2001; **103**:2897–902.

29. Rubiera M, Ribo M, Delgado-Mederos R, Santamarina E, Delgado P, Montaner J, et al. Tandem internal carotid artery/middle cerebral artery occlusion: an independent predictor of poor outcome after systemic thrombolysis. *Stroke* 2006; **37**:2301–05.

30. Alexandrov AV, Molina CA, Grotta JC, Garami Z, Ford SR, Alvarez-Sabin J, et al. For the CLOTBUST Investigators: Ultrasound-enhanced thrombolysis for acute ischemic stroke. *N Engl J Med* 2004; **351**:2170–8.

31. Molina CA, Ribo M, Rubiera M, Montaner J, Santamarina E, Delgado-Mederos R, et al. Microbubbles administration accelerates clot lysis during continuous 2-MHz ultrasound monitoring in stroke patients treated with intravenous tPA. *Stroke* 2006; **37**:425–9.

32. Markus HS, Harrison MJ. Estimation of cerebrovascular reactivity using transcranial Doppler, including the use of breath-holding as the vasodilatory stimulus. *Stroke* 1992; **23**:668–73.

33. Silvestrini M, Vernieri F, Pasqualetti P, Matteis M, Passarelli F, Troisi E. Impaired cerebral

vasoreactivity and risk of stroke in patients with asymptomatic carotid stenosis. *JAMA* 2000; **283**:2122–7.

34. Droste DW, Silling K, Stypmann J, Grude M, Kemeny V, Wichter T, et al. Contrast transcranial Doppler ultrasound in the detection of right-to-left shunts: time window and threshold in microbubble numbers. *Stroke* 2000; **31**:1640–5.

35. Belvis R, Leta RG, Marti-Fabregas J, Cocho D, Carreras F, Pons-Llado G, et al. Almost perfect concordance between simultaneous transcranial Doppler and transesophageal echocardiography in the quantification of right-to-left shunts. *J Neuroimaging* 2006; **16**:133–8.

5

Basic epidemiology of stroke and risk assessment

Jaakko Tuomilehto, Markku Mähönen and Cinzia Sarti

Definition of stroke

In epidemiological studies, stroke is defined by clinical findings and symptoms [1]: rapidly developed signs of focal (or global) disturbance of cerebral function lasting more than 24 hours (unless interrupted by surgery or death), with no apparent cause other than a vascular origin. This approach is supplemented with neuroimaging but even with advanced imaging techniques the diagnosis is based on clinical signs. Therefore, precise definitions of clinical signs are needed. WHO definitions are [1]:

Definite focal signs:

- unilateral or bilateral motor impairment (including dyscoordination)
- unilateral or bilateral sensory impairment
- aphasis/dysphasis (non-fluent speech)
- hemianopia (half-sided impairment of visual fields)
- diplopia
- forced gaze (conjugate deviation)
- dysphagia of acute onset
- apraxia of acute onset
- ataxia of acute onset
- perception deficit of acute onset.

Not acceptable as sole evidence of focal dysfunction:

- dizziness, vertigo
- localized headache
- blurred vision of both eyes
- dysarthria (slurred speech)
- impaired cognitive function (including confusion)
- impaired consciousness
- seizures.

(Although strokes can present in this way, these signs are not specific and cannot therefore be accepted as definite evidence of stroke.)

Neuroimaging studies are needed for classification of stroke by subtypes: subarachnoid hemorrhage, intracerebral hemorrhage and brain infarction (necrosis). Although there may be large variations in stroke subtype distributions between populations, thrombotic and embolic strokes are responsible for about 80–85% of all strokes in the Indo-European populations, and as low as 65% in some Asian populations. Subarachnoid hemorrhage represents 5–10% of all strokes, and occurs more often in younger subjects, while both intracerebral and especially thrombotic and embolic stroke increase markedly with age.

The scope of the problem

Stroke is the second leading cause of death worldwide in the adult population, the first being coronary heart disease [2]. Of note, stroke is an increasing problem in developing countries, 87% of stroke deaths occurring in low- and middle-income countries [2–4]. Stroke is the fourth leading cause of disease burden (as measured in disability-adjusted life years [DALYs]) after heart disease, HIV/AIDS and unipolar depressive disorders [2]. In the 1990s, it caused about 4.4 million deaths worldwide in 1990 and 5.4 million in 1999, with two-thirds of these deaths occurring in less-developed countries [5, 6]. While in high-income countries 9.9% of all deaths could be attributed to stroke, in low-and-middle-income countries this proportion was 9.5%, almost equal; because the total number of deaths in low- and middle-income countries is much greater than in high-income countries, globally the highest burden of stroke is among people living in low- and middle-income countries. DALYs due to stroke were 62.67 per million person-years in high-income countries, corresponding to 4.5% of the total DALYs, when the corresponding estimate for low-and-middle-income countries was 9.35 per

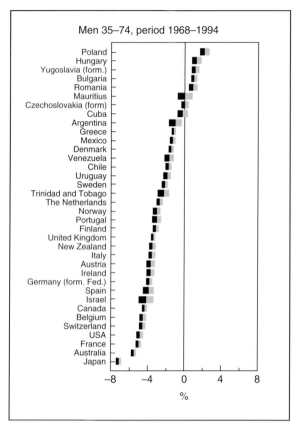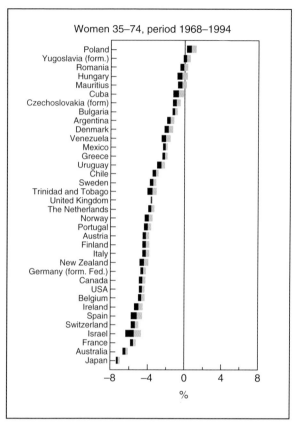

Figure 5.1. Annual percentage change in mortality from stroke in men (left) and women (right) aged 35–74 years in selected countries during the entire study period, 1968–1994. (Source and copyright, see reference 3.)

million person-years, and this translated to 6.3% of the total DALYs.

Incidence, mortality and case fatality

There are several issues related to the occurrence of stroke that are important from an epidemiological (and clinical) perspective. While it would be useful to know the incidence (occurrence of first stroke events), in most populations data may be available on mortality from stroke only, but not on non-fatal events. The case fatality at the stroke event, usually determined as the proportion of deaths occurring during the first 4 weeks after the onset of stroke event, gives information about the severity of stroke and may also reflect the efficacy of early management of acute stroke. The relative frequency of different sub-types of stroke varies among populations, and in particular among different ethnic groups. This variation may be in part due to genetic differences or due to differences in risk-factor profiles.

A comparison of routinely collected stroke mortality data from many countries shows that, in general, mortality rates have declined over recent decades, most notably in Japan, Australia, North America and Western Europe [7] (Figure 5.1). Mortality from stroke was highest in the world in Finland in the 1970s, together with Japan.

There are few studies with validated data from stroke registers or other sources. The incidence of stroke has declined sharply in Finland during the last decades [8], and in 1998 it was 241/100 000, not far from other Western industrialized countries, after a steady fall of about 3% per year throughout the 15 years studied. Mortality from stroke declined even more steeply, around 4% per year, with a standardized mortality rate in 1998 of 50/100 000 among men and 30/100 000 among women [8]. Other countries that already had comparatively lower stroke incidence rates in the 1980s, for example New Zealand [9], the USA [10], or Denmark [11], have reported no fall in stroke incidence, while an increase in the incidence of stroke has been observed in Eastern Europe and Russia [6, 7, 12]. In Shanghai, China, almost no decline in incidence of stroke but a clear decline in stroke mortality was reported [13]. The differences observed between countries in mortality rates, and even more in incidence rates, are, however, difficult to interpret, as they depend largely on the study design, the accuracy of the data collection, and the time point when the measurements were made.

The overall case fatality (the proportion of deaths among all strokes) is roughly 20% within the first month, and increases around 5% per year. There is, however, a large variation in case fatality of stroke among populations; in the WHO Monitoring of Trends and Determinants in Cardiovascular Disease (MONICA) Stroke Study among men, the case fatality of stroke ranged from 12% in northern Sweden to 53% in Moscow in Russia [14]. Overall, the case fatality was high in all eastern European countries. In women, the difference in case fatality of stroke between populations was larger than in men, ranging from 16% in Kuopio to 57% in Moscow.

Trends in stroke event rates, case fatality and mortality of stroke

Table 5.1 shows the trends, separately for each MONICA population, in stroke event rates, case fatality and mortality of stroke, both in the register and in routine mortality statistics. Stroke event rates declined in nine of 14 populations in men and eight of 14 populations in women. In men, the case fatality of stroke declined in seven populations, increased in eight, and fluctuated only slightly in two. Among women, a decline in case fatality was seen in eight populations, no obvious change was seen in three, and an increase was observed in three. The trends in case fatality were statistically significant among men in only two populations with declining trends and in two with increasing trends. Among women, there was a significant downward trend in four populations. Within each population, the CIs for the case fatality trends were larger than those for the trends in stroke event rates. Of the 14 populations, stroke mortality declined in eight populations among men and 10 populations among women. Stroke mortality increased in all the eastern European populations except in Warsaw, Poland. In Beijing, China and

in the nine western European populations, stroke mortality declined.

Changes in incidence and improved survival on the downward trend in stroke mortality are not easy to quantify, due to the difficulty of measuring accurately the incidence of stroke. The MONICA Stroke Study, for example, compared stroke incidence (or more precisely attack rate, which included various proportions of recurrent strokes), mortality and case fatality in 14 populations aged 35–64 years (mostly located in Europe except two – one in China and one in Novosibirsk in Asian Russia). The study confirmed the above observed trends in stroke incidence and mortality, and reported a large geographical variation also in case fatality. In most populations, changes in stroke mortality, whether declining or increasing, were principally attributable to changes in case fatality rather than changes in event rates [7].

> In many epidemiological studies strokes have been defined without confirmation by neuroimaging. Definitions by clinical means alone can be imprecise and sometimes misleading. Robust data have shown that the overall case fatality is roughly 20% within the first month and increases about 5% per year. Large variations occur between countries. On a global scale, stroke is the second most frequent cause of mortality world-wide and a leading cause of disability. It is especially prevalent in low- and middle-income countries.

Risk factors

Stroke has a multifactorial origin and a plethora of putative and confirmed risk factors have been listed and tested in various types of studies. The assessment of the global epidemiology is severely hindered by the lack of any kind of data on stroke occurrence and risk factors in most populations in the world. Although over 65% of all deaths due to stroke occur in developing countries, studies of stroke epidemiology in these populations hardly exist.

The American Heart Association Stroke Council's Scientific Statement Oversight Committee guideline has provided an overview of the evidence on various established and potential stroke risk factors and proposed recommendations for the reduction of stroke risk [15]. The committee used systematic literature reviews published during 2001 to January 2005, reference to previously published guidelines, personal files and expert opinions to summarize existing evidence

79

Table 5.1. Age standardized stroke attack rate, case fatality and mortality in the WHO MONICA Stroke Study populations [14].

Population	Attack Rate per 100 000		Case Fatality, %		Mortality Rate per 100 000	
	First 3 Years	Last 3 Years	First 3 Years	Last 3 Years	First 3 Years	Last 3 Years
Men						
CHN-BEI	248	241	27	26	67	63
	(234–264)	(226–255)	(24–29)	(23–29)	(59–75)	(56–71)
CEN-ELO	218	160	16	20	34	31
	(197–241)	(143–179)	(12–20)	(15–25)	(26–44)	(24–40)
FIN-KUO	572	510	19	16	72	50
	(340–407)	(292–340)	(16–23)	(13–20)	(58–88)	(30–63)
FIN-NKA	258	257	22	20	60	51
	(254–325)	(226–290)	(17–28)	(15–25)	(53–89)	(38–68)
FIN-TUL	236	228	23	17	54	37
	(209–267)	(201–257)	(18–29)	(12–21)	(41–70)	(27–50)
ITA-FR	129	121	35	24	45	29
	(120–139)	(112–130)	(32–39)	(21–27)	(41–52)	(25–34)
LTU-KAU	309	347	23	24	60	54
	(234–335)	(322–374)	(19–25)	(21–27)	(58–83)	(72–97)
POL-WAR	171	171	52	40	89	69
	(166–188)	(166–187)	(47–57)	(35–44)	(77–101)	(50–79)
RUS-MOC	270	216	32	53	86	111
	(241–302)	(190–245)	(26–37)	(45–59)	(70–105)	(93–153)
RUS-MOI	249	237	38	51	96	122
	(231–269)	(220–259)	(34–42)	(43–55)	(54–108)	(110–135)
RUS-NOI	438	449	27	35	122	190
	(382–500)	(409–500)	(21–33)	(30–40)	(93–159)	(132–192)
SWE-GOT	129	149	17	18	22	27
	(115–145)	(133–165)	(13–21)	(14–22)	(17–27)	(21–34)
SWE-NSW	221	219	16	12	35	26
	(205–230)	(203–235)	(12–19)	(10–15)	(29–42)	(21–33)
YUG-NOS	222	211	37	41	82	87
	(109–248)	(100–238)	(31–42)	(36–47)	(58–98)	(74–100)
Women						
CHN-BEI	175	182	30	27	64	50
	(163–188)	(160–195)	(27–34)	(24–31)	(47–81)	(43–58)
DEM-ELO	90	90	19	22	20	19
	(95–114)	(77–104)	(14–25)	(15–28)	(14–28)	(13–26)

Table 5.1. (cont.)

Population	Attack Rate per 100 000		Case Fatality, %		Mortality Rate per 100 000	
	First 3 Years	Last 3 Years	First 3 Years	Last 3 Years	First 3 Years	Last 3 Years
FIN-KUO	139	130	27	16	48	21
	(167–213)	(113–140)	(22–32)	(11–21)	(38–61)	(14–30)
FIN-NKA	124	117	23	20	29	23
	(103–148)	(97–140)	(16–31)	(13–27)	(19–41)	(15–34)
FIN-TUL	117	108	24	24	29	27
	(90–137)	(91–128)	(17–31)	(17–31)	(20–30)	(18–37)
ITA-FRI	68	50	42	31	26	18
	(57–70)	(53–65)	(37–47)	(26–36)	(22–30)	(15–22)
LTU-KAU	154	152	24	26	35	46
	(139–170)	(166–190)	(19–23)	(22–30)	(23–44)	(38–55)
POL-WAR	90	93	54	44	49	40
	(79–101)	(83–104)	(48–60)	(38–49)	(40–56)	(38–47)
RUS-MOC	146	94	39	47	53	44
	(120–165)	(79–110)	(31–44)	(30–55)	(43–65)	(35–55)
RUS-MOI	135	107	30	57	52	61
	(122–145)	(29–118)	(35–44)	(52–68)	(45–60)	(54–60)
RUS-MOI	341	391	25	23	87	82
	(303–383)	(352–433)	(20–31)	(18–27)	(58–109)	(65–106)
SWE-GOT	71	72	24	25	17	18
	(61–82)	(65–84)	(17–30)	(18–32)	(12–23)	(13–24)
SWE-MSW	119	136	21	17	25	23
	(107–132)	(123–150)	(17–25)	(13–20)	(20–31)	(18–20)
YUG-NOS	114	127	49	42	55	53
	(99–132)	(112–144)	(40–65)	(35–48)	(44–67)	(43–64)

Note: Values in parentheses are 95% CIs.

on standard criteria. Risk factors or risk markers for a first stroke were classified according to their potential for modification (non-modifiable, modifiable, or potentially modifiable) and strength of evidence (well-documented or less well-documented). Non-modifiable risk factors include age, sex, low birth weight, race/ethnicity and genetic factors. Well-documented and modifiable risk factors include hypertension, exposure to cigarette smoke, diabetes, atrial fibrillation and certain other cardiac conditions, dyslipidemia, carotid artery stenosis, sickle-cell disease, postmenopausal hormone therapy, poor diet, physical inactivity and obesity and central body fat distribution. Less well-documented or potentially modifiable risk factors include the metabolic syndrome, alcohol abuse, drug abuse, oral contraceptive use, sleep-disordered breathing, migraine headache, hyperhomocysteinemia, elevated lipoprotein(a), elevated lipoprotein-associated phospholipase, hypercoagulability, inflammation and infection. This paper represents probably the most thorough assessment of the prediction and potential for the prevention of stroke.

Non-modifiable risk factors of stroke

Age is probably the most important determinant of stroke; the risk of stroke doubles for each successive decade after age 55 years [16, 17]. This is also true for ischemic stroke, while the age relation of intracerebral hemorrhage is less steep and the peak age of SAH incidence is around 45–55 years. Stroke is a common disease in both men and women, but it is more common in men within the age range of 45–84 years [18, 19].

Racial or ethnic specific stroke risk is difficult to interpret. While within a country such as the USA clear ethnic group differences exist, African Americans [18, 20] and some Hispanic Americans [21, 22] have higher stroke incidence and mortality rates as compared with European Americans, globally stroke mortality does not follow any ethnic patterns [23]. Nevertheless, it is well known that intracerebral bleeding is more common in oriental populations, and SAH most common in Finland and Sweden [7, 24].

Both paternal and maternal history of stroke are associated with an increased stroke risk [24–26]. It is not necessarily "stroke genes" that are behind this familial aggregation, but one or more of the mechanisms may contribute to it such as (i) familial occurrence of risk factors for stroke, (ii) genetic susceptibility to these risk factors, (iii) familial sharing of environmental/lifestyle factors associated with stroke and (iv) the interaction between genetic and environmental effects [26–28]. Currently, rapid advances in genetic research are taking place and have resulted in the identification of genes associated with stroke and its subtypes. Low birth weight is another risk factor for stroke [29, 30], as it is for cardiovascular disease in general. Although these risk factors themselves cannot be modified, it does not mean that the stroke risk in such individuals could not be modified. In them, it is particularly important to pay attention to the control of modifiable risk factors.

There are several well-documented medical conditions and diseases that have importance as risk factors for stroke. These are described in the next chapter by Brainin et al. In this chapter, some general observations are made on lifestyle factors, and their relative importance for stroke incidence or recurrence is reported.

Among the non-modifiable risk factors old age, racial or ethnic factors, low birth weight, and sometimes genetic susceptibility play a role. In individuals with non-modifiable risk factors, prevention focused on the modifiable ones is particularly important.

Overall lifestyle patterns and stroke risk

Recently, in the analysis of the data from the Health Professionals Follow-up Study and from the Nurses' Health Study the impact on stroke risk of a combination of healthy lifestyle characteristics was evaluated and the burden of stroke that may be attributed to these unhealthy lifestyle choices was calculated [31]. Diet and other lifestyle factors were updated from self-reported questionnaires. A low-risk healthy lifestyle was defined as: (i) not smoking, (ii) a body mass index <25 kg/m^2, (iii) ≥ 30 min/day of moderate activity, (iv) modest alcohol consumption (men, 5 to 30 g/day; women, 5 to 15 g/day), and (v) scoring within the top 40% of a healthy diet score. Women with all five low-risk factors had a relative risk of 0.21 for total and 0.19 for ischemic stroke compared with women who had none of these factors. Among men, the corresponding relative risks were 0.31 for total and 0.20 for ischemic stroke. Among women, 47% of total and 54% of ischemic stroke cases were attributable to lack of adherence to a low-risk lifestyle, and among men the corresponding proportions were 35% and 52%, respectively. Low-risk lifestyle was not significantly associated with risk of hemorrhagic stroke, nor was it in the Women's Health Study [32]. Other studies have also evaluated joint effects of multiple lifestyle-related risk profiles on stroke risk. In the German EPIC Potsdam study, almost 60% of ischemic stroke cases could be attributed to hypertension, diabetes, hypercholesterolemia, smoking, and heavy alcohol consumption (>15 g alcohol/day in women, >30 g alcohol/day in men) [33]. Stamler et al. found that a low-risk lifestyle, defined as cholesterol <200 mg/dl, blood pressure $<120/80$ mmHg, and not smoking, was associated with 52% to 76% lower risk of total stroke mortality [34]. In the Women's Health Study, women with the healthiest lifestyle score, defined as never smoking, having a BMI <22 kg/m^2, exercising ≥ 4 times a week, consuming 0.5 to 1.5 drinks a day, and following a healthy diet, had 71% lower risk of ischemic stroke compared with women with the least healthy lifestyle [32]. Thus, a low-risk healthy lifestyle that is associated with a reduced risk of multiple chronic diseases also seems to be beneficial in the prevention of ischemic stroke.

In the WHO MONICA Project, repeated population surveys of cardiovascular risk factors and continuous monitoring of stroke events was conducted in 35–64-year-old people over a 7–13-year period in 15 populations in nine countries. Stroke trends were compared with trends in individual risk factors and their combinations [35]. A 3–4-year time lag between changes in risk factors and change in stroke rates was considered. Population-level trends in systolic blood pressure showed a strong association with stroke event trends in women, but there was no association in men. In women, 38% of the variation in stroke event trends was explained by changes in systolic blood pressure. Combining trends in daily cigarette smoking, serum cholesterol and BMI with systolic blood pressure into a risk score explained only a small additional fraction of the variation in stroke event trends.

Prediction of stroke in patients with TIA

Ischemic stroke is often preceded by early symptoms, i.e. a transient ischemic attack (TIA) [36]. The risk of stroke after a TIA attack has been underestimated for many years due to issues in study designs [37, 38]. Hospital-based and population-based cohort studies have reported 7-day risks of stroke of up to 10% [39–43]. Models with predictors for long-term risk of stroke after TIA or minor stroke have been developed [39–42, 44–46]. A substantial international variation exists as to how patients with suspected TIA are managed in the acute phase.

Rothwell et al. have developed and validated a simple risk score to predict stroke during the first 7 days after a TIA attack [47]. A six-point score derived (age [>60 years = 1], blood pressure [systolic ≥ 140 mmHg and/or diastolic ≥ 90 mmHg = 1], clinical features [unilateral weakness = 2, speech disturbance without weakness = 1, other = 0], and duration of symptoms in min [$\geq 60 = 2$, 10–59 = 1, <10 = 0]) was highly predictive of 7-day risk of stroke in patients with probable or definite TIA ($p < 0.0001$), in the Oxford Vascular Study population-based cohort of all referrals with suspected TIA ($p < 0.0001$), and in the hospital-based weekly TIA clinic-referred cohort ($p = 0.006$). In the suspected TIA cohort, 95% of strokes occurred in 101 (27%) patients with a score of 5 or greater: 7-day risk was 0.4% in 274 (73%) patients with a score less than 5, 12.1% in 66 (18%) with a score of 5, and 31.4% in 35 (9%) with a score of 6. In the hospital-referred clinic cohort, 14 (7.5%) patients had a stroke before their scheduled

appointment, all with a score of 4 or greater. The authors concluded that the risk of stroke during the 7 days after TIA seems to be highly predictable. While they call for further validations and refinements of this score, it is robust enough to be used in routine clinical practice to identify high-risk individuals in European populations who need emergency investigation and treatment.

> Transient ischemic attacks carry a high risk of early recurrence especially within the first days. Patients who suffered a TIA lasting longer than 1 hour carry a very high risk of suffering a lasting stroke as opposed to those whose TIA lasted only a few minutes. Simple risk scores to assess high versus low stroke risk in TIA patients are clinically useful.

Prediction of stroke in the general population

Various multivariable models can be generated to estimate a person's risk for stroke in the populations where prospective studies have been carried out. On the other hand, only a few such attempts exist, while plenty of risk prediction scores for coronary heart disease have been developed. This imbalance is mainly due to the fact that most prospective studies of cardiovascular disease have been carried out in the middle-aged populations (men) in whom coronary heart disease is a more common outcome than stroke. In addition, many risk prediction models have included mostly biological risk factors. It has been repeatedly pointed out that the major risk factors for coronary heart disease, stroke, peripheral vascular disease, type 2 diabetes and certain types of cancer all share the same lifestyle background. The reason why one person gets a stroke and another one type 2 diabetes etc. is not clear. Variations in genetic factors or interactions between lifestyle-related factors may provide some answers, but it is certainly not possible to make any use of such information for the individual risk assessment.

For stroke risk-assessment tools, complex interactions of risk factors and the effects of certain risk factors stratified by non-modifiable factors such as age, gender, ethnicity and geography are incompletely captured by such tools. Some risk-assessment tools are gender-specific and give one-, five-, or 10-year stroke risk estimates. The Framingham Stroke Profile (FSP) uses a Cox proportional-hazards model with risk factors as covariates and points calculated according

Table 5.2. Framingham stroke risk profile, modified [49].

	Points										
	0	+1	+2	+3	+4	+5	+6	+7	+8	+9	+10
Men											
Age, years	54–56	57–59	60–62	63–65	66–68	69–72	73–75	76–78	79–81	82–84	85
Untreated systolic blood pressure, mmHg	97–105	106–115	116–125	126–135	136–145	146–155	156–165	166–175	176–185	186–195	196–205
Treated systolic blood pressure, mmHg	97–105	106–112	113–117	118–123	124–129	130–135	136–142	143–150	151–161	162–176	177–205
History of diabetes	No		Yes								
Cigarette smoking	No			Yes							
Cardiovascular disease	No				Yes						
Atrial fibrillation	No				Yes						
Left ventricular hypertrophy on electrocardiogram	No					Yes					
Women											
Age, years	54–56	57–59	60–62	63–64	65–67	68–70	71–73	74–76	77–78	79–81	82–84
Untreated systolic blood pressure, mmHg		95–106	107–118	119–130	131–143	144–155	156–167	168–180	181–192	193–204	205–216
Treated systolic blood pressure, mmHg		95–106	107–113	114–119	120–125	126–131	132–139	140–148	149–160	161–204	205–216
History of diabetes	No			Yes							
Cigarette smoking	No			Yes							
Cardiovascular disease	No		Yes								
Atrial fibrillation	No						Yes				
Left ventricular hypertrophy on electrocardiogram	No				Yes						

to the weight of the model coefficients [48–50]. Independent stroke predictors are shown in Table 5.2. It is widely used, but its validity among various subgroups other than the Framingham cohort has not been adequately studied. Nevertheless risk-prediction tools based on clinical data have been developed [51, 52].

In a clinical setting, simple risk assessment tools that have been developed for instance for type 2 diabetes [53] might be useful since they do not require any laboratory testing. Similar tools have been now developed for dementia [54], but unfortunately we do not have such a simple risk-assessment tool for stroke. Yet it is not difficult to design such given the large number of prospective studies using stroke as the outcome. In both men and women the FINDRISC predicted the stroke incidence well [55]. This avenue in risk assessment needs to be further pursued in order to identify people at risk of stroke as early as possible.

> Stroke risk assessment leans on risk profiles in a population. The Framingham Stroke Profile is widely used but has so far not been validated in many populations.

New risk factors for stroke

As many as 60% to 80% of ischemic stroke events can be attributed to high blood pressure, dyslipidemia, smoking and diabetes, and also to atrial fibrillation and valvular heart disease (cardiogenic and embolic ischemic stroke) [56]. A recent review indicated that about 10% to 20% of atherosclerotic ischemic strokes can probably be attributed to recently established, probably causal risk factors for ischemic heart disease: raised apoB/apoA1 ratio, obesity, physical inactivity, psychosocial stress and low fruit and vegetable intake [57]. However, their causal role remains to be proven. While the importance of genes predisposing to stroke cannot be denied [58], the contribution of any single gene towards ischemic stroke is likely to be modest and to apply in selected patients only and in combination with environmental factors or via other epistatic (gene–gene or gene–environmental) effects.

Hankey proposed, based on the well-known Bradford Hill criteria on causality, a practical way to consider the causal significance of a risk factor for ischemic stroke [57]:

- Is there evidence from experiments in *humans*?
- Is the association between exposure to the risk factor and ischemic stroke shown by means of multiple variable regression analysis to be *independent* of other risk factors that may interact with the risk factor or be a confounding risk factor?
- Is the association *strong*?
- Is the association *consistent* from study to study?
- Is the *temporal relation* correct (exposure to the risk factor occurred before the stroke)?
- Is there a *dose–response relation* (increasing risk or severity of stroke associated with increasing dose or duration of exposure to the risk factor)?
- Is the association biologically plausible?
- Is the association epidemiologically plausible?
- Is there evidence that *reducing* exposure to the risk factor (e.g. by RCTs) leads to a reduction in the risk of stroke?

It needs to be pointed out that certain issues such as smoking and alcohol drinking, and many other dietary factors, can never be properly tested in real life, and if such experiments would appear, they can only be considered as cross-sectional in a particular population. Therefore, it is very important to understand the inferences that can be drawn from various studies. Techniques such as meta-analysis will help, but only if the original studies were done properly and were comparable. Therefore, resources should not be allocated disproportionately to emerging novel risk factors that may account for up to only 20% of all strokes at the expense of researching the determinants of the relatively few established causal factors that account for up to 80% of all strokes. The evidence is strong to suggest that the control of the established risk factors for stroke will result in prevention of a very large number of stroke events and premature deaths.

Chapter Summary

> On a global scale, stroke is the second most frequent cause of mortality world-wide and a leading cause of disability. It is especially prevalent in low- and middle-income countries. The WHO Monitoring of Trends and Determinants in Cardiovascular Disease (MONICA) stroke study compared the stroke incidence (or more precisely attack rate), mortality, and case fatality in 14 populations aged 35–64 years. The study confirmed the large geographical variation in stroke incidence and mortality, and also in case

fatality. The relative frequency of different subtypes of stroke varies among populations, and in particular among different ethnic groups. This variation may be in part due to genetic differences or due to differences in risk-factor profiles. In most populations, changes in stroke mortality, whether declining or increasing, have been principally attributable to changes in case fatality rather than changes in event rates. In many epidemiological studies strokes have been defined without confirmation by neuroimaging. Definitions by clinical means alone can be imprecise and sometimes misleading. Robust data have shown that the overall case fatality is roughly 20% within the first month and increases about 5%/year. Large variations occur between countries. Stroke has a multifactorial origin and a plethora of putative and confirmed risk factors have been listed and tested in various types of studies. Well-known modifiable risk factors for stroke are virtually the same as those for cardiovascular disease in general: hypertension, smoking, dyslipidemia, diabetes, etc. Among non-modifiable risk factors old age, racial or ethnic factors, low birth weight, and genetic susceptibility play a role. In individuals with non-modifiable risk factors prevention focused on the modifiable ones is particularly important. Stroke risk assessment and prevention rely on risk profiles in a population. The Framingham Stroke Profile is widely used but hitherto has not been validated in many populations. A recent review indicated that about 10% to 20% of atherosclerotic ischemic strokes can probably be attributed to more recently established, probably causal risk factors for ischemic heart disease: raised apolipoprotein B/A1 ratio, obesity, physical inactivity, psychosocial stress and low fruit and vegetable intake. However, their causal role remains to be proven. While the importance of genes predisposing to stroke cannot be denied, the contribution of any single gene towards ischemic stroke is likely to be modest and apply in selected patients only and in combination with environmental factors or via other epistatic (gene–gene or gene–environmental) effects. The evidence is strong to state that the control of the established risk factors for stroke will result in prevention of a very large number of stroke events and premature deaths.

References

1. MONICA Manual, Part IV:Event Registration. Section 2: Stroke event registration data component. Office of Cardiovascular Diseases, World Health Organization; 1999 [cited 16 Oct 2008]. Available from: http://www.ktl.fi/publications/monica/manual/part4/iv-2.htm.

2. Lopez AD, Mathers CD, Ezzati M, Jamison DT, Murray CJL. Global and regional burden of disease and risk factors, 2001: systematic analysis of population health data. *Lancet* 2006; **367**(9524):1747–57.

3. Strong K, Mathers C, Bonita R. Preventing stroke: saving lives around the world. *Lancet Neurol* 2007; **6**(2):182–7.

4. Beaglehole R, Ebrahim S, Reddy S, Voute J, Leeder S. Prevention of chronic diseases: a call to action. *Lancet* 2007; **370**(9605):2152–7.

5. Feigin VL, Lawes CM, Bennett DA, Anderson CS. Stroke epidemiology: a review of population-based studies of incidence, prevalence, and case-fatality in the late 20th century. *Lancet Neurol* 2003; **2**(1):43–53.

6. Feigin VL, Wiebers DO, Whisnant JP, O'Fallon WM. Stroke incidence and 30-day case-fatality rates in Novosibirsk, Russia, 1982 through 1992. *Stroke* 1995; **26**(6):924–9.

7. Sarti C, Rastenyte D, Cepaitis Z, Tuomilehto J. International trends in mortality from stroke, 1968 to 1994. *Stroke* 2000; **31**(7):1588–601.

8. Sivenius J, Tuomilehto J, Immonen-Raiha P, Kaarisalo M, Sarti C, Torppa J, et al. Continuous 15-year decrease in incidence and mortality of stroke in Finland: the FINSTROKE study. *Stroke* 2004; **35**(2):420–5.

9. Bonita R, Broad JB, Beaglehole R. Changes in stroke incidence and case-fatality in Auckland, New Zealand, 1981–91. *Lancet* 1993; **342**(8885):1470–3.

10. Derby CA, Lapane KL, Feldman HA, Carleton RA. Trends in validated cases of fatal and nonfatal stroke, stroke classification, and risk factors in southeastern New England, 1980 to 1991: data from the Pawtucket Heart Health Program. *Stroke* 2000; **31**(4):875–81.

11. Truelsen T, Prescott E, Gronbaek M, Schnohr P, Boysen G. Trends in stroke incidence. The Copenhagen City Heart Study. *Stroke* 1997; **28**(10):1903–7.

12. Korv J, Roose M, Kaasik AE. Changed incidence and case-fatality rates of first-ever stroke between 1970 and 1993 in Tartu, Estonia. *Stroke* 1996; **27**(2):199–203.

13. Hong Y, Bots ML, Pan X, Hofman A, Grobbee DE, Chen H. Stroke incidence and mortality in rural and urban Shanghai from 1984 through 1991. Findings from a community-based registry. *Stroke* 1994; **25**(6):1165–9.

14. Sarti C, Stegmayr B, Tolonen H, Mahonen M, Tuomilehto J, Asplund K. Are changes in mortality from stroke caused by changes in stroke event rates

or case fatality? Results from the WHO MONICA Project. *Stroke* 2003; **34**(8):1833–40.

15. Goldstein LB, Adams R, Alberts MJ, Appel LJ, Brass LM, Bushnell CD, et al. Primary Prevention of Ischemic Stroke: A Guideline From the American Heart Association/American Stroke Association Stroke Council: Cosponsored by the Atherosclerotic Peripheral Vascular Disease Interdisciplinary Working Group; Cardiovascular Nursing Council; Clinical Cardiology Council; Nutrition, Physical Activity, and Metabolism Council; and the Quality of Care and Outcomes Research Interdisciplinary Working Group: The American Academy of Neurology affirms the value of this guideline. *Circulation* 2006; **113**(24):e873–923.

16. Brown RD, Whisnant JP, Sicks JD, O'Fallon WM, Wiebers DO. Stroke incidence, prevalence, and survival: secular trends in Rochester, Minnesota, through 1989. *Stroke* 1996; **27**(3):373–80.

17. Wolf PA, D'Agostino RB, O'Neal MA, Sytkowski P, Kase CS, Belanger AJ, et al. Secular trends in stroke incidence and mortality. The Framingham Study. *Stroke* 1992; **23**(11):1551–5.

18. Sacco RL, Boden-Albala B, Gan R, Chen X, Kargman DE, Shea S, et al. Stroke incidence among white, black, and Hispanic residents of an urban community: the Northern Manhattan Stroke Study. *Am J Epidemiol* 1998; **147**(3):259–68.

19. Immonen-Raiha P, Sarti C, Tuomilehto J, Torppa J, Lehtonen A, Sivenius J, et al. Eleven-year trends of stroke in Turku, Finland. *Neuroepidemiology* 2003; **22**(3):196–203.

20. Broderick J, Brott T, Kothari R, Miller R, Khoury J, Pancioli A, et al. The Greater Cincinnati/Northern Kentucky Stroke Study: preliminary first-ever and total incidence rates of stroke among blacks. *Stroke* 1998; **29**(2):415–21.

21. Gorelick PB. Cerebrovascular disease in African Americans. *Stroke* 1998; **29**(12):2656–64.

22. Howard G, Anderson R, Sorlie P, Andrews V, Backlund E, Burke GL. Ethnic differences in stroke mortality between non-Hispanic whites, Hispanic whites, and blacks. The National Longitudinal Mortality Study. *Stroke* 1994; **25**(11):2120–5.

23. Rosamond WD, Folsom AR, Chambless LE, Wang CH, McGovern PG, Howard G, et al. Stroke incidence and survival among middle-aged adults: 9-year follow-up of the Atherosclerosis Risk in Communities (ARIC) cohort. *Stroke* 1999; **30**(4):736–43.

24. Ingall T, Asplund K, Mahonen M, Bonita R. A multinational comparison of subarachnoid hemorrhage epidemiology in the WHO MONICA stroke study. *Stroke* 2000; **31**(5):1054–61.

25. Welin L, Svardsudd K, Wilhelmsen L, Larsson B, Tibblin G. Analysis of risk factors for stroke in a cohort of men born in 1913. *N Engl J Med* 1987; **317**(9):521–6.

26. Kiely DK, Wolf PA, Cupples LA, Beiser AS, Myers RH. Familial aggregation of stroke. The Framingham Study. *Stroke* 1993; **24**(9):1366–71.

27. Jousilahti P, Rastenyte D, Tuomilehto J, Sarti C, Vartiainen E. Parental history of cardiovascular disease and risk of stroke. A prospective follow-up of 14371 middle-aged men and women in Finland. *Stroke* 1997; **28**(7):1361–6.

28. Liao D, Myers R, Hunt S, Shahar E, Paton C, Burke G, et al. Familial history of stroke and stroke risk. The Family Heart Study. *Stroke* 1997; **28**(10):1908–12.

29. Barker DJ, Lackland DT. Prenatal influences on stroke mortality in England and Wales. *Stroke* 2003; **34**(7):1598–602.

30. Eriksson JG, Forsen T, Tuomilehto J, Osmond C, Barker DJ. Early growth, adult income, and risk of stroke. *Stroke* 2000; **31**(4):869–74.

31. Chiuve SE, Rexrode KM, Spiegelman D, Logroscino G, Manson JE, Rimm EB. Primary prevention of stroke by healthy lifestyle. *Circulation* 2008; **118**(9):947–54.

32. Kurth T, Moore SC, Gaziano JM, Kase CS, Stampfer MJ, Berger K, et al. Healthy lifestyle and the risk of stroke in women. *Arch Intern Med* 2006; **166**(13):1403–9.

33. Weikert C, Berger K, Heidemann C, Bergmann MM, Hoffmann K, Klipstein-Grobusch K, et al. Joint effects of risk factors for stroke and transient ischemic attack in a German population: the EPIC Potsdam Study. *J Neurol* 2007; **254**(3):315–21.

34. Stamler J, Stamler R, Neaton JD, Wentworth D, Daviglus ML, Garside D, et al. Low risk-factor profile and long-term cardiovascular and noncardiovascular mortality and life expectancy: findings for 5 large cohorts of young adult and middle-aged men and women. *JAMA* 1999; **282**(21):2012–8.

35. Tolonen H, Mahonen M, Asplund K, Rastenyte D, Kuulasmaa K, Vanuzzo D, et al. Do trends in population levels of blood pressure and other cardiovascular risk factors explain trends in stroke event rates? Comparisons of 15 populations in 9 countries within the WHO MONICA Stroke Project. World Health Organization Monitoring of Trends and Determinants in Cardiovascular Disease. *Stroke* 2002; **33**(10):2367–75.

36. Rothwell PM, Warlow CP. Timing of TIAs preceding stroke: time window for prevention is very short. *Neurology* 2005; **64**(5):817–20.

37. Coull AJ, Rothwell PM. Underestimation of the early risk of recurrent stroke: evidence of the need for a standard definition. *Stroke* 2004; **35**(8):1925–9.

38. Rothwell PM. Incidence, risk factors and prognosis of stroke and TIA: the need for high-quality, large-scale epidemiological studies and meta-analyses. *Cerebrovasc Dis* 2003; **16** Suppl 3:2–10.

39. Johnston SC, Gress DR, Browner WS, Sidney S. Short-term prognosis after emergency department diagnosis of TIA. *JAMA* 2000; **284**(22):2901–6.

40. Lovett JK, Dennis MS, Sandercock PA, Bamford J, Warlow CP, Rothwell PM. Very early risk of stroke after a first transient ischemic attack. *Stroke* 2003; **34**(8):e138–40.

41. Coull AJ, Lovett JK, Rothwell PM. Population based study of early risk of stroke after transient ischaemic attack or minor stroke: implications for public education and organisation of services. *BMJ* 2004; **328**(7435):326.

42. Hill MD, Yiannakoulias N, Jeerakathil T, Tu JV, Svenson LW, Schopflocher DP. The high risk of stroke immediately after transient ischemic attack: a population-based study. *Neurology* 2004; **62**(11):2015–20.

43. Lisabeth LD, Ireland JK, Risser JM, Brown DL, Smith MA, Garcia NM, et al. Stroke risk after transient ischemic attack in a population-based setting. *Stroke* 2004; **35**(8):1842–6.

44. Hankey GJ, Slattery JM, Warlow CP. Transient ischaemic attacks: which patients are at high (and low) risk of serious vascular events? *J Neurol Neurosurg Psychiatry* 1992; **55**(8):640–52.

45. Kernan WN, Viscoli CM, Brass LM, Makuch RW, Sarrel PM, Roberts RS, et al. The stroke prognosis instrument II (SPI-II): a clinical prediction instrument for patients with transient ischemia and nondisabling ischemic stroke. *Stroke* 2000; **31**(2):456–62.

46. Rothwell PM, Mehta Z, Howard SC, Gutnikov SA, Warlow CP. Treating individuals 3: from subgroups to individuals: general principles and the example of carotid endarterectomy. *Lancet* 2005; **365**(9455):256–65.

47. Rothwell PM, Giles MF, Flossmann E, Lovelock CE, Redgrave JN, Warlow CP, et al. A simple score (ABCD) to identify individuals at high early risk of stroke after transient ischaemic attack. *Lancet* 2005; **366**(9479):29–36.

48. Wolf PA, D'Agostino RB, Belanger AJ, Kannel WB. Probability of stroke: a risk profile from the Framingham Study. *Stroke* 1991; **22**(3):312–8.

49. D'Agostino RB, Wolf PA, Belanger AJ, Kannel WB. Stroke risk profile: adjustment for antihypertensive medication. The Framingham Study. *Stroke* 1994; **25**(1):40–3.

50. Wang TJ, Massaro JM, Levy D, Vasan RS, Wolf PA, D'Agostino RB, et al. A risk score for predicting stroke or death in individuals with new-onset atrial fibrillation in the community: the Framingham Heart Study. *JAMA* 2003; **290**(8):1049–56.

51. Zhang XF, Attia J, D'Este C, Yu XH, Wu XG. A risk score predicted coronary heart disease and stroke in a Chinese cohort. *J Clin Epidemiol* 2005; **58**(9):951–8.

52. Lumley T, Kronmal RA, Cushman M, Manolio TA, Goldstein S. A stroke prediction score in the elderly: validation and Web-based application. *J Clin Epidemiol* 2002; **55**(2):129–36.

53. Saaristo T, Peltonen M, Lindstrom J, Saarikoski L, Sundvall J, Eriksson JG, et al. Cross-sectional evaluation of the Finnish Diabetes Risk Score: a tool to identify undetected type 2 diabetes, abnormal glucose tolerance and metabolic syndrome. *Diab Vasc Dis Res* 2005; **2**(2):67–72.

54. Kivipelto M, Ngandu T, Laatikainen T, Winblad B, Soininen H, Tuomilehto J. Risk score for the prediction of dementia risk in 20 years among middle aged people: a longitudinal, population-based study. *Lancet Neurol* 2006; **5**(9):735–41.

55. Silventoinen K, Pankow J, Lindstrom J, Jousilahti P, Hu G, Tuomilehto J. The validity of the Finnish Diabetes Risk Score for the prediction of the incidence of coronary heart disease and stroke, and total mortality. *Eur J Cardiovasc Prev Rehabil* 2005; **12**(5):451–8.

56. Whisnant JP. Modeling of risk factors for ischemic stroke. The Willis Lecture. *Stroke* 1997; **28**(9):1840–4.

57. Hankey GJ. Potential new risk factors for ischemic stroke: what is their potential? *Stroke* 2006; **37**(8):2181–8.

58. Casas JP, Hingorani AD, Bautista LE, Sharma P. Meta-analysis of genetic studies in ischemic stroke: thirty-two genes involving approximately 18,000 cases and 58,000 controls. *Arch Neurol* 2004; **61**(11):1652–61.

Common risk factors and prevention

Michael Brainin, Yvonne Teuschl and Karl Matz

The aim of primary prevention is to reduce the risk of first-ever stroke in asymptomatic people. Seven factors are regarded as potentially modifiable risk factors for vascular diseases: high blood pressure, high cholesterol, smoking, excessive or heavy regular alcohol consumption, physical inactivity, overweight and dietary factors. The strategy in primary prevention is to lower stroke risk attributed to these factors through education, lifestyle changes and medication. Non-modifiable risk factors arising from diseases such as atrial fibrillation or diabetes mellitus can be lowered by controlling and treating the underlying disorder. Targets of primary stroke prevention can be the entire population or high-risk – but stroke-free – individuals partly suffering from disorders such as hypertension or diabetes mellitus.

Lifestyle factors

Stroke prevalence has been associated with individual lifestyle factors (e.g. smoking, exercise, body mass index (BMI), alcohol consumption) in several studies. Healthy lifestyle in general was considered in one large prospective cohort study of healthy women. In this study, healthy lifestyle, consisting of abstinence from smoking, low-normal body mass index, moderate alcohol consumption, regular exercise and healthy diet, was found to be associated with a reduction in ischemic stroke (RR 0.3; 95% CI 0.1–0.6) [1]. Using the data of two large cohort studies, the Nurses' Health Study (71 243 women) and the Health Professionals Follow-up Study (43 685 men), Chiuve et al. [2] defined a low-risk lifestyle score based on the five lifestyle components non-smoking, moderate activity $\geq$ 30 min/day, healthy diet, body mass index < 25 kg/m^2 and modest alcohol consumption (men 5–30 g/day, women 5–15 g/day). The total number of low-risk factors was associated with a significantly reduced risk of total and ischemic stroke in men and women. Persons with low-risk lifestyle (all five low-risk

lifestyle factors) had a decreased risk of stroke compared to persons fulfilling none of the low-risk lifestyle factors, RR 0.2 (95% CI 0.1–0.4) and RR 0.3 (95% CI 0.2–0.5) for women and men respectively. However, only 2% of women and 4% of men were at low risk for all five factors.

Lifestyle modifications have a high potential to prevent at low cost and low risk the development of stroke risk factors such as diabetes, dyslipidemia, obesity and hypertension. Thus, they should be an important issue in stroke prevention.

> Five low-risk lifestyle factors with a high potential to prevent stroke:
> * non-smoking
> * moderate activity $\geq$ 30 min/day
> * healthy diet
> * body mass index < 25 kg/m^2
> * modest alcohol consumption.

Cigarette smoking

Smoking is a leading cause of burden of disease. Projections estimate the mortality attributed to tobacco will rise from 5.4 million to 6.4 million in 2015 and to 8.3 million in 2030 [3]. Nearly one-third of these deaths are caused by cardiovascular diseases and 8% by cerebrovascular diseases [3].

Smoking is a well-documented preventable risk factor of stroke. Large observational studies have shown cigarette smoking to be an independent risk factor for stroke in both men and women [e.g. 4–7]. A meta-analysis of 22 studies indicates an overall risk increase for stroke (RR 1.5; 95% CI 1.4–1.6) [8]. Smoking causes changes in blood pressure and weight; adjusted for age, blood pressure and obesity stroke risk was RR 2.6 (95% CI 2.3–2.9). A dose–response relationship was identified ranging from RR 2.5 (1–14 cigarettes/day) to RR 3.8 ($\geq$25 cigarettes/day) [8].

Stroke risk for smokers as compared to non-smokers differed between stroke types, being highest for subarachnoid hemorrhages (OR 2.9; 95% CI 2.5–3.5), nearly 2-fold for ischemic stroke (OR 1.9; 95% CI 1.7–2.2) and no clear relationship for intra-cerebral hemorrhages (OR 0.7; 95% CI 0.6–1.0) [8]. Smoking is a well-established risk factor for ischemic stroke [8]. A meta-analysis focusing only on subar-achnoid hemorrhages (SAH) found a relative risk of 1.9 (95% CI 1.5–2.3) for two longitudinal studies and an odds ratio of 3.5 (95% CI 2.9–4.3) for seven case-control studies [9]. In a study including young and middle-aged patients (18–49 years) and with the risk of aneurysmal SAH adjusted for other risk factors such as family history, hypertension and BMI, the OR was 3.66 (95% CI 2.64–5.07) [10]. Another population-based case-controlled study including 432 cases of first-ever SAH found an increased risk of SAH as high as 7.8 (adjusted OR; 95% CI 3.9–15.7) for heavy smokers (>20 cigarettes/day), and OR 4.2 (95% CI 2.4–7.2) for light smokers [11].

Association of smoking and intracerebral hemor-rhages (ICH) is less well established. One meta-analysis studying the risk factors for ICH found an adjusted relative risk for current smokers of 1.3 (95% CI 1.1–1.6; 13 studies) and an adjusted relative risk of 1.1 (95% CI 0.9–1.3; 12 studies) for ever having smoked [12]. Two large prospective studies, the Phys-icians' Health Study [13] and the Women's Health Study [14], found a positive dose-dependent associ-ation of ICH risk and smoking in men and women. The age and risk factors adjusted RR were 2.1 (95% CI 1.1–4.1) and 2.9 (95% CI 1.1–7.5) for heavy smokers (≥20 cigarettes/day), 1.8 (95% CI 0.6–5.7) and 2.4 (95% CI 0.7–8.3) for light smokers (<20 cigarettes/day), and 0.8 (95% CI 0.5–1.2) and 1.3 (95% CI 0.6–2.6) for past smokers compared to never smokers, for men and women respectively.

Non-smokers exposed to tobacco smoke were estimated to absorb only the equivalent of 0.1–1 ciga-rette based on urine cotinine. Nevertheless passive smoking was associated with a greater progression in atherosclerosis [15]. Never smokers exposed to tobacco smoke had in the period of 3 years a mean increase of intimal media thickness (IMT) of the carotid artery of 31.6 μm (SD ± 2.0) compared to 25.9 μm (SD ± 2.1; p = 0.010) for non-smokers not exposed to smoke. The mean increase of IMT for current smokers was 43.0 μm (SD ± 1.9) [15]. Only a few studies investigated stroke risk due to environ-mental tobacco smoke exposure. A meta-analysis of 16 studies of variable design and quality suggests that

spousal cigarette smoking is associated with an increased stroke risk (RR 1.3; 95% CI 1.2–1.4). The relative risk of stroke found for the highest level of exposure was 1.6 (95% CI 1.3–1.8) [16].

Smoking may have additive effects and potentiate the effects of other risk factors. In the Oslo study, a large cohort study, blood pressure of fatal stroke cases was higher than blood pressure of other participants, but the absolute difference was larger for non-smokers than for smokers. This may suggest a lower tolerance for high blood pressure in smokers [17]. Similar effects were found for BMI and blood glucose level. Differences in BMI and blood glucose level between fatal stroke cases and other men were only found for non-smokers [17]. An interaction between smoking and the use of oral contraceptives was noted for women. Compared to non-smoking women not using oral contraceptives, smoking women not using oral contraceptives had an increased risk of ischemic stroke OR 1.2 (95% CI 0.7–2.1); non-smoking women using oral contraceptives had a 2.1 increased risk (95% CI 1.0–4.5), but smoking women using oral contraceptives had a 7.2 higher risk (95% CI 3.2–16.1) [18]. A similar but weaker synergistic effect was observed for hemorrhagic stroke. The risk for hemor-rhagic stroke was 1.2 (OR; 95% CI 0.6–2.4) higher for non-smoking women using oral contraceptives, 2.1 times higher (OR; 95% CI 1.5–3.0) for smoking women not using oral contraceptives and 3.1 (OR; 95% CI 1.7–5.8) for smoking women using oral con-traceptives [19].

Smoking cessation reduces stroke risk rapidly. In a meta-analysis total stroke risk was 1.2 (95% CI 1.1–1.3) in former smokers [8]. In the Framingham Study stroke risk had decreased 5 years after quitting smoking to the level of non-smokers [4]. In the Nurses' Health Study total and ischemic stroke excess risk nearly disappeared after 2 years and relative risk for former smokers compared to never smokers was 1.4 (95% CI 1–1.7) while it was 2.6 (95% CI 2.1–3.2) in current smokers [5]. In a Japanese cohort relative risk for stroke mortality had declined 2–4 years after smoking cessation by 27% and after 10–15 years it was decreased by 52% and no longer differed from people who had never smoked [7].

The benefits of quitting smoking are evident; how-ever, due to its addictive effect the success in smoking cessation is only modest. Several behavioral and pharmacological therapies are available to assist smokers in quitting and their effects are the subject of a number of Cochrane reviews (e.g. [20–24]). All forms of nicotine replacement therapy (nicotine gum, transdermal patches, nasal spray, inhalers, tablets) are effective in increasing abstinence from smoking (RR 1.6; 95% CI 1.5–1.7) [20]. The antidepressants bupropion (OR 1.9; 95% CI 1.7–2.2) and nortriptyline (OR 2.3; 95% CI 1.6–3.4) are also successful for smoking cessation. Their effect seems, however, to be independent of their antidepressant effect and they are of similar efficacy to nicotine replacements [21]. The nicotine receptor partial agonist varenicline was also found to be more effective in 12 months abstinence when compared to a placebo or to bupropion [22]. Currently not enough evidence has been found for the efficacy of cannabinoid type 1 receptor antagonists [23]. Psychosocial intervention such as behavioral therapy, self-help or telephone counseling are effective but have to be intensive [24].

> Stroke risk for smokers is 2.9-fold for subarachnoid hemorrhages and nearly 2-fold for ischemic stroke. Even passive smoking was associated with increased risk for stroke.

Alcohol consumption

Excessive alcohol drinking increases all-cause mortality, as well as the risk of coronary heart disease and stroke [25]. A meta-analysis including 35 observational studies found for a consumption of more than 60 g of ethanol/day (approximately six drinks) an increased risk of ischemic stroke (RR 1.7; 95% CI 1.3–2.2) and hemorrhagic stroke (RR 2.2; 95% CI 1.5–3.2) [26].

The relationship between alcohol and overall and ischemic stroke risk was described as J-shaped [25, 26]. This suggests that benefits overcome the harmful effect of alcohol at light-moderate alcohol consumption. Light alcohol consumption (<12 g/day) was associated with a reduction in all stroke (RR 0.83; 95% CI 0.75–0.91) and ischemic stroke (RR 0.80; 95% CI 0.67–0.96), and moderate consumption (12–24 g/day) with a reduction in ischemic stroke (RR 0.72; 95% CI 0.57–0.91) [26]. A positive linear relationship was found between alcohol consumption and hemorrhagic stroke [25, 26]. The relative risk reduction for total stroke for light alcohol drinking (<12 g/day) seems to be larger for women (RR 0.7; 0.6–0.7) than for men (RR 0.9; 95% CI 0.8–1) [26].

The apparently positive effect of light to moderate alcohol consumption is still under discussion.

Beneficial effects on lipids and hemostatic factors have been reported [27]. Especially the flavonoids of red wine have been presumed to be involved in preventing the formation of atherosclerotic plaques [28]. Comparing the type of alcoholic beverage consumed, wine seems to be associated with the lowest ischemic stroke and vascular risk [29–31]. The pattern of drinking seems to influence the vascular risk; binge drinking, even when alcohol consumption was otherwise light, increases the risk of ischemic and total stroke [32, 25].

Heavy alcohol intake and binge drinking increase blood pressure and the risk of hypertension, thereby increasing stroke risk; this seems to be especially true for hemorrhagic stroke [33–35]. In hypertensive subjects stroke risk was increased significantly by heavy drinking. In a 26-year Japanese prospective cohort study hemorrhagic stroke risk (RR 3.1; 95% CI 1.1–9.1) and to a lesser extent ischemic stroke risk (RR 2.0; 95% CI 1.1–3.6) were increased significantly in hypertensive heavy drinkers compared to non-drinking and light-drinking hypertensive subjects, whereas for non-hypertensive persons the increased risks of hemorrhagic stroke (RR 1.7; 95% CI 0.6–4.9) and ischemic stroke (RR 1.4; 95% CI 0.8–2.5) attributed to heavy drinking were not significant [34]. Reducing excessive alcohol intake was found to reduce systolic blood pressure by 3.8 mmHg in four randomized controlled intervention studies [36].

Heavy long-term alcohol consumption (>36 g/day or more than three drinks/day) and episodic heavy drinking increase the risk of atrial fibrillation, a major risk factor of stroke [37].

> Excessive alcohol drinking increases all-cause mortality, as well as the risk of coronary heart disease and stroke, but benefits overcome the harmful effect at light-moderate alcohol consumption levels.

Obesity

A high body mass index (BMI ≥25) is associated with an increased risk of stroke in men [38, 39] and women [40, 41]. Ischemic stroke rate increases in a dose-dependent manner with body mass index (BMI) [38, 41–45]. The relationship between hemorrhagic stroke and BMI is less clear. Some studies found no influence of BMI on hemorrhagic stroke risk [39, 40, 41, 43], whereas others found an increased risk of hemorrhagic stroke for people with elevated body mass index [38, 44].

Abdominal adiposity (measured by waist-to-hip ratio) has been suggested to be a better indicator for stroke risk than overall body mass (measured by BMI). Even when accounting for BMI, abdominal adiposity was found to be associated with increased stroke rate [41, 46, 47].

Obesity is associated with an increased risk of hypertension, diabetes and dyslipidemia. Adjusting for these confounding risk factors often attenuates the effect of body mass without eliminating it [38–40, 42, 44, 47]. Nevertheless it is still under discussion whether obesity is an independent risk factor of stroke or mediated through blood pressure, diabetes and cholesterol levels.

No randomized controlled trial has tested the effect of weight reduction in obese adults on stroke risk [48]. However, in a meta-analysis systolic blood pressure was reduced by 4.4 mmHg and diastolic blood pressure by 3.6 mmHg for an average weight loss of 5.1 kg [49].

Combined interventions including dietary and exercise strategies with cognitive-behavioral therapy were the most successful for weight loss [50]. Increasing the intensity of psychological intervention resulted in greater weight reduction [50].

> Obesity (high body mass index or high waist-to-hip ratio) is associated with an increased risk of stroke.

Physical inactivity

Several prospective longitudinal population studies have shown the protective effect of regular physical activity for stroke in women and men. In a meta-analysis of 18 cohort and five case–control studies, physically highly active individuals had a lower risk of stroke and lower stroke mortality than those with low activity (RR 0.7; 95% CI 0.7–0.8). Similarly, moderately active individuals had a lower risk of stroke, compared with those who were inactive (RR 0.8; 95% CI 0.7–0.9) [51].

A similar relationship was found in ischemic stroke for high versus low activity (RR 0.8; 95% CI 0.7–0.9) and for moderate versus low activity (RR 0.9; 95% CI 0.8–1.1) [51]. Only a few studies investigated the effect of activity on hemorrhagic stroke. However, in a meta-analysis high and moderate activity significantly decreased hemorrhagic stroke risk when compared with low activity (RR 0.7; 95% CI 0.5–0.9 and RR 0.9; 95% CI 0.6–1.1) [51].

Additionally, leisure-based physical activity (2 to 5 hours per week) has been independently associated with a reduced severity of ischemic stroke at admission and better short-term outcome [52].

Some studies found a dose–response relationship between stroke risk and different levels of activity [e.g. 53, 54–56]; others found a U-shaped relationship or no difference between moderate and high physical activity [e.g. 57, 58]. This may be explained by different definitions of physical activity and levels of activity. Additionally there may be different metabolic effects of different types of exercise. Overall only a few studies have evaluated the influence of occupational physical activity; the definitions of activity levels and activity types vary considerably and the amount of activity is generally self-assessed. Commuting physical activity (walking or cycling to work) may also reduce stroke risk [56]. Study results on the influence of the type of activity on stroke risk are inconsistent (a meta-analysis distinguishing between leisure and occupational physical activity found a protective effect of both activity types) [59]. People active at work had a decreased risk for ischemic (RR 0.6; 95% CI 0.4–0.8) and hemorrhagic stroke (RR 0.3; 95% CI 0.1–0.8), and those physically active during leisure time had a decreased risk for ischemic (RR 0.8; 95% CI 0.7–0.9) and hemorrhagic stroke (RR 0.7; 95% CI 0.6–1.0). No randomized controlled trial has studied the effect of regular controlled exercises on stroke risk. There is not enough evidence for the type and intensity of fitness training protecting best against stroke.

The favorable effect of physical activity is at least partly mediated through beneficial effects on other risk factors. Physical activity decreases body weight and blood pressure, and increases HDL serum cholesterol, plasma tissue and glucose tolerance [60, 61]. Additionally physically more active people were found to be more often non-smokers [e.g. 58].

> Regular physical activity has a protective effect for stroke, probably mediated through beneficial effects on other risk factors.

Dietary factors

Poor dietary habits contribute to the development of other stroke risk factors such as obesity, diabetes, hypertension and dyslipidemia. The Global Burden of Disease study 2000 estimates that in Europe 4.4% of total disability-adjusted life years (DALYs) lost are attributed to low fruit and vegetable intake and another 7.8% to overweight and obesity [62]. Changes in dietary habits therefore have high potential for reducing stroke risk. Different foods and nutrients have been suggested to influence stroke risk via several mechanisms, e.g. by influencing blood pressure, insulin resistance, inflammation risk, platelet function, endothelial function and oxidation [63].

In large epidemiological studies, high fruit and vegetable intake was associated in a dose-dependent fashion with decreased risk of stroke. A meta-analysis including nine cohort studies found that persons eating more than five servings of fruit or vegetables per day had a decreased relative risk of stroke RR 0.7 (95% CI 0.7–0.8) compared to people eating fewer than three servings. This effect was significant for both ischemic and hemorrhagic stroke [64]. In the Nurses' Health study including 75 596 women and the Health Professionals' Follow-up Study including 38 683 men ischemic and total stroke risk were reduced respectively by 7% and 3% in women and by 4% and 5% in men for each increment of one serving of fruits and vegetables per day [65]. Combining both studies the quintile with the highest intake of fruits and vegetables had a decreased relative risk of stroke RR 0.69 (95% CI 0.52–0.92) compared to the lowest quintile. In a meta-analysis of seven cohort studies whole grain intake was associated with a reduction in cardiovascular disease but not stroke [66]. Generally, persons with higher fruit and vegetable intake were more likely to be non-smokers, engaged in more physical activity and more highly educated [e.g. 65, 67, 68].

The consumption of oily fish or $n-3$ fatty acids has been suggested to decrease the risk of vascular disease by lowering serum lipids, decreasing blood pressure, decreasing platelet aggregation, improving vascular reactivity, and decreasing inflammation. Ecological studies raised the concern that high fish consumption may increase the risk of hemorrhagic stroke. A meta-analysis of eight cohort studies suggested a lower risk of ischemic stroke in people who consumed fish at least once per month (RR 0.7; 95% CI 0.5–1.0), but no association for hemorrhagic stroke [69]. However, several studies did not distinguish between stroke subtypes. Another concern was raised on the negative effect of methyl mercury contamination in fish. An evaluation of all risks and benefits of fish intake indicates that for modest fish consumption (1–2 servings/week) the benefits of fish intake exceed the potential risks; people with very

high consumption should limit some fish species with high mercury levels [70]. A quantitative analysis of fish consumption and stroke risk including six studies found that any fish consumption had greater relative risk reduction than no fish consumption [71].

Observational studies found an association between sodium intake and stroke mortality [72]. This association is at least partly mediated by the well-studied positive relationship between salt intake and blood pressure [73]. A reduction in salt intake in hypertensive persons (median urinary sodium reduction by 78 mmol/day or 4.6 g/day) reduced systolic blood pressure by 5.1 mmHg and diastolic blood pressure by 2.7 mmHg. In normotensive individuals systolic and diastolic blood pressure were reduced by 2.0 mmHg and 1.0 mmHg respectively for a median reduction of 74 mmol/day or 4.4 g urinary sodium [74]. The Dietary Approaches to Stop Hypertension (DASH) trial, a randomized controlled study including 412 participants, found strong evidence for the benefit of low sodium intake [75]. Participants were randomized to one of three sodium intake levels and either the DASH diet (rich in vegetables and fruits and low in dairy fat products, and total and saturated fat and cholesterol) or a control diet (a typical American diet). Both sodium reduction and the DASH diet reduced blood pressure significantly.

Epidemiological studies found an inverse relationship between intake of potassium and risk of stroke [76, 77]. Potassium intake can attenuate salt sensitivity and may thus prevent or delay hypertension [78].

Dietary calcium, especially from dairy sources and dietary magnesium have been found to be inversely associated with blood pressure and with lower incidence of stroke in prospective cohort studies; however, the evidence is only moderate [63].

Different nutrients and aliments cannot be seen independently of each other and thus the effect of different diets has been investigated. The DASH diet (see above) was associated with a significant decrease in blood pressure [75]. Fung et al. used the individual information on food intake of the Nurses' Health Study to classify individuals' alimentation according to the DASH-style diet. Women with a dietary pattern more similar to the DASH diet had a lower relative stroke risk, and this effect increased linearly with an adjusted RR of 0.8 (95% CI 0.7–1.0) for the quintile with the highest intake of a DASH-style diet compared to the quintile with the lowest intake of a DASH-style diet [79]. A Mediterranean-style diet rich in α-linolenic acid, olive oil, canola oil, fish, fruits, vegetables and whole grains and low in saturated fat has been found to be successful in secondary prevention of coronary heart disease [80]. However, a randomized controlled trial including 48 835 women with dietary interventions consisting of total fat reduction to 20% of energy intake, an increased intake of fruits, vegetables and grain did not result in a reduced incidence of coronary events and stroke [81].

Reviewing the current evidence Ding and Mozaffarian suggest that a diet low in sodium, high in potassium, and rich in fruits and vegetables, whole grains, cereal fiber, and fatty fish has the highest potential to reduce stroke risk [63].

> A diet low in sodium, high in potassium, and rich in fruits and vegetables, whole grains, cereal fiber, and fatty fish has the highest potential to reduce stroke risk.

Postmenopausal estrogen replacement therapy

Until menopause women generally suffer from a lower rate of vascular diseases, including ischemic stroke. This has been attributed to a protective effect of estrogen and thus research has focused on the beneficial effect of postmenopausal hormone therapy for the prevention of cardiovascular diseases and stroke. However, a meta-analysis of nine observational studies indicated an increased risk of stroke – especially of ischemic stroke – in women using hormone replacement therapy, with RR for overall and ischemic stroke respectively of 1.1 (95% CI 1.0–1.2) and 1.2 (95% CI 1.0–1.4) [82]. Another meta-analysis including 28 randomized controlled trials found a significant increase in total stroke RR of 1.3 (95% CI 1.1–1.5) and ischemic stroke RR of 1.3 (95% CI 1.1–1.6) for women using hormone replacement therapy [83]. A Cochrane systematic review came to the same conclusion and found hormone replacement therapy to be associated with an increased risk of stroke in primary prevention trials (RR 1.4; 95% CI 1.1–1.9) [84]. Two meta-analyses suggest that hormone therapy (estrogen alone or with progesterone) increases the risks of venous thromboembolism, heart attack, stroke (after 3 years of use), breast cancer, gallbladder disease and dementia, and the only benefits are that it reduces the risks of fracture and colorectal cancer after 4 or 5 years of treatment [82, 85].

Selective estrogen receptor modulators (SERM) are a class of drugs used for hormone replacement therapy lacking the steroid structure of estrogens but able to bind directly to estrogen receptors [86]. SERMs have estrogen-agonist effects on bone and lipid metabolism but not in the breasts and uterus, and they may therefore prevent cardiovascular risk and osteoporosis without increased risk of breast cancer. To date few studies have investigated the effect of SERMs on stroke risk. The Multiple Outcomes of Raloxifene Evaluation (MORE) trial including 7705 osteoporotic postmenopausal women found no overall effect on cardiovascular events (including stroke) but a decreased risk of stroke (RR 0.4; 95% CI 0.2–0.9) and cardiovascular events in a subset of women with increased cardiovascular risk at baseline [87]. In the Raloxifene Use for The Heart (RUTH) trial including 10 101 postmenopausal women with coronary heart disease or multiple risk factors for coronary heart disease no effect of raloxifene on the risk of coronary events or stroke incidence was found, but the risk of fatal stroke was increased (RR 1.5; 95% CI 1.0–2.2) [88]. A meta-analysis (nine trials) investigating the risk of ischemic stroke in tamoxifen treatment for breast cancer found an increase of overall (RR 1.4; 95% CI 1.1–1.7) and ischemic stroke risk (RR 1.8; 95% CI 1.4–2.4) [89].

> Hormone replacement therapy is associated with an increased risk of stroke.

Diseases and pathological conditions
Hypertension

Elevated blood pressure is the best-documented treatable risk factor for stroke. Worldwide, about 54% of strokes and 13.5% of deaths are attributed to high blood pressure (systolic blood pressure >115 mmHg; [90]). High blood pressure (BP >115/75 mmHg) is strongly and directly related to vascular and overall mortality without evidence of any threshold [91]. Starting at a BP of 115/75 mmHg, stroke mortality risk increases steeply in an approximately log-linear relationship with BP [91]. Age attenuates this relationship and stroke risk increases with every 10 mmHg of systolic BP by 40–50%, 30–40% and 20–30% for the age groups <60, 60–69 and ≥70 respectively [92].

Lowering BP substantially reduces stroke and coronary risks. A meta-analysis of randomized controlled trials comparing antihypertensive drugs to placebo showed an overall stroke risk reduction of 30% when BP was lowered. A meta-regression of these data suggests a risk reduction of 31% for every 10 mmHg reduction of systolic BP [92]. The benefit of BP reduction suggested by the results of clinical trials is therefore consistent with the relationship found in cohort studies.

As a consequence guidelines recommend lowering BP to 140/85 mmHg or below [93]. The antihypertensive treatment should be more aggressive in diabetic patients (see below) [94]. A combination of two or more antihypertensive agents is often necessary and preferable to achieve these targets [93].

To compare the effect of the different classes of blood pressure lowering drugs (angiotensin-converting enzyme (ACE) inhibitors, calcium antagonists, angiotensin-receptor blockers (ARBs), and thiazide diuretics and/or β-adrenergic receptor blockers) the Blood Pressure Lowering Treatment Trialists' (BPLTT) Collaboration performed a large meta-analysis including 29 randomized trials and more than 160 000 participants [95, 96]. No antihypertensive drug class was found to be superior in reducing stroke risk [92, 95, 96]. A meta-analysis comparing "old" (diuretics and/or β-blockers) with "new" hypertensive drugs (calcium-channel blockers, ACE inhibitors, AR1 blockers and α-blockers) suggests a small benefit of calcium-channel blockers [97].

A meta-analysis comparing the effect of β-blockers to other hypertensive drugs suggests that the relative risk of stroke is 16% higher for β-blockers [98]. However, despite reporting different amounts of BP reduction for different drugs, the analysis did not account for it. Due to the association between BP reduction and stroke incidence, the inferiority of β-blockers may reflect lesser BP reduction, especially in central BP, and they may still be considered an option for initial and subsequent antihypertensive treatment [93].

As the strength in the association between BP and stroke risk attenuates with age, one might expect differences in the effect of BP-lowering drugs in older patients. Additionally the prevalence of systolic hypertension (systolic blood pressure >140 mmHg and diastolic blood pressure <90 mmHg) increases with age. In elderly subjects controlling hypertension regardless of whether it is isolated systolic hypertension or not has been shown to be beneficial [99]. A recent meta-analysis including 31 trials with more than 190 000 participants found no evidence for the advantage of a specific antihypertensive drug class according to age (younger or older than 65 years) [100].

The Hypertension in the Very Elderly Trial (HYVET), a randomized controlled trial, showed that even hypertensive patients older than 80 years benefit from blood pressure lowering therapy by a reduction in non-fatal stroke rate (RR 0.7; 95% CI 0.5–1.0) and stroke mortality (RR 0.6; 95% CI 0.4–1.0) [101].

> Elevated blood pressure is the best-documented treatable risk factor for stroke. Lowering BP reduces stroke risk by 31% for every 10 mmHg systolic BP reduction.

Diabetes mellitus

There is insufficient evidence from randomized trials that improving glucose control reduces stroke [102, 103]. Maintaining the target glucose level reduced the risk of microvascular complication but not the risk of macrovascular events, including stroke [103]. However, findings from a small prospective cohort study, the Northern Manhattan Study (NOMAS), provide new evidence for a possible advantage of tight glucose control in diabetic subjects. Participants with a history of diabetes showed an increased risk of stroke only when fasting blood glucose was elevated [104]. On the other hand, two recent large randomized controlled studies – the Action to Control Cardiovascular Risk in Diabetes Study (ACCORD) [105] and the Action in Diabetes and Vascular Disease: Preterax and Diamicron Modified Release Controlled Evaluation study (ADVANCE) [106] – found no effect of intensive blood glucose control on major vascular events. Both studies were partly secondary prevention trials. The ACCORD study included more than 10 000 diabetic persons with cardiovascular diseases or at high risk for cardiovascular disease. No differences in major macrovascular events (RR 0.9; 95% CI 0.8–1.0) or non-fatal stroke rate (RR 1.1; 95% CI 0.8–1.5) were found for intensive as compared to standard blood glucose control. At the same time the overall death rate was higher for the intensive control group (1.2; 95% CI 1.0–1.5). The ADVANCE trial included more than 11 000 patients with type 2 diabetes with a history of major macro- or microvascular disease and another vascular risk factor. Compared to the standard glucose control group, an effect of intensive glucose control was only found on the risk of major microvascular events – especially on nephropathy (RR 0.9; 95% CI 0.8–1.0) but not on major macrovascular events (RR 0.9; 95% CI 0.8–1.1). In both trials hypoglycemia occurred more frequently in the intensive control group as compared to the standard therapy group.

In addition to an increased stroke risk subjects with type 2 diabetes have an increased prevalence of other stroke risk factors such as obesity, hyperlipidemia and hypertension. Hypertension and diabetes are highly correlated and diabetic persons have an increased prevalence of hypertension [107]. Lowering blood pressure has been shown to decrease the risk for all cardiovascular events regardless of the drug used [94]. In diabetic patients blood pressure should be lowered to below 130/80 mmHg [92].

Dyslipidemia in type 2 diabetes is characterized by an increased blood triglyceride concentration and reduced HDL cholesterol concentration. However, total and LDL cholesterol concentrations do not differ from the general population [108]. Treatment with statins reduces LDL cholesterol and stroke risk similarly to results seen in non-diabetic persons [109, 110]. Statin therapy reducing LDL cholesterol on average by 1.0 mmol/l was found to reduce stroke by 24% (95% CI 6%–39%) and major vascular events by 22% (95% CI 13%–30%) in 5963 diabetic participants. This was comparable to risk reduction in non-diabetic participants [109]. Similarly, statin therapy reduced stroke risk by 33% in diabetic and by 24% in non-diabetic participants in the lipid-lowering arm of the ASCOT study [110]. The difference between the effects in diabetic and non-diabetic persons was not significant.

There is insufficient evidence that improving glucose control reduces stroke. Treatment of diabetic patients with statins reduced the risk of stroke by 24–33%.

Dyslipidemia

Older epidemiological studies found no relationship between total serum cholesterol level and overall stroke incidence [111]. This might be due to different relationships for ischemic and intracerebral hemorrhages. In prospective cohort studies stroke risk was found to be positively associated with serum cholesterol level in ischemic stroke but negatively for intracerebral hemorrhages [112].

Age, sex and vascular risk factors can modify the relationship between blood cholesterol and vascular mortality. A meta-analysis of 61 observational prospective studies analyzed the influence of blood cholesterol on vascular mortality by distinguishing different age classes, sex and different levels of blood pressure [112]. Overall the association between total blood cholesterol and stroke mortality was weak; a positive association was only found in the age group 45–59. For ischemic stroke this association was weakly positive in middle age (40–59) and may be accounted for by an association between total cholesterol and blood pressure. For hemorrhagic stroke the association was negative and only found for older participants (70–79). The relationship between total blood cholesterol and stroke mortality is highly dependent on blood pressure. For systolic blood pressure levels below 145 mmHg this association was positive, for higher blood pressure levels the relationship was negative. These relationships are similar for both stroke types but stronger in hemorrhagic stroke.

Insufficient data are available to identify a relationship between low-density lipoprotein (LDL) cholesterol and stroke incidence [113]. High-density lipoprotein (HDL), in contrast, was found to be negatively associated with total and ischemic stroke incidence in several prospective cohort studies [112]. No such relationship was found for hemorrhagic stroke.

In contrast to the partly inconsistent findings from epidemiological studies, randomized controlled trials found a clear positive effect of cholesterol-lowering statin (3-hydroxy-3-methylglutaryl coenzyme A (HMG-CoA) reductase inhibitors) therapy on the incidence of ischemic stroke. In a review of 26 randomized trials of statins including more than 95 000 patients, the incidence of stroke was reduced from 3.4% to 2.7% (OR 0.8; 95% CI 0.7–0.9) [114]. This was mainly due to a reduction in non-fatal stroke, from 2.7% to 2.1%. Contrary to what might be expected from observational studies, the incidence of hemorrhagic stroke was not higher in the statins group than in the control group (OR 0.9; 95% CI 0.7–1.2); however, the numbers were only 78 compared to 84 patients. The effect of statins was clearly associated with LDL; for every 10% decrease in LDL cholesterol stroke rate was reduced by 15.6%. A more recent review including 42 trials assessing statin therapy found similar results [115]: stroke incidence was significantly decreased by statin therapy (RR 0.8; 95% CI 0.8–0.9). Similarly, the incidence of non-hemorrhagic stroke was decreased (eleven trials; RR 0.8; 95% CI 0.7–0.9). However, the incidence of hemorrhagic stroke (eleven trials; RR 0.9; 95% CI 0.7–1.3) did not differ between statin and non-statin treatment.

The event rate for hemorrhagic stroke was not reported. The effect of statin treatment on bleeding risk remains unclear. A prospective cohort study including 629 patients with intracerebral hemorrhages studied the effect of statin treatment before the event. No effect of statins was found on 30-day mortality, 90-day mortality or functional independency [116].

Because of the linear relationship between risk reduction in stroke and LDL cholesterol level, a more intensive statin therapy might be indicated. A meta-analysis of seven partly secondary prevention trials including more than 29 000 patients with coronary artery disease found a significant reduction of stroke (OR 0.8; 95% CI 0.7–1.0) and myocardial infarction (OR 0.8; 95% CI 0.8–0.9) for more intensive statin therapy compared to less intensive therapy [117]. The LDL levels achieved varied between 1.6 and 2.2 mmol/l and between 2.1 and 3.2 mmol/l for the more and less intensive statin regimes, respectively. Intensive therapy found a significant excess of elevated aminotransferase levels compared to less intensive therapy (1.5% vs. 0.4%; OR 1.1; 95% CI 2.3–7.4).

On the other hand the secondary prevention trial Stroke Prevention with Aggressive Reduction in Cholesterol Levels (SPARCL) showed an increased risk for recurrent hemorrhagic stroke in patients treated with high-dose atorvastin ($n = 55$ vs. 33 for placebo). This effect of atorvastin was independent of other factors influencing intracerebral hemorrhage, such as age, sex and blood pressure, and was not related to LDL cholesterol levels [118].

Among other lipid-lowering therapies used in primary stroke prevention were niacin, gemfibrozil, clofibrate, bezafibrate and lifestyle modifications. In a meta-analysis including 38 primary and secondary stroke prevention trials using different lipid-lowering therapies, the most effective in reducing stroke risk were statins [119]. For non-statin drugs no significant effect on stroke incidence was found [119]. The effect of diet (seven trials) was strongest, but highly variable and therefore insignificant (OR 0.6; 95% CI 0.3–1.1; $p = 0.11$). At the same time the cholesterol-lowering effect was highest for statins (21.8% in statins compared to 8.3% non-statin drugs). Taking all lipid-lowering therapies together a strong correlation was found between stroke incidence and final cholesterol level ($r^2 = 0.48$). The threshold for a final cholesterol level that could clearly separate between risk reduction and no risk reduction was 232 mg/dl or 6.0 mmol/l [119].

Randomized controlled trials found a clear positive effect of cholesterol-lowering statin therapy on the incidence of ischemic stroke.

Atrial fibrillation

Atrial fibrillation (AF) is a strong independent risk factor for ischemic stroke [120]. The prevalence of atrial fibrillation (AF) increases with age, ranging from 0.1% among persons younger than 55 years to 9% among persons older than 80 years; it is almost 4% for persons older than 60 years [121]. AF is therefore primarily a risk factor in the older population. A long-term increase in AF has been projected until 2050 [121]. This is not caused only by the aging population but probably also by a higher prevalence of obesity in the Western world.

Strokes associated with AF generally have a higher mortality and poorer functional outcome [122, 123]. In the Framingham Study the risk of ischemic stroke was nearly 5-fold for subjects with AF [120]. However, stroke risk is highly variable in patients with atrial fibrillation and depends on sex, age and the presence of other stroke risk factors; for those older than 75 years without prior stroke or TIA the stroke rate ranged from 3.2% to 5.2% per year [124].

Risk assessment is particularly important to balance potential benefits and risks of chronic antithrombotic therapy. Risk stratification should be used to determine whether patients should be given oral anticoagulation, aspirin, or nothing. Several schemes to stratify stroke risk in patients with atrial fibrillation have been proposed and tested [125]. A review comparing 12 stratification schemes found substantial differences between them [125]. Observed rates for the low stroke risk class ranged from 0% to 2.3% per year and those for the high-risk class from 2.5% per year to 7.9% per year. Using eleven different schemes to classify individual stroke risk in a common test cohort resulted in 7% to 42% of the patients being categorized as at low risk, and 11 to 77% being at high risk [125]. These differences between risk stratification schemes probably contribute to confusion and the inconsistent use of anticoagulant treatment. All stratification schemes include the occurrence of a previous stroke or TIA as powerful identification element. This makes risk assessment in primary prevention even more difficult. Despite some clear benefit of anticoagulants in patients with atrial fibrillation they are still underused, partly because of a high perceived risk of bleeding and fears about being responsible for hemorrhages [126, 127].

Stroke risk in patients with AF is markedly decreased by the use of oral anticoagulation. A meta-analysis of 29 randomized trials including more than 28 000 participants with at least 3 months' follow-up showed that antiplatelet agents compared to a placebo or no treatment reduced relative stroke risk by 22% (95% CI 6%–35%) in patients with non-valvular AF [128]. For primary prevention this corresponds to an absolute risk reduction of 0.8% per year. Compared to the control group, adjusted-dose warfarin (target INR 2.0–3.0) reduced stroke risk relatively by 64% (95% CI 49%–74%); this corresponds to an absolute risk reduction of 2.7% in primary prevention. In direct comparison adjusted-dose warfarin proved to be more effective than anti-platelet therapy at reducing stroke (relative risk reduction 39%; 95% CI 18%–52%) [128]. Major extracranial bleeding events and intracranial hemorrhages were rare and therefore risk estimates are imprecise. However, the increase in absolute risk of major extracranial hemorrhage was less than the absolute reduction in stroke risk [128]. A recent Cochrane review including patients with non-valvular atrial fibrillation and no history of stroke or TIA found a risk reduction of ischemic stroke of OR 0.5 (95% CI 0.4–0.7) for oral anticoagulants compared to antiplatelet therapy and an increased risk of intracranial hemorrhages of OR 2.0 (95% CI 1.2–3.3) [129]. There have been concerns because participants of clinical trials are usually highly selected and especially very old persons, with the highest risk of AF, stroke and hemorrhages, are generally not included. However, the results of these randomized trials have been found to translate well into clinical practice. Warfarin therapy compared to no treatment or aspirin was associated with a 51% reduced risk of thromboembolism (95% CI 39%–60%) in a cohort of persons with non-valvular AF [130]. Intracranial hemorrhages were rare but slightly higher for warfarin (adjusted hazard ratio 2.0; 95% CI 1.2–3.1; 0.46 vs. 0.23 per 100 person-years). The risk of non-intracranial major hemorrhages was not increased [130]. The risk of major hemorrhages increases with older age; however, this was independent of the use of warfarin [131]. The WASPO (Warfarin vs. Aspirin for Stroke Prevention in Octogenarians) [132] and BAFTA (Birmingham Atrial Fibrillation Treatment of the Aged) [133] trials

showed that warfarin was safe and effective in older individuals.

Stroke risk for patients with paroxysmal or persistent AF is comparable to the risk in patients with permanent AF [134]. Patients with rheumatic mitral valve disease with AF are at high risk of systemic embolism and therapy with oral anticoagulation (target INR 2–3) is recommended [135]. Patients with a prosthetic heart valve, with or without AF, should receive long-term anticoagulation with a target INR based on the prosthesis type [136].

> Atrial fibrillation is a strong independent risk factor for ischemic stroke, which is markedly decreased by oral anticoagulation.

Chapter Summary

Five low-risk **lifestyle factors** with a high potential to prevent stroke:

- Non-smoking – stroke risk for smokers increases 2.9-fold for subarachnoid hemorrhages and 2-fold for ischemic stroke, but there is no clear relationship for intracerebral hemorrhages. The relative risk of passive smoking for stroke can be as high as 1.6.
- Modest alcohol consumption – excessive alcohol drinking increases all-cause mortality, as well as the risk of coronary heart disease and stroke. But benefits overcome the harmful effect of alcohol at light-moderate alcohol consumption.
- Body mass index <25 kg/m² – a high body mass index is associated with an increased risk of stroke. Abdominal adiposity (as measured by waist-to-hip ratio) has been suggested to be an even better indicator for stroke risk than overall body mass (as measured by BMI).
- Moderate activity ≥30 min/day – regular physical activity has a protective effect for stroke.
- Healthy diet – a diet low in sodium, high in potassium, and rich in fruits and vegetables, whole grains, cereal fiber, and fatty fish has the highest potential to reduce stroke risk.

These five lifestyle modifications contribute to the reduction of other stroke risk factors such as diabetes, hypertension and dyslipidemia.

Diseases and pathological conditions
- Elevated blood pressure is the best-documented treatable risk factor for stroke. Lowering BP

substantially reduces stroke with a risk reduction of 31% for every 10 mmHg reduction of systolic BP. Guidelines recommend lowering BP to 140/85 mmHg or below. No antihypertensive drug class was found to be superior in reducing stroke risk.

- There is insufficient evidence from randomized trials that improving glucose control reduces stroke. Cardiovascular mortality associated with different blood cholesterol levels was three times higher in diabetic compared to non-diabetic men. Treatment of diabetic patients with statins reduced the risk of stroke by 24–33%.

- In prospective cohort studies stroke risk was found to be weakly positively associated with serum cholesterol level in ischemic stroke but negatively for intracerebral hemorrhages. High-density lipoprotein (HDL) was found to be negatively associated with total and ischemic stroke incidence. Randomized controlled trials found a clear positive effect of cholesterol-lowering statin therapy on the incidence of ischemic stroke.

- Atrial fibrillation (AF, permanent, paroxysomal or persistent) is a strong independent risk factor for ischemic stroke (risk = nearly 5-fold). Stroke risk in patients with AF is markedly decreased by the use of oral anticoagulation (primary prevention: absolute risk reduction of 0.8% per year, warfarin being more effective than anti-platelet therapy).

References

1. Kurth T, Moore S, Gaziano J, Kase C, Stampfer M, Berger K, Buring J. Healthy lifestyle and the risk of stroke in women. *Arch Intern Med* 2006; **166**: 1403–9.

2. Chiuve SE, Rexrode KM, Spiegelman D, Logroscino G, Manson JE, Rimm EB. Primary prevention of stroke by healthy lifestyle. *Circulation* 2008; **118**:947–54.

3. Mathers CD, Loncar D. Projections of global mortality and burden of disease from 2002 to 2030. *PLoS Med* 2006; **3**:e442.

4. Wolf PA, D'Agostino RB, Kannel WB, Bonita R, Belanger AJ. Cigarette smoking as a risk factor for stroke. The Framingham Study. *JAMA* 1988; **259**:1025–9.

5. Kawachi I, Colditz GA, Stampfer MJ, Willett WC, Manson JE, Rosner B, et al. Smoking cessation in relation to total mortality rates in women. A prospective cohort study. *Ann Intern Med* 1993; **119**:992–1000.

6. Wannamethee SG, Shaper AG, Whincup PH, Walker M. Smoking cessation and the risk of stroke in middle-aged men. *JAMA* 1995; **274**:155–60.

7. Iso H, Date C, Yamamoto A, Toyoshima H, Watanabe Y, Kikuchi S, et al. JACC Study Group. Smoking cessation and mortality from cardiovascular disease among Japanese men and women: the JACC Study. *Am J Epidemiol* 2005; **161**:170–9.

8. Shinton R, Beevers G. Meta-analysis of relation between cigarette smoking and stroke. *BMJ* 1989; **298**:789–94.

9. Teunissen LL, Rinkel GJ, Algra A, van Gijn J. Risk factors for subarachnoid hemorrhage: a systematic review. *Stroke* 1996; **27**:544–9.

10. Broderick JP, Viscoli CM, Brott T, Kernan WN, Brass LM, Feldmann E, et al. Hemorrhagic Stroke Project Investigators. Major risk factors for aneurysmal subarachnoid hemorrhage in the young are modifiable. *Stroke* 2003; **34**:1375–81.

11. Anderson CS, Feigin V, Bennett D, Lin RB, Hankey G, Jamrozik K. Australasian Cooperative Research on Subarachnoid Hemorrhage Study (ACROSS) Group. Active and passive smoking and the risk of subarachnoid hemorrhage: an international population-based case-control study. *Stroke* 2004; **35**:633–7.

12. Ariesen MJ, Claus SP, Rinkel GJ, Algra A. Risk factors for intracerebral hemorrhage in the general population: a systematic review. *Stroke* 2003; **34**:2060–5.

13. Kurth T, Kase CS, Berger K, Schaeffner ES, Buring JE, Gaziano JM. Smoking and the risk of hemorrhagic stroke in men. *Stroke* 2003; **34**:1151–5.

14. Kurth T, Kase CS, Berger K, Gaziano JM, Cook NR, Buring JE. Smoking and risk of hemorrhagic stroke in women. *Stroke* 2003; **34**:2792–5.

15. Howard G, Wagenknecht LE, Burke GL, Diez-Roux A, Evans GW, McGovern P, et al. Cigarette smoking and progression of atherosclerosis: The Atherosclerosis Risk in Communities (ARIC) Study. *JAMA* 1998; **279**:119–24.

16. Lee PN, Forey BA. Environmental tobacco smoke exposure and risk of stroke in nonsmokers: a review with meta-analysis. *J Stroke Cerebrovasc Dis* 2006; **15**:190–201.

17. Håheim LL, Holme I, Hjermann I, Leren P. Smoking habits and risk of fatal stroke: 18 years follow up of the Oslo Study. *J Epidemiol Community Health* 1996; **50**:621–4.

18. WHO Collaborative Study of Cardiovascular Disease and Steroid Hormone Contraception. Ischemic stroke and combined oral contraceptives: results of an international, multicentre, case-control study. *Lancet* 1996; **348**:498–505.

19. WHO Collaborative Study of Cardiovascular Disease and Steroid Hormone Contraception. Haemorrhagic

stroke, overall stroke risk, and combined oral contraceptives: results of an international, multicentre, case-control study. *Lancet* 1996; **348**:505–10.

20. Stead LF, Perera R, Bullen C, Mant D, Lancaster T. Nicotine replacement therapy for smoking cessation. *Cochrane Database Syst Rev* 2008; CD000146.

21. Hughes JR, Stead LF, Lancaster T. Antidepressants for smoking cessation. *Cochrane Database Syst Rev* 2007; CD000031.

22. Cahill K, Stead LF, Lancaster T. Nicotine receptor partial agonists for smoking cessation. *Cochrane Database Syst Rev* 2007; CD006103.

23. Cahill K, Ussher M. Cannabinoid type 1 receptor antagonists (rimonabant) for smoking cessation. *Cochrane Database Syst Rev* 2007; CD005353.

24. Barth J, Critchley J, Bengel J. Psychosocial interventions for smoking cessation in patients with coronary heart disease. *Cochrane Database Syst Rev* 2008; CD006886.

25. Mazzaglia G, Britton AR, Altmann DR, Chenet L. Exploring the relationship between alcohol consumption and non-fatal or fatal stroke: a systematic review. *Addiction* 2001; **96**:1743–56.

26. Reynolds K, Lewis B, Nolen JD, Kinney GL, Sathya B, He J. Alcohol consumption and risk of stroke: a meta-analysis. *JAMA* 2003; **289**:579–88.

27. Rimm EB, Williams P, Fosher K, Criqui M, Stampfer MJ. Moderate alcohol intake and lower risk of coronary heart disease: meta-analysis of effects on lipids and haemostatic factors. *BMJ* 1999; **319**:1523–8.

28. de Lange DW, Hijmering ML, Lorsheyd A, Scholman WL, Kraaijenhagen RJ, Akkerman JW, et al. Rapid intake of alcohol (binge drinking) inhibits platelet adhesion to fibrinogen under flow. *Alcohol Clin Exp Res* 2004; **28**:1562–8.

29. Truelsen T, Gronbaek M, Schnohr P, Boysen G. Intake of beer, wine, and spirits and risk of stroke: the Copenhagen city heart study. *Stroke* 1998; **29**:2467–72.

30. Malarcher AM, Giles WH, Croft JB, Wozniak MA, Wityk RJ, Stolley PD, et al. Alcohol intake, type of beverage, and the risk of cerebral infarction in young women. *Stroke* 2001; **32**:77–83.

31. Mukamal K, Ascherio A, Mittleman M, Conigrave K, Camargo C, Kawachi I, et al. Alcohol and risk for ischemic stroke in men: the role of drinking patterns and usual beverage. *Ann Intern Med* 2005; **142**:11–19.

32. Hillbom M, Numminen H, Juvela S. Recent heavy drinking of alcohol and embolic stroke. *Stroke* 1999; **30**:2307–12.

33. Wannamethee SG, Shaper AG. Patterns of alcohol intake and risk of stroke in middle-aged British men. *Stroke* 1996: 1033–9.

34. Kiyohara Y, Kato I, Iwamoto H, Nakayama K, Fujishima M. The impact of alcohol and hypertension on stroke incidence in a general Japanese population. The Hisayama Study. *Stroke* 1995; **26**:368–72.

35. Bazzano LA, Gu D, Reynolds K, Wu X, Chen CS, Duan X, et al. Alcohol consumption and risk for stroke among Chinese men. *Ann Neurol* 2007; **62**:569–78.

36. Dickinson HO, Mason JM, Nicolson DJ, Campbell F, Beyer FR, Cook JV, et al. Lifestyle interventions to reduce raised blood pressure: a systematic review of randomized controlled trials. *J Hypertens* 2006; **24**:215–33.

37. Djoussé L, Levy D, Benjamin EJ, Blease SJ, Russ A, Larson MG, et al. Long-term alcohol consumption and the risk of atrial fibrillation in the Framingham Study. *Am J Cardiol* 2004; **93**:710–3.

38. Kurth T, Gaziano J, Berger K, Kase C, Rexrode K, Cook N, et al. Body mass index and the risk of stroke in men. *Arch Intern Med* 2002; **162**:2557–62.

39. Jood K, Jern C, Wilhelmsen L, Rosengren A. Body mass index in mid-life is associated with a first stroke in men: a prospective population study over 28 years. *Stroke* 2004; **35**:2764–9.

40. Kurth T, Gaziano J, Rexrode K, Kase C, Cook N, Manson J, et al. Prospective study of body mass index and risk of stroke in apparently healthy women. *Circulation* 2005; **111**:1992–8.

41. Hu G, Tuomilehto J, Silventoinen K, Sarti C, Mannisto S, Jousilahti P. Body mass index, waist circumference, and waist-hip ratio on the risk of total and type-specific stroke. *Arch Intern Med* 2007; **167**:1420–7.

42. Abbott RD, Behrens GR, Sharp DS, Rodriguez BL, Burchfiel CM, Ross GW, et al. Body mass index and thromboembolic stroke in nonsmoking men in older middle age. The Honolulu Heart Program. *Stroke* 1994; **25**:2370–6.

43. Rexrode KM, Hennekens CH, Willett WC, Colditz GA, Stampfer MJ, Rich-Edwards JW, et al. A prospective study of body mass index, weight change, and risk of stroke in women. *JAMA* 1997; **277**:1539–45.

44. Song YM, Sung J, Davey Smith G, Ebrahim S. Body mass index and ischemic and hemorrhagic stroke: a prospective study in Korean men. *Stroke* 2004; **35**:831–6.

45. Park JW, Lee SY, Kim SY, Choe H, Jee SH. BMI and stroke risk in Korean women. *Obesity* 2008; **16**:396–401.

46. Walker SP, Rimm EB, Ascherio A, Kawachi I, Stampfer MJ, Willett WC. Body size and fat

distribution as predictors of stroke among US men. *Am J Epidemiol* 1996; **144**:1143–50.

47. Suk SH, Sacco RL, Boden-Albala B, Cheun JF, Pittman JG, Elkind MS, et al. Northern Manhattan Stroke Study. Abdominal obesity and risk of ischemic stroke: the Northern Manhattan Stroke Study. *Stroke* 2003; **34**:1586–92.

48. Curioni C, Andre C, Veras R. Weight reduction for primary prevention of stroke in adults with overweight or obesity. *Cochrane Database Syst Rev* 2006; CD006062.

49. Neter J, Stam B, Kok F, Grobbee D, Geleijnse J. Influence of weight reduction on blood pressure: A meta-analysis of randomized controlled trials. *Hypertension* 2003; **42**:878–84.

50. Shaw K, Gennat H, O'Rourke P, Del Mar C. Exercise for overweight or obesity. *Cochrane Database Syst Rev* 2006; CD003817.

51. Lee C, Folsom A, Blair S. Physical activity and stroke risk: A meta-analysis. *Stroke* 2003; **34**:2475–81.

52. Deplanque D, Masse I, Lefebvre C, Libersa C, Leys D, Bordet R. Prior TIA, lipid-lowering drug use, and physical activity decrease ischemic stroke severity. *Neurology* 2006; **67**:1403–10.

53. Wannamethee G, Shaper AG. Physical activity and stroke in British middle aged men. *BMJ* 1992; **304**:597–601.

54. Thrift AG, Donnan GA, McNeil JJ. Reduced risk of intracerebral hemorrhage with dynamic recreational exercise but not with heavy work activity. *Stroke* 2002; **33**:559–64.

55. Hu FB, Stampfer MJ, Colditz GA, Ascherio A, Rexrode KM, Willett WC, et al. Physical activity and risk of stroke in women. *JAMA* 2000; **283**: 2961–7.

56. Hu G, Sarti C, Jousilahti P, Silventoinen K, Barengo NC, Tuomilehto J. Leisure time, occupational, and commuting physical activity and the risk of stroke. *Stroke* 2005; **36**:1994–9.

57. Lee IM, Paffenbarger RS Jr. Physical activity and stroke incidence: the Harvard Alumni Health Study. *Stroke* 1998; **29**:2049–54.

58. Lee IM, Hennekens CH, Berger K, Buring JE, Manson JE. Exercise and risk of stroke in male physicians. *Stroke* 1999; **30**:1–6.

59. Wendel-Vos GC, Schuit AJ, Feskens EJ, Boshuizen HC, Verschuren WM, Saris WH, et al. Physical activity and stroke: A meta-analysis of observational data. *Int J Epidemiol* 2004; **33**:787–98.

60. Cornelissen VA, Fagard RH. Effects of endurance training on blood pressure, blood pressure-regulating mechanisms, and cardiovascular risk factors. *Hypertension* 2005; **46**:667–75.

61. Shaw K, Gennat H, O'Rourke P, Del Mar C. Exercise for overweight or obesity. *Cochrane Database Syst Rev* 2006; CD003817.

62. Pomerleau J, McKee M, Lobstein T, Knai C. The burden of disease attributable to nutrition in Europe. *Public Health Nutr* 2003; **6**:453–61.

63. Ding EL, Mozaffarian D. Optimal dietary habits for the prevention of stroke. *Semin Neurol* 2006; **26**:11–23.

64. He FJ, Nowson CA, MacGregor GA. Fruit and vegetable consumption and stroke: meta-analysis of cohort studies. *Lancet* 2006; **367**:320–6.

65. Joshipura KJ, Ascherio A, Manson JE, Stampfer MJ, Rimm EB, Speizer FE, et al. Fruit and vegetable intake in relation to risk of ischemic stroke. *JAMA* 1999; **282**:1233–9.

66. Mellen PB, Walsh TF, Herrington DM. Whole grain intake and cardiovascular disease: a meta-analysis. *Nutr Metab Cardiovasc Dis* 2008; **18**:283–90.

67. Sauvaget C, Nagano J, Allen N, Kodama K. Vegetable and fruit intake and stroke mortality in the Hiroshima/Nagasaki Life Span Study. *Stroke* 2003; **34**:2355–60.

68. Johnsen SP, Overvad K, Stripp C, Tjønneland A, Husted SE, Sørensen HT. Intake of fruit and vegetables and the risk of ischemic stroke in a cohort of Danish men and women. *Am J Clin Nutr* 2003; **78**:57–64.

69. He K, Song Y, Daviglus ML, Liu K, Van Horn L, Dyer AR, et al. Fish consumption and incidence of stroke: a meta-analysis of cohort studies. *Stroke* 2004; **35**:1538–42.

70. Mozaffarian D, Rimm EB. Fish intake, contaminants, and human health: evaluating the risks and the benefits. *JAMA* 2006; **296**:1885–99.

71. Bouzan C, Cohen JT, Connor WE, Kris-Etherton PM, Gray GM, König A, et al. A quantitative analysis of fish consumption and stroke risk. *Am J Prev Med* 2005; **29**:347–52.

72. Nagata C, Takatsuka N, Shimizu N, Shimizu H. Sodium intake and risk of death from stroke in Japanese men and women. *Stroke* 2004; **35**:1543–7.

73. Stamler J. The INTERSALT Study: background, methods, findings, and implications. *Am J Clin Nutr* 1997; **65**:626S–42S.

74. He FJ, MacGregor GA. Effect of longer-term modest salt reduction on blood pressure. *Cochrane Database Syst Rev* 2004; CD004937.

75. Sacks FM, Svetkey LP, Vollmer WM, Appel LJ, Bray GA, Harsha D, et al. DASH-Sodium Collaborative Research Group. Effects on blood pressure of reduced dietary sodium and the Dietary Approaches to Stop Hypertension (DASH) diet. DASH-Sodium

Collaborative Research Group. *N Engl J Med* 2001; **344**:3–10.

76. Ascherio A, Rimm EB, Hernán MA, Giovannucci EL, Kawachi I, Stampfer MJ, et al. Intake of potassium, magnesium, calcium, and fiber and risk of stroke among US men. *Circulation* 1998; **98**:1198–204.

77. Bazzano LA, He J, Ogden LG, Loria C, Vupputuri S, Myers L, et al. Dietary potassium intake and risk of stroke in US men and women: National Health and Nutrition Examination Survey I epidemiologic follow-up study. *Stroke* 2001; **32**:1473–80.

78. Morris RC Jr, Sebastian A, Forman A, Tanaka M, Schmidlin O. Normotensive salt sensitivity: effects of race and dietary potassium. *Hypertension* 1999; **33**:18–23.

79. Fung TT, Chiuve SE, McCullough ML, Rexrode KM, Logroscino G, Hu FB. Adherence to a DASH-style diet and risk of coronary heart disease and stroke in women. *Arch Intern Med* 2008; **168**:713–20.

80. de Lorgeril M, Salen P. The Mediterranean diet in secondary prevention of coronary heart disease. *Clin Invest Med* 2006; **29**:154–8.

81. Howard B, Van Horn L, Hsia J, Manson J, Stefanick M, Wassertheil-Smoller S, et al. Low-fat dietary pattern and risk of cardiovascular disease: the women's health initiative randomized controlled dietary modification trial. *JAMA* 2006; **295**:655–666.

82. Nelson HD, Humphrey LL, Nygren P, Teutsch SM, Allan JD. Postmenopausal hormone replacement therapy: scientific review. *JAMA* 2002; **288**:872–81.

83. Bath PM, Gray LJ. Association between hormone replacement therapy and subsequent stroke: a meta-analysis. *BMJ* 2005; **330**:342.

84. Gabriel-Sánchez R, Carmona L, Roque M, Sánchez-Gómez GL, Bonfill X. Hormone replacement therapy for preventing cardiovascular disease in post-menopausal women. *Cochrane Database Syst Rev* 2005: CD002229.

85. Farquhar CM, Marjoribanks J, Lethaby A, Lamberts Q, Suckling JA. Cochrane HT Study Group. Long term hormone therapy for perimenopausal and postmenopausal women. *Cochrane Database Syst Rev* 2005; CD004143.

86. Riggs BL, Hartmann LC. Selective estrogen-receptor modulators – mechanisms of action and application to clinical practice. *N Engl J Med* 2003; **348**:618–29.

87. Barrett-Connor E, Grady D, Sashegyi A, Anderson PW, Cox DA, Hoszowski K, et al. MORE Investigators (Multiple Outcomes of Raloxifene Evaluation). Raloxifene and cardiovascular events in osteoporotic postmenopausal women: four-year results from the MORE (Multiple Outcomes of Raloxifene Evaluation) randomized trial. *JAMA* 2002; **287**:847–57.

88. Barrett-Connor E, Mosca L, Collins P, Geiger MJ, Grady D, Kornitzer M, et al. Raloxifene Use for The Heart (RUTH) Trial Investigators. Effects of raloxifene on cardiovascular events and breast cancer in postmenopausal women. *N Engl J Med* 2006; **355**:125–37.

89. Bushnell CD, Goldstein LB. Risk of ischemic stroke with tamoxifen treatment for breast cancer: a meta-analysis. *Neurology* 2004; **63**:1230–3.

90. Lawes CM, Vander Hoorn S, Rodgers A. International Society of Hypertension. Global burden of blood-pressure-related disease, 2001. *Lancet* 2008; **371**:1513–8.

91. Lewington S, Clarke R, Qizilbash N, Peto R, Collins R. Age-specific relevance of usual blood pressure to vascular mortality: a meta-analysis of individual data for one million adults in 61 prospective studies. *Lancet* 2002; **360**:1903–13.

92. Lawes CM, Bennett DA, Feigin VL, Rodgers A. Blood pressure and stroke: an overview of published reviews. *Stroke* 2004; **35**:1024.

93. Mancia G, De Backer G, Dominiczak A, Cifkova R, Fagard R, Germano G, et al. Guidelines for the management of arterial hypertension: The Task Force for the Management of Arterial Hypertension of the European Society of Hypertension (ESH) and of the European Society of Cardiology (ESC). *Eur Heart J* 2007; **28**:1462–536.

94. Mancia G. Optimal control of blood pressure in patients with diabetes reduces the incidence of macro- and microvascular events. *J Hypertens Suppl* 2007; **25** Suppl 1:S7–12.

95. Neal B, MacMahon S, Chapman N. Effects of ACE inhibitors, calcium antagonists, and other blood-pressure-lowering drugs: results of prospectively designed overviews of randomised trials. Blood Pressure Lowering Treatment Trialists' Collaboration. *Lancet* 2000; **356**:1955–64.

96. Turnbull F. Blood Pressure Lowering Treatment Trialists' Collaboration. Effects of different blood-pressure-lowering regimens on major cardiovascular events: results of prospectively-designed overviews of randomised trials. *Lancet* 2003; **362**:1527–35.

97. Staessen JA, Li Y, Thijs L, Wang JG. Blood pressure reduction and cardiovascular prevention: an update including the 2003–2004 secondary prevention trials. *Hypertens Res* 2005; **28**:385–407.

98. Lindholm LH, Carlberg B, Samuelsson O. Should beta blockers remain first choice in the treatment of primary hypertension? A meta-analysis. *Lancet* 2005; **366**:1545–53.

99. Staessen J, Fagard R, Thijs L, Celis H, Arabidze G, Birkenhager W, et al. Randomised double-blind comparison of placebo and active treatment for older patients with isolated systolic hypertension. The systolic hypertension in Europe (syst-eur) trial investigators. *Lancet* 1997; **350**:757–64.

100. Blood Pressure Lowering Treatment Trialists' Collaboration, Turnbull F, Neal B, Ninomiya T, Algert C, Arima H, Barzi F, et al. Effects of different regimens to lower blood pressure on major cardiovascular events in older and younger adults: meta-analysis of randomised trials. *BMJ* 2008; **336**:1121–3.

101. Beckett NS, Peters R, Fletcher AE, Staessen JA, Liu L, Dumitrascu D, et al. HYVET Study Group. Treatment of hypertension in patients 80 years of age or older. *N Engl J Med* 2008; **358**:1887–98.

102. Turner RC, Cull CA, Frighi V, Holman RR. Glycemic control with diet, sulfonylurea, metformin, or insulin in patients with type 2 diabetes mellitus: progressive requirement for multiple therapies (UKPDS 49). UK Prospective Diabetes Study (UKPDS) Group. *JAMA* 1999; **281**:2005–12.

103. UK Prospective Diabetes Study (UKPDS) Group. Intensive blood-glucose control with sulphonylureas or insulin compared with conventional treatment and risk of complications in patients with type 2 diabetes (UKPDS 33). *Lancet* 1998; **352**:837–53.

104. Boden-Albala B, Cammack S, Chong J, Wang C, Wright C, Rundek T, et al. Diabetes, fasting glucose levels, and risk of ischemic stroke and vascular events: findings from the Northern Manhattan Study (NOMAS). *Diabetes Care* 2008; **31**:1132–7.

105. Gerstein HC, Miller ME, Byington RP, Goff DC Jr, Bigger JT, Buse JB, et al. Action to Control Cardiovascular Risk in Diabetes Study Group. Effects of intensive glucose lowering in type 2 diabetes. *N Engl J Med* 2008; **358**:2545–59.

106. Patel A, MacMahon S, Chalmers J, Neal B, Billot L, Woodward M, et al. ADVANCE Collaborative Group. Intensive blood glucose control and vascular outcomes in patients with type 2 diabetes. *N Engl J Med* 2008; **358**:2560–72.

107. Kannel WB, Wilson PW, Zhang TJ. The epidemiology of impaired glucose tolerance and hypertension. *Am Heart J* 1991; **121**:1268–73.

108. UK Prospective Diabetes Study 27. Plasma lipids and lipoproteins at diagnosis of NIDDM by age and sex. *Diabetes Care* 1997; **20**:1683–7.

109. Collins R, Armitage J, Parish S, Sleigh P, Peto R. Heart Protection Study Collaborative Group. MRC/BHF Heart Protection Study of cholesterol-lowering with simvastatin in 5963 people with diabetes: a randomised placebo-controlled trial. *Lancet* 2003; **361**:2005–16.

110. Sever PS, Poulter NR, Dahlof B, Wedel H, Collins R, Beevers G, et al. Reduction in cardiovascular events with atorvastatin in 2,532 patients with type 2 diabetes: Anglo-Scandinavian Cardiac Outcomes Trial–lipid-lowering arm (ASCOT-LLA). *Diabetes Care* 2005; **28**:1151–7.

111. Prospective studies collaboration. Cholesterol, diastolic blood pressure, and stroke: 13,000 strokes in 450,000 people in 45 prospective cohorts. *Lancet* 1995; **346**:1647–53.

112. Lewington S, Whitlock G, Clarke R, Sherliker P, Emberson J, Halsey J, et al. Prospective Studies Collaboration. Blood cholesterol and vascular mortality by age, sex, and blood pressure: a meta-analysis of individual data from 61 prospective studies with 55,000 vascular deaths. *Lancet* 2007; **370**:1829–39.

113. Shahar E, Chambless LE, Rosamond WD, Boland LL, Ballantyne CM, McGovern PG, et al. Atherosclerosis Risk in Communities Study. Plasma lipid profile and incident ischemic stroke: the Atherosclerosis Risk in Communities (ARIC) study. *Stroke* 2003; **34**:623–31.

114. Amarenco P, Labreuche J, Lavallee P, Touboul P. Statins in stroke prevention and carotid atherosclerosis: Systematic review and up-to-date meta-analysis. *Stroke* 2004; **35**:2902–9.

115. O'Regan C, Wu P, Arora P, Perri D, Mills EJ. Statin therapy in stroke prevention: a meta-analysis involving 121,000 patients. *Am J Med* 2008; **121**:24–33.

116. Fitzmaurice E, Wendell L, Snider R, Schwab K, Chanderraj R, Kinnecom C, et al. Effect of statins on intracerebral hemorrhage outcome and recurrence. *Stroke* 2008; **39**:2151–4.

117. Josan K, Majumdar SR, McAlister FA. The efficacy and safety of intensive statin therapy: a meta-analysis of randomized trials. *CMAJ* 2008; **178**:576–84.

118. Goldstein LB, Amarenco P, Szarek M, Callahan A 3rd, Hennerici M, Sillesen H, et al. SPARCL Investigators. Hemorrhagic stroke in the Stroke Prevention by Aggressive Reduction in Cholesterol Levels study. *Neurology* 2008; **70**:2364–70.

119. Corvol JC, Bouzamondo A, Sirol M, Hulot JS, Sanchez P, Lechat P. Differential effects of lipid-lowering therapies on stroke prevention: a meta-analysis of randomized trials. *Arch Intern Med* 2003; **163**:669–76.

120. Wolf PA, Abbott RD, Kannel WB. Atrial fibrillation as an independent risk factor for stroke: the Framingham Study. *Stroke* 1991; **22**:983–8.

121. Go AS, Hylek EM, Phillips KA, Chang Y, Henault LE, Selby JV, et al. Prevalence of diagnosed atrial fibrillation in adults: national implications for rhythm management and stroke prevention: the AnTicoagulation and Risk Factors in Atrial Fibrillation (ATRIA) Study. *JAMA* 2001; **285**:2370–5.

103

122. Steger C, Pratter A, Martinek-Bregel M, Avanzini M, Valentin A, Slany J, et al. Stroke patients with atrial fibrillation have a worse prognosis than patients without: data from the Austrian Stroke registry. *Eur Heart J* 2004; **25**:1734–40.

123. Roquer J, Rodríguez-Campello A, Gomis M, Ois A, Martínez-Rodríguez JE, Munteis E, et al. Comparison of the impact of atrial fibrillation on the risk of early death after stroke in women versus men. *J Neurol* 2006; **253**:1484–9.

124. Stroke Risk in Atrial Fibrillation Working Group. Independent predictors of stroke in patients with atrial fibrillation: a systematic review. *Neurology* 2007; **69**:546–54.

125. Stroke Risk in Atrial Fibrillation Working Group. Comparison of 12 risk stratification schemes to predict stroke in patients with nonvalvular atrial fibrillation. *Stroke* 2008; **39**:1901–10.

126. Gross CP, Vogel EW, Dhond AJ, Marple CB, Edwards RA, Hauch O, et al. Factors influencing physicians' reported use of anticoagulation therapy in nonvalvular atrial fibrillation: a cross-sectional survey. *Clin Ther* 2003; **25**:1750–64.

127. Stafford RS, Radley DC. The underutilization of cardiac medications of proven benefit, 1990 to 2002. *J Am Coll Cardiol* 2003; **41**:56–61.

128. Hart RG, Pearce LA, Aguilar MI. Meta-analysis: antithrombotic therapy to prevent stroke in patients who have nonvalvular atrial fibrillation. *Ann Intern Med* 2007; **146**:857–67.

129. Aguilar MI, Hart R, Pearce LA. Oral anticoagulants versus antiplatelet therapy for preventing stroke in patients with non-valvular atrial fibrillation and no history of stroke or transient ischemic attacks. *Cochrane Database Syst Rev* 2007; CD006186.

130. Go AS, Hylek EM, Chang Y, Phillips KA, Henault LE, Capra AM, et al. Anticoagulation therapy for stroke prevention in atrial fibrillation: how well do randomized trials translate into clinical practice? *JAMA* 2003; **290**:2685–92.

131. Fang MC, Go AS, Hylek EM, Chang Y, Henault LE, Jensvold NG, et al. Age and the risk of warfarin-associated hemorrhage: the anticoagulation and risk factors in atrial fibrillation study. *J Am Geriatr Soc* 2006; **54**:1231–6.

132. Rash A, Downes T, Portner R, Yeo W, Morgan N, Channer K. A randomised controlled trial of warfarin versus aspirin for stroke prevention in octogenarians with atrial fibrillation (WASPO). *Age Ageing* 2007; **36**:151–6.

133. Mant J, Hobbs FD, Fletcher K, Roalfe A, Fitzmaurice D, Lip GY, et al. Warfarin versus aspirin for stroke prevention in an elderly community population with atrial fibrillation (the Birmingham Atrial Fibrillation Treatment of the Aged Study, BAFTA): a randomised controlled trial. *Lancet* 2007; **370**:493–503.

134. Hart RG, Pearce LA, Rothbart RM, McAnulty JH, Asinger RW, Halperin JL. Stroke with intermittent atrial fibrillation: incidence and predictors during aspirin therapy. Stroke Prevention in Atrial Fibrillation Investigators. *J Am Coll Cardiol* 2000; **35**:183–7.

135. Salem DN, Stein PD, Al-Ahmad A, Bussey HI, Horstkotte D, Miller N, et al. Antithrombotic therapy in valvular heart disease – native and prosthetic: the Seventh ACCP Conference on Antithrombotic and Thrombolytic Therapy. *Chest* 2004; **126**:457S–82S.

136. Bonow RO, Carabello BA, Kanu C, de Leon AC Jr, Faxon DP, Freed MD, et al. American College of Cardiology/American Heart Association Task Force on Practice Guidelines; Society of Cardiovascular Anesthesiologists; Society for Cardiovascular Angiography and Interventions; Society of Thoracic Surgeons. ACC/AHA 2006 guidelines for the management of patients with valvular heart disease: a report of the American College of Cardiology/American Heart Association Task Force on Practice Guidelines (writing committee to revise the 1998 Guidelines for the Management of Patients With Valvular Heart Disease): developed in collaboration with the Society of Cardiovascular Anesthesiologists: endorsed by the Society for Cardiovascular Angiography and Interventions and the Society of Thoracic Surgeons. *Circulation* 2006; **114**:e84–231.

Cardiac diseases relevant to stroke

Claudia Stöllberger and Josef Finsterer

Introduction

Cardiac diseases can be relevant to stroke in different respects:

- In embolic stroke, cardiac diseases may be the cause of embolism, such as atrial fibrillation (AF), endocarditis, left ventricular aneurysm or left ventricular hypertrabeculation/non-compaction (LVHT).
- Brady- and tachyarrhythmias may compromise cerebral blood flow.
- Cardiac diseases may coexist, and influence the clinical course and rehabilitation, such as coronary heart disease or dilatative cardiomyopathy (dCMP).
- In some instances, cardiac diseases may be the consequence of the stroke, such as stroke-induced transient left ventricular dysfunction, also referred to as Takotsubo syndrome (TTS).
- Congenital abnormalities such as patent foramen ovale (PFO) or atrial septal aneurysm (ASA) may implicate paradoxical embolism.

Several diseases may coexist in a single patient, such as coronary heart disease and AF. Thus, from a pragmatic point of view, this chapter aims to focus on the most frequent and controversially discussed cardiac abnormalities in stroke patients.

Rhythm disturbances

Atrial fibrillation

AF is a cardiac arrhythmia, defined by the absence of P waves and varying RR distances in the electrocardiogram. AF is a common arrhythmia and its prevalence increases with age up to 9% at age 80–89 years (Figure 7.1). Approximately 85% of the individuals with AF are between 65 and 85 years of age [1]. Apart from hemodynamic consequences due to the loss of atrial contraction and symptoms, such as palpitations,

AF may lead to embolic stroke or peripheral or mesenteric embolism. Compared to patients with sinus rhythm, patients with AF due to rheumatic heart disease, particularly mitral stenosis, have a 17-fold increased risk of stroke, whereas patients with non-rheumatic AF have a 5-fold increased risk of stroke [2]. Among all ischemic strokes 17–31% occur because of embolic complications of AF [3–5]. Effective methods of detecting AF in stroke patients are warranted since patients with AF after ischemic stroke are at high risk of suffering recurrent strokes, irrespective of whether AF is permanent or paroxysmal.

Diagnosing paroxysmal atrial fibrillation

Whereas diagnosis of permanent AF is easily feasible from the 12-lead electrocardiogram, identifying paroxysmal AF in stroke patients is still a challenge. A review comprising five studies analyzed the diagnostic yield of monitoring devices to detect paroxysmal AF in 736 stroke patients: Holter monitoring over 24–72 hours detected AF in 4.6%, whereas 4-day or 7-day event loop recorders detected AF in an additional 6–8% after negative Holter monitoring [6]. A further study applied 7-day event recording at 0, 3, and 6 months and detected AF in 14% of patients with an initial negative Holter [7]. Interestingly, frequent supraventricular ectopic beats (>70 during a 24-hour Holter) were predictors of AF [7]. Another study found that the combined use of Holter and serial electrocardiograms within the first 3 days gave a better rate of AF detection (14%) than serial electrocardiograms alone (11%) [8].

Future developments for detection of paroxysmal atrial fibrillation

Detection of paroxysmal AF is impeded by the available monitoring devices. The electrodes may cause skin irritation, making it difficult to wear

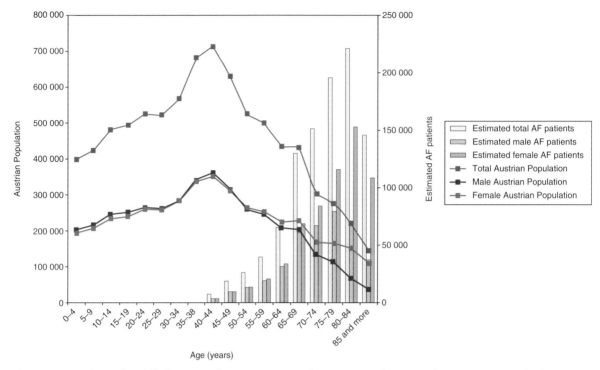

Figure 7.1. Prevalence of atrial fibrillation according to age ranges in the Austrian population according to an estimation for the US population [1].

them for long periods. Event loop recorders miss asymptomatic AF because they rely on the patient's recognition of symptoms. Improved methods for detecting AF are currently being evaluated in pilot trials, such as a 30-day cardiac event monitoring belt in the EMBRACE study or the Reveal XT [9]. The Reveal XT (Medtronic Inc.) is an implantable event-triggered recorder which detects and monitors atrial and ventricular tachycardias. Using a special algorithm, the device is able to detect AF episodes, and their time of onset and duration (Figure 7.2). Ongoing studies are evaluating the use of this implantable loop recorder for the diagnosis of paroxysmal AF in patients with stroke.

Left atrial appendage occlusion for stroke prevention in atrial fibrillation

Surgical or percutaneous closure of the left atrial appendage (LAA) is considered an alternative to oral anticoagulation (OAC) to prevent strokes in AF [10]. However, there are several concerns about the rationale and safety of LAA occlusion.

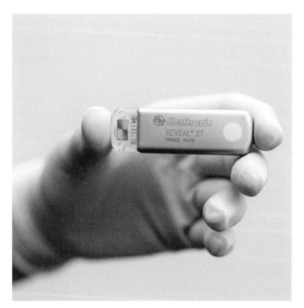

Figure 7.2. The Reveal XT (Medtronic Inc.) is an implantable device recording the cardiac rhythm for up to 3 years. Ongoing studies are evaluating these implantable loop recorders for the diagnosis of paroxysmal atrial fibrillation in patients with stroke.

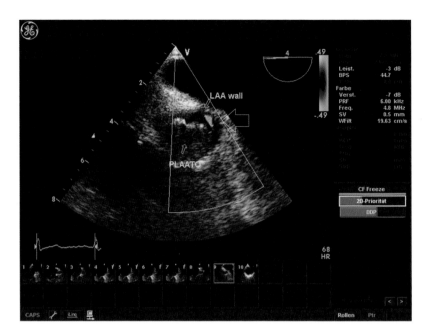

Figure 7.3. Transesophageal echocardiographic picture of the left atrium and left atrial appendage with a percutaneously implanted left atrial appendage occluder (PLAATO device) showing a small jet by color Doppler sonography (arrow) between the PLAATO device and the left atrial appendage wall. This jet was not visible at PLAATO implantation but was only detected after 24 months.

There is no evidence that embolism in AF exclusively derives from LAA thrombi. When prospectively investigating clinically stable outpatients with AF and with no recent embolism by transesophageal echocardiography, the prevalence of LAA thrombi was only 2.5%, and during a follow-up of 58 months LAA thrombus did not predict stroke/embolism [11].

The LAA has properties which may impede the completion of the occlusion. The LAA myocardium has a higher distensibility than the left atrial myocardium. Progressive dilatation of the LAA occurs in AF, possibly leading to leakage of a primarily completely closed LAA. Incomplete LAA closure creates a pouch with stagnant blood flow, which enhances thrombus formation (Figure 7.3).

Even if technical improvements lead to a more effective LAA occlusion, potential further side-effects have to be considered. The LAA plays an important role in hemodynamic and body fluid regulation. LAA elimination may impede physiological regulation of heart failure and thirst-perception [12]. The LAA is a place of secretion of atrial natriuretic peptide (ANP). ANP contributes to physiological control of lipid mobilization in humans so LAA elimination might promote development of obesity [13]. In view of global warming and the obesity epidemic, LAA elimination is a highly questionable procedure for stroke prevention.

Ablation of atrial fibrillation for stroke prevention

Radiofrequency catheter ablation (RFA) of AF is a recently proposed interventional method to cure AF. There are concerns, however, whether RFA is a safe and effective therapy to prevent strokes.

The targets of RFA are myocardial sleeves near the junction of the pulmonary veins with the left atrium and autonomic ganglia in the left atrial posterior wall, all located epicardially. The RFA catheter, however, is introduced into the left atrium and thus radiofrequency energy is delivered from the endocardial surface with the aim of creating transmural lesions. Thus, RFA can only be performed successfully when affecting the epicardial side of the left atrial wall. Therefore the rate of procedural complications, including pericardial tamponade and life-threatening atrio-esophageal fistula, is considerably high [14].

Since AF is not only an electrical problem, the targets of RFA are not well defined. AF results from long-standing arterial hypertension, and ischemic and valvular heart disease leading to structural abnormalities such as atrial myocardial fibrosis. Since RFA does not abolish myocardial fibrosis it can be expected that ectopic activity may arise from other non-ablated regions and that AF may recur. These considerations are supported by the low long-term efficacy of RFA, especially in permanent AF and structural heart disease [14].

The mean age of patients in whom RFA has been performed so far is 50–63 years [14]. The success rate of RFA is low when the patient is over 65 years [15]. The prevalence of AF, however, increases with advancing age (Figure 7.1) [1]. Thus, the proportion of AF patients who might profit from RFA is much lower than the proportion of those who might not.

Possible candidates for RFA tend to have a low risk of embolic stroke since they are under 65 years and mostly have AF without cardiovascular diseases. RFA, however, increases the risk of stroke periprocedurally due to endocardial lesions. OAC for at least 3 months is usually recommended to prevent thrombus formation on the ablation lines [14]. It has also been emphasized that recurrent AF is more frequently clinically silent after than before RFA [16]. As a consequence it is uncertain whether OAC can be stopped at all after RFA. Furthermore, the transseptal puncture during RFA creates interatrial shunts, and it is at present unknown whether these shunts are clinically relevant in terms of paradoxical embolism. Thus, RFA may create new potential sources of arterial embolism.

We doubt that RFA prevents stroke in AF for the following reasons:

- The majority of AF patients are too old for RFA.
- Candidates for RFA belong to a subgroup with a low risk of embolism.
- The RFA procedure itself may increase the embolic risk.
- At present it is uncertain how long this embolic risk persists after the procedure.

Atrial fibrillation (AF) may lead to embolic stroke. Patients with AF have a 5-fold (non-rheumatic AF) to 17-fold increased risk of stroke (embolism due to rheumatic heart disease).

Bradycardia and tachycardia

If brady- or tachycardia is observed in a stroke patient, the initial diagnostic steps are very similar and aim to assess the clinical severity and to differentiate between cardiac and non-cardiac causes. A suggested practical approach to stroke patients with brady- or tachycardia is given in Table 7.1.

Brady- or tachycardia causes symptoms such as dizziness, light-headedness, spells or fainting. These symptoms may erroneously be interpreted as epileptic seizures. Thus, Holter monitoring to detect recurrent episodes of brady- or tachycardia may be useful in

Table 7.1. Practical approach to stroke patients with brady- or tachycardia.

Assessment of vital signs
Measurement of blood pressure
Registration of a 12-lead electrocardiogram
Measurement of the QT interval according to Bazett's formula: $QTc = QT/\sqrt{RR}$
Registration of the body temperature
Blood tests (electrolytes, blood cell count, D-dimer, C-reactive protein, thyroid function tests)
Assessment of current and previous medication

patients with suggestive symptoms. The electroencephalogram is usually normal in these patients.

Bradycardia

Bradycardia is defined as a heart rate <50 beats per minute, and becomes symptomatic only when the rate drops significantly. Bradycardia may be due to cardiac and non-cardiac causes. Non-cardiac causes comprise side-effects of drugs, and disorders such as hypothyroidism, hypothermia, electrolyte disturbances and increased parasympathetic tone. Furthermore, the brain may be involved in cardiovascular regulation, and the insular cortex is assumed to play a role in rhythm control [17]. Cardiac causes of bradycardia include acute or chronic coronary heart disease, valvular heart disease, and degenerative primary electrical disease. Performing a standard electrocardiogram enables one to diagnose more precisely the type of bradycardia as sinus bradycardia, atrioventricular block, sinus arrest, or AF, and to look for signs of acute myocardial ischemia and to assess whether QT prolongation is present, which is a potentially life-threatening situation [18].

Tachycardia

Tachycardia is defined as a heart rate >100 beats per minute. Like bradycardia, tachycardia may be caused by non-cardiac and cardiac causes. Non-cardiac causes of tachycardia in stroke patients comprise fever, hypovolemia, anemia, hyperthyroidism, pulmonary embolism, pain, alcohol withdrawal, bronchospasm, side-effects of drugs and rebound in patients previously treated with beta-blocking agents. Cardiac causes of tachycardia are the same as for bradycardia, and the clinical consequences range from palpitations to sudden cardiac death.

Brady- or *tachycardia* causes symptoms such as dizziness, light-headedness, spells or fainting. These symptoms may erroneously be interpreted as epileptic seizures.

QT prolongation

Prolongation of ventricular repolarization manifests as a prolongation of the QT interval on the electrocardiogram. QT prolongation may be associated with torsades de pointes tachycardia. Torsades de pointes are often self-limited and are associated with palpitations, dizziness or syncope. Degeneration into ventricular fibrillation and sudden cardiac death can occur. In addition to the congenital long QT syndrome many drugs, such as antiarrhythmic drugs class IA and III, antibiotics, antihistamines, neuroleptics and antidepressants, are known to prolong the QT interval. Information about QT-prolonging drugs can be obtained from the internet (www.torsades.org). Most of these drugs block a specific potassium channel substantially involved in ventricular repolarization. Cardiovascular diseases induce a higher susceptibility to drug-induced prolongation of the QT interval. Correctable factors include hypokalemia, concomitant administration of different QT-prolonging drugs and bradycardia. Stroke is another condition associated with QT prolongation in 30–40% of patients [19, 20]. QT prolongation in stroke may be due to cardiovascular comorbidity, concomitant drug intake and metabolic disturbances, but may also originate from ischemic cerebral region, especially the insular region [17, 19].

If QT prolongation is observed in a stroke patient, triggering factors should be screened and, if possible, corrected. Special care should be taken with patients with QT prolongation associated with bradycardia because it entails the risk of torsades de pointes [18]. In these patients the heart rate should be raised to >80 beats per minute and implantation of a pacemaker should be strongly considered.

Stroke is associated with QT prolongation in 30–40% of patients.

Coronary heart disease
Coexistence of coronary heart disease and stroke

There is a frequent coexistence of coronary heart disease and stroke, most probably due to common atherosclerotic risk factors such as arterial hypertension, diabetes mellitus, smoking, and hypercholesterolemia. A history of symptomatic coronary heart disease, either myocardial infarction or angina pectoris, is found in up to 33% of patients with ischemic stroke [21]. An autopsy study of patients with fatal stroke found coronary plaques in 72%, coronary stenosis in 38% and myocardial infarction in 41% [22]. Two-thirds of the myocardial infarctions in that study were clinically silent [22]. Coronary heart disease, however, is not only a frequent finding at autopsy but also influences the prognosis of patients surviving a stroke. Five-year follow-up studies have shown that survivors of ischemic stroke are more likely to die of cardiac causes than of recurrent stroke [21, 23]. These results stress the importance for the neurologist to be aware of cardiac symptoms of stroke patients and for the cardiologist to develop cardioprotective measures for stroke patients.

There is a frequent coexistence of coronary heart disease and stroke, most probably due to common atherosclerotic risk factors.

Diagnosis of coronary heart disease in stroke patients

When caring for stroke patients in the acute or rehabilitation phase, it is necessary to be aware of clinical symptoms of myocardial ischemia such as chest pain or exertional dyspnea, or electrocardiographic abnormalities such as ST-depression, T-wave abnormalities or newly developing Q-waves [20]. The detection of myocardial injury can be improved by measuring serum levels of troponin T or troponin I, biomarkers which are found to be highly specific for myocardial necrosis [24]. Elevated troponin levels in stroke patients with signs or symptoms of myocardial ischemia should entail rhythm monitoring and cardiological consultation regarding further therapeutic and diagnostic measures, including coronary angiography and percutaneous coronary intervention. Stroke patients with normal troponin levels but signs and symptoms suggestive of myocardial ischemia should also be referred to the cardiologist, because stress testing might be indicated. In acute stroke patients without a history or signs of coronary heart disease, however, elevated troponin levels are not indicators of silent coronary heart disease, but rather of a bad prognosis due to heart and renal failure [25].

Troponin positivity may also indicate myocardial involvement in neuromuscular disease [26].

Myocardial infarction as a cause of embolism

Cardiogenic embolism from a left ventricular thrombus may occur as a complication of acute or subacute myocardial infarction or due to a ventricular aneurysm in the chronic phase of a large, mainly anterior wall infarction [27]. The incidence of left ventricular thrombi early after myocardial infarction has declined in recent years, most probably due to changes in the acute therapy of myocardial infarction, which now comprises intensive anticoagulant therapy and percutaneous coronary interventions [28]. However, left ventricular thrombi may still be detected in patients after myocardial infarction, especially if revascularization in the acute phase has not been performed or was unsuccessful or if the myocardial infarction affected large parts of the left ventricle. Thus, imaging studies to look for left ventricular thrombi, preferentially transthoracic echocardiography, should be performed in all stroke patients with a history or electrocardiographic signs of previous myocardial infarction.

> Acute or subacute myocardial infarction and ventricular aneurysms can be a cause of embolic stroke.

Valvular heart disease
Infective endocarditis and stroke

Ischemic and hemorrhagic strokes occur in 10 to 23% of patients with endocarditis and cluster during the period of untreated infection [29–31]. Among patients with endocarditis and stroke, the mitral valve seems to be more frequently affected than the aortic valve [30, 31]. Native valves as well as prosthetic valves may be affected by endocarditis, leading to stroke. Stroke patients with prosthetic valves have a worse prognosis than patients with native valves [32, 33].

Diagnosis of infective endocarditis

Despite the availability of echocardiography, laboratory and microbiological investigations, considerable delay occurs until infective endocarditis is diagnosed. Between onset of the symptoms and diagnosis a mean interval of 31 days has been reported [34]. This is due to the unspecific symptoms of endocarditis such as prolonged flu-like disease, generalized weakness and fatigue. Embolic events such as stroke are frequently the cause of hospital admission in these patients [29]. Thus, endocarditis has to be considered as a differential diagnosis in all stroke patients, and symptoms suggestive of endocarditis should be asked for at admission. The suspicion of endocarditis should increase if laboratory signs such as elevated blood sedimentation rate, leukocytosis or elevated C-reactive protein are found or if the patient is febrile. Blood cultures should be taken in these patients before initiation of antibiotic therapy. In most of the cases with stroke and suspected endocarditis transesophageal echocardiography is necessary because of its better visualization of the valves, valve prosthesis and vegetation to confirm or exclude the diagnosis (Figure 7.4).

Therapy of infective endocarditis

Antibiotic therapy is the main measure in therapy for infective endocarditis. The risk of stroke in infective endocarditis has been shown to decrease rapidly within 1 week after the initiation of antibiotic therapy [29]. However, if there are large vegetations or destruction of the valves leading to heart failure cardiac surgery may be necessary. In the past, cardiac surgeons have frequently been reluctant to operate on infective endocarditis patients with acute stroke because of concerns about cerebral bleeding complications because of anticoagulation during the cardiopulmonary bypass. However, delay in surgical intervention can lead to the death of patients who might have benefited from surgery [35]. Although no prospective data are available, a recent retrospective study of patients with infective endocarditis and stroke undergoing cardiac surgery has shown that mortality was 18%, complete neurological recovery was achieved in 70% of the survivors and secondary cerebral hemorrhage due to cardiac surgery occurred less frequently than was previously thought [36]. Based on these findings we recommend that in the event of infective endocarditis in a stroke patient the neurologist, cardiologist, microbiologist and cardiac surgeon should discuss together the optimal therapeutic management. The therapy should be planned with consideration of the clinical course, the echocardiographic findings, the microorganism involved, the response to antibiotic therapy and the neurological condition.

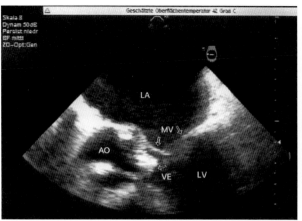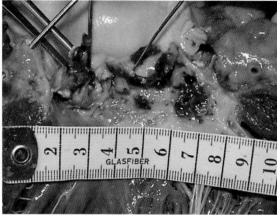

Figure 7.4. Transesophageal echocardiographic picture (left) and autopsy specimen (right) of a patient with embolic stroke and aortic valve endocarditis. LA = left atrium, MV = mitral valve, LV = left ventricle, VE = vegetation, AO = aortic valve.

Strokes occur in 10 to 23% of patients with endo-carditis, especially of the mitral valve. Endocarditis must be considered as a differential diagnosis in all stroke patients if laboratory signs of inflammation are present.

Stroke after heart valve surgery

After heart valve surgery patients are at increased risk of thromboembolism, due to either thrombus forma-tion on the artificial valve, infective endocarditis or AF. The embolic risk varies according to the type of surgery (repair versus replacement), the type of replaced valve (bioprosthesis versus mechanical pros-thesis) and the affected valve (mitral versus aortic valve). Approximately 20% of patients with an aortic or mitral valve prosthesis have an embolic stroke within 15 years after valve replacement [37].

Valve repair

Valve repair is nowadays the preferred surgical cor-rection of mitral regurgitation. Long-term follow-up studies have shown that after mitral repair, the risk of ischemic stroke is similar to that in the general popu-lation [38]. However, mitral repair is not always tech-nically feasible, and AF may develop postoperatively, especially when the left atrium is already enlarged before surgery.

Bioprosthesis

Generally, the embolic risk is lower in patients with bioprostheses than with mechanical prostheses. Pros-theses in the aortic position have a lower embolic risk

than in the mitral position [37]. A disadvantage of bioprostheses is their propensity to degenerate, neces-sitating reoperation [39]. Furthermore, as in patients after valve repair, AF may develop, especially after mitral valve surgery, and increase embolic risk.

Mechanical valve prosthesis

Patients with mechanical prostheses have a higher embolic risk with mitral than with aortic valve replacement [37]. Preoperative left ventricular dys-function has been identified as an additional risk factor for stroke in patients with mitral prostheses. Patients with a mechanical valve prosthesis and poorly controlled OAC are at increased risk of ische-mic stroke as well as bleeding, including cerebral bleeding [39, 40].

After heart valve surgery patients are at increased risk of thromboembolism.

Patent foramen ovale

In utero, the foramen ovale serves as a physiological conduit for right-to-left shunting. Once the pulmon-ary circulation is established after birth, left atrial pressure increases and allows functional closure of the foramen ovale. This is followed by anatomical closure of the septum primum and septum secun-dum. In about 25% of humans, the closure is incom-plete, and patent foramen ovale (PFO) remains as a flap-like opening, permitting right-to-left shunting when the right atrial pressure exceeds the left atrial pressure. Transesophageal echocardiography (TEE) is considered the method of choice for diagnosing

Table 7.2. Studies investigating the venous system in suspected paradoxical embolism.

Author (year)	Patients	Technique	Days between event and investigation	Prevalence of thrombosis, %	Location of thrombosis, n
[77] (1991)	23	V	2–210	26	Femoral, 3
					Iliac, 3
[78] (1993)	42	V	0–90	60	Calf, 13
					Popliteal, 2
					Femoral, 8
					Iliac, 1
[79] (1993)	13	V	0–28	0	0
[80] (1994)	17	R	ND	35	ND
[81] (1994)	16	V or D	ND	31	ND
[82] (1994)	27	V or D	ND	11	ND
[83] (1994)	18	V	1–300	11	ND
[84] (1997)	53	V	1–15	9	ND
[85] (2004)	46	MRV	2 ± 0.67	20	Pelvic, 9

Notes: V = venography, R = radioisotope venography, ND = data not given, D = duplex sonography, MRV = magnetic resonance venography.

PFO, although there is considerable interobserver ($\kappa = 0.77$) and intraobserver ($\kappa = 0.82$) variability in the diagnosis [41].

Paradoxical embolism

PFO does not manifest clinically, but several retrospective and case–control studies in patients with cryptogenic stroke found that the prevalence of PFO is 30–46% and thus higher than in the general population [42–44]. Paradoxical embolism has been assumed to be the pathomechanism. However, only few of the reported cases of cryptogenic stroke in patients with PFO meet the criteria for the diagnosis of paradoxical embolism, which are: systemic embolism without a cardiac source, presence of venous thrombosis or pulmonary embolism and an intracardiac defect which will permit right-to-left shunting. Screening especially for venous thromboembolism has been performed only rarely. The results of these studies highlight the importance of searching for venous thromboembolism early after stroke (Table 7.2). Delays in venous diagnostic evaluation may account for negative or confusing results.

There are indications that paradoxical embolism is enhanced by right atrial structures such as Chiari's network or Eustachian valves. These congenital remnants may maintain an embryonic right atrial flow pattern into adult life and direct the blood from the inferior vena cava preferentially toward the interatrial septum [45, 46].

Stroke risk and PFO

It is uncertain whether the recurrence rate of stroke in patients with cryptogenic stroke is dependent on the presence of a PFO. In one observational study of patients treated with aspirin, the incidence of recurrent stroke was higher in patients with than without PFO [47]. In a further prospective randomized study, the recurrence rate of stroke was the same in those with or without PFO in those treated with either warfarin or aspirin [44]. The question of whether subjects from the general population with PFO have an increased risk of ischemic stroke has been studied by two prospective cohort studies, which unanimously found that PFO was not a risk factor for future cerebrovascular events [48, 49]. Overall, it has not been demonstrated that patients with PFO are at increased risk of recurrent stroke. Furthermore, it is uncertain how many strokes in PFO patients are due to paradoxical embolism and how to treat paradoxical embolism. Results from randomized clinical trials on these issues are urgently needed.

Patent foramen closure and risk of recurrent stroke

Surgical or interventional closure of PFO is increasingly performed as a measure to prevent recurrent stroke in patients with suspected paradoxical embolism. However, no randomized trial examining the efficacy of PFO device closure exists [50]. Given the potential risks and costs associated with PFO closure, it would be prudent to await the results of diligently designed randomized clinical trials before recommending this unproven procedure.

Interventional PFO closure might even create new cardiac sources for embolism. Thrombus formation may occur on the left side of the occlusion device and lead to arterial embolism, especially in patients with coagulopathies [51].

> In patients with cryptogenic stroke the prevalence of patent foramen ovale is 30–46%, but patients with PFO are not at increased risk of recurrent stroke.

Atrial septal aneurysm

An atrial septal aneurysm (ASA) is diagnosed echocardiographically if the atrial septum appears abnormally redundant and mobile. Unfortunately, there are no uniform echocardiographic criteria for this abnormality. The etiology of ASA is unknown. ASA is frequently associated with PFO. It is uncertain whether strokes in ASA are due to paradoxical embolism or other mechanisms. The prevalence of ASA, as assessed by echocardiography in the general population, is 1–2% and depends on the echocardiographic criteria. Furthermore, interobserver ($\kappa = 0.45$) and intraobserver ($\kappa = 0.74$) variability in diagnosing ASA is high [41]. Similarly to PFO, ASA has been found to be closely associated with cryptogenic stroke in retrospective and case–control studies, but failed to be identified as a risk factor for future stroke in prospective randomized or population-based studies [44, 47–49]. Due to the rarity of ASA it will be difficult to perform adequately powered studies. Development of uniformly accepted diagnostic criteria would facilitate research into ASA.

> Atrial septal aneurysm has been found to be closely associated with cryptogenic stroke but is not a risk factor for future stroke.

Dilatative cardiomyopathy

Dilatative cardiomyopathy (dCMP) is a cardiac condition characterized by dilatation of the cardiac cavities (LVEDD >57 mm), reduced systolic function (FS <25%), and normal coronary angiography [52]. dCMP is frequently associated with cardiac rhythm abnormalities and intraventricular thrombus formation. Whether dCMP without AF is associated with an increased risk of stroke or embolism is under debate. At least in patients with dCMP and documented intracardiac thrombus formation the risk of stroke or embolism is regarded as being increased. The prevalence of intra-atrial thrombi in patients with dCMP is estimated to be 20–25% and the prevalence of intraventricular thrombi 50% [53]. During an observational period of 31 months 5% of the patients with dCMP developed a stroke [54]. Among 846 patients with ischemic stroke dCMP was found in 19%, who all had benefits from OAC [55]. Single cases with dCMP who developed ischemic stroke have also been reported, such as two patients with dCMP from cardiac involvement in Duchenne muscular dystrophy [56]. Although OAC is recommended for secondary stroke prevention in patients with dCMP and intracardiac thrombus formation [53, 57], the efficacy of OAC for dCMP has never been proved in a prospective clinical study [58].

Restrictive cardiomyopathy

Restrictive cardiomyopathy (rCMP) is diagnosed echocardiographically if there is enlargement of both atria, normal systolic function and wall thickness and a restrictive filling pattern (deceleration time <150 ms) [59]. The cause of rCMP may be idiopathic or rCMP may be a cardiac manifestation of amyloidosis, sclerodermia, sarcoidosis, hemochromatosis, Churg-Strauss syndrome, hypereosinophilic syndrome, hyperoxaluria, cystinosis, Gaucher's disease, Fabry's disease, Noonan's syndrome, Werner's syndrome, reactive arthritis, pseudoxanthoma elasticum, various neuromuscular disorders, carcinoid or lymphoma [59, 60]. Compared to dCMP, patients with rCMP are assumed to have a worse prognosis regarding morbidity and mortality [60]. Whether rCMP is associated with an increased risk of ischemic stroke is unknown, but single cases with rCMP have been described who developed an ischemic stroke [61]. In a study of 15 patients with amyloidosis 60% developed an arterial thromboembolic event, three

113

of whom had an ischemic stroke and two transitory ischemic attacks [62]. Most probably these embolic events have their source in the enlarged left atrium and are aggravated by AF, which develops frequently in rCMP patients [59].

Takotsubo syndrome

Takotsubo syndrome (TTS), also known as apical ballooning, is a reversible neuromyocardial failure which resembles acute myocardial infarction clinically and electrophysiologically in patients with normal coronary arteries [63]. TTS is clinically characterized by sudden onset of anginal chest pain, dyspnea or syncope. Initially, the ECG shows ST elevation, which turns into negative T-waves a few hours or days later, which may persist for months [64, 65]. Reversible akinesia or hypokinesia affects most frequently the left ventricular apex but rarely also the midventricular segments: the non-affected ventricular segments show hyper-contractility. Cardiac enzymes such as creatine phosphokinase and troponin might be slightly elevated. Coronary angiography shows no stenoses of the coronary arteries. The cause and pathogenesis of TTS are unknown, but it may be triggered by physical or emotional stress and catecholamine toxicity [66]. TTS has been described in association with pheochromocytoma, lymphoma, alcohol withdrawal, plasmapheresis, intestinal perforation, severe knee joint pain, overexertion, amyotrophic lateral sclerosis, subarachnoidal hemorrhage, anesthesia, ventricular tachycardia, pneumothorax, pulmonary embolism, maline myopathy, tracheostomy, and metabolic

myopathy [67]. TTS results in significantly reduced systolic function, and wall motion abnormalities, which may give rise to thrombus formation and lastly cardioembolic events. However, cerebral stroke or transient ischemic attack have been only rarely reported during a TTS episode [68, 69].

Left ventricular hypertrabeculation/ non-compaction

Left ventricular hypertrabeculation/noncompaction (LVHT) is characterized by a meshwork of interwoven myocardial strings, lined with endocardium, which constitutes a spongy myocardial layer clearly distinct from the normal compacted myocardium (Figure 7.5) [70]. The noncompacted to compacted layer ratio required to fulfill the diagnostic criteria is >2, although there is no consensus about the echocardiographic criteria to define LVHT [70]. Consensus, however, exists that LVHT is most easily diagnosed on echocardiography. LVHT is most frequently located in the apex of the left ventricle and over the lateral wall, but usually spares the middle and basal parts of the septum. LVHT is frequently associated with heart failure and systolic dysfunction, which have been also identified as prognostic factors in LVHT [71]. Because of the heterogeneous genetic background of LVHT it does not seem to represent a distinct cardiomyopathy but is rather the result of an attempt to compensate for an insufficiently contracting myocardium or possibly the result of myocarditis. LVHT is associated with neuromuscular disorders

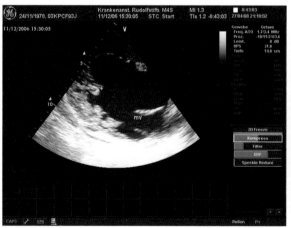
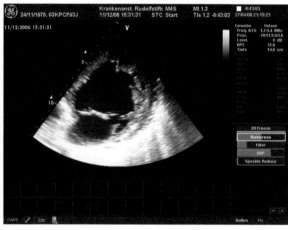

Figure 7.5. Transthoracic echocardiographic parasternal long axis view (left) and apical four-chamber view (right) showing left ventricular hypertrabeculation/non-compaction involving the posterobasal and lateral wall (left).

(NMDs) in up to 82% of the cases, if systematically searched for [72]. Among all NMDs, Barth syndrome is the one most frequently associated with LVHT [73].

No consensus has been reached so far as to whether LVHT is associated with an increased risk of stroke/embolism or not. In a study on 62 patients with LVHT no increased risk of these patients developing stroke/embolism as compared with age, sex, and left ventricular fractional shortening matched controls was found [70]. In a retrospective study of 104 patients with LVHT stroke was found on imaging studies in 16% of them [74]. Though stroke/embolism has been reported in single patients with LVHT, we regard it as not justified to generally propose OAC for LVHT patients, unless there is concomitant AF, severely reduced left ventricular systolic function, or any other established indication of OAC. So far there is no evidence for a general clotting defect in LVHT patents requiring OAC [70].

Endomyocardial fibrosis

Endomyocardial fibrosis is a rare disease in European countries and is more prevalent in women than in men. Clinically, endomyocardial fibrosis is characterized by severe congestive heart failure with only moderately increased heart size. Systolic performance is normal or only slightly depressed despite severe restriction on filling, atrioventricular valve regurgitation, or both. Echocardiography may reveal partial obliteration of the right or left ventricle [75]. Endocardial resection with atrioventricular valve replacement is the treatment of choice, with appreciable postoperative improvement and a 10-year survival of approximately 70% [75]. Whether there is a generally increased risk of stroke in patients with endomyocardial fibrosis is unknown, but single patients have been reported who developed an ischemic stroke. Among these is one who developed multiple ischemic strokes in association with endomyocardial fibrosis from schistosomiasis and one with multiple cerebellar and cerebral infarctions from endomyocardial fibrosis associated with hypereosinophilic syndrome [76].

Chapter Summary

Rhythm disturbances
Atrial fibrillation (AF) may lead to embolic stroke or peripheral or mesenteric embolism. Patients with AF have a 5-fold (non-rheumatic AF) to 17-fold

increased risk of stroke (embolism due to rheumatic heart disease). Diagnosis of permanent AF is feasible from the 12-lead electrocardiogram, and paroxysomal AF can be diagnosed with 24–72-hour Holter monitoring or 7-day event loop recorders. Surgical or percutaneous closure of the left atrial appendage is considered as an alternative to oral anticoagulation to prevent strokes in AF.

Brady- or tachycardia causes symptoms such as dizziness, light-headedness, spells or fainting. These symptoms may erroneously be interpreted as epileptic seizures.

QT prolongation: stroke is associated with QT prolongation in 30–40% of patients. QT prolongation in stroke may be due to cardiovascular comorbidity, concomitant drug intake and metabolic disturbances, but may also be due to the affected brain region, especially the insular region. QT prolongation may be associated with torsades de pointes tachycardia, which is associated with palpitations, dizziness or syncope. Degeneration into ventricular fibrillation and sudden cardiac death can occur.

Coronary heart disease
There is a frequent coexistence of coronary heart disease and stroke, most probably due to common atherosclerotic risk factors. Suspected coronary heart disease should lead to cardiological consultation for further therapeutic and diagnostic measures, including coronary angiography and percutaneous coronary intervention. Acute or subacute myocardial infarction and ventricular aneurysms can also be a cause of embolic stroke.

Valvular heart disease
Ischemic and hemorrhagic strokes occur in 10 to 23% of patients with endocarditis, especially of the mitral valve. Diagnosis of infective endocarditis is difficult. Thus, endocarditis has to be considered as a differential diagnosis in all stroke patients if laboratory signs of inflammation are present.

After heart valve surgery patients are at increased risk of thromboembolism. The embolic risk varies according to the type of surgery (repair versus replacement), the type of replaced valve (bioprosthesis versus mechanical prosthesis) and the affected valve (mitral versus aortic valve).

Patent foramen ovale (PFO)
In about 25% of humans the foramen ovale remains open, permitting right-to-left shunting when the right atrial pressure exceeds the left atrial pressure. In patients with cryptogenic stroke the prevalence of

PFO is 30–46% (paradoxical embolism from venous thrombosis), but it has not been demonstrated that patients with PFO are at increased risk of recurrent stroke and no randomized trials exist examining the efficacy of PFO device closure to prevent recurrent stroke.

Atrial septal aneurysms

An atrial septal aneurysm is diagnosed echo-cardiographically if the atrial septum appears abnormally redundant and mobile. Similarly to PFO, atrial septal aneurysm has been found to be closely associated with cryptogenic stroke in retrospective and case–control studies, but failed to be identified as a risk factor for future stroke in prospective randomized or population-based studies.

It is unknown whether conditions such as **dilative cardiomyopathy, restrictive cardiomyopathy, Takotsubo syndrome** (a reversible neuromyocardial failure, which resembles acute myocardial infarction clinically and electrophysiologically in patients with normal coronary arteries), **left ventricular hypertrabeculation** or **endomyocardial fibrosis** raise the risk of stroke independently of the presence of atrial fibrillation.

References

1. Feinberg WM, Blackshear JL, Laupacis A, et al. Prevalence, age distribution, and gender of patients with atrial fibrillation. *Arch Intern Med* 1995; **155**:469–73.

2. Wolf PA, Dawber TR, Thomas HE Jr, Kannel WB. Epidemiologic assessment of chronic atrial fibrillation and risk of stroke: The Framingham Study. *Neurology* 1978; **28**:973–77.

3. Saxena R, Lewis S, Berge E, et al., for the International Stroke Trial Collaborative Group. Risk of early death and recurrent stroke and effect of heparin in 3169 patients with acute ischemic stroke and atrial fibrillation in the international stroke trial. *Stroke* 2001; **32**:2333–7.

4. Marini C, De Santis F, Sacco S, et al. Contribution of atrial fibrillation to incidence and outcome of ischemic stroke. Results from a population-based study. *Stroke* 2005; **36**:1115–9.

5. Steger C, Pratter A, Martinek-Bregel M, et al. Stroke patients with atrial fibrillation have a worse prognosis than patients without: data from the Austrian Stroke registry. *Eur Heart J* 2004; **25**: 1734–40.

6. Liao J, Khalid Z, Scallan C, et al. Noninvasive cardiac monitoring for detecting paroxysmal atrial fibrillation or flutter after acute ischemic stroke. A systematic review. *Stroke* 2007; **38**:2935–40.

7. Wallmann D, Tüller D, Wustmann K, et al. Frequent atrial premature beats predict paroxysmal atrial fibrillation in stroke patients. An opportunity for a new diagnostic strategy. *Stroke* 20007; **38**:2292–4.

8. Douen AG, Pageau N, Medic S. Serial electrocardiographic assessments significantly improve detection of atrial fibrillation 2.6-fold in patients with acute stroke. *Stroke* 2008; **39**:480–2.

9. Spring M, Dorian P, Fry B, et al. A 30-day cardiac event monitor belt for recording paroxysmal atrial fibrillation after a cerebral ischemic event. The EMBRACE Pilot Study. *Stroke*; 2008; **39**:571–2.

10. Sick PB, Schuler G, Hauptmann KE, et al. Initial worldwide experience with the WATCHMAN left atrial appendage system for stroke prevention in atrial fibrillation. *J Am Coll Cardiol* 2007; **49**:1490–5.

11. Stöllberger C, Chnupa P, Kronik G, et al. Transesophageal echocardiography to assess embolic risk in patients with atrial fibrillation. *Ann Intern Med* 1998; **128**:630–8.

12. Stöllberger C, Schneider B, Finsterer J. Elimination of the left atrial appendage to prevent stroke or embolism? Anatomic, physiologic, and pathophysiologic considerations. *Chest* 2003; **124**:2356–62.

13. Moro C, Crampes F, Sengenes C, et al. Atrial natriuretic peptide contributes to physiological control of lipid mobilization in humans. *FASEB J* 2004; **18**:908–10.

14. Natale A, Raviele A, Arentz T, et al. Venice Chart international consensus document on atrial fibrillation ablation. *J Cardiovasc Electrophysiol* 2007; **18**:560–80.

15. Lee SH, Tai CT, Hsieh MH, et al. Predictors of early and late recurrence of atrial fibrillation after catheter ablation of paroxysmal atrial fibrillation. *J Interv Card Electrophysiol* 2004; **10**:221–6.

16. Hindricks G, Piorkowski C, Tanner H, et al. Perception of atrial fibrillation before and after radiofrequency catheter ablation: relevance of asymptomatic arrhythmia recurrence. *Circulation* 2005; **112**:307–13.

17. Oppenheimer S. Cerebrogenic cardiac arrhythmias: cortical lateralization and clinical significance. *Clin Auton Res* 2006; **16**:6–11.

18. Topilski I, Rogowski O, Rosso R, et al. The morphology of the QT interval predicts torsade de pointes during acquired bradyarrhythmias. *J Am Coll Cardiol* 2007; **49**:320–8.

19. Tatschl C, Stöllberger C, Matz K, et al. Insular involvement is associated with QT prolongation:

ECG abnormalities in patients with acute stroke. *Cerebrovasc Dis* 2006; **21**:47–53.

20. Fure B, Bruun Wyller T, Thommessen B. Electrocardiographic and troponin T changes in acute ischaemic stroke. *J Intern Med* 2006; **259**:592–7.

21. Dhamoon MS, Tai W, Boden-Albala B, et al. Risk of myocardial infarction or vascular death after first ischemic stroke. The Northern Manhattan Study. *Stroke* 2007; **38**:1752–8.

22. Gongora-Rivera F, Labreuche J, Jaramillo A, et al. Autopsy prevalence of coronary atherosclerosis in patients with fatal stroke. *Stroke* 2007; **38**:1203–10.

23. Hankey GJ, Majrozik K, Broadhurst RJ, et al. Five-year survival after first-ever stroke and related prognostic factors in the Perth Community Stroke Study. *Stroke* 2000; **31**:2080–6.

24. Barber M, Morton JJ, Macfarlane PW, et al. Elevated troponin levels are associated with sympathoadrenal activation in acute ischaemic stroke. *Cerebrovasc Dis* 2007; **23**:260–6.

25. Jensen JK, Kristensen SR, Bak S, et al. Frequency and significance of troponin T elevation in acute ischemic stroke. *Am J Cardiol* 2007; **99**:108–12.

26. Finsterer J, Stöllberger C, Krugluger W. Cardiac and noncardiac, particularly neuromuscular, disease with troponin-T positivity. *Neth J Med* 2007; **65**:289–95.

27. Vaitkus PT, Barnathan EX. Embolic potential, prevention and management of mural thrombus complicating anterior myocardial infarction: a meta-analysis. *J Am Coll Cardiol* 1993; **22**:1004–9.

28. Zielinska M, Kaczmarek K, Tylkowski M. Predictors of left ventricular thrombus formation in acute myocardial infarction treated with successful primary angioplasty with stenting. *Am J Med Sci* 2008; **335**:171–6.

29. Dickerman SA, Abrutyn E, Barsic B, et al. The relationship between the initiation of antimicrobial therapy and the incidence of stroke in infective endocarditis: an analysis from the ICE prospective cohort study (ICE-PCS). *Am Heart J* 2007; **154**: 1086–94.

30. Cabell CH, Pond KK, Peterson GE, et al. The risk of stroke and death in patients with aortic and mitral valve endocarditis. *Am Heart J* 2001; **142**:75–80.

31. Anderson DJ, Goldstein LB, Wilkinson WE, et al. Stroke location, characterization, severity, and outcome in mitral vs aortic valve endocarditis. *Neurology* 2003; **61**:1341–6.

32. Thuny F, Avierinos JF, Tribouilloy C, et al. Impact of cerebrovascular complications on mortality and neurologic outcome during infective endocarditis:

a prospective multicentre study. *Eur Heart J* 2007; **28**:1155–61.

33. Wang A, Athan E, Pappas PA, et al. Contemporary clinical profile and outcome of prosthetic valve endocarditis. *JAMA* 2007; **297**:1354–61.

34. Schulz R, Werner GS, Fuchs JB, et al. Clinical outcome and echocardiographic findings of native and prosthetic valve endocarditis in the 1990s. *Eur Heart J* 1996; **17**:281–8.

35. Parrino PE, Kron IL, Ross SD, et al. Does a focal neurologic deficit contraindicate operation in a patient with endocarditis? *Ann Thorac Surg* 1999; **67**:59–64.

36. Ruttmann E, Willeit J, Ulmer H, et al. Neurological outcome of septic cardioembolic stroke after infective endocarditis. *Stroke* 2006; **37**:2094–9.

37. Ruel M, Masters RG, Rubens FD, et al. Late incidence and determinants of stroke after aortic and mitral valve replacement. *Ann Thorac Surg* 2004; **78**:77–84.

38. Russo A, Grigioni F, Avierinos JF, et al. Thromboembolic complications after surgical correction of mitral regurgitation. *J Am Coll Cardiol* 2008; **51**:1203–11.

39. Kulik A, Bédard P, Lam BK, et al. Mechanical versus bioprosthetic valve replacement in middle-aged patients. *Eur J Cardio-thorac Surg* 2006; **30**:485–91.

40. Will MB, Bernacca GM, Bell EF, et al. Our inability to predict thromboembolic events after prosthetic valve surgery. *J Heart Valve Dis* 2006; **15**:570–80.

41. Cabanes L, Coste J, Derumeaux G, et al. Interobserver and intraobserver variability in detection of patent foramen ovale and atrial septal aneurysm with transesophageal echocardiography. *J Am Soc Echocardiogr* 2002; **15**:441–6.

42. Lechat P, Mas JL, Lascault G, et al. Prevalence of patent foramen ovale in patients with stroke. *N Engl J Med* 1988; **318**:1148–52.

43. Lamy C, Giannesini C, Zuber M, et al. Clinical and imaging findings in cryptogenic stroke patients with and without patent foramen ovale. The PFO-ASA Study. *Stroke* 2002; **33**:706–11.

44. Homma S, Sacco RL, Di Tullio MR, et al., for the PFO in Cryptogenic Stroke Study (PICSS) Investigators. Effect of medical treatment in stroke patients with patent foramen ovale. Patent Foramen Ovale in Cryptogenic Stroke Study. *Circulation* 2002; **105**: 2625–31.

45. Schneider B, Hofmann T, Justen MH, et al. Chiari's network: normal anatomic variant or risk factor for arterial embolic events? *J Am Coll Cardiol* 1995; **26**:203–10.

46. Schuchlenz HW, Saurer G, Weihs W, et al. Persisting Eustachian valve in adults: relation to patent foramen

ovale and cerebrovascular events. *J Am Soc Echocardiogr* 2004; **17**:231–3.

47. Mas JL, Arquizan C, Lamy C, et al. Patent Foramen Ovale and Atrial Septal Aneurysm Study Group. Recurrent cerebrovascular events associated with patent foramen ovale, atrial septal aneurysm, or both. *N Engl J Med* 2001; **345**:1740–6.

48. Di Tullio MR, Sacco RL, Sciacca RR, et al. Patent foramen ovale and the risk of ischemic stroke in a multiethnic population. *J Am Coll Cardiol* 2007; **49**:797–802.

49. Meissner I, Khandheria BK, Heit JA, et al. Patent foramen ovale: innocent or guilty? Evidence from a prospective population-based study. *J Am Coll Cardiol* 2006; **47**:440–5.

50. Slottow TL, Steinberg DH, Waksman R. Overview of the 2007 Food and Drug Administration Circulatory System Devices Panel meeting on patent foramen ovale closure devices. *Circulation* 2007; **116**:677–82.

51. Stöllberger C, Finsterer J, Krexner E, et al. Stroke and peripheral embolism from an Amplatzer septal occluder 5 years after implantation. *J Neurol* 2008; **255**:1270–1.

52. Burkett EL, Hershberger RE. Clinical and genetic issues in familial dilated cardiomyopathy. *J Am Coll Cardiol* 2005; **45**:969–81.

53. Gibelin P. Anticoagulant treatment and dilated cardiomyopathy. *Arch Mal Coeur Vaiss* 1995; **88**(suppl 4):617–21.

54. Crawford TC, Smith WT 4th, Velazquez EJ, et al. Prognostic usefulness of left ventricular thrombus by echocardiography in dilated cardiomyopathy in predicting stroke, transient ischemic attack, and death. *Am J Cardiol* 2004; **93**:500–3.

55. Tribolet de Abreu TT, Mateus S, et al. Therapy implications of transthoracic echocardiography in acute ischemic stroke patients. *Stroke* 2005; **36**:1565–6.

56. Ikeniwa C, Sakai M, Kimura S, et al. Two cases of Duchenne muscular dystrophy complicated with dilated cardiomyopathy and cerebral infarction. *No To Shinkei* 2006; **58**:250–5.

57. McCabe DJ, Rakhit RD. Antithrombotic and interventional treatment options in cardioembolic transient ischaemic attack and ischaemic stroke. *J Neurol Neurosurg Psychiatry* 2007; **78**:14–24.

58. Stokman PJ, Nandra CS, Asinger RW. Left ventricular thrombus. *Curr Treat Options Cardiovasc Med* 2001; **3**:515–21.

59. Stöllberger C, Finsterer J. Extracardiac medical and neuromuscular implications in restrictive cardiomyopathy. *Clin Cardiol* 2007; **30**:375–80.

60. Artz G, Wynne J. Restrictive cardiomyopathy. *Curr Treat Options Cardiovasc Med* 2000; **2**:431–8.

61. Salih MA, Al-Jarallah AS, Abdel-Gader AG, et al. Cardiac diseases as a risk factor for stroke in Saudi children. *Saudi Med J* 2006; **27**(suppl 1):S61–8.

62. Hausfater P, Costedoat-Chalumeau N, Amoura Z, et al. AL cardiac amyloidosis and arterial thromboembolic events. *Scand J Rheumatol* 2005; **34**:315–9.

63. Stöllberger C, Finsterer J, Schneider B. Tako-tsubo-like left ventricular dysfunction: clinical presentation, instrumental findings, additional cardiac and non-cardiac diseases and potential pathomechanisms. *Minerva Cardioangiol* 2005; **53**:139–45.

64. Abe Y, Kondo M, Matsuoka R, et al. Assessment of clinical features in transient left ventricular apical ballooning. *J Am Coll Cardiol* 2003; **41**: 737–42.

65. Gianni M, Dentali F, Grandi AM, et al. Apical ballooning syndrome or takotsubo cardiomyopathy: a systematic review. *Eur Heart J* 2006; **27**:1523–9.

66. Ueyama T, Senba E, Kasamatsu K, et al. Molecular mechanism of emotional stress-induced and catecholamine-induced heart attack. *J Cardiovasc Pharmacol* 2003; **41**(suppl 1):S115–8.

67. Finsterer J, Stöllberger C, Sehnal E, et al. Apical ballooning (Takotsubo syndrome) in mitochondrial disorder during mechanical ventilation. *J Cardiovasc Med (Hagerstown)* 2007; **8**:859–63.

68. Lemke DM, Hussain SI, Wolfe TJ, et al. Takotsubo cardiomyopathy associated with seizures. *Neurocrit Care* 2008; (in press)

69. Matsuoka K, Nakayama S, Okubo S, et al. Transient cerebral ischemic attack induced by transient left ventricular apical ballooning. *Eur J Intern Med* 2004; **15**:393–5.

70. Stöllberger C, Finsterer J. Left ventricular hypertrabeculation/noncompaction. *J Am Soc Echocardiogr* 2004; **17**:91–100.

71. Stöllberger C, Winkler-Dworak M, Blazek G, et al. Prognosis of left ventricular hypertrabeculation/ noncompaction is dependent on cardiac and neuromuscular comorbidity. *Int J Cardiol* 2007; **121**:189–93.

72. Stöllberger C, Finsterer J, Blazek G. Left ventricular hypertrabeculation/noncompaction and association with additional cardiac abnormalities and neuromuscular disorders. *Am J Cardiol* 2002; **90**:899–902.

73. Finsterer J, Stöllberger C, Blazek G. Prevalence of Barth syndrome in adult left ventricular hypertrabeculation /noncompaction. *Scand Cardiovasc J* 2008; **42**:157–60.

74. Finsterer J, Stöllberger C, Mölzer G, et al. Cerebrovascular events in adult left ventricular hypertrabeculation/noncompaction with and without myopathy. *Int J Cardiol* 2007; December 17, Epub.

75. Schneider U, Jenni R, Turina J, et al. Long-term follow up of patients with endomyocardial fibrosis: effects of surgery. *Heart* 1998; **79**:362–7.

76. Sarazin M, Caumes E, Cohen A, et al. Multiple microembolic borderzone brain infarctions and endomyocardial fibrosis in idiopathic hypereosinophilic syndrome and in *Schistosoma mansoni* infestation. *J Neurol Neurosurg Psychiatry* 2004; **75**:305–7.

77. Gautier JC, Dürr A, Koussa S, et al. Paradoxical cerebral embolism with a patent foramen ovale. A report of 29 patients. *Cerebrovasc Dis* 1991; **1**:193–202.

78. Stöllberger C, Slany J, Schuster I, et al. The prevalence of deep venous thrombosis in patients with suspected paradoxical embolism. *Ann Intern Med* 1993; **119**:461–5.

79. Ranoux D, Cohen A, Cabanes L, et al. Patent foramen ovale: is stroke due to paradoxical embolism? *Stroke* 1993; **24**:31–4.

80. Itoh T, Matsumoto M, Handa N, et al. Paradoxical embolism as a cause of ischemic stroke of uncertain etiology. A transcranial Doppler sonographic study. *Stroke* 1994; **25**:771–5.

81. Hanna JP, Sun JP, Furlan AJ, et al. Patent foramen ovale and brain infarct. Echocardiographic predictors, recurrence, and prevention. *Stroke* 1994; **25**:782–6.

82. Klötzsch C, Janßen G, Berlit P. Transesophageal echocardiography and contrast-TCD in the detection of a patent foramen ovale: experiences with 111 patients. *Neurology* 1994; **44**:1603–6.

83. Rohr-Le Floch J. Foramen ovale perméable et embolie paradoxale: une hypothèse controversée. *Rev Neurol (Paris)* 1994; **150**:282–5.

84. Lethen H, Flachskampf FA, Schneider R, et al. Frequency of deep vein thrombosis in patients with patent foramen ovale and ischemic stroke or transient ischemic attack. *Am J Cardiol* 1997; **80**:1066–9.

85. Cramer SC, Rordorf G, Maki JH, et al. Increased pelvic vein thrombi in cryptogenic stroke. Results of the Paradoxical Emboli From Large Veins in Ischemic Stroke (PELVIS) Study. *Stroke* 2004; **35**:46–50.

8

Common stroke syndromes

Céline Odier and Patrik Michel

Introduction

The approach to neurovascular disease has considerably changed over the last decade. With advances in neuroimaging, localization of the lesion has become easier. However, clinical recognition of stroke syndromes is still very important for several reasons.

First, in the acute phase, it enables diagnosis, exclusion of stroke imitators (migraine, epilepsy, PRES, anxiety, psychogenic, etc.), and recognition of rare manifestations of stroke, such as cognitive-behavioral presentations which are easily misdiagnosed.

Second, it contributes to the planning of acute interventions by localizing the stroke (anterior versus posterior circulation or cortical versus subcortical involvement) and by interpretation of imaging abnormalities. Each subtype of stroke may benefit from intravenous thrombolysis for example, but only some subtypes, such as proximal intracranial occlusion, may be appropriate candidates for acute endovascular recanalization.

Third, during hospitalization, localization helps to direct the subsequent work-up. If a cardioembolic etiology is suspected, for instance, it would lead to more intensive cardiac investigations, such as transesophageal echography or repeated 24-hour cardiac rhythm recording. In contrast, if a lacunar etiology is presumed, the cardiac investigation may remain limited.

Fourth, it also allows the clinician to anticipate, recognize and treat complications related to a specific stroke type, such as large fluctuations in the lacunar "capsular warning syndrome" or brainstem compression from cerebellar edema.

Finally, making the correct diagnosis means choosing the appropriate secondary prevention. In the presence of a significant carotid stenosis, endarterectomy may be very effective if the recent stroke occurred in the territory distal to the stenosis, but of limited effectiveness if another territory is involved.

Several classifications for stroke territory, mechanism and etiology exist. The TOAST classification [1] is most frequently used for stroke mechanism, but is partially outdated (Table 8.1). A modification of it (SS-TOAST) adds a variety of clinical and radiological criteria and seems more accurate [2]. The greater difficulty in using it has been improved by a recently published computer algorithm. The Oxfordshire method defines four subtypes of strokes according to clinical presentation attributed to a vascular territory: lacunar infarcts (LACI), total anterior circulation infarcts (TACI), partial anterior circulation infarcts (PACI), and posterior circulation infarcts (POCI).

In this chapter, we will discuss classic presentations of anterior circulation, posterior circulation, lacunar, watershed, and hemorrhagic strokes and try to identify clinical clues which can improve the diagnosis.

Anterior circulation syndromes

The anterior circulation refers to the part of the brain perfused by the carotid arteries. There are five main intracranial branches, which are from proximal to distal: ophthalmic, posterior communicating (PCoA), anterior choroidal (AChA), anterior cerebral (ACA) and middle cerebral (MCA) arteries. In some individuals, 2–10% according to different authors [3, 4], the posterior cerebral artery (PCA) comes from the carotid artery, via a large PCoA, while the proximal PCA originating from the basilar artery is hypo- or aplastic. In these cases, the anterior circulation irrigates the PCA territory. This variant of the circle of Willis is also known as a fetal origin of the PCA.

The anterior circulation can be subdivided into two systems, the leptomeningeal artery system vascularizing the cortex, the adjacent white matter and the AChA, and the deep perforating artery system, perfusing the basal ganglia, the centrum semiovale and the parts of internal capsule.

Table 8.1. Stroke categories according to the TOAST classification.

1. Large-vessel disease

2. Small-vessel disease

3. Cardioembolism

4. Other etiology

5. Undetermined or multiple possible etiologies

Middle cerebral artery (MCA)

The middle cerebral artery (MCA) is also designated the Sylvian artery, from Jacques Dubois, known as Jacobus Sylvius (1489–1555), a linguist and anatomist in Paris. The artery is subdivided into the M1 segment, from which start the deep perforating lenticulostriate arteries, the M2 segment, corresponding to the segment after the bifurcation into superior and inferior divisions, and the M3 segment, including the insular part. The M4 segments, the leptomeningeal arteries, arise from the M3 segments and are named orbito-frontal, prefrontal, precentral, central sulcus, anterior parietal, posterior parietal, angular and temporal arteries, with important variations in their territories.

The MCA territory is the one most frequently affected by acute strokes. MCA territory infarcts can be subtle or a devastating clinical syndrome, depending on the site of the occlusion, the extent of ischemia, the etiology, and the collateral arterial network. As collateral networks are highly variable, an occlusion of the same artery at the same place may lead to quite variable severity of the stroke and of prognosis. Large infarcts are defined as involvement of two of the three MCA territories (deep, superior and inferior divisions) and "malignant MCA stroke" as complete or near complete MCA territory infarction with ensuing mass effect from brain edema.

Clinically, a patient with an *acute complete MCA* infarction presents contralateral hemiparesis, hemihypesthesia, hemianopsia, and ipsilateral conjugated eye and head deviation (the patient looks at his/her lesion). The patient is usually awake or presents mild drowsiness or agitation, particularly with a right infarct. Cognitive signs are always present: in the case of a left lesion, aphasia, and most of the time global, ideomotor apraxia. In the case of a right lesion, contralateral multimodal hemineglect (visual, motor, sensitive, visual, spatial, auditive), anosognosia (denial of illness), anosodiaphoria (indifference to illness),

asomatognosia (lack of awareness of a part of one's own body) and confusional state are seen. This picture suggests an M1 occlusion with or without carotid occlusion and is associated with a rather unfavorable prognosis. Particularly in younger people, malignant stroke with brain edema may develop, leading to high intracranial pressure and subsequent subfacial, uncal and transtentorial herniation. The clinical deterioration occurs typically within 48–72 hours, when vigilance decreases and initial signs worsen. New cortical symptoms may occur because of infarction of ACA or PCA arteries, which become compressed against interhemispheric falx and cerebellar tentorium, respectively. When the herniation of the medial temporal lobe continues, the uncus compresses the third cranial nerve, leading to an ipsilateral fixed mydriasis and the contralateral cerebral peduncle is compressed against the cerebellar tentorium, leading to ipsilateral corticospinal signs, such as Babinski's sign and paresis (Kernohan notch). A bilateral ptosis has also been described as an imminent sign of temporal herniation, mostly in a right malignant MCA infarct [5]. Early recognition of patients at risk enables the medical team to propose a hemicraniectomy for selected patients, a treatment which has proved highly effective if performed within 48 hours and before those signs occur [6].

A *complete superficial MCA* infarct, sparing the lenticulostriated arteries, suggests a thrombus in a distal part of the MCA trunk, at the bifurcation of the artery (proximal M2 segment). Motor and sensitive functions of the lower limbs are less involved than the face and arms. If leg involvement is important and persistent, concomitant ischemia in the internal capsule (AChA) or in the ACA territory should be suspected. The visual field deficit may be a contralateral homonymous hemianopia or a quadrantanopsia. The deviation of the head and the eyes is more transitory and the sensitive deficit is less severe. Cognitive deficits are similar to an M1 occlusion but often less pronounced or rapidly improving.

An infarct of the *superior* (sometimes called *anterior*) M2 division of the MCA manifests itself clinically with contralateral isolated brachiofacial paresis, partial brachiofacial sensitive loss (mainly tactile and discriminative modalities), transient conjugate ipsilateral eye and head deviation and aphasia (aphemia or Broca aphasia) frequently associated with buccolingual apraxia in the case of left infarcts and various degrees of multimodal hemineglect, anosognosia, anosodiaphoria, confusion and monotone language in right lesions. Visual fields are usually spared.

In the presence of an infarct of the *inferior* (sometimes called *posterior*) M2 division of the MCA, less frequent than superior division infarction, the presentation includes contralateral homonymous hemianopsia or upper quadrantanopsia, mild or transient brachiofacial paresis and cognitive disturbances, which are the dominant part of the picture. With a left lesion, Wernicke's aphasia or conduction aphasia are observed and with a right lesion, hemineglect, constructional and clothing dyspraxia, spatial disorientation, behavioral changes, confusional state, hallucination, delusions and amusia may be present.

Involvement of one of the *leptomeningeal branches* (M3 or M4) can produce highly circumscribed infarcts accompanied by specific neurological deficits and is most of the time related to embolism. For example, an isolated Wernicke's aphasia occurs with occlusion of the left posterior temporal branch and suggests strongly a cardioembolic mechanism, particularly in the elderly.

The lenticulostriate arteries vascularize the basal ganglia and parts of the internal capsule. Ischemia in their territory can therefore produce severe deficits with a very small-volume lesion. Cortical signs are absent or minor, except in the case of deafferentation of the cortex by interruption of subcortical cortical pathways. Clinical signs include proportional hemiparesis, hemihypesthesia, dysarthria, hypophonia, and occasionally abnormal movements in the case of involvement of basal ganglia.

The centrum ovale receives its blood supply from medullary perforating arteries coming principally from leptomeningeal arteries. Small infarcts (less than 1.5 cm) usually present as lacunar syndromes but deficits are often less proportional than in pontine or internal capsule lacunes.

Etiology in the deep perforator territories of the MCA is mostly lipohyalinosis and local arteriolosclerosis, in contrast with larger and multiple infarcts, which are embolic from an arterial or cardiac source. Both small and larger lesions may occur in the border-zone area between the deep (leptomeningeal) and superficial (meningeal) arteries from hemodynamic mechanisms (see below).

> The MCA territory is the one most frequently affected by acute strokes. Symptoms of an *acute complete MCA* infarction: contralateral hemiparesis, hemihypesthesia, hemianopsia, ipsilateral conjugated eye and head deviation (the patient looks at his/her lesion); plus, in the case of a left lesion, aphasia, and in the case of a right lesion, contralateral multimodal hemineglect. Malignant stroke with brain edema

may develop, leading to high intracranial pressure and subsequent herniation.

Infarctions of the lower arterial segments show similar symptoms, but not the complete picture.

Anterior cerebral artery (ACA)

The ACA is subdivided into the A1 segment (before the anterior communicating artery (ACoA)), followed by the A2 segment (after the ACoA), then A3 segments. The A1 segment has deep perforating arteries, named the medial lenticulostriate arteries, and gives rise to the recurrent artery of Heubner (raH), which supplies the caudate head, the genu and anterior arm of the internal capsule and the supero-anterior putamen. Both the lenticulostriate arteries and the raH are particularly vulnerable during aneurysm surgery of the ACoA.

The clinical presentation of ACA infarcts includes weakness predominantly of the distal lower limb and to a lesser degree of the upper limb, motor hemineglect, transcortical motor aphasia and behavioral disturbances (with involvement of the supplementary motor area). Sensory hemisyndromes affecting mainly the contralateral leg are also described. Sphincter dysfunction, mutism, anterograde amnesia, grasping, and behavioral disturbances are particularly frequent in ischemia of the deep perforating arteries and the raH. Involvement of the corpus callosum can produce the callosal disconnection syndrome, secondary to interruption of the connection of physical information from the right hemisphere to cognitive center in the left hemisphere. Therefore, it is restricted to the left hand, which presents ideomotor apraxia, agraphia, tactile anomia (inability to name objects placed into the left palm) and the alien-hand syndrome.

> *ACA infarcts cause* weakness predominantly of the distal lower limb and to a lesser degree of the upper limb, motor hemineglect and transcortical motor aphasia.

Anterior choroidal artery (AChA)

The boundaries of the territory supplied by the AChA are still controversial [7], probably reflecting interpersonal variants. The artery vascularizes to a variable degree the inferior posterior and retrolenticular part of the internal capsule, the tail of the caudate nucleus, part of the lenticular nucleus, the posterior corona radiata, the lateral geniculate body and the beginning of the optic radiations. Clinically less important are variable contributions to the vascular supply of the uncus, amygdala, hippocampus, optic tract, parts of midbrain (substantia nigra, cerebral peduncle), sub-thalamic region, and choroid plexus.

In the majority of patients, the presentation is a lacunar syndrome: pure motor or sensorimotor hemiparesis and less frequently a pure sensory deficit or an ataxic hemiparesis syndrome.

A rarer but typical presentation of AChA infarcts is the triad of contralateral severe hemiparesis, hemihypesthesia and upper quadrantanopsia or contralateral versus ipsilateral hemianopsia (in the case of lateral geniculate body or optic tract, respectively) without cognitive disturbances, in contrast with MCA infarction. A rare but specific visual field defect is a homonymous defect in the upper and lower quadrants with sparing of a horizontal sector [8].

Rarely, cognitive signs occur in AChA infarcts secondarily to involvement of thalamocortical pathways, including hemineglect and constructional apraxia with right lesion and thalamic aphasia (fluent language with relatively preserved comprehension and repetition but anomia, jargon speech and semantic paraphasic errors) with left infarct. AchA infarct may therefore imitate incomplete MCA strokes.

> Lacunar syndrome within AChA territory causes most frequently pure motor or sensorimotor hemiparesis. A rarer but typical presentation of AChA infarcts is the triad of contralateral severe hemiparesis, hemihypesthesia and upper quadrantanopsia.

Internal carotid artery (ICA)

The manifestations of acute internal carotid occlusion are quite variable, depending on the collateral status and preexisting carotid stenosis. *Embolic occlusion of the ICA*, either proximally or distally, usually leads to severe stroke, showing concomitant signs of all anterior circulation arteries. Consciousness is usually more decreased and leg weakness more severe and persistent than in isolated proximal MCA occlusion.

In contrast, a progressive atherosclerotic occlusion is usually less severe, with a classic subacute two-phase presentation. It may even be asymptomatic. Retinal ischemia from carotid emboli may be transient (amaurosis fugax) or persistent (central retinal artery occlusion or branch retinal artery occlusion). It often occurs in isolation and requires urgent work-up including detailed ophthalmological examination, carotid imaging and a search for Horton's arteritis.

In the case of a chronic ICA stenosis or occlusion, hemodynamic stress such as hypotension can lead to a watershed stroke.

In rare situations, an individual can present a *limb-shaking TIA*, which manifests as a choreic or a coarse tremor-like abnormal movement of variable frequency and several minutes duration, mostly of the upper extremity. It typically occurs when an orthostatic stress leads to a hypoperfusion of the brain [9] secondary to carotid severe stenosis.

> *Embolic occlusion of the ICA*, either proximally or distally, usually leads to severe stroke, showing concomitant signs of all anterior circulation arteries. *A progressive atherosclerotic occlusion* is usually less severe, with a classic subacute two-phase presentation or even asymptomatic. Retinal ischemia from carotid emboli may be transient (amaurosis fugax) or persistent.

Posterior circulation syndromes

The posterior circulation is also called the vertebrobasilar circulation. The two vertebral arteries leave the subclavian arteries, pass through transverse foramina in the apophysis of the sixth to the second cervical vertebra, enter the cranium through the foramen magnum, and join together to form the basilar artery (BA). The BA gives several paramedian and circumferential branches as well as four cerebellar arteries, and then splits into two PCAs at the level of the cerebellar tentorium. There exist numerous individual variations, the clinically most important being the fetal origin of the PCAs from the carotid arteries (via the PCoA).

Clinical clues to differentiate posterior from anterior circulation strokes

Important clinical symptoms and signs point to a posterior circulation stroke and should be recognized. Preceding TIAs and strokes in the days and hours before are more frequent in the posterior circulation. Similarly, headache is more frequent in the posterior circulation, is typically ipsilateral to the infarct, and may have features of primary headaches such as migraine [10].

Past diplopia, tilt of the vision, true rotatory or linear vertigo, drunken-type gait, hiccup, bilateral or crossed motor or sensory symptoms, initial decreased level of consciousness and amnesia should be actively searched for in the history of stroke patients.

On exam, a disconjugate gaze strongly suggests a brainstem lesion. It may occur as a fixed misalignment of the ocular axis, such as in vertical skew deviation of the eyes as part of the ocular tilt reaction. Alternatively, it is due to a paresis of one or several orbital muscles as a result of an infarct of a single nucleus or its intra-axial fascicle (cranial nerves III, IV or VI), or from connections in between these nuclei (such as in internuclear ophthalmoplegia).

Gaze paresis may also be conjugate in brainstem lesions. If the eyes are deviated toward the hemiparesis, i.e. there is "wrong-way eye deviation" if compared to a hemispheric lesion in the MCA territory, the eyes cannot be directed to the other side because the command centers allowing this action are damaged in the pons (for saccades: parapontine reticular formation, PPRF; and for pursuit: parts of the nucleus of the VI) or the midbrain (parts of the nucleus of the VI). Contrarily to most supratentorial infarcts, this eye deviation cannot be overcome with oculovestibular reflexes ("doll's eyes maneuver"). A lateral medullary lesion (Wallenberg syndrome) leads to an ipsilateral deviation of the eyes, however, and is usually accompanied by a marked horizontal or horizonto-rotatory nystagmus.

A vertical gaze paresis (upwards, downwards, or both) points to a dorsal mesencephalic lesion and may be associated with a caudal paramedian thalamic infarct, especially if downgaze palsy is also present.

A nystagmus of central origin may be recognized by its direction (vertical, multidirectional gaze-evoked or pendular), the absence of nausea despite clear-cut nystagmus with primary gaze, and its lack of improvement with fixation. However, it should be underlined that a medullary or a cerebellar stroke can mimic a peripheral nystagmus and that vestibular ischemia from AICA may result in a peripheral vestibular lesion.

An ocular tilt reaction is characterized by the triad of skew deviation (downward displacement of the axis of the globe ipsilateral to the lesion), conjugate ocular torsion towards the side of the lesion and head tilt to the side of the lesion. Visual tilt of the environment towards the side of the lesion is frequently associated and may result in "upside-down vision". The ocular tilt reaction may be caused by peripheral lesion of the vestibular apparatus or the central vestibular connections including vestibular nuclei, vestibulocerebellum, and the medial longitudinal fascicle (MLF) up to the interstitial nucleus of Cajal.

Another visual sign is Horner's syndrome, consisting of myosis, mild ptosis of the upper and lower eyelid, and hemifacial anhydrosis. It occurs with an ipsilateral dorsolateral brainstem, upper cervical, or thalamic lesion, but may also occur due to a carotid dissection, the peripheral sympathetic fibers surrounding the carotid artery.

Motor, cerebellar and sensitive signs are less specific in brainstem lesions, but the presence of bilateral or crossed signs is suggestive. The former is due to the bilateral supply of the brainstem by one midline artery (the BA). The latter is caused by ischemia of cranial nerves and fascicles that produce ipsilateral signs and simultaneous damage to the long sensory and motor tracts that cross in the caudal parts of the brainstem. Truncular ataxia is quite characteristic of brainstem lesions, and acute unilateral deafness (with or without vertigo) suggests ischemia in the AICA territory.

Despite these clinical clues, lacunar brainstem infarcts may be indistinguishable from supratentorial ones, and proximal PCA occlusion may mimic MCA infarction. In the latter situation, hemiparesis results from ischemia to the cerebral peduncles, cognitive signs and eye deviation from thalamic involvement, and hemianopia from thalamic or hemispheric PCA ischemia. If somnolence, early anisocoria or vertical gaze palsy are present, posterior circulation stroke is more probable than carotid territory stroke.

> Clinical symptoms and signs that point to a posterior circulation stroke: preceding TIAs and strokes in the days and hours before the infarct, headache, typically ipsilateral to the infarct, a disconjugate gaze or a conjugate gaze paresis with the eyes deviated toward the hemiparesis (brainstem lesion), a vertical gaze paresis (dorsal mesencephalic lesion), nystagmus, ocular tilt reaction (triad of skew deviation, conjugate ocular torsion towards the side of the lesion and head tilt to the side of the lesion), Horner's syndrome (myosis, mild ptosis of the upper and lower eyelid, and hemifacial anhydrosis), bilateral or crossed motor, cerebellar and sensitive signs, truncular ataxia, acute unilateral deafness, somnolence and early anisocoria.

The vertebral artery (VA) and the posterior inferior cerebellar artery (PICA)

The vertebral arteries give origin to two arteries before joining to form the basilar artery: the anterior spinal artery, which supplies the medial medulla oblongata and the upper cervical cord, and the PICA, which supplies the inferior cerebellum and the dorsolateral medulla. The latter structure may also receive direct (long circumferential) branches from the vertebral artery. Three classic clinical syndromes are recognized in their territory: the medial medullary stroke (or Déjerine syndrome); the dorsolateral medullary stroke (or Wallenberg syndrome); and the hemimedullary stroke (or Babinski-Nageotte syndrome).

The medial medullary stroke is a rare stroke syndrome and classically includes contralateral hemiparesis sparing the face (corticospinal tract), contralateral lemniscal sensory loss (medial lemniscus) and ipsilateral tongue paresis (nucleus of hypoglossal nerve and tract). The laterodorsal medullary stroke is the most common of those three syndromes and is named the Wallenberg syndrome, after Adolf Wallenberg (1862–1946), a German neurologist. Wallenberg syndrome and an infarct in the inferior cerebellum stroke can be seen in isolation or together, the latter being usually the case if the vertebral artery is occluded. Wallenberg's syndrome includes ipsilateral thermoalgesic facial deficit (spinal trigeminal nucleus and tract), contralateral thermoalgesic deficit (spinothalamic tract), dysphagia, dysphonia due to palatal and vocal cord weakness (ambiguous nucleus), ipsilateral ataxia (inferior cerebellar peduncle), severe nausea, vomiting, nystagmus, ocular and truncular ipsipulsion (vestibular nuclei) and ipsilateral Horner's sign (descending sympathetic tract). Hiccup is common, and may be refractory to treatment. If a Wallenberg's syndrome is present, the presence or absence of an inferior cerebellar lesion cannot be determined clinically.

Inferior cerebellar lesions in the PICA territory without involvement of the dorsolateral medulla present with vertigo, nausea, vomiting, nystagmus, ipsilateral limb ataxia, severe gait ataxia and ocular/truncular ipsipulsion. A deceptive appearance of PICA stroke is the isolated vertigo presentation, which can mimic a vestibular neuronitis. One clue which can help to make the correct diagnosis is the presence of an unusual nystagmus, which will be purely horizontal or direction-changing, and preservation of the vestibulo-ocular reflex with the head thrust (Halmagyi) maneuver. This maneuver should not be applied in patients with suspected vertebral artery dissection.

Isolated inferior cerebellar infarcts usually have a good outcome. However, in the case of large PICA infarcts, a post-infarct edema can provoke brainstem compression, obstruction of the fourth ventricle with subsequent hydrocephalus and tonsillar (downward) or transtentorial (upward) herniation. In the first case, the patient develops paresthesia in the shoulder, neck stiffness up to opisthotonos, no motor responses, small and unreactive pupils, ataxic then superficial respiratory pattern, Cushing's triad (hypertension, bradycardia, apnea) and finally cardio-respiratory arrest. With transtentorial herniation, lethargy and coma are accompanied by central hyperventilation, upward gaze paralysis, unreactive, mid-position pupils and decerebration.

The hemimedullary syndrome is very rare and includes Wallenberg's presentation with Déjerine's syndrome, leading to contralateral motor and all-modalities sensory deficits, ipsilateral tongue, pharynx and vocal cord weakness and facial thermoalgesic deficit, ipsilateral ataxia and Horner's syndrome.

> Dorsolateral medullary stroke (or Wallenberg syndrome) is the most common brainstem syndrome of vertebral artery involvement.

The anterior inferior cerebellar artery (AICA)

The AICA vascularizes the dorsolateral inferior pons, the antero-inferior cerebellum, the cochlea, the labyrinth, and the VIIIth cranial nerve. Major variations of the extent of cerebellar supply by the three cerebellar arteries may make localization to the AICA difficult unless certain cranial nerve deficits are present.

The classic AICA syndrome includes vertigo with vomiting and nystagmus (vestibular nuclei, vestibular nerve or labyrinthine artery), ipsilateral deafness with tinnitus (cochlear nerve or cochlear artery), ipsilateral peripheral-type facial palsy (facial nucleus or fascicle of VII), ipsilateral facial hypesthesia (trigeminal nuclei or fascicle), ipsilateral Horner's syndrome (descending sympathetic tract), ipsilateral ataxia, dysarthria (middle cerebellar peduncle and cerebellum) and contralateral thermoalgesic sensory deficit (spinothalamic tract). It is frequently misdiagnosed as Wallenberg syndrome, but the main clinical distinctions are the hearing loss and the peripheral-type facial palsy. Occasionally, horizontal ipsilateral gaze palsy or dysphagia are also present. More rarely, AICA territory stroke can present as an isolated vertigo or isolated cerebellar syndrome.

The superior cerebellar artery (SCA)

An isolated SCA syndrome is rare, but the territory is regularly involved in distal basilar artery occlusion. The SCA syndrome includes ipsilateral limb and gait ataxia and important dysarthria. Nystagmus (middle and/or superior cerebellar peduncle, superior cerebellum and vermis), ipsilateral Horner's syndrome (descending sympathetic tract), contralateral fourth palsy (IV nucleus), and contralateral thermoalgesic sensory deficit (spinothalamic tract) may be present. Other signs have been described, such as ipsilateral choreiform abnormal movements or palatal myoclonus (superior cerebellar peduncle interrupting the dentatorubral pathway), sleep abnormalities, and partial contralateral deafness (lateral lemniscus). Given its close relationship to the distal basilar artery, SCA strokes are very frequently embolic (from an arterial or cardiac source).

The basilar artery (BA)

The BA lies on the ventral surface of the brainstem and vascularizes the pons, the mesencephalon and the middle and upper cerebellum through the AICA and SCA. Its territory can be subdivided into three parts on a ventro-dorsal level [11]. The anteromedial territory receives its blood supply from the paramedian arteries, the anterolateral territory from the short circumferential arteries (or anterolateral arteries) and the dorsolateral territory from the long circumferential arteries (or posterolateral arteries) as well as from the cerebellar arteries. In ventral paramedian lesions, hemiparesis is the most severe. In anterolateral lesions, the motor deficit is mild and can predominate in the leg (crural dominant hemiparesis), reflecting the topographical orientation of the fibers (leg – lateral, arm – medial) [12]. Dorsolateral lesions often involve the spinothalamic tract and lateral part of the medial lemniscus, while paramedian infarcts involve the medial part of the medial lemniscus. Involvement of the tegmentum implies more sensory, cranial nerves and oculomotor deficits.

Stroke severity in the BA territory is highly variable: it can present with isolated neurological deficits in the case of penetrator occlusions of lacunar origin or can be devastating when the artery itself is acutely occluded. Different eponym syndromes have been described in the literature, corresponding to circumscribed lesions and precise deficits (see Table 8.2)

Occlusion of the basilar artery mostly results in a devastating stroke with severe disability or death. About half of individuals present premonitory signs and symptoms, especially if atherosclerosis of the vertebral or basilar artery is the cause. Some symptoms are nonspecific, such as paresthesias, dysarthria, ("herald") hemiparesis or dizziness. More specific prodromes are mentioned above, and also include pathological laughter ("fou rire prodromique") [13] as well as pseudoseizures with tonic spasm of the side which will become paretic [14]. Rapid identification of basilar artery ischemia can help to provide aggressive therapy by i.v. or i.a. thrombolysis before a catastrophic picture of a locked-in syndrome or coma. Indeed, it has been shown that vessel recanalization and low NIHSS on admission were independent predictors of favorable outcome [15].

Less severe pontine stroke syndromes are listed in Table 8.2. Severe pontine strokes are characterized by a locked-in syndrome that involves quadriplegia, bilateral face palsy, and horizontal gaze palsy. Consciousness and vertical gaze are usually spared unless the midbrain is involved. Therefore, careful examination of voluntary up- and downgaze in a seemingly comatose patient may establish preserved consciousness and communication.

Distal basilar territory stroke usually leads to midbrain ischemia and is therefore characterized by ocular manifestations, such as disorders of reflex and voluntary vertical gaze, skew deviation, disorder of convergence with pseudosixth palsy in the presence of hyperconvergence, Collier sign (upper eyelid retraction), and small pupils with diminished reaction to light because of interruption of the afferent limb of the pupillary reflex. Small midbrain lesions may result in nuclear or fascicular third nerve palsies. Nuclear palsy is recognizable by bilateral upgaze paresis and bilateral ptosis as the medial subnucleus of the III innervates the contralateral superior rectus muscle and the central nucleus innervates both levator palpebrae superioris. Other classic midbrain syndromes can be found in Table 8.2. Hypersomnolence or coma usually requires extension of the ischemia into the thalamic territory as part of the "top of the basilar syndrome" [16].

Atherosclerosis and embolism are the two major mechanisms of basilar artery stroke and occlusion. Common sites of atherothrombotic stenosis are the origin of vertebral arteries (which can lead to artery-to-artery embolism), the intracranial part of the VA, where thrombus frequently extends into the caudal part of the BA, between the union of VA and AICA, and the midpart of the BA [17]. Embolic clots may arise from vertebral or basilar atherosclerosis or from aortic or cardiac sources. They are a regular cause of

Table 8.2. Selected brainstem syndromes with their eponyms.

Eponym	Site	Cranial nerves	Tracts	Signs
Weber	Base of midbrain	III	Corticospinal	Oculomotor palsy with crossed hemiplegia
Claude	Midbrain tegmentum	III	Red nucleus and brachium conjunctivum	Oculomotor palsy with contralateral cerebellar ataxia and tremor
Benedikt	Midbrain tegmentum	III	Red nucleus	Oculomotor palsy, contralateral abnormal movements
Nothnagel	Midbrain tectum	Unilateral or bilateral III	Superior cerebellar peduncles	Oculomotor palsy, ipsilateral cerebellar ataxia
Parinaud	Dorsal midbrain			Paralysis of upward gaze, light-near dissociation, retraction nystagmus, eyelid retraction, lid lag
Raymond	Ventral caudal pons	VI	Corticospinal tract	Abduction palsy and crossed hemiplegia
Millard-Gubler	Caudal ventral medial pons	VII, VI (fascicles)	Corticospinal tract	Abduction and peripheral facial palsy, contralateral hemiplegia
Foville	Caudal tegmental medial pons	VI nucleus, VII, PPRF	Corticospinal tract, medial lemniscus, MLF	Gaze and peripheral facial palsy, contralateral hemiparesis (and hypesthesia, INO)
Raymond-Cestan	Rostral dorsal pons	(PPRF and VI nucleus)	Spinothalamic tract and medial lemniscus (corticospinal tract)	Ataxia with "rubral" tremor, contralateral all sensory modalities deficit (contralateral hemiparesis, ipsilateral gaze palsy)
Marie-Foix	Lateral caudal pons (AICA)		Middle cerebellar peduncle, corticospinal, spinothalamic tracts	Ipsilateral ataxia, contralateral hemiparesis and spinothalamic sensory loss
Wallenberg	Medulla, lateral tegmentum	Spinal V, IX, X, XI	Lateral spinothalamic tract, descending sympathetic fibers, spino- and olivocerebellar tracts	Ipsi V, IX, X, XI palsy, Horner's, cerebellar ataxia. Contralateral pain and temperature deficit
Déjerine	Medial medullary syndrome	XII	Corticospinal, lemniscus median	Ipsilateral tongue palsy, contralateral hemiplegia and lemniscal sensory loss
Opalski	Submedullary syndrome	V, IX, X, XI	Corticospinal tract below the pyramid	Ipsilateral hemiplegia with Wallenberg syndrome
Babinski-Nageotte	Hemimedullary syndrome			Combination of Wallenberg's, Déjerine's and Opalsi's syndromes

distal vertebral and proximal BA occlusions, and the predominant cause of distal BA occlusions.

Another less common cause of BA strokes is the dolichoectasic basilar or vertebral arteries. They have been documented in up to 10% and are related to the presence of vascular risk factors and an increased risk for lacunar stroke [18].

Rapid identification of basilar artery ischemia can help to provide timely aggressive therapy by i.v. or i.a. thrombolysis before a catastrophic picture develops.

The posterior cerebral artery (PCA)

The PCA is subdivided into four segments with associated clinical presentation. An occlusion of the proximal segment (P1 or precommunal) usually causes a total PCA infarction, including upper midbrain, variable parts of the thalamus and posterior hemispheric territory. Occlusions of the P2 (or postcommunal) segment before the branching of the thalamogeniculate arteries provoke ischemic lesions in the lateral thalamus and the hemispheric PCA territory. Lastly, cortical PCA branch occlusion causes diverse cortical lesions in the superficial PCA territory, including the occipital, postero-inferior temporal and variable part of the posterior parietal lobes.

Sensory symptoms are quite common in PCA infarcts and are usually related to laterothalamic involvement. Motor symptoms are infrequent and minor [19] and are mostly related to laterothalamic edema affecting the posterior internal capsule or to ischemia of the cerebral peduncles. In the latter situation, a patient may present severe contralateral hemiplegia, hypesthesia and hemianopsia, mimicking an MCA stroke as mentioned above.

Bilateral PCA infarcts are typical of the "top of the basilar syndrome", which may also include dyschromatopsia, visual agnosia or alexia-without agraphia with a left lesion, spatial disorientation (topographagnosia), palinopsia, amusia, Balint syndrome (asimultanognosia or incapacity to see a scene as a whole, ocular apraxia or poor hand–eye coordination and optic ataxia or apraxia of gaze), metamorphosia, and prosopagnosia [16]. The syndrome of bilateral PCA strokes must be distinguished from PRES (posterior reversible encephalopathy syndrome) and venous thrombosis, all of which can cause headaches, central visual loss and decreased level of consciousness.

The source of PCA strokes is embolic in the majority of cases, i.e. from cardiac sources, and proximal vertebrobasilar and aortic atherothrombotic disease. Rarer causes include dissections, fetal origin of PCA and migrainous stroke.

> Sensory symptoms (visual loss, hemianopsia) are quite common in PCA infarcts, while motor symptoms are infrequent and minor. The "top of the basilar syndrome" causes headaches, central visual loss and decreased level of consciousness.

The thalamus

The thalamus is a centrally situated structure with extensive reciprocal connections with the cortex, basal

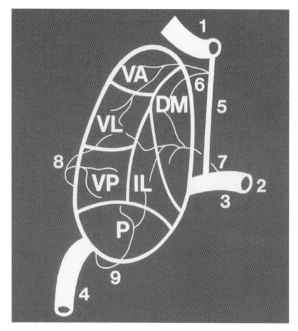

Figure 8.1. Carotid artery (1); basilar artery (2); posterior cerebral segment P1 (3); segment P2 (4); posterior communicating artery (5); tuberothalamic artery (6); paramedian arteries (7); thalamogeniculate artery (8); posterior choroidal artery (9). Source: Barth et al. in: Bogousslavsky J, Caplan L, eds. *Stroke Syndromes.* Cambridge: Cambridge University Press; 2001: 461.

ganglia and brainstem nuclei. Therefore it can mimic cortical and subcortical strokes in the anterior or posterior circulation and is also called "the great imitator". Its vascularization is subdivided into four territories correlated with the organization of the thalamic nuclei [20] (Figure 8.1):

- the tuberothalamic (or polar) artery
- the thalamogeniculate (or inferolateral) artery
- the paramedian arteries
- the posterior choroidal artery (PChA).

The thalamus is essentially fed by the posterior circulation via branches from the PCA (P1 and P2 segments), the PCoA and the PChA. Only blood going to the lateral geniculate body (via the AChA) and the anterior thalamus (via the PCoA) may stem from the carotid system.

There are inter-individual variations in thalamic supply, leading to variable clinical presentations and prognosis. For example, Percheron reported that the paramedian arteries may arise from a unique P1 segment or from a vascular arcade connecting both P1 segments.

The tuberothalamic (or polar) artery arises from the PCoA and irrigates the anterior nuclei, the ventral anterior nucleus, amygdalofugal pathway, mamillothalamic tract, rostral part of the ventrolateral nucleus, ventral pole of the medial dorsal nucleus and ventral part of the internal medullary lamina. It is absent in about a third of the population, in which case the paramedian arteries vascularize its territory. Infarction results in anterograde amnesia (mostly reversible if unilateral), automatic-voluntary dissociation with facial paresis for emotional movement, personality changes, mild contralateral hemiparesis or clumsiness. Cognitive and behavioral disturbances include temporospatial disorientation, euphoria, misjudgment, lack of spontaneity, apathy, emotional unconcern, and a unique behavioral pattern, named palipsychism [21]. Individuals present a disorganized speech with grammatically correct phrases, but with intrusions of unrelated themes, which have usually been discussed previously. With a left lesion, buccofacial or limb apraxia and thalamic aphasia can occur with reduced fluency, anomia, phonological and semantic paraphasia, perseveration, impaired comprehension, acalculia with preservation of reading and repetition. Visual-spatial disturbances are present with a right lesion.

The thalamogeniculate (or inferolateral) arteries are a group of 5–10 arteries arising from the P2 segment of the PCA. The principal branches supply the ventrolateral nucleus and the ventroposterior nuclei, while the medial branches supply the medial geniculate body and the inferior branches the rostral and lateral pulvinar, as well as the laterodorsal nucleus. The clinical presentation can include contralateral hemihypesthesia, involving one or several sensory modalities. It may be associated with choreoathetoid movements, hemiataxia, slight transient hemiparesis and thalamic astasia. Thalamic astasia is characterized by disequilibrium backwards or toward the side contralateral to the lesion in the absence of significant motor deficit and is thought to result from interruption of the dentatorubrothalamic pathway. Sensory deficits are heterogeneous. Individuals describe paresthesias without objective deficit, particularly in the cheiro-oral region, or a "mid-line split", defined by a subjective sensation of an abrupt stopping of the deficit on the midline of the trunk. Pseudoradicular sensory deficit is also suggestive of a thalamic involvement. Subsequent to, or rarely in the acute phase of, an inferolateral infarct,

some individuals develop paroxysmal stimulus-sensitive, severe and refractory pain in the affected hemibody side with vasomotor disturbances and choreoathetoid movements, named the thalamic pain syndrome of Déjerine-Roussy. The "thalamic hand", described by Foix and Hillemand, is flexed, pronated and the thumb is buried beneath the other fingers [20]. Behavioral disturbances are infrequent in inferolateral stroke and include soft executive dysfunction and affective changes, resembling those found after cerebellar stroke [21].

The paramedian arteries arise from the P1 segment of the PCA. The inferior and middle rami irrigate parts of the midbrain and the pons, while the superior ramus irrigates a variable extent of thalamus but mostly the dorsomedial nucleus, the intralaminar nuclei and internal medullary lamina. Infarctions also tend to involve the medial midbrain. The classic features consist of a triad with an initial decreased level of consciousness with or without fluctuations, vertical gaze abnormalities and cognitive impairment, which become more obvious after the resolution of the somnolence. Bilateral involvement is evidently more severe. Cognitive disturbances consist mostly of personality changes with disinhibited behavior, impulsivity, apathy and even loss of psychic self-activation associated with amnesia similar to Korsakoff syndrome. This picture of amnesia and behavioral disturbances is recognized as a "thalamic dementia". However, severe persistent amnestic syndrome is observed only with concomitant lesion of the anterior nucleus. With unilateral infarction, a left–right asymmetry is obvious in language versus visual-spatial impairment. The aphasia, named adynamic aphasia [20], is characterized by a reduced verbal fluency, with perseveration and paraphasic errors but with a relatively preserved syntax, comprehension and repetition. Hypophonia and dysarthria can be associated.

The fourth territory is irrigated by the PChA, arising from the P2 segment of the PCA, and is subdivided into medial and lateral branches. They supply the pulvinar, part of the lateral and medial geniculate body, the posterior parts of the intralaminar nuclei, and lateral dorsal and lateral posterior nuclei. They also irrigate posterior portions of medial temporal structures, parts of midbrain and probably the subthalamic nucleus. The clinical syndrome is characterized by visual field defects, decreased optokinetic nystagmus contralaterally to the lesion, contralateral hemisensory loss with mild hemiparesis, and transcortical aphasia. Visual field deficits include homonymous quadrantanopsia, superior or inferior, and a homonymous horizontal wedge-shaped sectoranopsia, which is highly suggestive of a lateral geniculate body lesion irrigated by the PChA. On the other hand, a homonymous visual defect in the upper and lower quadrants sparing a horizontal sector is highly characteristic of vascular lesions in the lateral geniculate body irrigated by the AChA [22]. Some individuals, in the event of pulvinar involvement, develop delayed contralateral hyperkinetic movements, including ataxia, rubral tremor, dystonia, myoclonus and chorea, a syndrome named the "jerky dystonic unsteady hand". No specific behavioral disturbance is described, but some spatial neglect was associated with right pulvinar lesions.

> Ischemia in the thalamus can mimic cortical and subcortical strokes in the anterior or posterior circulation. Depending on the location there can be additional symptoms (e.g. amnesia, cognitive impairment, decreased level of consciousness, personality changes, hemiataxia, pain).

Lacunar stroke syndromes

Lacunes are defined as small subcortical infarcts less than 1.5 cm in diameter occurring in perforator territories. Together with leukoaraiosis, microbleeds, and "hypertensive" (deep) intracerebral hemorrhages, they are part of the spectrum of small-vessel disease. This disease is tightly related to chronic hypertension, but diabetes, male gender, increasing age, smoking, previous lacunar TIA or stroke, and coronary artery disease are also risk factors. About 20% of all strokes are considered to be of lacunar origin, and it is estimated that only one of five lacunes is symptomatic. Lacunes result most frequently from occlusion of a single penetrating artery from lipohyalinosis within the artery. Other mechanisms include microatheromas, occlusion of the penetrator orifice from a large plaque in the mother artery, microembolism, vasculitis, hypercoagulable states or genetic disease (CADASIL) and are present in up to a third of patients [23].

Five main classical lacunar syndromes are recognized:
- pure motor hemiparesis
- pure sensory stroke
- sensorimotor stroke
- dysarthria–clumsy hand syndrome
- ataxic hemiparesis.

Pure motor hemiparesis and ataxic hemiparesis are most frequently due to an infarct in the internal capsule, corona radiata or basis pontis. The deficit is usually proportional, involving face, arm and leg to the same extent. Pure sensory stroke is usually related to a lesion in the ventroposterior nucleus of the thalamus, and less frequently the corona radiata. Sensorimotor stroke may result from a lesion of the internal capsule, and rarely from the paramedian pons. Dysarthria–clumsy hand syndrome is due most of the time to a lacunar infarct in the basis pontis, less frequently to a lesion in the internal capsule or cerebral peduncle. Therefore, a lacunar stroke in a specific location may lead to different lacunar stroke syndromes. Similarly, it has to be repeated that non-lacunar strokes and small intracerebral hemorrhages may present as lacunar syndromes, underlining the need for appropriate neuroimaging of all patients suspected of stroke.

Many other lacunar syndromes have been described. They include isolated dysarthria, facial paresis, pure motor hemiparesis with internuclear ophthalmoplegia, isolated third nerve palsy, pure motor hemiparesis with transient subcortical aphasia, isolated ataxia and hemichorea-hemiballismus [24], and many of the syndromes in Table 8.2. Hemichorea-hemiballismus is a classic presentation of a lacunar infarct in the subthalamic nucleus, but lesions in the basal ganglia may also cause it.

Ischemic lacunar strokes have some characteristic clinical features. They often progress during the first 24–48 hours after onset or can fluctuate considerably. If a severe hemiplegia alternates repeatedly with normal function, the phenomenon is called "capsular warning syndrome", resulting usually from a lacune in the internal capsule. About half of these fluctuating patients will end with a lacunar stroke within 24–48 hours. The pathogenesis is not clear but seems to be rather electrophysiological, given its stereotyped fluctuations, and the absence of response to antithrombotic medication and to elevation of perfusion pressure. In the acute setting, individuals with presumed lacunar strokes should be treated with intravenous thrombolysis whenever possible, as overall they respond as well as do patients with other stroke subtypes.

Although lacunar infarcts have better recovery and lower mortality rate during the first year, small-vessel disease carries a high risk of vascular death, recurrent stroke and development of cognitive disturbances [25].

131

Lacunes are small subcortical infarcts less than 1.5 cm in diameter occurring in perforator territories. Five main classic lacunar syndromes are recognized:

- pure motor hemiparesis
- pure sensory stroke
- sensorimotor stroke
- dysarthria–clumsy hand syndrome
- ataxic hemiparesis.

Watershed infarcts (WS)

Watershed (or borderzone) infarcts represent about 5% of all strokes. They involve the junction of distal regions of two arterial systems. Pathophysiologically, systemic hemodynamic failure, tight stenosis (or occlusion) of a cervical or intracranial artery [26], or embolic occlusion of an intracerebral artery are implicated. Recently, a combination of these mechanisms has been proposed [27]: hypoperfusion due to severe arterial stenosis or occlusion would impair the reserve of brain areas becoming more susceptible to the effect of microemboli, and low flow with stagnation of blood would increase clot formation and decrease wash-out of emboli.

WS infarcts have been studied best in the anterior circulation in relationship to severe stenosis or occlusion of the ICA. Two typical patterns are observed: cortical WS (CWS) and the internal WS (IWS) strokes. The CWS area is located superficially in the cortex between the MCA, ACA and PCA territories. Strokes appear radiologically as wedges extending from the prefrontal or parieto-occipital cortex down to the frontal and occipital horns of the lateral ventricle respectively. The IWS area is situated in an anterior–posterior orientation in the centrum semi-ovale and along the lateral ventricle [28]. Incomplete IWS strokes may appear as a small single lesion or as a chain-like (or rosary-like) pattern in this deep territory. There is better evidence that IWS stroke, particularly rosary-like infarction in the centrum semi-ovale, has an association with hemodynamic failure rather than with embolic mechanisms.

Clinical presentation of WS infarction is heterogeneous and depends on the location of ischemic changes. Signs and symptoms may be bilateral in the case of systemic hypotension or unilateral in the case of unilateral carotid severe stenosis or occlusion. The classic picture of a bilateral deep anterior IWS stroke, the "man-in-the-barrel" with proximal weakness of upper and lower limbs, is rare. Posterior infarction is classically associated with Balint's syndrome (asimultagnosia, optic ataxia and ocular apraxia). If an arterial pathology is present, onset can be less abrupt than in embolic strokes and can fluctuate with changes of blood pressure and body position. Infratentorially, WS strokes are not well investigated.

The watershed area in the upper spinal cord is thought to be on the thoracic level T4 to T6 because of paucity of blood supply [29] and in the lumbosacral segments due to the high concentration of neurons and higher metabolic demands [30].

> Watershed (or borderzone) infarcts involve the junction of distal regions of two arterial systems. The clinical presentation is heterogeneous and depends on the location of ischemic changes.

Chapter Summary

Anterior circulation syndromes
The anterior circulation refers to the part of the brain perfused by the carotid arteries.

Middle cerebral artery (MCA)
The MCA territory is the one most frequently affected by acute strokes. MCA territory infarcts can be subtle or a devastating clinical syndrome, depending on the site of the occlusion, the extent of ischemia, the etiology, and the collateral arterial network.

Symptoms of an *acute complete MCA* infarction: contralateral hemiparesis, hemihypesthesia, hemianopsia, ipsilateral conjugated eye and head deviation (the patient looks at his/her lesion); plus, in the case of a left lesion, aphasia, and in the case of a right lesion, contralateral multimodal hemineglect. Malignant stroke with brain edema may develop, leading to high intracranial pressure and subsequent herniation.

Infarctions of the lower arterial segments show similar symptoms, but not the complete picture (e.g. isolated brachiofacial paresis with or without visual field symptoms).

Internal carotid artery (ICA)
Embolic occlusion of the ICA, either proximally or distally, usually leads to severe stroke, showing concomitant signs of all anterior circulation arteries. *A progressive atherosclerotic occlusion* is usually less severe, with a classic subacute two-phase presentation, or even asymptomatic. Retinal ischemia from carotid emboli may be transient (amaurosis fugax) or persistent (central retinal artery occlusion or branch retinal artery occlusion).

Posterior circulation syndromes

The two vertebral arteries leave the subclavian arteries and join together to form the basilar artery.

Clinical symptoms and signs that point to a posterior circulation stroke: preceding TIAs and strokes in the days and hours before the infarct, headache, typically ipsilateral to the infarct, a disconjugate gaze or a conjugate gaze paresis with the eyes deviated toward the hemiparesis (brainstem lesion), a vertical gaze paresis (dorsal mesencephalic lesion), nystagmus, ocular tilt reaction (triad of skew deviation, conjugate ocular torsion towards the side of the lesion and head tilt to the side of the lesion), Horner's syndrome (myosis, mild ptosis of the upper and lower eyelid, and hemifacial anhydrosis), bilateral or crossed motor, cerebellar and sensitive signs, truncular ataxia, acute unilateral deafness, somnolence and early anisocoria.

Lacunar stroke syndromes

Lacunes = small subcortical infarcts less than 1.5 cm in diameter occurring in perforator territories. Five main classic lacunar syndromes are recognized:

- pure motor hemiparesis
- pure sensory stroke
- sensorimotor stroke
- dysarthria–clumsy hand syndrome
- ataxic hemiparesis.

Ischemic lacunar strokes have some characteristic clinical features. They often progress during the first 24–48 hours after onset or can fluctuate considerably.

Watershed infarcts

Watershed (or borderzone) infarcts involve the junction of distal regions of two arterial systems. The clinical presentation is heterogeneous and depends on the location of ischemic changes. The classic picture of a bilateral deep anterior IWS stroke, the "man-in-the-barrel" with proximal weakness of upper and lower limbs, is rare.

References

1. Rovira A, Grive E, Rovira A, Alvarez-Sabin J. Distribution territories and causative mechanisms of ischemic stroke. *Eur Radiol* 2005; **15**(3):416–26.

2. Ay H, Furie KL, Singhal A, Smith WS, Sorensen AG, Koroshetz WJ. An evidence-based causative classification system for acute ischemic stroke. *Ann Neurol* 2005; **58**(5):688–97.

3. van der Lugt A, Buter TC, Govaere F, Siepman DA, Tanghe HL, Dippel DW. Accuracy of CT angiography in the assessment of a fetal origin of the posterior cerebral artery. *Eur Radiol* 2004; **14**(9):1627–33.

4. Brandt T, Steinke W, Thie A, Pessin MS, Caplan LR. Posterior cerebral artery territory infarcts: clinical features, infarct topography, causes and outcome. Multicenter results and a review of the literature. *Cerebrovasc Dis* 2000; **10**(3):170–82.

5. Averbuch-Heller L, Leigh RJ, Mermelstein V, Zagalsky L, Streifler JY. Ptosis in patients with hemispheric strokes. *Neurology* 2002; **58**(4):620–4.

6. Vahedi K, Hofmeijer J, Juettler E, Vicaut E, George B, Algra A, et al. Early decompressive surgery in malignant infarction of the middle cerebral artery: a pooled analysis of three randomised controlled trials. *Lancet Neurol* 2007; **6**(3):215–22.

7. Hamoir XL, Grandin CB, Peeters A, Robert A, Cosnard G, Duprez T. MRI of hyperacute stroke in the AChA territory. *Eur Radiol* 2004; **14**(3):417–24.

8. Helgason CM. A new view of anterior choroidal artery territory infarction. *J Neurol* 1988; **235**(7):387–91.

9. Baumgartner RW, Baumgartner I. Vasomotor reactivity is exhausted in transient ischaemic attacks with limb shaking. *J Neurol Neurosurg Psychiatry* 1998; **65**(4):561–4.

10. Brandt T, Steinke W, Thie A, Pessin MS, Caplan LR. Posterior cerebral artery territory infarcts: clinical features, infarct topography, causes and outcome. Multicenter results and a review of the literature. *Cerebrovasc Dis* 2000; **10**(3):170–82.

11. Tatu L, Moulin T, Bogousslavsky J, Duvernoy H. Arterial territories of human brain: brainstem and cerebellum. *Neurology* 1996; **47**(5):1125–35.

12. Kataoka S, Miaki M, Saiki M, Saiki S, Yamaya Y, Hori A, et al. Rostral lateral pontine infarction: neurological/topographical correlations. *Neurology* 2003; **61**(1):114–7.

13. Wali GM. "Fou rire prodromique" heralding a brainstem stroke. *J Neurol Neurosurg Psychiatry* 1993; **56**(2):209–10.

14. Bassetti C, Bogousslavsky J, Barth A, Regli F. Isolated infarcts of the pons. *Neurology* 1996; **46**(1):165–75.

15. Arnold M, Nedeltchev K, Schroth G, Baumgartner RW, Remonda L, Loher TJ, et al. Clinical and radiological predictors of recanalisation and outcome of 40 patients with acute basilar artery occlusion treated with intra-arterial thrombolysis. *J Neurol Neurosurg Psychiatry* 2004; **75**(6):857–62.

16. Caplan LR. "Top of the basilar" syndrome. *Neurology* 1980; **30**(1):72–9.

17. Idicula TT, Joseph LN. Neurological complications and aspects of basilar artery occlusive disease. *Neurologist* 2007; **13**(6):363–8.

18. Pico F, Biron Y, Bousser MG, Amarenco P. Concurrent dolichoectasia of basilar and coronary arteries. *Neurology* 2005; **65**(9):1503–4.

19. Brandt T, Steinke W, Thie A, Pessin MS, Caplan LR. Posterior cerebral artery territory infarcts: clinical features, infarct topography, causes and outcome. Multicenter results and a review of the literature. *Cerebrovasc Dis* 2000; **10**(3):170–82.

20. Schmahmann JD. Vascular syndromes of the thalamus. *Stroke* 2003; **34**(9):2264–78.

21. Carrera E, Bogousslavsky J. The thalamus and behavior: effects of anatomically distinct strokes. *Neurology* 2006; **66**(12):1817–23.

22. Brazis PW, Masdeu JC, Biller J. *Localization in Clinical Neurology*. Lippincott Williams & Wilkins; 2006: 155.

23. Baumgartner RW, Sidler C, Mosso M, Georgiadis D. Ischemic lacunar stroke in patients with and without potential mechanism other than small-artery disease. *Stroke* 2003; **34**(3):653–9.

24. Arboix A, Lopez-Grau M, Casasnovas C, Garcia-Eroles L, Massons J, Balcells M. Clinical study of 39 patients with atypical lacunar syndrome. *J Neurol Neurosurg Psychiatry* 2006; **77**(3):381–4.

25. Norrving B. Lacunar infarcts: no black holes in the brain are benign. *Pract Neurol* 2008; **8**(4):222–8.

26. Bogousslavsky J, Regli F. Unilateral watershed cerebral infarcts. *Neurology* 1986; **36**(3):373–7.

27. Caplan LR, Hennerici M. Impaired clearance of emboli (washout) is an important link between hypoperfusion, embolism, and ischemic stroke. *Arch Neurol* 1998; **55**(11):1475–82.

28. Momjian-Mayor I, Baron JC. The pathophysiology of watershed infarction in internal carotid artery disease: review of cerebral perfusion studies. *Stroke* 2005; **36**(3):567–77.

29. Novy J, Carruzzo A, Maeder P, Bogousslavsky J. Spinal cord ischemia: clinical and imaging patterns, pathogenesis, and outcomes in 27 patients. *Arch Neurol* 2006; **63**(8):1113–20.

30. Duggal N, Lach B. Selective vulnerability of the lumbosacral spinal cord after cardiac arrest and hypotension. *Stroke* 2002; **33**(1):116–21.

Less common stroke syndromes

Wilfried Lang

Introduction

This chapter deals with focal brain ischemia, either TIA or ischemic stroke. Causes, mechanisms and clinical syndromes of brain hemorrhage are described elsewhere. This chapter is divided into three parts. The first part focuses on an uncommon mechanism of focal brain ischemia, which is low flow. Most TIA and ischemic strokes are caused by embolism or in situ artery occlusion. Hemodynamic causes of focal brain ischemia are less common. Secondly, uncommon clinical presentations of focal brain ischemia are described. In the third part, uncommon causes of TIA and ischemic stroke are presented together with associated clinical syndromes.

Uncommon mechanism of stroke: low flow

Ischemic strokes and transient ischemic attacks caused by low cerebral flow – anterior circulation

Most ischemic strokes and transient ischemic attacks are caused by embolic and acute, in situ (usually thrombotic) occlusion of an artery in the brain. However, in some patients severe stenosis or occlusion of carotid or vertebral arteries may cause a critical reduction of blood flow, particularly when collateral circulation is compromised because the circle of Willis is incomplete or diseased. Mechanisms to compensate for the reduction of blood flow are vasodilatation by autoregulation and an increase of the oxygen extraction fraction. If the vascular bed is maximally dilated the supplied brain is particularly vulnerable to any fall in perfusion pressure. Under these circumstances a small drop in systemic blood pressure may cause transient or permanent focal ischemia.

Boundary-zone infarcts

The evidence that at least some boundary-zone infarcts are caused by low flow rather than acute arterial occlusion is that a sudden, profound and relatively prolonged hypotension (e.g. as a result of cardiac arrest or cardiac surgery) sometimes causes infarction bilaterally in the posterior boundary zones between the supply territories of the middle cerebral artery (MCA) and the posterior cerebral artery in the parieto-occipital regions. The clinical features include visual disorientation and agnosia, and amnesia.

Hemianopia is the most common symptom in unilateral posterior boundary-zone infarction, usually with macular sparing and predominating in the lower quadrant. Brachiofacial hypoesthesia is frequent, while motor weakness is rare and remains mild. In the dominant hemisphere, lesions manifest as either isolated word-finding difficulty or transcortical sensory aphasia (impaired comprehension but preserved word repetition and speech output). In the non-dominant hemisphere contralateral hemispatial neglect and anosognosia are usually found.

Anterior boundary-zone infarction is recognized in severe carotid stenosis or occlusion. The boundary zone is located in the frontoparasagittal region, between the supply territories of the MCA and the anterior cerebral artery in the frontoparasagittal region. The clinical features are contralateral weakness of the leg, more than the arm and sparing the face, some impaired sensation of the same distribution and transcortical motor aphasia (intact comprehension and repetition with impaired speech output), which may be preceded by mutism if in the dominant hemisphere.

There is an internal or subcortical boundary zone in the corona radiate and centrum semiovale, lateral and/or above the lateral ventricle. This lies between the supply areas of the lenticulostriate perforating branches from the MCA trunk and the medullary perforating arteries which arise from the cortical branches of the MCA and the anterior and, perhaps, posterior cerebral arteries. Infarction can occur within this internal boundary zone, usually causing lacunar or partial anterior circulation syndrome, in association with severe carotid disease and sometimes an obvious hemodynamic precipitating cause.

A sudden and profound hypotension sometimes causes **boundary-zone infarction**.

A fall in cerebral perfusion pressure as a cause of focal brain ischemia should be suspected if the symptoms start under certain circumstances [1]:

- on standing up very quickly, even if postural hypotension cannot be demonstrated in the clinic
- immediately after a heavy meal
- in very hot weather
- with exercise, coughing or hyperventilation
- during Valsalva maneuver (but embolism is another possibility)
- during a clinically obvious episode of cardiac dysrhythmia (chest pain, palpitations, etc.) but embolism from heart is also possible
- during operative hypotension
- if the patient has recently been started on or increased the dose of any drug likely to cause hypotension.

Limb-shaking TIA

A transient ischemic attack which is typically associated with severe large artery disease with exhausted hemodynamic reserve is "limb shaking TIA". It is characterized by 30–60 sec episodes of repetitive jerking movements of contralateral arm and/or leg and has been described with carotid occlusion but also with stenosis of intracranial vessels, e.g. middle cerebral artery or anterior cerebral artery. "Limb shaking TIA" is elicited in situations which dispose to low flow, e.g. orthostatic dysregulation, hyperventilation in Moyamoya disease, or by carotid compression. The symptoms usually point towards a seizure-like activity and are often misdiagnosed as focal seizures. In contrast to seizure activity, limb shaking shows no somatotopic spread of movement activity (no Jacksonian march) and usually has a low frequency (about 3 Hz). It is reported that limb shaking disappears with revascularization, e.g. carotid endarterectomy or extracranial–intracranial bypass (Figure 9.1).

A transient ischemic attack which is typically associated with severe large artery disease with exhausted hemodynamic reserve is **"limb-shaking TIA"**.

Ischemic ophthalmopathy

Another symptom of low flow is monocular transient retinal ischemia occurring when looking into bright light. Objects appear bleached and a brief visual loss may follow. This symptom has been related to retinal claudication: an increase in the metabolic demand during exposure to bright light cannot be met because of an already marginal perfusion. Ischemic ophthalmopathy is a specific, concomitant disorder of uncompensated, critically reduced perfusion pressure due to internal carotid artery occlusive disease. Quite characteristic is the history of a gradual, progressive loss of visual acuity, occasionally with bouts of obscuration, leading to a slowly progressive, irreversible damage of the retinal neuronal layer. Further typical findings are neovascularization of the retina and iris (rubeosis iris) [2].

Ischemic strokes and transient ischemic attacks caused by low cerebral flow, posterior circulation

Rotational vertebral artery occlusion (RVAO) and stroke

Rotational vertebral artery occlusion (RVAO) is caused by mechanical compression of vertebral arteries during head rotation. The vertebral artery is usually compressed at the atlantoaxial C1–C2 level. Tendinous insertions, osteophytes or degenerative changes resulting from cervical spondylosis may be the cause of compression. Most RVAO patients exhibit an ipsilateral stenosis or vessel malformation (e.g. hypoplasia) and a contralateral dominant vertebral artery. With ispilateral head rotation, the (contralateral) dominant vertebral artery is compressed. The leading symptom is vertigo, followed by tinnitus. Video-oculography showed that RVAO is associated with a mixed downbeat torsional and horizontal beating nystagmus which may spontaneously reverse direction [3]. The labyrinth is predominantly supplied by the internal auditory artery, which is usually a branch of the anterior inferior cerebellar artery (AICA). As AICA usually takes off the basilar artery at its lower portion, reduced blood flow from the vertebral artery would result in ischemia. Approximately 50% of RVAO patients treated conservatively

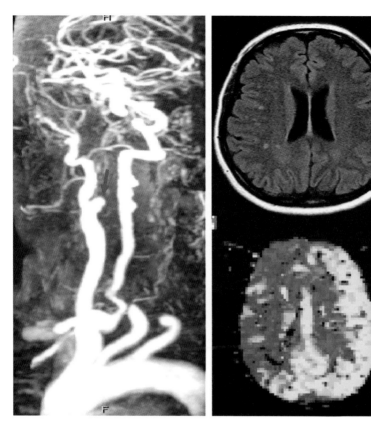

Figure 9.1. Limb-shaking TIA. A 55-year-old woman with risk factors (metabolic syndrome, smoking) presented with a limb shaking of the left leg when standing. The right internal carotid artery (ICA) was occluded. Occlusion was presumably acute. Territory of the ICA was supplied from the left ICA via the anterior communicating artery. There was no collateral blood flow from the posterior communicating artery. Initially, the symptom was considered to be focal epileptic. Perfusion MR showed reduction of blood flow in the anterior territory of the right middle cerebral artery and the right anterior cerebral artery.

suffered from infarction or residual neurological deficits [4]. Brief episodes of rotational vertigo can also be caused by compression of the vestibular nerve as caused by close contact with intracranial vessels, particularly the posterior inferior cerebellar artery (PICA).

> **Rotational vertebral artery occlusion** (RVAO) is caused by mechanical compression of vertebral arteries during head rotation. The leading symptom is vertigo, followed by tinnitus.

Drop attack and vertebrobasilar ischemia

"Drop attacks" are episodes of sudden loss of postural tone which cause the subject to fall to the ground without apparent loss of consciousness, vertigo or other sensation. The attack occurs without warning and is not induced by a change of posture or movement of the head. The patient may be unable to rise immediately after the fall despite being uninjured. Not a single patient in the New England Medical Center Posterior Circulation Registry had a drop attack as the only symptom of posterior circulation ischemia [5]. With vertebrobasilar ischemia, sudden

falls are usually preceded by and associated with symptoms such as vertigo, diplopia or blurred vision (Figure 9.2). A "drop attack" has been described in a patient with parasagittal motor cortex/subcortex ischemia in the territory of both anterior cerebral arteries [6].

> In "drop attacks" a sudden loss of postural tone causes a fall to the ground without loss of consciousness.

Subclavian steal syndrome and hemodynamic effects of proximal vertebral artery disease

Most patients with subclavian artery stenosis or occlusion are asymptomatic. In a large series, only 15 out of 324 patients (4.8%) had objective signs of brachial ischemia such as aching after exercise or coolness of the arm. Among 116 patients with unilateral steal as shown by ultrasonography none had symptoms of brain ischemia [7]. Among more than 400 patients with posterior circulation TIAs or ischemic stroke only two had symptoms (TIAs) attributable to significant subclavian or innominate artery

137

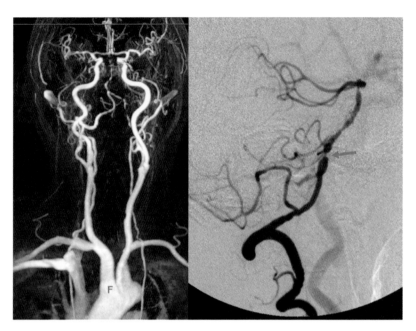

Figure 9.2. Drop attack. An 82-year-old woman with insulin-dependent diabetes mellitus suffered from recurrent short episodes with nausea, vertigo (sensation of being turned around), sweating, blurred vision, weakness and sudden falling without losing consciousness. Episodes were particularly frequent after reduction of elevated blood pressure. Stenosis of the basilar artery proximal to the AICA (anterior inferior cerebellar artery) was assumed to be the cause of these drop attacks. Symptoms disappeared after stent-PTA of the stenosis.

disease [8]. Symptoms which have been associated with decreased anterograde flow or retrograde flow in the vertebral artery are episodes with dizziness, diplopia, decreased vision or oszillopsia. The attacks are brief and may be elicited by exercise of the arm. A difference in the wrist or the antecubital pulses and a difference of blood pressure between the two arms are reliable signs which indicate subclavian steal syndrome. Causes of stenosis or occlusion of the vertebral artery are: arteriosclerosis, Takayashu disease and temporal arteritis or mechanical trauma, as have been reported by bowlers or baseball pitchers.

> Most patients with subclavian artery stenosis or occlusion are asymptomatic. Associated symptoms may include episodes with dizziness, diplopia, decreased vision or oszillopsia.

Severe stenosis or occlusion of the proximal vertebral artery is more likely to be a cause of embolism than to have hemodynamic effects: among 407 patients in the New England Medical Center Posterior Circulation Registry 80 of 407 patients had severe stenosis or occlusion of the proximal vertebral artery. In 45 of the 80 (56%) embolization was the most likely cause of cerebral ischemia. Only in 13 of 80 were hemodynamic effects considered to be the cause of cerebral ischemia. Twelve of these 13 patients had severe bilateral occlusive disease of the vertebral artery [8].

Hyperviscosity and low flow

Blood flow in the brain is determined by the size of blood vessels, blood pressure and hemorrheological factors of the blood. Abnormal changes of blood plasma with hematological disease (e.g. Waldenstrom's macroglobulinemia or paraproteinemia), increase in cell counts (e.g. in diseases such as polycythemia vera, erythrocytosis or hyperleukotic leukemias), and decreased red cell deformability (sickle-cell anemia, spherocytosis, hemoglobinopathies) lead to a hyperviscous state [9].

Cerebral blood flow is diminished with high hematocrit as found in polycythemia vera. Symptoms are often unspecific, such as headache, dizziness or vertigo, paresthesias, blurred vision or tinnitus. Low flow and/or increased coagulability may be the cause of focal brain ischemia. Different ischemic patterns have been described, such as lacunar infarction, boundary infarction, Binswanger's disease or large artery (territorial) infarction. In sickle-cell anemia, deformability of red cells is decreased. This may cause damage in the microcirculation, particularly in the boundary zones between major arterial territories. But large-artery occlusive disease, occasionally with the development of moyamoya, was also found. Plasma hyperviscosity syndrome is a clinical entity with mucous membrane bleeding, blurred vision, visual loss, lethargy, headache, dizziness, vertigo, tinnitus, paresthesias, and occasionally seizures.

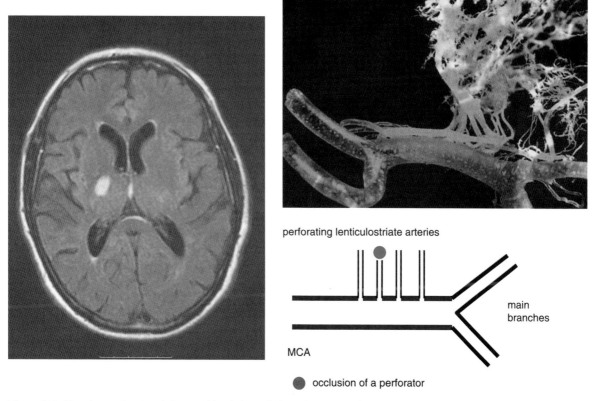

perforating lenticulostriate arteries

main branches

MCA

occlusion of a perforator

Figure 9.3. Capsular warning sign. A 65-year-old with hypercholesterolemia was referred to the hospital because of a sudden weakness of left face, arm and leg. He was unable to walk. He was dysarthric. Symptoms disappeared after about 10 minutes but over the next 5 hours he had four further identical episodes lasting for several minutes. The next day he suffered a lacunar stroke in the internal capsule with persisting pure motor hemiparesis. It is assumed that the occlusion of a single perforating artery (lenticulostriate artery) was the cause of the lacunar infarct.

Abnormal changes of blood plasma lead to a **hyperviscous state** and cerebral blood flow can be diminished. Symptoms are often unspecific, such as headache, dizziness or vertigo, paresthesias, blurred vision or tinnitus.

Uncommon clinical presentations of stroke

The capsular warning syndrome

A small infarct in the internal capsule is considered to be caused by the occlusion of a single lenticulostriate artery which arises from the mainstem of the middle cerebral artery (MCA). This infarct typically presents with "pure motor hemiparesis". The term "capsular warning syndrome" describes the phenomenon in which the infarct may be preceded by repetitive, stereotypic transient ischemic attacks with "pure motor hemiparesis" ("lacunar TIAs"). This burst of hemiplegic TIAs is limited in time and lasts about 24–48 hours. The risk of developing a lacunar infarct is about 40% within the next few days. In situ small-vessel disease (microatheroma or lipohyalinosis) is considered to be the most likely mechanism. Alternatively, it has been suggested that an atheroma in the MCA may cause a high-grade obstruction at the origin of the single lenticulostriate artery [10] (Figure 9.3).

Bilateral blindness: "top of the basilar artery"

Sudden cortical blindness is a rare symptom of TIA or stroke and has been explained by an occlusion of the "top of the basilar artery" at the origin of the posterior cerebral arteries [11]. The visual field defects may be

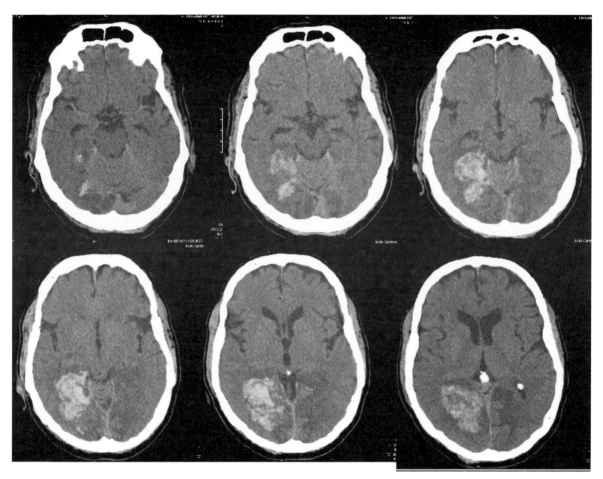

Figure 9.4. "Blind sight". A 65-year-old patient with known Parkinson's disease and vascular risk factors (diabetes mellitus, hypertension, obesity and smoking) suddenly lost muscle tone and consciousness. On admission he was awake, responded to verbal commands and was partially oriented. Pupils were mid-dilated, response to light was reduced. He reported not seeing anything with either eye. There was no weakness of the limbs. Although without conscious visual perception he was able to unconsciously prevent himself from bumping into objects when walking. When showing him different numbers of fingers he mentioned not seeing the fingers but his performance of rating the number of presented fingers was much above chance. CCT showed a bilateral infarction in the territory of the posterior cerebral artery with hemorrhage on the right side. The primary visual cortex of each side was damaged.

quite asymmetric and variable. Symptoms may be transient (TIA) or persisting. Even when severe cortical blindness is present, patients may retain some ability to avoid bumping into objects and may blink to visual threat. This so-called blind sight is probably explained by some sparing of the visual cortex and by preservation of the so-called second visual system, which is composed of the superior colliculi and their projections to peristriate cortex (Figure 9.4). Embolism from the heart or the proximal vertebrobasilar artery is the cause of this sign [12]. Other symptoms of bilateral ischemia in the territory of the PCA may be: memory loss, usually involving both anterograde and retrograde amnesia, and agitated delirium. In

cases of persistent amnesia, bilateral infarction of the mesial temporal lobe was described [8].

> Bilateral blindness can be due to occlusion of the basilar artery at the bifurcation to the posterior cerebral arteries.

Amnesia

Personal (autobiographical) memories depend on the ability to encode, store and retrieve information which we consciously experience ("autobiographic episodes"). The cognitive system representing this ability is termed episodic memory. It can be tested by questions about recent personal history or more systematically by presenting a list of words and by testing free recall of them after a few minutes. The anatomical structures underlying episodic memory are the Papez circle (hippocampus, parahippocampus, ento- and perirhinal cortex, cingulate gyrus, fornix, nucleus anterior thalami, mamillothalamic tracts and mammillary bodies), the basolateral limbic circuit (dorso-medial thalamic nucleus and amygdala) and the basal forebrain. Input from this system is necessary to ensure that the multimodal information from the environment which is processed and integrated in the neocortical association areas becomes memorable and retrievable. A disorder of the system underlying episodic memory causes ante-rograde amnesia. The arterial blood supply of the anatomical structures subserving episodic memory has many sources, particularly the anterior cerebral artery and the anterior communicating artery (basal forebrain and fornix), posterior communicating artery (parts of the thalamus), posterior cerebral artery (hippocampus and parahippocampal gyrus), anterior choroidal artery (anterior hippocampus and adjacent cortex) and posterior choroidal artery (parts of the fornix).

There are three uncommon but relevant stroke syndromes which cause amnesia:

- bilateral infarcts of the medio-basal temporal lobe
- bilateral thalamic infarcts and
- subarachnoid hemorrhage from aneurysm of the anterior communicating artery.

Memory defects can follow unilateral or bilateral infarcts of the medio-basal temporal lobe but are more common with left-sided and bilateral lesions. Recall of memories is mainly based on two processes, judgements that something is familiar and the conscious recollection of an episode with all attributes. Depending on the site of the lesion, recognition of familiarity or conscious recollection may be more disturbed. Further-more, left-sided infarcts are known to cause predomin-antly verbal amnesia whereas right-sided lesions may disturb visuo-spatial memories. Embolism from the heart or proximal vertebrobasilar artery is typically found to be the cause of bilateral infarcts.

Infarcts in the anterior and dorsomedial thalamus can produce severe memory deficits which are almost always accompanied by other neurological and neuropsychological symptoms such as attentional deficits, language disturbance, neglect or executive dysfunctions. If amnesia is the leading clinical symptom TIA or stroke has to be distinguished from transient global amnesia (TGA). TIA and stroke are either accompanied by other neuropsychological symptoms or can be demonstrated with brain imaging.

> Amnesia can be caused by temporal lobe or thalamic infarcts.

Reduced vigilance or coma as the leading symptom

Bilateral paramedian thalamic infarction can result from an occlusion of a single thalamic-subthalamic artery which branches from the posterior cerebral artery (PCA). Patients can be hypersomnolent or comatose as if being in an anoxic or metabolic coma without local-izable neurological signs. After regaining consciousness, disturbance of vertical gaze function (upgaze palsy, combined up- and downgaze palsy or skew deviation) and neuropsychological deficits may become apparent.

Coma is more frequently found in patients with acute occlusion of the basilar artery in whom ischemia involves the bilateral pontine tegmentum. But here, additional neurological signs such as ophthalmoplegia and bilateral extensor plantar reflexes indicate brainstem ischemia.

> Coma is frequently found in basilar artery occlusion.

Agitation and delirium as the presenting symptom

According to the American Psychiatric Association (1987) delirium is defined as a clinical symptom with the following symptoms and signs:

- reduced ability to maintain attention to external stimuli and to appropriately shift attention to new stimuli
- disorganized thinking as indicated by irrelevant or incoherent speech
- symptoms such as reduced level of consciousness, perceptual disturbances (misinterpretations, illusions or hallucinations), disturbances of sleep–wake cycle, increased or decreased psychomotor activity, disorientation to time, place, or person, memory impairment
- clinical features developing over a short time and tending to fluctuate over the course of a day.

Agitation and/or delirium may be the leading or the only symptom of acute stroke. It is uncommon

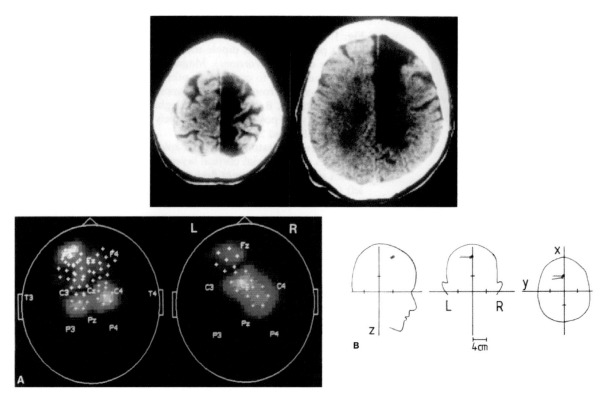

Figure 9.5. Contralateral akinesia/hypokinesia. A patient suffered from a large infarction in the territory of the right anterior cerebral artery (ACA). His left arm was spontaneously not used but showed forced grasping reflexes to visual and tactile stimuli. The patient participated in an experiment with measurements of magnetic fields of the brain preceding spontaneous movements of the right index finger. With movements of the right finger an activation in the intact left supplementary motor area (SMA) preceding the onset of movement by more than 1 second was shown [17].

and may not be considered a clinical manifestation of stroke. In a retrospective analysis, 19 of 661 stroke patients (3%) presented with delirium [13]. Right hemisphere infarcts that include the hippocampus, amygdala, entorhinal and perirhinal cortex and their underlying white matter have been found to be most frequently associated with agitation and delirium.

Isolated cranial nerves

Stroke in the brainstem is typically indicated by (a) ipsilateral cranial nerve (III–XII) palsy (single or multiple) together with contralateral motor or sensory deficit, (b) bilateral motor and/or sensory deficits or (c) disorders of conjugate eye movements. Rarely, cranial nerve palsy without any sensory or motor deficits may indicate a focal brainstem ischemia. Two out of 22 patients with focal ischemic lesions in the mesencephalon had an isolated palsy of the oculomotor nerve [14]. Thömke et al. [15] studied 29 patients with diabetes mellitus and oculomotor nerve

palsy. In five patients a focal ischemic lesion in the mesencephalon was causal for the deficit. Isolated palsy of the trochlear nerve has been described with focal hemorrhage or ischemia in the mesencephalon. Isolated palsy of the abducens, trigeminal, facial nerve and even of the vestibular part of the vestibulocochlear nerve is caused by focal hemorrhage or ischemia in the pons [16]. Ischemia may be caused by low flow in boundary zones.

> Focal brainstem ischemia may cause isolated cranial nerve palsy.

Akinesia or involuntary movements

Acute hypokinetic or hyperkinetic movement disorders are an uncommon but sometimes the leading symptom of stroke.

Acute akinesia or hypokinesia of the contralateral part of the body is found after ischemic lesions of the medial part of the frontal lobe [17] (Figure 9.5). The supplementary motor area (SMA) is the medial part of the premotor cortex and is supplied by the anterior cerebral artery. It is part of a neuronal loop which involves frontal cortex, basal ganglia and thalamus. The SMA receives excitatory input from the ventro-lateral thalamus. Lesions of the SMA in the left hemisphere cause a lack of spontaneous speech (transcortical motor aphasia) with preserved comprehension and repetition and a hypokinesia/akinesia of contralateral body. Usually, these symptoms are transient. Lesions of the right SMA are associated with hypokinesia/akinesia of the left part of the body. Bilateral lesions of the mesial frontal cortex are known to cause severe akinetic states. Typically there is a marked contrast between the paucity or absence of spontaneous movements and the preserved or even exaggerated ability to respond to external visual or tactile clues ("forced grasping"). Response to external stimuli helps to distinguish motor hypokinesia/akinesia from motor neglect. Motor (hemi-) neglect may be an isolated symptom but is mainly part of a neglect syndrome which is characterized by a reduction of focal attention.

Hemichorea-hemiballism is the most frequently reported acute involuntary movement disorder in acute stroke. It has classically been described after an acute small deep infarct in the subthalamic nucleus [18].

> Akinesia can be caused by lesions in the medial frontal lobe.

Focal paresis

Weakness of one side of the body is the most frequent symptom of TIA or stroke. Typically either one part or several parts of the body are involved (face, arm, leg, face + arm, face + arm + leg). It is more uncommon in focal brain ischemia for isolated movements such as extension of fingers and hand or movements of the tongue to be the only symptom (Figure 9.6).

Uncommon causes of stroke and associated clinical syndromes

Stroke manifestations of systemic disease

Infective and non-infective endocarditis: multi-territorial pattern of ischemic stroke

Endocarditis of the heart and its valves in particular can be classified into infective and non-infective types. The vast majority of endocarditis is secondary to infections caused by bacterial (*Staphylococcus aureus*,

coagulase-negative *Staphylococcus* or *Enterococcus*) or, rarely, fungal (*Candida*, *Aspergillus*) organisms [19]. Cerebral embolism from infected valves is the central mechanism of neurological injury in patients with infective endocarditis. Embolic debris from infected valves typically lodges in the distal branches of the middle cerebral artery [20]. Over 50% of patients had infarcts involving more than one arterial territory [21]. Besides brain and retinal ischemia, other cerebrovascular complications include intracranial hemorrhage and subarachnoid hemorrhage [22]. Mycotic aneurysms are often assumed to be the cause of cerebral hemorrhage. They are thought to develop after septic microembolism to the vaso vasorum of cerebral vessels. But mycotic aneurysms are found in less than 3% of hemorrhages. More common mechanisms of hemorrhage include hemorrhagic transformation of the ischemic infarction, septic endarteritis and non-aneurysmal arterial erosion at the site of the previous embolic occlusion, and concurrent antithrombotic medication use [23].

Non-infective endocarditis is termed non-bacterial thrombotic endocarditis (NBTE). It is characterized by the accumulation of sterile platelet and fibrin aggregates on the heart valves to form small vegetations. About 50% of NBTE cases occur in association with cancer, especially mucin-producing adenocarcinomas (particularly pancreatic carcinoma and non-small-cell lung cancer) and hematological malignancies (lymphoma and leukemia [24]). Although only less than 2% of patients with cancer have NBTE, up to 50% of these patients with NBTE suffer from stroke [25]. A significant proportion of patients with NBTE have other disorders, including rheumatic heart disease, rheumatological diseases such as lupus (where it is referred to as Lipman-Sacks endocarditis), AIDS, gastrointestinal diseases such as cirrhosis, and severe systemic illness, such as burns or sepsis [26]. Small and large multi-territorial infarction is a radiographic sign in NBTE [27]. Thus, encephalopathy rather than focal deficits may be the initial clinical presentation.

> Endocarditis of various origins typically causes multi-territorial infarctions.

Inflammatory vasculopathies and connective tissue disease: a chronic and multisystemic disease

Inflammatory vasculopathies and connective tissue disease are Takayashu's arteritis, systemic lupus

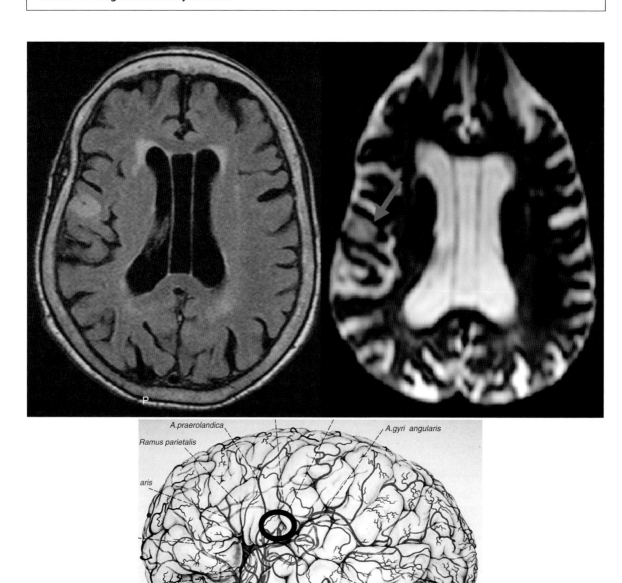

Figure 9.6. Focal paresis. A 95-year-old woman suffered from slurred speech. There was a shift of the tongue to the left side. Diffusion-weighted imaging showed a small cortical lesion in the frontal operculum which was most likely caused by a cardiac embolism because of atrial fibrillation.

erythematosus (SLE), antiphospholipid antibody syndrome, Sneddon syndrome, primary systemic vasculitis (classic polyarteritis nodosa, microscopic polyangiitis, Churg-Strauss syndrome, Wegener's granulomatosis), Sjögren syndrome, Behcet disease, primary angiitis of the central nervous system, and paraneoplastic vasculitis. Warlow et al. [1] have summarized clinical clues which may in general indicate inflammatory vasculopathies and connective tissue disease. Patients may present with TIA and stroke but also with encephalopathy:

- preceding or accompanying systemic features such as weight loss, headache, malaise, skin rash, livedo reticularis, arthropathy, renal failure and fever
- lack of any other obvious or more common cause of stroke
- younger patient in most cases (an exception being giant cell arteritis)
- a raised ESR and C-reactive protein
- anemia and leukocytosis in the routine blood screening tests
- when there is diagnostic suspicion, specified immunological tests such as raised serum antiphospholipid, double-stranded DNA and antineutrophil cytoplasmic antibodies (ANCA).

Among those diseases, giant cell arteritis and systemic lupus erythematosus are uncommon but not rare and will be presented in more detail.

Giant cell arteritis is also known as temporal arteritis, cranial arteritis or Horton's disease. The annual incidence increases with age from 2.6/100 000 for those aged between 50 and 59 years to 44.6/100 000 for those older than 80 years. Headache, especially in the night, located in the temporal region, fever, weight loss, fatigue and malaise or arthralgia and jaw claudication are the predominating symptoms. Most patients with giant cell arteritis have symptoms of polymyalgia rheumatica, which may precede the headache. A raised ESR (over 50 or even 100 mm in the first hour) is also indicative.

Ischemic symptoms of the retina and the brain usually develop late in the course of disease. But stroke may even be the first indication of disease. Giant cell arteritis involves the ophthalmic, posterior ciliary and central retinal arteries, which causes infarction of the optic nerve. It may also involve intracranial vessels, particularly the extradural vertebral arteries, which may cause stroke. Diplopia and ophthalmoplegia may develop but are mainly caused by necrosis of the extraocular muscles and not by brainstem ischemia.

Systemic lupus erythematosus is a chronic auto-immune disease affecting mainly young women. It much more often causes a generalized subacute or chronic encephalopathy than focal ischemic or hemorrhagic cerebral episodes. Intimal proliferation involving small vessels may represent florid or healed vasculitic lesions. Large artery occlusions can be explained in some patients by cardiac sources (NBTE:

non-bacterial thrombotic embolism). Most patients have circulating antinuclear antibodies. A raised antinuclear factor is highly sensitive but not specific. Double-stranded DNA and anti-Sm antibodies are much more specific but are found in less than half of cases. A high proportion of patients also have antiphospholipid antibodies, which seem to be particularly associated with cardiac valvular vegetations and arterial thrombosis. The antiphospholipid syndrome cannot be diagnosed on the basis of a raised single titer of antibody in the serum. The titer must be substantially raised on several occasions and must be associated not only with ischemic stroke but also with other manifestations of disease such as deep venous thrombosis, recurrent miscarriage, livedo reticularis, cardiac valvular vegetations, migraine-like headache, thrombocytopenia, or hemolytic anemia.

Inflammatory vasculopathies require special diagnostic tests.

Intracranial vasculopathies caused by virus and bacterial infection

Varicella zoster virus vasculopathy

Varicella zoster virus (VZV) vasculopathy may often be clinically silent but may present with stroke and can be diagnosed because of the following symptoms, signs and findings (for review: Nagel et al. [28]). (1) About two-thirds of patients have a history of zoster rash, particularly ophthalmic-distribution zoster or a history of chicken pox. There is a delay between the onset of zoster/chicken pox and the onset of stroke averaging 4.1 months (range between same day and 2.5 years). But about one-third of patients with a pathologically and virologically verified disease have no history of zoster rash or chicken pox. (2) Angiographic evidence of narrowing in cerebral arteries may be found in MR angiography. In vascular studies 70% had vasculopathies. Different patterns of vascular lesions have been found. There was pure large artery disease in 13%, pure small artery disease in 37% and a mixed vascular pathology in most patients (50%). (3) Varicella zoster virus as the cause of stroke can be proven by examinations of the cerebrospinal fluid: 67% of patients have a pleocytosis (>5 white blood cells/mm^3). Thus, some patients may even have no pleocytosis. Specific antibodies (anti-VZV-IgG) with proven intrathecal synthesis were found in 93% of patients, and VZV-DNA in 30%.

A negative result for both VZV DNA and anti-VZV-IgG antibody in CSF can reliably exclude the diagnosis of VZV vasculopathy.

Chronic bacterial, meningeal infections

Ischemic stroke complicates chronic meningeal infections which cause inflammation and thrombosis of arteries and veins on the surface of the brain. With tuberculous meningitis, infection is predominantly located at the base of the brain and vasculitis causes thrombosis in the large intracranial arteries and territorial infarction. Different vascular territories may be involved depending on the spatial extent of the meningeal infection. Tuberculous meningitis has to be considered as a clinical syndrome when one of the following criteria accompanies ischemic stroke [29]:

- medical history with manifestation of tuberculosis in the lungs or in a different organ (this manifestation may have been many decades ago)
- one or more symptoms indicating chronic meningeal infection such as headache or subfebrile temperature preceding stroke
- other signs indicating a process in the basal meninges such as lesion of cranial nerves or development of hydrocephalus as a consequence of an obstruction of the basal cisterns.

In addition there may be more unspecific signs as well, such as loss of appetite, drowsiness or myalgia. Contrast-enhanced magnetic resonance imaging may show up the basal meningitis. The cerebrospinal fluid shows mild to moderate pleocytosis with white blood cells up to $300/mm^3$, the glucose is reduced with subacute infections and protein is elevated as a sign of the disturbed circulation of the cerebrospinal fluid. Infection with tuberculosis can be proven by cytology (Ziehl–Neelsen), culture, detection of DNA (PCR) or antigen.

Syphilitic meningovasculitis

Syphilitic meningovasculitis may be the first clinical presentation of an infection with *Treponema pallidum*. The primary infection with a syphilitic lesion in the mucosa may have been months to years ago. Syphilitic meningovasculitis presents with an obliteration of small or middle-large vessels; rarely are large arteries involved. The territory of the middle cerebral artery is mainly involved. Infected vessels and their vasa vasorum together with lymphocytic infiltration cause a slow progression of stenosis leading to occlusion.

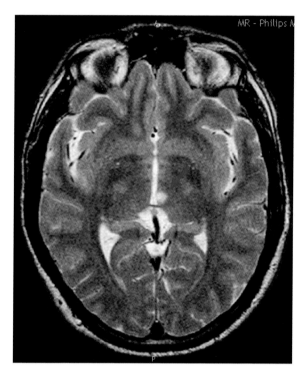

Figure 9.7. Meningovascular syphilis. The patient presented with the following signs: awake but apathic, decreased episodic memory, complete upgaze palsy, incomplete downgaze palsy, disturbed converge of eyes, contraversive ocular tilt reaction (tendency to fall to the right side and skew deviation). Pupils were reactive to light. There was a minimal hemiparesis shown up by a tendency to pronate with the right arm. MR shows a vascular lesion in the territory of the left thalamic-subthalamic artery. This lesion was caused by meningovascular syphilis proved by intrathecal production of specific antibodies (FTA-Abs) and mild pleocytosis.

Patients may present with signs of meningeal (meningo-encephalitic) inflammation such as headache, dizziness, feeling sick, sleep disorder, change of personality, apathy and deficits of episodic memory. Ischemic stroke can be preceded by TIA. Usually, the size of ischemic infarcts is small. There may be lesions of the cranial nerves because of the associated meningitis (Figure 9.7). Documentation of the intrathecal production of specific antibodies is required for a definite diagnosis of syphilitic meningovasculitis. Pleocytosis in the CSF together with specific antibodies in the serum can be taken as evidence of a likely syphilitic meningovasculitis. Other mechanisms of stroke associated with syphilis are mesaaortitis luetica with aortic dissection and endocarditis.

Viral and bacterial infections can cause specific vasculopathies.

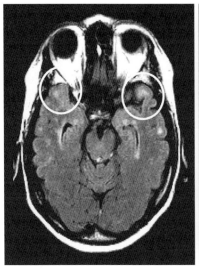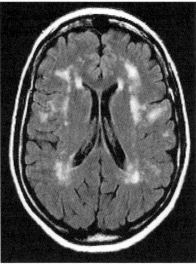

Figure 9.8. CADASIL. Extensive morphological abnormalities are found in CADASIL despite the absence of vascular risk factors, particularly in younger patients. White matter hyperintensities (WMHs) are characteristically located in the white matter of the anterior temporal lobe and the external capsule, which is unusual for other small-vessel diseases. (Courtesy of Professor Franz Fazekas, University of Graz.)

Hereditary causes of stroke (single gene disorders) and their clinical presentation

CADASIL (cerebral autosomal dominant arteriopathy with subcortical infarcts and leukoencephalopathy), Fabry disease and MELAS (mitochondrial encephalopathy lactic acidosis and stroke) are genetic disorders associated with their own clinical and radiological presentation.

CADASIL

Genetic and pathological research suggests that the accumulation of the ectodomain of the NOTCH 3 protein is associated with severe ultrastructural alterations of the arteriolar wall [30]. The earliest clinical manifestation of CADASIL is migraine with aura at a mean age of 28 years. The aura may be visual or sensory but the frequency of attacks with basilar, hemiplegic and prolonged aura is high. At a mean age of 41 years, stroke becomes manifest in the course of disease. Two-thirds of patients present with lacunar syndromes such as pure motor, ataxic hemiparesis, pure sensory or sensory motor stroke. With increasing load of subcortical white matter lesion, vascular dementia with deficits of executive functions, and attentional and memory deficits develops (mean age of 50 years). Twenty percent of patients have severe mood disorders, and focal or generalized seizures have been observed in about 8% of patients.

Microangiopathy or small-vessel disease (SVD) is the morphological presentation of the disease with multiple lacunar lesions and extensive white matter hyperintensities (WMHs), which may be accompanied by evidence of microbleeds (MBs). A first hint for CADASIL is the presence of extensive morphological abnormalities with SVD in the absence of vascular risk factors, especially in younger patients. Not infrequently, such a constellation may lead to a false suspicion of multiple sclerosis. Further evidence comes from the distribution of WMHs. In CADASIL, WMHs are characteristically located in the white matter of the anterior temporal lobe and the external capsule as early as in the third decade [31]. Location of WMHs and age of onset are unusual for other SVDs (Figure 9.8).

> CADASIL is a rare genetic disorder causing small-vessel disease and multiple white matter lesions in young adults.

Fabry disease

Fabry's disease, also Anderson-Fabry's disease or angiokeratomy corporis diffusum, is an X-linked lysosomal storage disorder. Alpha-galactosidase deficiency leads to accumulation of glycolipids, mainly in endothelial and smooth muscle cells. A more recent study of 721 sufferers from acute cryptogenic stroke aged 18 to 55 years showed a rare but not negligible frequency of Fabry disease, which was 4.9% in male and 2.4% in female stroke patients [32]. The patients are mainly young and present with a variety of symptoms and signs which are caused by deposition

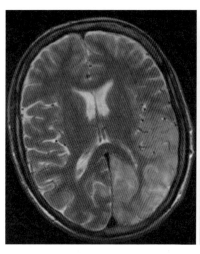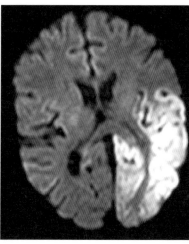

Figure 9.9. MELAS. MELAS-related brain lesions appear bright on diffusion-weighted imaging (right-hand picture). A hint towards the correct diagnosis is that MELAS lesions usually tend to cross the known borders of the vascular territories of the brain. In this patient, the two vascular territories, posterior cerebral artery and middle cerebral artery, of the left hemisphere are involved. (Courtesy of Professor Franz Fazekas, University of Graz.)

of glycolipids in the tissue: skin manifestation with angiokeratomas (mainly in the bathing-trunk area) and hypohydrosis, small fiber neuropathy with burning pain and paresthesias in hands and feet, renal dysfunction or failure, vessel ectasia (particular basilar artery), corneal dystrophy, cardiomyopathy and stroke.

The early presence of incidental WMHs has been observed and there appears to be a predisposition for infarction to occur in the vertebrobasilar system. Vascular ectasia up to the megadolichobasilar artery has also been reported. The most specific abnormality, however, appears to be a hyperintense signal of the pulvinar thalami on T1-weighted images [33]. Up to one-quarter of patients with Fabry disease may show this abnormality, which could be a consequence of microvascular calcification. Clinically silent or manifest strokes, both cortical and subcortical, are caused by occlusion of small vessels or by extasia of larger vessels, embolism from the heart, and rarely by intracranial hemorrhage.

> Fabry disease presents with a variety of symptoms, including stroke.

MELAS (mitochondrial encephalopathy lactic acidosis and stroke)

MELAS is a mitochondrial disorder that causes stroke-like syndromes in young patients, occurring as early as the teenage years, with transient or permanent hemianopia, aphasia or hemiparesis. Sudden episodes of headache and seizure or vomiting occur.

Blood lactate levels are elevated, indicating dysfunction of the respiratory chain. Most commonly, MELAS is associated with a mitochondrial DNA point mutation at position 3243 within the tRNA encoding gene. Many different phenotypes, alone or in combinations, have been reported with this mutation (hearing impairment, cognitive decline, progressive external ophthalmoplegia, or epilepsy).

MELAS-related brain lesions appear bright on diffusion-weighted imaging with reduced diffusity on corresponding ADC maps and are thus frequently mistaken for acute infarction [34]. A hint towards the correct diagnosis comes from the fact that MELAS lesions usually tend to cross the known borders of the vascular territories of the brain and have a variable ADC. Posterior parietal and occipital locations appear to be most frequent (Figure 9.9). The lesions may also subside without remaining signal changes, which would be quite unusual for infarction, and have a tendency to slowly progress or to reoccur at other sites, sometimes within relatively short intervals of days to weeks [35]. Besides increased levels of lactate in the CSF during the attack, MR spectroscopy may also serve to demonstrate increased lactate in the brain parenchyma and cerebral lesions as well as in the CSF [36]. The most likely origin of stroke-like episodes is a sudden metabolic failure with loss of function and transient or persistent cellular damage.

> MELAS is a mitochondrial disorder causing stroke-like syndromes, red-ragged fibers, myopathy and lactacidosis.

Arterial dissection: uncommon clinical presentations

Bogousslavsky et al. [37] found an incidence of arterial dissection of 2.5% in 1200 consecutive first stroke patients. Under the age of 45 the incidence of cervical artery dissection (CAD) is much higher at 10–25% and CAD is the second leading cause of stroke in younger adults [38]. Most patients with dissections are between 30 and 50 years of age, and the mean age is approximately 40 years. The annual incidence of cervical internal carotid artery dissection was found to be 3.5 per 100 000 in those older than 20 years, and the annual incidence of vertebral artery dissection 1.5 per 100 000 [39]. Extracranial ICA dissection typically occurs about 2 cm distal to the bifurcation, near the C2/C3 vertebral level, and extends superiorly for a variable distance. The vertebral artery is most mobile and susceptible to mechanical injury at the C1/C2 level.

Predisposing factors for CAD are trauma (mild or trivial, major, iatrogenic), arteriopathies (e.g. fibromuscular dysplasia, Ehlers Danlos syndrome, Marfan syndrome), migraine, recent infection or drugs (cocaine). Estimates of dissection risk after chiropractic manipulation vary widely with the study methodology but range from 1 in 5.85 million manipulations to as many as 1 in 20 000 manipulations. One study found connective tissue disorders in one-fourth of patients with cervical artery dissections after chiropractic manipulations [40].

Arterial dissections usually arise from an intimal tear that allows the development of an intramural hematoma (false lumen). In some patients, no communication between the true and the false lumen can be demonstrated, suggesting that some dissections are the result of a primary intramedial hematoma. Subintimal dissections are more likely to cause luminal stenosis. Subadventitial dissections may cause arterial dilatation (aneurysms). Mechanisms of ischemic stroke are either hemodynamic compromise secondary to luminal narrowing or occlusion or embolism from thrombus within the true lumen. The absence of an external elastic lamina and a thin adventitia makes intracranial arteries prone to subadventitial dissection and subsequent subarachnoid hemorrhage. SAH is reported in about one-fifth of intracranial ICA dissections and in more than half of intracranial vertebral artery dissections [41].

Saver and Easton [42] summarized symptoms and signs of ICA dissection:

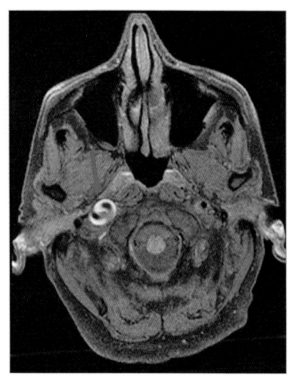

Figure 9.10. Collet Sicard syndrome in dissection of the internal carotid artery. A 60-year-old man noticed right-sided neck pain, ipsilateral headache, problems with swallowing and tongue movements and dysarthria (hoarseness). Some weeks later he was admitted to a neurological department and presented with right-sided glossopharyngeal and spinal accessory nerve lesions (moderate paresis of the upper portion of the trapezius and the sternocleidomastoid muscles), hypoglossus and recurrent nerve palsies. MRI showed a dissection of the right internal carotid artery in its very distal extracranial section with a prominent subadventitial wall hematoma and expansion of the vessel diameter but without relevant narrowing of the lumen. There was a prominent coiling of the internal carotid artery in the area of dissection. The combination of lower cranial nerve palsies (IX to XII) is commonly referred to as Collet Sicard syndrome. (Courtesy of Dr Michael Spiegel, University of Innsbruck.)

- ischemic stroke (46%)
- TIA (30%)
- unusual and sharp pain in the face or in the neck on the side ipsilateral to ICA dissection (21%)
- pulsatile tinnitus alone when carotid dissection spreads distally to the base of the skull (2%)
- partial Horner's syndrome as a result of damage to the sympathetic nerve fibers around the dissected ICA (32%) and
- ipsilateral palsies of one or more cranial nerves (IX, X, XI, XII), particularly the hypoglossus (XII), as a result of nerve compression (3%) at the base of the skull (Figure 9.10).

Baumgartner et al. [43] have reported that dissections causing ischemic events are more often associated with occlusion and stenosis greater than 80% and that dissections that do not cause ischemic events are more often associated with Horner's syndrome and lower cranial nerve palsies.

Cervical artery dissection is the second leading cause of stroke in young adults.

Symptoms and sign of extracranial vertebral dissection are [42]:

- ischemic stroke (75%)
- TIA (25%)
- head or neck pain (75%)
- rarely: cervical nerve root lesions (C5 and C6) as caused by ischemia or pressure from the bulging arterial wall.

Aortic arch dissection can cause generalized brain hypoxemia and low-flow infarction as a result of systemic hypotension caused by cardiac tamponade, acute aortic regurgitation or myocardial infarction. Dissection may spread out into the major neck arteries and may cause occlusion with low flow or TIA and ischemic stroke by embolism. Clues for the diagnosis of aortic dissection are [1]:

- sudden and severe anterior chest pain and/or interscapular pain which may move as the dissection extends
- syncope
- hypotension
- diminished, unequal or absent arterial pulses and blood pressure in the arms and sometimes legs
- acute aortic regurgitation and cardiac failure
- simultaneous or sequential ischemia in carotid, subclavian, vertebral, spinal, coronary and other aortic branches if the dissection extends over several centimeters.

Moyamoya

The first report of a patient was published in 1957 by Takeuchi and Shimizu [44] with the diagnosis "bilateral hypoplasia of the internal carotid arteries". This was a 29-year-old man who had been suffering from visual disturbance and hemiconvulsive seizures since the age of 10 years.

Moyamoya is defined by a pattern of severe stenosis or occlusion of one or more often of both internal carotid arteries with additional involvement of the circle of Willis. It may progress after diagnosis. Small collaterals develop from the lenticulostriate, thalamoperforating and pial arteries at the base of the brain, from leptomeningeal collaterals of the posterior cerebral artery or from branches of the external cerebral artery (orbital, ethmoidal or transdural). The pattern of collaterals looks like a puff of smoke (moyamoya in Japanese) in the basal ganglia region on the cerebral angiogram. Moyamoya is mostly, but not entirely, found in Japanese and other East Asian subjects. The annual incidence in Japan has been calculated to be 0.35/100 000 persons. It is mainly familial or congenital but can be caused by various disorders (meningeal or nasopharyngeal infection, vasculitis, irradiation, trauma, a generalized fibromuscular dysplasia, sickle-cell disease or neurofibromatosis, drugs such as cocaine).

The mechanism of brain ischemia is low flow. The vascular reserve capacity is exhausted and ischemia can be provoked by conditions which induce vasodilatation, such as hyperventilation, and are often precipitated by infection in the upper respiratory airway. Children present with recurrent focal cerebral ischemia and infarction, cognitive impairment, headache, seizure and, occasionally, involuntary movements. Adults can present with either focal brain ischemia (TIA, stroke; 63.4%), hemorrhage (21.6%), epileptic seizures (7.6%) or others (e.g. cognitive impairment, headache; 7.5%) [45].

Moyamoya is characterized by stenosis/occlusion of both internal carotid arteries and a network of collaterals ("haze"). It is mostly, but not exclusively, found in Japan.

Migraine and stroke

The prevalence of migraine with aura is about 4%. An aura is defined as a neurological symptom which is localizable in the brain, develops gradually over 5–20 minutes and lasts less than 1 hour. Aura can be classified into:

- typical aura with visual, hemiparesthetic, aphasic or hemiparetic (hemiplegic) symptoms and signs
- prolonged aura (lasting longer than 1 hour but less than 7 days with normal brain imaging)
- basilar aura
- migraine aura without headache
- migraine with acute aura onset.

With migrainous infarction the symptoms associated with the typical aura are not fully reversible after

7 days and/or there is an infarct on brain imaging. The following criteria have to be fulfilled:

- patient has previously fulfilled criteria for migraine with neurological aura
- the present attack is typical of previous attacks, but neurological deficits are not completely reversible within 7 days or/and neuroimaging demonstrates ischemic infarction in the relevant area
- other causes of infarction have been ruled out by appropriate investigations (particularly other causes which are associated with migraine, such as CADASIL, MELAS or antiphospholipid syndrome, or which may mimic migraine such as arterial dissection).

A migrainous stroke often results in a homonymous hemianopia and rarely causes persisting and severe disability. Arterial occlusion has rarely been demonstrated and it is not clear why it occurs. "Vasospasm" is often postulated and is said to have been observed in the retinal circulation during transient monocular blindness in a few patients. A migrainous stroke should never be a diagnosis of desperation when no other cause of ischemic stroke can be found, but a positive statement to describe a characteristic clinical syndrome in the absence of no more likely causes of stroke [1].

A migrainous stroke only rarely causes persisting deficits.

Chapter Summary

- An uncommon mechanism of brain ischemia: low flow.

  In some patients severe stenosis or occlusion of carotid or vertebral arteries may cause a critical reduction of blood flow; a drop in systemic blood pressure may cause transient or permanent focal ischemia. A sudden and profound hypotension sometimes causes **boundary-zone infarction**. A fall in cerebral perfusion pressure as a cause of focal brain ischemia should be suspected if the symptoms start under certain circumstances, such as after cardiac arrest or cardiac surgery, on standing up very quickly, or with exercise, coughing or hyperventilation. Syndromes of low flow may include **"limb-shaking TIA"**, **monocular transient retinal ischemia**, **rotational vertebral artery occlusion** and **"drop attacks"**. Abnormal changes of blood plasma

with hematological disease (e.g. paraproteinemia), increase of cell counts (e.g. polycythemia vera) and decreased red cell deformability (e.g. sickle cell anemia) lead to a **hyperviscous state** and cerebral blood flow can be diminished, causing unspecific symptoms such as headache, dizziness or vertigo, paresthesias, blurred vision or tinnitus.

- Uncommon clinical presentations of stroke
  - Include sudden cortical blindness, akinesia, agitation and delirium, as well as isolated cranial nerve palsy.
- Uncommon causes of stroke
  - Infective or non-infective **endocarditis** can lead to cerebral embolism from the valves of the heart, resulting in a multi-territorial pattern of stroke.
  - **Inflammatory vasculopathies** (e.g. giant cell arteritis, systemic lupus erythematodes, polyarteritis nodosa, paraneoplastic vasculitis). In giant cell arteritis infarction of the optic nerve can develop. Systemic lupus erythematodes more often causes a generalized subacute or chronic encephalopathy than focal ischemic or hemorrhagic cerebral episodes. A raised antinuclear factor, double-stranded DNA, anti-Sm antibodies or antiphospholipid antibodies can frequently be found.
  - **Varicella zoster virus (VZV) vasculopathy** may present with stroke. Diagnosis: history of zoster rash, particularly ophthalmic-distribution zoster or a history of chicken pox, MR angiographic evidence of narrowing in cerebral arteries, pleocytosis and anti-VZV-IgG and VZV DNA in the cerebrospinal fluid.
  - **Tuberculous meningitis** (inflammation and thrombosis of arteries and veins on the surface of the brain can lead to ischemic stroke). Diagnosis: medical history of tuberculosis, symptoms indicating chronic meningeal infection, lesion of cranial nerves or development of hydrocephalus, cytology (Ziehl–Neelsen), culture, detection of DNA (PCR) or antigen.
  - **Syphilitic meningovasculitis** presents with an obliteration of small or middle-large vessels; rarely are large arteries involved. Usually, the size of ischemic infarcts is small. Diagnosis: intrathecal production of specific antibodies or pleocytosis in the CSF with specific antibodies in the serum.
  - **CADASIL** (cerebral autosomal dominant arteriopathy with subcortical infarcts and leukoencephalopathy) manifests with migraine

with aura at a mean age of 28 years. At a mean age of 41 years, stroke (small-vessel disease with multiple lacunar lesions) becomes manifest.

- Patients with **Fabry's disease** (an X-linked alpha-galactosidase deficiency leads to an accumulation of glycolipids) are young and present with a variety of symptoms: angio-keratomas, small fiber neuropathy, renal failure, cardiomyopathy and stroke.

- **MELAS** (mitochondrial encephalomyopathy lactic acidosis and stroke) is a mitochondrial disorder that causes stroke-like syndromes in young patients, occurring as early as the teenage years, with transient or permanent hemianopia, aphasia or hemiparesis. The most likely origin of stroke-like episodes is a sudden metabolic failure with loss of function and transient or persistent cellular damage.

- **Cervical artery dissection** (CAD) is the second leading cause of stroke in younger adults. Ischemic stroke can also be a symptom of **extracranial vertebral dissection. Aortic arc dissection** can cause low-flow infarction or ischemic stroke by embolism.

- **Moyamoya** is mostly found in East Asians and shows a pattern of severe stenosis or occlusion of one or both internal carotid arteries; the mechanism of brain ischemia is low flow.

- A **migrainous** stroke often results in a homonymous hemianopia and rarely causes persisting and severe disability.

References

1. Warlow C, van Gijn J, Dennis M, Wardlaw J, Bamford J, Hankey G, et al. *Stroke*, 3rd ed. Oxford: Blackwell; 2008.

2. Ringelstein ER, Stögbauer F. Border zone infarcts. In: Bogousslavsky J, Caplan L, eds. *Stroke Syndromes*, 2nd ed. Cambridge: Cambridge University Press; 2001: 564–83.

3. Choi KD, Shin HY, Kim JS, Kim SH, Kwon OK, Koo JW, et al. Rotational vertebral artery syndrome: oculographic analysis of nystagmus. *Neurology* 2005; 65:1287–90.

4. Kuether TA, Nesbit GM, Clark GM, Barnell SL. Rotational vertebral artery occlusion: a mechanism of vertebrobasilar insufficiency. *Neurosurgery* 1997; 41:427–32.

5. Caplan LR, Wityk RJ, Glass TA, Tapia J, Pazdera L, Chang HM, et al. New England Medical Center

Posterior Circulation registry. *Ann Neurol* 2004; 56:389–98.

6. Gerstner E, Liberato B, Wright CB. Bi-hemispheric anterior cerebral artery with drop attack and limb shaking TIAs. *Neurology* 2005; 65:174.

7. Hennerici M, Klemm C, Rautenberg W. The subclavian steal phenomenon: a common vascular disorder with rare neurological deficits. *Neurology* 1988; 38:669–73.

8. Caplan LR. *Posterior Circulation Disease. Clinical Findings, Diagnosis, and Management.* Boston: Blackwell; 1996.

9. Dashe JF. Hyperviscosity and stroke. In: Bogousslavsky J, Caplan L, eds. *Uncommon Causes of Stroke* Cambridge: Cambridge University Press; 2001: 100–10.

10. Donnan GA, O'Malley HM, Quang L, Hurley S, Bladin PF. In: Donnan GA, Norrving B, Bamford J, Bogousslavsky J, eds. *Subcortical Stroke*, 2nd ed. Oxford: Oxford University Press; 2002: 175–84.

11. Caplan LR. "Top of the basilar" syndrome. *Neurology* 1980; 30:72–9.

12. Fisher CM. The posterior cerebral artery syndrome. *Can J Neurol Sci* 1986; 13:232–9.

13. Dunne JW, Leedman PJ, Edis RH. Inobvious stroke: a cause of delirium and dementia. *Austr N Z J Med* 1986: 16:771–8.

14. Bogousslavsky J, Maeder P, Regli F, Meuli R. Pure midbrain infarction: clinical syndromes, MRI, and etiologic patterns. *Neurology* 1994; 44:2032–40.

15. Thömke F, Tettenborn B, Hopf HC. Third nerve palsy as the sole manifestation of midbrain ischemia. *Neuro-ophthalmology* 1995; 15:327–35.

16. Thömke F. Brainstem diseases causing isolated ocular nerve palsies. *Neuro-ophthalmology* 2002; 28:53–67.

17. Lang W, Cheyne D, Kristeva R, Beisteiner R, Lindinger G, Deecke L. Three-dimensional localization of SMA activity preceding voluntary movement – A study of electric and magnetic fields in a patient with infarction of the right supplementary motor area. *Ex Brain Res* 1991; 87:688–95.

18. Gheka J, Bogousslavsky J. Abnormal movements. In: Bogousslavsky J, Caplan L, eds. *Stroke Syndromes*, 2nd ed. Cambridge: Cambridge University Press; 2001: 162–82.

19. Prabhakaran S. Neurologic complications of endocarditis. *Continuum* 2008; 14:53–74.

20. Jones HR, Siekert RG. Neurological manifestations of infective endocarditis. Review of clinical and therapeutic challenges. *Brain* 1989; 112:1295–315.

21. Anderson DJ, Goldstein LB, Wilkinson WE, et al. Stroke location, characterization, severity, and

outcome in mitral vs aortic valve endocarditis.
Neurology 2003; **61**:1341–6.

22. Hart RG, Foster JW, Luther MF, Kanter MC. Stroke in infective endocarditis. *Stroke* 1990; **21**:695–700.

23. Hart RG, Kagan-Hallett K, Joerns SE. Mechanisms of intracranial hemorrhage in infective endocarditis. *Stroke* 1987; **18**:1048–56.

24. Biller J, Challa VR, Toole JF, Howard VJ. Nonbacterial thrombotic endocarditis. A neurological perspective of clinicopathological correlations of 99 patients. *Arch Neurol* 1982; **39**:95–8.

25. Rogers LR, Cho ES, Kempin S, Posner JB. Cerebral infarction from non-bacterial thrombotic endocarditis. Clinical and pathological study including the effects of anticoagulation. *Am J Med* 1987; **83**:746–56.

26. Lopez JA, Ros RS, Fishbein MC, Siegel RJ. Nonbacterial thrombotic endocarditis: a review. *Am Heart J* 1987; **113**:773–84.

27. Singhal AB, Topcuoglu MA, Buonanno FS. Acute ischemic stroke patterns in infective and nonbacterial thrombotic endocarditis: a diffusion-weighted magnetic resonance imaging study. *Stroke* 2002; **33**:1267–73.

28. Nagel MA, Cohrs RJ, Mahalingam R, et al. The varizella zoster virus vasculopathies – clinical, CSF, imaging, and virologic features. *Neurology* 2008; **70**:853–60.

29. Schmutzhard E. *Entzündliche Erkrankungen des Nervensystems*. Stuttgart: Thieme; 2000.

30. Joutel A, Corpechot C, Ducros A, et al. Notch3 mutations in CADASIL, a hereditary adult-onset condition causing stroke and dementia. *Nature* 1996; **383**:707–10.

31. van den Boom, Lesnik Oberstein S, Ferrari M, Haan M. Cerebral autosomal dominant arteriopathy with subcortical infarcts and leukoencephalopathy: MR imaging findings at different ages – 3rd–6th decades. *Radiology* 2003; **229**:683–90.

32. Rolfs A, Böttcher T, Zschiesche M, et al. Prevalence of Fabry disease in patients with cryptogenic stroke: a prospective study. *Lancet* 2005; **366**:1794–6.

33. Takanashi J, Barkovich A, Dillon W, Sherr E, Hart K, Packman S. T1 hyperintensity in the pulvinar: a key imaging feature for diagnosis of Fabry disease. *Am J Neuroradiol* 2003; **24**:916–21.

34. Mizrachi I, Gomez-Hassan D, Blaivas M, Trobe J. Pitfalls in the diagnosis of mitochondrial encephalopathy with lactic acidosis and stroke-like episodes. *J Neuroophthalmol* 2006; **26**:38–43.

35. Iizuka T, Sakai F, Kan S, Suzuki N. Slowly progressive spread of the stroke-like lesions in MELAS. *Neurology* 2003; **61**:1238–44.

36. Möller H, Kurlemann G, Pützler M, Wiedermann D, Hilbich T, Fiedler B. Magnetic resonance spectroscopy in patients with MELAS. *J Neurol Sci* 2005; **229–230**:131–9.

37. Bogousslavsky J, Despland PA, Regli F. Spontaneous carotid dissection with acute stroke. *Arch Neurol* 1987; **44**:137–40.

38. Bogousslavsky J, Pierre P. Ischemic stroke in patients under age 45. *Neurol Clin* 1992; **10**:113.

39. Schievink WI. Spontaneous dissection of the carotid and vertebral arteries. *N Engl J Med* 2001; **344**:898.

40. Zweifler RM, Silverboard GS. Arterial dissections. In: Mohr JP, Choi DW, Grotta JC, et al., eds. *Stroke: Pathophysiology, Diagnosis, and Management*, 4th ed. New York: Churchill Livingstone; 2004: 549–73.

41. Friedman AH, Drake CG. Subarachnoid hemorrhage from intracranial dissecting aneurysm. *J Neurosurg* 1984; **60**:325.

42. Saver JL, Easton JD. Dissections and trauma of cervicocerebral arteries. In: Barnett HJM, Mohr JP, Stein BM, et al., eds. *Stroke: Pathophysiology, Diagnosis and Management*, 3rd ed. New York: Churchill Livingstone; 1998: 769.

43. Baumgartner RW, Arnold M, Baumgartner I, et al. Carotid dissection with and without events: local symptoms and cerebral artery findings. *Neurology* 2001; **57**:827.

44. Takeuchi K, Shimizu K. Hypoplasia of the bilateral internal carotid arteries. *No To Shinkei* 1957; **9**:37.

45. Adams HP. Moya-moya. In: Bogousslavsky J, Caplan J, eds. *Uncommon Causes of Stroke*. Cambridge: Cambridge University Press; 2001: 241.

Intracerebral hemorrhage

Michael Brainin and Raoul Eckhardt

Hemorrhages into the brain occur unexpectedly and are often lethal events. Typical warning signs are not known; rarely a feeling of unsteadiness, dizziness or a tingling sensation can precede an intracerebral hemorrhage (ICH), but such symptoms do not have localizing value such as in ischemia, where stroke-like warning signs (transient attacks) can occur days or weeks before the onset of a stroke. Often enough only a history of elevated blood pressure is known. Thus, for most patients, it comes "out of the blue". The volume of the hemorrhage into the brain is the most decisive prognostic component and when reaching a total volume (such as more than 60 ml within one cerebral hemisphere) that cannot be compensated by intracranial compartmental reserve capacity, the consequences are downward herniation of the medial temporal lobe and compression of the brainstem.

Primary intracerebral hemorrhage associated with hypertension most commonly occurs in deep brain structures (e.g. putamen, thalamus, cerebellum and pons). By contrast, primary intracerebral hemorrhages that occur in lobar regions, particularly in elderly patients, are commonly related to cerebral amyloid angiopathy but might also be associated with hypertension (Table 10.1). At many centers non-contrast CT is the imaging modality of choice for the assessment of intracerebral hemorrhage, owing to its widespread availability and rapid acquisition time. MRI has not been favored due to its higher costs and due to the fact that conventional T1-weighted and T2-weighted MRI pulse sequences are not sensitive to blood in the hyperacute stage. However, recent studies have impressively shown that blood-sensitive gradient echo (GRE) sequences are as accurate as CT for the detection of intraparenchymal hemorrhage and far superior to CT for the detection of chronic hemorrhage [1, 2]. (See Chapter 3 for a detailed discussion of imaging.)

More recently, some "new" aspects of hemorrhages have been discussed among clinicians and researchers, one being the fact that hemorrhages can grow within the first hours after onset [3]. This is well known in classic textbooks of neuropathology as *"Wühlblutung"* (the bleeding that penetrates or forces itself into the parenchyma), and has been described in cases of large hemorrhages extending into lobes or ganglia. It is also well known that hemorrhages into the thalamic region tend to rupture into the ventricles after some hours or days, and this is manifested as a dramatic clinical event with sudden deterioration and herniation signs.

The fact that many parenchymal hemorrhages have a tendency to "grow" has led to therapeutic efforts to inhibit this process by early artificial clotting. Thus, a chance to restrict blood volume in the brain has been seen and prevention of growth within a given time-constrained window has been designed as a therapeutic intervention [4].

Another issue arising from clinical practice comes from the increasing incidence of anticoagulation-associated ICH in elderly people with atrial fibrillation and other cardiac diseases. While in many cases it is often not evident whether anticoagulation (especially when within the therapeutic range) is the cause of ICH and thus can be rated as a "complication" of therapy, it might equally often be considered a failure of anticoagulation therapy resulting from insufficient protection of the brain. Then, an ischemic infarct turning into a secondary hemorrhage is visible upon first imaging. Due to the primary ischemic lesions rapidly turning hemorrhagic, the true incidence of secondary hemorrhagic infarcts is probably higher than was previously thought (for classification of secondary hemorrhages see Table 10.2). Genetic tests or markers of primary hemorrhage would in the future be helpful in making important distinctions between primary and secondary hemorrhages into the brain but are not yet applicable for routine use [5]. New MRI techniques, including

Table 10.1. Distribution by site of 1539 cases of ICH from the Austrian Stroke Registry seen at stroke units between 2003 and 2007.

	N	**(%)**
Putaminal/thalamic	704	(45.7)
Lobar	528	(34.3)
Cerebellar	72	(4.7)
Pontine	58	(3.8)
Miscellaneous	177	(11.5)

Table 10.2. CT classification of hemorrhagic transformation.

Hemorrhagic infarction type 1 (HI-1)
Petechiae along the margins of the infarct
Hemorrhagic infarction type 2 (HI-2)
Petechiae within the infarct region without space-occupying effect
Parenchymal hematoma type 1 (PH-1)
Hematoma in up to 30% of infarct region with some space-occupying effect
Parenchymal hematoma type 2 (PH-2)
Dense hematoma in more than 30% of infarct region with substantial space-occupying effect

Source: Adapted from Kidwell CS, Wintermark M. *Lancet Neurol* 2008; 7:256–67 [2].

magnetic resonance spectroscopy and diffusion tensor imaging, might have importance in the understanding of hemorrhagic injury and provide insights into the time course and pathophysiology of ICH [6].

Silent hemorrhages seen on blood-sensitive gradient echo sequences have also been found quite frequently and their clinical significance as risk factors has not been fully determined. They might be relevant markers of vascular risk factors or in patients already having suffered an ICH, and might signal an increased risk of further hemorrhage. This risk might also be increased in anticoagulation patients, but this has not yet been confirmed in controlled studies.

Today, patients with ICH represent a growing workload on any stroke emergency ward or stroke unit. Stroke physicians and stroke nurses should be trained to manage not only ischemic strokes but also ICH because of their differing risks, varying prognosis and high proportion of complications, and

therefore ICH patients often require a different intensity of observation and separate management.

A number of European and North American guidelines have been published in recent years with a focus on management, treatment or imaging [6–8], and, referring to these, one further chapter in this book is dedicated to treatment aspects. Therefore here the focus is limited to clinical aspects and diagnosis. Subarachnoid hemorrhages are not covered in this chapter as they are mainly caused by rupture of cerebral aneurysms, which in most European countries are not treated on stroke units but on neurosurgical wards or wards with extensive neurointensive care. For this, the reader is referred to textbooks of neurointensive or neurosurgical care.

> Intracerebral hemorrhage (ICH) comes "out of the blue sky"; typical warning signs are not known. The volume of the hemorrhage (>60 ml) is the most decisive prognostic component.

Incidence and prevalence rates

ICH, like ischemic stroke, has a clear age-dependent incidence rate, occurring slightly earlier in life than ischemic attacks. Most population-based registries report an incidence of 10 per 100 000 per year, and variations exist towards higher rates in some populations. A decrease of rates has been reported over time from several regions of the world. While the exact reasons for this decline are not known, it is reasonable to assume that a decline in rates as well as severity of arterial hypertension has significantly contributed to the declining rate of ICH [9–11].

Early mortality, which is mostly reported as 30-day mortality, is higher than in ischemic stroke and largely depends on bleeding volume. In the cerebral hemispheres, a volume of over 60 ml carries a unfavorable prognosis and is seen for deep hemorrhage (93%), and slightly less often for lobar bleeding (71%). Smaller bleedings show better prognosis and less early mortality. Overall, up to 50% of all ICH cases do not survive the first month [12–14].

One multivariate analysis showed that independent prognostic factors of 30-day mortality were ICH volume, Glasgow Coma Score on admission, age over 80 years, infratentorial origin of ICH and presence of intraventricular blood [15].

It is worth noting that in one study a decreased mortality rate was seen when such patients are cared for in a setting of a neurological/neurosurgical intensive care unit compared to treatment in general intensive care units (ICU) [16].

One randomized trial investigated the effect of an acute stroke unit in patients with primary intracranial hemorrhage [17]: 56 patients were allocated to an acute stroke unit and 65 to a general medical ward. The 30-day mortality rate was 39% in the acute stroke unit, compared with 63% in the general medical wards, and the 1-year mortality rates were 52% and 69%, respectively. Thus, the reduced mortality after primary intracranial hemorrhage seen in a stroke unit could be attributed to a large difference in survival during the first 30 days.

This is corroborated by another finding from the Austrian Stroke Registry reporting on 1539 cases of ICH treated on stroke units between 2003 and 2007. Though not controlled or randomized, the overall 3-month mortality seen in this cohort was 19%, and far lower than expected when compared to any other series or uncontrolled experiences reported from other regions or countries [18].

It is generally believed that ICH survivors have better neurological and functional prognoses than the survivors of ischemic stroke [19].

> The incidence of ICH is 10 per 100 000 per year; early mortality is up to 50% within the first month. Factors determining prognosis are ICH volume, Glasgow Coma Score on admission, age over 80 years, infratentorial origin of ICH and presence of intraventricular blood.

Risk factors

Genetics of spontaneous ICH

Monogenic disorders associated with spontaneously occurring ICH are not known. No genetic markers exist to date. But some disorders convey an increased risk of ICH, and have more frequent microscopic bleeding, such as hereditary cerebral amyloid angiopathy, CADASIL and collagen type IV A1-associated vasculopathy. Genetic screening and counseling might be reasonable for pedigrees of patients with some very rare and selected cases. Defining the more complex genetics of sporadic ICH, however, will probably require defining multiple common genetic variants with weaker effects. While investigations of genetic risk factors for sporadic ICH have thus far been limited to candidate gene polymorphisms, whole-genome association studies are being undertaken in

sporadic ICH. They are likely to generate novel insights into cerebral bleeding risks and strategies for prevention [20].

Hypertension, smoking, alcohol, cholesterol and drugs

Hypertension is the most common risk factor for spontaneous intracerebral hemorrhage and the frequency has been estimated to be between 70 and 80%. The causative role of hypertension is supported by the high frequency of left ventricular hypertrophy in autopsy of patients with ICH. The role of hypertension and the beneficial effect of antihypertensive treatment with regard to risk of ICH were verified in several large clinical trials. In the PROGRESS trial [21] the relative risk of ICH was reduced by 76% in comparison with the placebo-treated group after 4 years of follow-up.

Other risk factors for ICH in addition to old age, hypertension and ethnicity include cigarette smoking and excessive alcohol consumption. Both the Physicians' Health Study and the Women's Health Study [22, 23] confirmed the role of smoking as a risk factor for ICH. For men smoking 20 cigarettes or more the relative risk of ICH was 2.06 (95% CI 1.08–3.96) and for women smoking 15 cigarettes or more the relative risk was 2.67 (95% CI 1.04–6.90).

Several studies document an increased risk of ICH in relation to regular alcohol consumption and that spontaneous ICH can also be triggered by binge drinking [24].

Anticoagulation increases the risk of ICH 8 to 11 times compared to patients of similar age who are not on anticoagulation [25, 26].

While elevated cholesterol levels play a less significant role in ICH than in ischemia, statin use and/or very low levels of cholesterol have been questionable factors in increasing the risk of ICH. In one series of 629 ICH patients the effect of statin use was investigated. Statins were used by 149/629 (24%) before ICH. There was no effect of pre-ICH statin use on the rates of functional independence (28% versus 29%, $P = 0.84$) or mortality (46% versus 45%, $P = 0.93$). Conversely, ICH survivors treated with statins after discharge did not have a higher risk of recurrence (adjusted HR 0.82, 95% CI 0.34–1.99, $P = 0.66$). Thus, inferences made from observational data show that statin use prior to ICH does not influence mortality or functional outcome and statin use following

ICH is not associated with an increased risk of ICH recurrence [27].

A variety of illicit drugs, such as amphetamine and cocaine, are known to cause ICH and this possibility should be kept in mind in young patients in whom other causes such as arteriovenous malformation or trauma have been excluded [26, 28]. Previous medications, such as thrombolytics, also increase the risk of ICH. Brain tumors, vasculitis and various vasculopathies, including sinus thrombosis, are important causes of ICH. They have been described in detail elsewhere [26, 29].

> Hypertension is the most common risk factor for spontaneous ICH. Further risk factors include old age, cigarette smoking, excessive alcohol consumption, anticoagulation, and illicit drugs such as amphetamine and cocaine.

Etiology

Intracerebral hemorrhage (ICH) is classified into primary (80–85%) and secondary (15–20%) causes. More than 50% of primary ICH events are associated with hypertension, and 30% are found in association with cerebral amyloid angiopathy (CAA).

Intracerebral hemorrhages predominantly occur at certain locations, which are associated with specific underlying diseases. Thus deep basal ganglia bleedings are often found in patients with hypertensive disease, whereas lobar bleedings are often seen in elderly patients with CAA [30, 31].

Secondary ICH may be caused by aneurysms, arteriovenous malformations, oral anticoagulants, antiplatelets, coagulopathies, neoplasms, trauma, vasculitis, moyamoya disease or sinus venous thrombosis.

Underlying vascular lesions are more common in patients with intracerebral hemorrhages located in lobar lesions, and larger hematomas are more commonly associated with arteriovenous malformations. With an underlying arteriovenous malformation, characteristic flow voids can be seen in the brain parenchyma on MRI. CT angiography or MR angiography might reveal the underlying vascular lesion; however, in some cases, catheter angiography is required and might need to be repeated if the results were initially negative owing to the mass effect of the hematoma. Findings from imaging such as pathological calcifications, presence of subarachnoid blood, vessel abnormalities or an unusual location of hemorrhage can be considered to support an indication for direct catheter angiography. Cavernous malformation can usually be reliably diagnosed by means of GRE MRI, where one or more hypointense rings show due to hemosiderin from a previous bleeding.

> Intracerebral hemorrhages (ICH) are classified into primary (80–85%, mainly associated with hypertension and cerebral amyloid angiopathy) and secondary (15–20%) causes.

Small-vessel disease

The 'miliary aneurysms' described by Charcot and Bouchard in the small penetrating vessels of patients with intracerebral bleeding have been shown to be 'false' aneurysms. The aneurysmal feature was based on the impression of irregularity of the penetrating vessels due to their intramural blood accumulation denoting penetration, leakage and intima destruction. It was C. M. Fisher who concluded from the detailed study of two brains that hypertensive ICH most likely results from rupture of lipohyalinoic arteries followed by secondary arterial ruptures at the periphery of the enlarging hematoma in a cascade or avalanche fashion [26]. This observation of mechanical disruption and tearing of smaller vessels might account for the gradual development of ICH and can probably be considered the most relevant neuropathological correlate for the 'growing' properties of hemorrhages. The main histological findings in vessels of ICH patients include lipohyalinosis and media hypertrophy, as well as elongation of the deep penetrating arterioles of the brain. The lenticulostriate, thalamoperforating and basilar artery rami and pontem are affected most often. In the cerebellum the arterioles supplying the area of the dentate nucleus are often involved, the rami of the superior and posterior inferior cerebellar arteries.

> Hypertensive ICH most likely results from rupture of lipohyalinoic arteries followed by secondary arterial ruptures at the periphery of the enlarging hematoma.

Cerebral amyloid angiopathy (CAA)

CAA refers to the deposition of amyloid proteins into the cerebral vessel walls with degenerative changes. Hereditary forms of CAA are known but CAA is most commonly sporadic and related to amyloid β (Aβ) peptide deposition. This deposition is seen in the

157

walls of small arteries and arterioles of the lepto-meninges, cerebral and cerebellar cortices, and less often in capillaries and veins. Overlaps with Alzheimer's disease are known and therefore old age and positive ApoE ε4 allele are major risk factors for both conditions. Although the metabolism and pathological triggers for CAA production and deposition are not well understood, CAA is now recognized as a major cause of non-hypertensive lobar cerebral hemorrhage in the elderly. Its overlaps with dementia are recognized though also less well understood.

CAA is a frequent finding particularly over the age of 70 years, differing only in amount and distribution. In elderly persons over the age of 90 years it is present in 50% of individuals and in AD patients it is present in over 80% of all neuropathological cases.

The biological and neuropathological interaction between amyloid β (Aβ) deposition in primary degenerative diseases of the brain as well as in elderly patients with a high risk of parenchymal bleeding is a major focus of research. In one rare hereditary form with excessive CAA deposits, cognitive decline was independent of other Alzheimer-related pathological criteria, such as neurofibrillary tangles. Mounting evidence shows that drugs able to inhibit amyloid deposition seem to be an avenue for clinical therapy options for amyloid-associated progressive cognitive decline [32].

The "Boston criteria" proposed for the clinical diagnosis of CAA-ICH include "definite", "probable" (with or without supporting neuropathology) and "possible" diagnostic categories. Whereas the "definite" category is based on neuropathological workup of the brain, the "probable" category includes at least two acute or chronic lobar hemorrhagic lesions without any other definite cause for this hemorrhage, including current anticoagulation treatment with an INR >3.0, head injury, stroke, neoplasm or other disease that can mimic such a condition. The criteria for "possible" CAAH are a single lobar hemorrhage in a person older than 55 years and no other obvious cause of this bleed [31]. Whereas the "probable" cases have an accuracy of 100%, the possible category was only confirmed to have a 62% accuracy. One study showed that patients with CAA deposits more often have cerebral hemorrhages associated with anticoagulant, antiplatelet or thrombolysis treatment [33, 34].

CAA-associated hemorrhages account for the second largest group of hemorrhages after hypertensive bleedings and their rate depends on the case mix of elderly people at one stroke unit. Gradient echo MRI can be useful to detect silent hemorrhages in typical (cortical) areas and thus help to determine the diagnosis of CAA. Amyloid PET imaging is currently being tested as a tool for direct diagnosis but so far no peripheral blood markers for CAA or CAA-related risk of ICH have been found; only some hereditary forms can be diagnosed from blood or other tissue samples [34].

> Cerebral amyloid angiopathy (CAA) refers to the deposition of amyloid proteins into the cerebral vessel walls with degenerative changes.

Microbleeds

MRI visualizes acute and chronic hematomas, but also old, clinically non-apparent cerebral microbleeds that are not detected on CT. Microbleeds have a hypointense appearance on MRI and are usually smaller than 5–10 mm. Pathological studies have shown that microbleeds seen with GRE MRI usually correspond to hemosiderin-laden macrophages adjacent to small vessels and are indicative of previous extravasation of blood [35]. One review [36] included 53 case series studies involving 9073 participants, 4432 of whom were people with cerebrovascular diseases. Significant variations in MRI magnet strength, flip angle, slice gap and slice thickness were found as well as inconsistent definitions of microbleed size (44% chose a diameter of ≤5 mm). The authors found a 5% prevalence of microbleeds in healthy adults, rising to 34% (95% CI 31–36) in people with ischemic stroke, and to 60% (95% CI 57–64) in people with non-traumatic intracerebral hemorrhage (ICH). Microbleeds were seen in 83% (95% CI 71–90) of ICH cases with recurrent ICH [36].

Hypertension, cerebral amyloid angiopathy, getting older, and, less commonly, cerebral autosomal dominant arteriopathy with silent infarcts and leukoaraiosis (CADASIL) have been identified as important risk factors for microbleeds [37–39]. Microbleeds have been suggested as markers of a bleeding-prone angiopathy [40, 41]. The results of several case reports and small series suggest that patients with microbleeds might be at increased risk of hemorrhage when on antithrombotic or thrombolytic therapy. By contrast, the results of two large studies did not show an increased risk of hemorrhage in patients with microbleeds who were treated with intravenous tissue plasminogen activator [42, 43].

Although there are still many studies ongoing, microbleeds are considered to bear prognostic significance for any future bleeding event and have been confirmed as a common finding in patients with cerebral amyloid angiopathy. There they are most commonly found in lobar brain regions [32]. By contrast, in patients with intracerebral hemorrhage due to hypertensive disease, microbleeds are most commonly found in deep and infratentorial regions, although hypertension can also contribute to lobar microbleeds. A pattern of multiple hemorrhages without an underlying cause and restricted to lobar regions in an elderly patient is highly indicative of a diagnosis of cerebral amyloid angiopathy according to the Boston Criteria. A particularly noteworthy finding is that the total number of microbleeds predicts the risk of future symptomatic intracerebral hemorrhage in patients with lobar hemorrhage and probable cerebral amyloid angiopathy [44].

> Old, clinically non-apparent cerebral microbleeds can be visualized on MRI, and have been suggested as markers of a bleeding-prone angiopathy.

Clinical syndromes

Clinical presentation of spontaneous ICH depends on site and size. Therefore, clinical investigation as well as neuroimaging are both important for a reliable diagnosis. All attempts to make a probabilistic diagnosis on clinical grounds alone to differentiate between ischemic and hemorrhagic stroke have not been considered satisfactory [45].

In our series of 1539 ICH cases we have located 45% in the putaminal region and in the thalamus, 34% in a lobar location, 5% in the cerebellum, about 4% in the pons, and 11% were not classifiable (Table 10.1).

Putaminal hemorrhages are the most frequent ones. If the hemorrhage spreads from the putamen into the thalamic region, they are called putaminothalamic. Then they show a large volume extending over the area of the basal ganglia and deep white matter of one hemisphere. Such an ICH can rupture into the lateral or third ventricles, giving rise to sudden posturing and coma. More often, progression is not abrupt but gradual and can be seen occurring over several hours, showing an increase of sensorimotor hemiparesis and a gradual decrease of alertness. Usually transition into drowsiness and stupor occurs in parallel with a decrease in motor function. If a progressive deterioration of consciousness is seen in

a hemiparetic patient with a sensorimotor hemiparesis, this can give rise to suspicion of a growing hematoma. Noting such a progression is vital and contrasts with ischemic strokes, most of which tend to remain stable. If no deterioration or progression occurs in the first hours or days, hemorrhages such as small or medium-sized putaminal bleedings also tend to remain stable after the first few days and cannot be distinguished from ischemic infarcts in the basal ganglia and capsular region on clinical grounds alone. They both present with sudden onset of sensorimotor hemiparesis of varying degree and can both be associated with additional hemispheric symptoms such as aphasia or neglect. This contradicts the prevailing opinion at some centers that "typical" hemiparetic strokes that remain stable can be reliably considered to be caused by ischemia and therefore do not need confirmation with neuroimaging. In general, there is also no medical rationale to restrict imaging to young patients or to patients with some other demographic or clinical feature.

ICH can also occur extremely abruptly and loss of consciousness can occur within minutes after onset. This is the case in large putaminal or thalamic hematomas that rupture into the ventricles, or in pontine hemorrhages extending over the midline.

Contralateral limb weakness and hemisensory symptoms are typical of mid-sized putaminal hemorrhages, whereas bleeding into the thalamus causes a distinct and total hemisensory loss and dense hemiplegia.

Conjugate eye deviation to the side of the bleeding signals extension into the frontal lobe. This is a sign either of frontal lobar hemorrhage or of a putaminal hemorrhage extending into the deep frontal white matter. In contrast, thalamic hemorrhage can be accompanied by a conjugate spasm of both eyes, appearing as convergent downward gaze (the patient looks at his/her nose tip). The pupil which is smaller denotes the hemispheric side of the bleeding, and, when present, this invariably denotes involvement of subthalamic structures. Such cases have to be monitored closely because of the likelihood of rupture into the ventricles. This is the case when sudden, bilateral localizing signs appear and loss of consciousness is the rule.

Vomiting is a frequent sign of ICH but can also indicate ischemic stroke. It can be a prominent sign in posterior fossa hemorrhage, and, although patients with cerebellar hemorrhages almost always vomit

159

early in the clinical course, it is not a reliable sign with either localizing or etiological value. Many patients with posterior fossa hemorrhage show severe impairment of sitting balance and ataxia that can be pronounced ipsilaterally. Close observation of vital parameters is crucial, as deterioration can be sudden or progressive over the first few days after onset. Evacuation of the hematoma can also become necessary after some days.

Contrasting with lay beliefs, headache is also not a cardinal symptom of ICH. Headache can occur in large hematomas and has no localizing value unless it is very severe and then indicates rupturing in cerebrospinal fluid space. In patients with loss of consciousness meningeal irritation must not be apparent.

Clinical presentation of spontaneous ICH depends on site and size. The most frequent putaminal hemorrhages show a sudden onset. Progressive deterioration of consciousness points to a growing hematoma, and sudden posturing and coma to a rupture of the bleeding into the lateral or third

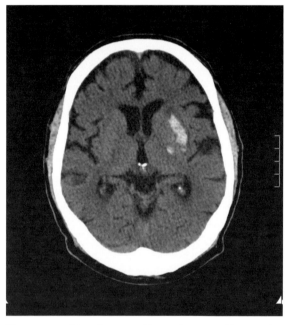

Figure 10.1. CT: small putaminal hemorrhage (possibly secondary to ischemic infarction).

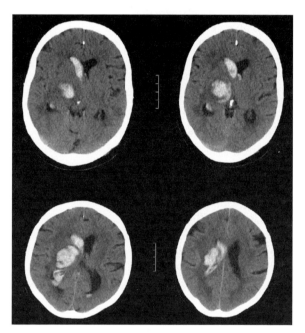

Figure 10.3. CT: large putaminothalamic hemorrhage with rupture into lateral and third ventricles. The estimated blood volume is 60 ml.

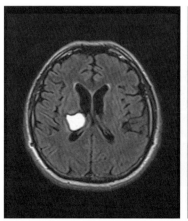
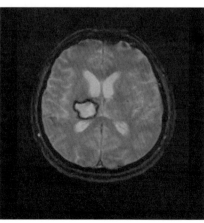

Figure 10.2. MRI: subacute thalamic hemorrhage with gradient echo (GRE) sequence (left).

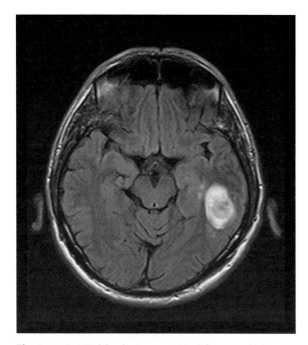

Figure 10.4. MRI: lobar hematoma in the left temporal lobe.

ventricle. Vomiting and headache are frequent, but not reliable, signs. See Figures 10.1–10.6.

Complications

An increase in the bleeding volume is an early complication of ICH. The frequency of increased bleeding is high, though it might not be clear in all cases whether growth of volume is due to rebleeding or continuous bleeding. Brott et al. showed that "growth", defined as a 33% increase of hematoma volume on CT, occurred in 26% of 103 patients within 4 hours after the first symptoms. Another 12% had growth within the following 20 hours. Hemorrhage growth was significantly associated with clinical deterioration [46]. Enlargement of ICH is also seen when observation periods are extended up to 48 hours, though the frequency diminishes with time from onset of symptoms. Predictors of hemorrhage expansion include initial hematoma volume, early presentation, irregular shape, liver disease,

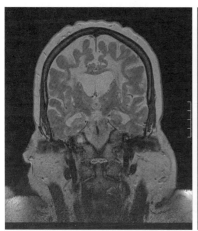
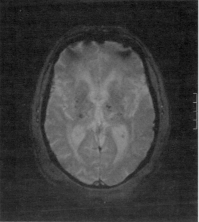

Figure 10.5. MRI: coronal slice though lateral ventricles (T2 weighted) showing extensive lacunar infarctions and widespread leukoaraiosis. The transverse horizontal slice (GRE) shows multiple punctuate hemorrhages within the putamen and central white matter indicative of advanced vascular (hypertensive) encephalopathy.

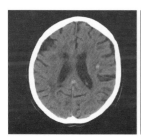
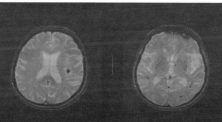
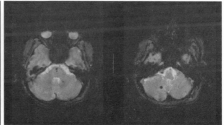

Figure 10.6. CT: left shows only one larger intracerebral hematoma, whereas on MRI additional multiple punctuate hematomas are seen indicative of amyloid encephalopathy.

hypertension, hyperglycemia, alcohol use and hypo-fibrinogenima [47].

Between 36% and 50% of patients with spontaneous ICH suffer additional intraventricular hemorrhage (IVH) and the 30-day mortality rate was reported as 43% for patients with ICH and IVH compared with 9% in patients with isolated IVH [48]. Tuhrim et al. [48] found that location of parenchymal origin of ICH, distribution of ventricular blood and total volumes are predictors of outcome in patients with spontaneous ICH and intraventricular extension. Furthermore, hydrocephalus was found to be an independent predictor of mortality.

Edema after ICH is observed in the acute and subacute phase and may increase up to 14 days [49]. Shrinking of the hematoma due to clot retraction leads to an accumulation of serum in the early phase [50]. Thrombin and several serum proteins were found to be involved in the inflammatory reaction of the perihematomal zone [51, 52]. Factors released from activated platelets at the site of bleeding, such as vascular endothelial growth factor, may interact with thrombin to increase vascular permeability and contribute to the development of edema [53]. Several studies in spontaneous ICH suggest that the role of perihematomal ischemia is small and has no great clinical importance [54].

> Frequent complications are an increase of the bleeding volume, intraventricular hemorrhage, hydrocephalus and edema.

Chapter Summary

Intracerebral hemorrhage (ICH) comes "out of the blue sky"; typical warning signs are not known. The volume of the hemorrhage into the brain is the most decisive prognostic component. More than 60 ml within one cerebral hemisphere leads to herniation of the medial temporal lobe and compression of the brainstem.

Incidence: 10 per 100 000 per year. Early mortality: up to 50% within the first month (prognostic factors: ICH volume, Glasgow Coma Score on admission, age over 80 years, infratentorial origin of ICH, and presence of intraventricular blood).

Risk factors: hypertension is the most common risk factor. Further risk factors: old age, cigarette smoking, excessive alcohol consumption, anticoagulation and illicit drugs such as amphetamine and cocaine.

Etiology: intracerebral hemorrhage (ICH) is classified into primary (80 to 85%) and secondary (15 to 20%) causes. Hypertensive ICH (more than 50% of primary ICH typically in basal ganglia) most likely results from rupture of lipohyalinoic arteries followed by secondary arterial ruptures at the periphery of the enlarging hematoma. Thirty percent are found in association with cerebral amyloid angiopathy. Cerebral amyloid angiopathy (CAA 30% at primary ICH, typically lobar bleedings) refers to the deposition of amyloid proteins into the cerebral vessel walls with degenerative changes. Secondary ICH may be caused by aneurysms, arterio-venous malformations, oral anticoagulants, antiplatelets, coagulopathies, neoplasms, trauma, vasculitis, moyamoya disease or sinus venous thrombosis.

Clinical presentation of spontaneous ICH depends on site and size. Imaging (non-contrast CT) is necessary to differentiate ischemic infarcts from hemorrhage. Putaminal hemorrhages show a sudden onset of sensorimotor hemiparesis of varying degree and can be associated with additional hemispheric symptoms such as aphasia or neglect. Progressive deterioration of consciousness points to a growing hematoma, and sudden posturing and coma to a rupture of the bleeding into the lateral or third ventricle. Conjugate eye deviation to the side of the bleeding signals extension into the frontal lobe; a conjugate spasm of both eyes appearing as convergent downward gaze signals thalamic hemorrhage. Vomiting and headache are frequent, but not reliable, signs with neither localizing or etiological value.

Complications are due to increase of the bleeding, intraventricular hemorrhage, hydrocephalus and edema.

References

1. Becker K, Tirschwell D. Intraparenchymal hemorrhage, bleeding, hemostasis, and the utility of CT angiography. *Int J Stroke* 2008; 3:11–13.

2. Kidwell CS, Wintermark M. Imaging of intracranial haemorrhage. *Lancet Neurol* 2008; 7:256–67.

3. Brott T, Broderick J, Kothari R, Barsan W, Tomsick T, Sauerbeck L, et al. Early hemorrhage growth in patients with intracerebral hemorrhage. *Stroke* 1997; 28:1–5.

4. Xi G, Keep RF, Hoff JT. Mechanisms of brain injury after intracerebral haemorrhage. *Lancet Neurol* 2006; 5:53–63.

5. Rosell A, Cuadrado E, Ortega-Aznar A, Hernández-Guillamon M, Lo EH, Montaner J. MMP-9-positive

neutrophil infiltration is associated to blood-brain barrier breakdown and basal lamina type IV collagen degradation during hemorrhagic transformation after human ischemic stroke. *Stroke* 2008; **39**:1121–6.

6. Steiner T, Kaste M, Forsting M, Mendelow D, Kwiecinski H, Szikora I, et al. Recommendations for the management of intracranial haemorrhage – part I: spontaneous intracerebral haemorrhage. The European Stroke Initiative Writing Committee and the Writing Committee for the EUSI Executive Committee. *Cerebrovasc Dis* 2006; **22**:294–316.

7. Masdeu JC, Irimia P, Asenbaum S, Bogousslavsky J, Brainin M, Chabriat H, et al. EFNS. EFNS guideline on neuroimaging in acute stroke. Report of an EFNS task force. *Eur J Neurol* 2006; **13**:1271–83.

8. Broderick J, Connolly S, Feldmann E, Hanley D, Kase C, Krieger D, et al. American Heart Association; American Stroke Association Stroke Council; High Blood Pressure Research Council; Quality of Care and Outcomes in Research Interdisciplinary Working Group. Guidelines for the management of spontaneous intracerebral hemorrhage in adults: 2007 update: a guideline from the American Heart Association/ American Stroke Association Stroke Council, High Blood Pressure Research Council, and the Quality of Care and Outcomes in Research Interdisciplinary Working Group. *Stroke* 2007; **38**:2001–23.

9. Sacco RL, Boden-Albala B, Gan R, Chen X, Kargman DE, Shea S, et al. Stroke incidence among white, black, and Hispanic residents of an urban community: the Northern Manhattan Stroke Study. *Am J Epidemiol* 1998; **147**:259–68.

10. Islam MS, Anderson CS, Hankey GJ, Hardie K, Carter K, Broadhurst R, et al. Trends in incidence and outcome of stroke in Perth, Western Australia during 1989 to 2001: the Perth Community Stroke Study. *Stroke* 2008; **39**(3):776–82.

11. Fang J, Alderman MH, Keenan NL, Croft JB. Declining US stroke hospitalization since 1997: National Hospital Discharge Survey, 1988–2004. *Neuroepidemiology* 2007; **29**(3–4):243–9.

12. Fujii Y, Takeuchi S, Sasaki O, Minakawa T, Tanaka R. Multivariate analysis of predictors of hematoma enlargement in spontaneous intracerebral hemorrhage. *Stroke* 1998; **29**:1160–6.

13. Broderick J, Brott T, Duldner JE, Tomsick T, Huster G. Volume of intracerebral hemorrhage: a powerful and easy-to-use predictor of 30-day mortality. *Stroke* 1993; **24**:987–93.

14. Counsell C, Boonyakarnkul S, Dennis M, Sandercock P, Bamford J, Burn J, et al. Primary intracerebral haemorrhage in the Oxfordshire community stroke project, 2: prognosis. *Cerebrovasc Dis* 1995; **5**:26–34.

15. Hemphill JC, 3rd, Bonovich DC, Besmertis L, Manley GT, Johnston SC. The ICH score: a simple, reliable grading scale for intracerebral hemorrhage. *Stroke* 2001; **32**:891–7.

16. Diringer MN, Edwards DF. Admission to a neurologic/ neurosurgical intensive care unit is associated with reduced mortality rate after intracerebral hemorrhage. *Crit Care Med* 2001; **29**:635–40.

17. Rønning OM, Guldvog B, Stavem K. The benefit of an acute stroke unit in patients with intracranial haemorrhage: a controlled trial. *J Neurol Neurosurg Psychiatry* 2001; **70**:631–4.

18. Eckhardt R, Schnabl S, Brainin M. Management of hemorrhages on Austrian stroke units. *Wiener Med Wschr* (in press).

19. Paolucci S, Antonucci G, Grasso MG, Bragoni M, Coiro P, De Angelis D, et al. Functional outcome of ischemic and hemorrhagic stroke patients after inpatient rehabilitation: a matched comparison. *Stroke* 2003; **34**:2861–5.

20. Rost NS, Greenberg SM, Rosand J. The genetic architecture of intracerebral hemorrhage. *Stroke* 2008 May 8. [Epub ahead of print].

21. PROGRESS Collaborative Group: Randomised trial of a perindopril-based blood-pressure-lowering regimen among 6,105 individuals with previous stroke or transient ischaemic attack. *Lancet* 2001; **358**:1033–41.

22. Kurth T, Kase CS, Berger K, Schaeffner ES, Buring JE, Gaziano JM. Smoking and the risk of hemorrhagic stroke in men. *Stroke* 2003; **34**:1151–5.

23. Kurth T, Kase CS, Berger K, Gaziano JM, Cook NR, Buring JE. Smoking and risk of hemorrhagic stroke in women. *Stroke* 2003; **34**:2792–5.

24. Juvela S, Hillbom M, Palomaki H. Risk factors for spontaneous intracerebral hemorrhage. *Stroke* 1995; **26**:1558–64.

25. Rosand J, Hylek EM, O'Donnell HC, Greenberg SM. Warfarin-associated hemorrhage and cerebral amyloid angiopathy: a genetic and pathologic study. *Neurology* 2000; **55**:947–51.

26. Kase CS, Mohr JP, Caplan LR. Intracerebral hemorrhage. In: Mohr JP, Choi DC, Grotta JC, et al., eds. *Stroke: Pathophysiology, Diagnosis, and Management*, 4th ed. Philadelphia: Churchill Livingstone; 2004: 327–76.

27. Fitzmaurice E, Wendell L, Snider R, Schwab K, Chanderraj R, Kinnecom C, et al. Effect of statins on intracerebral hemorrhage outcome and recurrence. *Stroke* 2008 Apr 24. [Epub ahead of print]PMID: 18436876.

28. He J, Whelton PK, Vu B, Klag MJ. Aspirin and risk of hemorrhagic stroke: a meta-analysis of randomized controlled trials. *JAMA* 1998; **280**:1930–1935.

29. Caplan LR. Intracerebral hemorrhage. In: Caplan LR, ed. *Caplan's Stroke: a Clinical Approach*, 3rd ed. Boston: Butterworth-Heinemann; 2000: 383–418.

30. Lang EW, Ren Ya Z, Preul C, Hugo HH, Hempelmann RG, Buhl R, et al. Stroke pattern interpretation: the variability of hypertensive versus amyloid angiopathy hemorrhage. *Cerebrovasc Dis* 2001; **12**:121–30.

31. Knudsen KA, Rosand J, Karluk D, Greenberg SM. Clinical diagnosis of cerebral amyloid angiopathy: validation of the Boston criteria. *Neurology* 2001; **56**:537–9.

32. Greenberg SM, Briggs ME, Hyman BT, Kokoris GJ, Takis C, Kanter DS, et al. Apolipoprotein E epsilon 4 is associated with the presence and earlier onset of hemorrhage in cerebral amyloid angiopathy. *Stroke* 1996; **27**:1333–7.

33. McCarron MO, Nicoll JA. Apolipoprotein E genotype and cerebral amyloid angiopathy-related hemorrhage. *Ann N Y Acad Sci* 2000; **903**:176–9.

34. Revesz T, et al. Cerebral amyloid angiopathy. In: Kalimo H, ed. *Pathology and Genetics, Cerebrovascular Diseases*. Basel: ISN Neuropath Press; 2005: 94–102.

35. Fazekas F, Kleinert R, Roob G, Kleinert G, Kapeller P, Schmidt R, et al. Histopathologic analysis of foci of signal loss on gradient-echo T2*-weighted MR images in patients with spontaneous intracerebral hemorrhage: evidence of microangiopathy-related microbleeds. *Am J Neuroradiol* 1999; **20**(4):637–42.

36. Cordonnier C, Al-Shahi Salman R, Wardlaw J. Spontaneous brain microbleeds: systematic review, subgroup analyses and standards for study design and reporting. *Brain* 2007; **130**:1988–2003.

37. Kinoshita T, Okudera T, Tamura H, Ogawa T, Hatazawa J. Assessment of lacunar hemorrhage associated with hypertensive stroke by echo-planar gradient-echo T2*-weighted MRI. *Stroke* 2000; **31**:1646–50.

38. Tsushima Y, Tamura T, Unno Y, Kusano S, Endo K. Multifocal low-signal brain lesions on T2*-weighted gradient-echo imaging. *Neuroradiology* 2000; **42**:499–504.

39. Tsushima Y, Aoki J, Endo K. Brain microhemorrhages detected on T2*-weighted gradient-echo MR images. *Am J Neuroradiol* 2003; **24**:88–96.

40. Kidwell CS, Saver JL, Villablanca JP, et al. Magnetic resonance imaging detection of microbleeds before thrombolysis: an emerging application. *Stroke* 2002; **33**:95–8.

41. Wong KS, Chan YL, Liu JY, Gao S, Lam WW. Asymptomatic microbleeds as a risk factor for aspirin-associated intracerebral hemorrhages. *Neurology* 2003; **60**:511–13.

42. Kakuda W, Thijs VN, Lansberg MG, et al. Clinical importance of microbleeds in patients receiving IV thrombolysis. *Neurology* 2005; **65**:1175–8.

43. Fiehler J, Albers GW, Boulanger JM, et al. Bleeding risk analysis in stroke imaging before thrombolysis (BRASIL): pooled analysis of T2*-weighted magnetic resonance imaging data from 570 patients. *Stroke* 2007; **38**:2738–44.

44. Greenberg SM, Eng JA, Ning M, Smith EE, Rosand J. Hemorrhage burden predicts recurrent intracerebral hemorrhage after lobar hemorrhage. *Stroke* 2004; **35**:1415–20.

45. Weir CJ, Murray GD, Adams FG, Muir KW, Grosset DG, Lees KR. Poor accuracy of stroke scoring systems for differential clinical diagnosis of intracranial haemorrhage and infarction. *Lancet* 1994; **344**:999–1002.

46. Brott T, Broderick J, Kothari R, Barsan W, Tomsick T, Sauerbeck L, et al. Early hemorrhage growth in patients with intracerebral hemorrhage. *Stroke* 1997; **28**:1–5.

47. Fujii Y, Takeuchi S, Sasaki O, Minakawa T, Tanaka R. Multivariate analysis of predictors of hematoma enlargement in spontaneous intracerebral hemorrhage. *Stroke* 1998; **29**:1160–6.

48. Tuhrim S, Horowitz DR, Sacher M, Godbold JH. Volume of ventricular blood is an important determinant of outcome in supratentorial intracerebral hemorrhage. *Crit Care Med* 1999; **27**:617–21.

49. Gebel JM Jr, Jauch EC, Brott TG, Khoury J, Sauerbeck L, Salisbury S, et al. Relative edema volume is a predictor of outcome in patients with hyperacute spontaneous intracerebral hemorrhage. *Stroke* 2002; **33**:2636–41.

50. Xi G. Intracerebral hemorrhage: pathophysiology and therapy. *Neurocritical Care* 2004; **1**:5–18.

51. Lee KR, Colon GP, Betz AL, Keep RF, Kim S, Hoff JT. Edema from intracerebral hemorrhage: the role of thrombin. *J Neurosurg* 1996; **84**:91–96.

52. Castillo J, Davalos A, Alvarez-Sabin J, Pumar JM, Leira R, Silva Y, Montaner J, Kase CS. Molecular signatures of brain injury after intracerebral hemorrhage. *Neurology* 2002; **58**:624–629.

53. Sansing LH, Kaznatcheeva EA, Perkins CJ, Komaroff E, Gutman FB, Newman GC. Edema after intracerebral hemorrhage: correlations with coagulation parameters and treatment. *J Neurosurg* 2003; **98**:985–992.

54. Schellinger PD, Fiebach JB, Hoffmann K, Becker K, Orakcioglu B, Kollmar R, et al. Stroke MRI in intracerebral hemorrhage: is there a perihemorrhagic penumbra? *Stroke* 2003; **34**:1674–1679.

Cerebral venous thrombosis

Jobst Rudolf

Introduction

Acute thrombosis of the cerebral sinuses and veins (cerebral venous thrombosis, CVT) is considered to be the cause of an acute stroke in approximately 1% of all stroke patients. However, the incidence of CVT is not known, as population-based studies are lacking. It has been estimated that annually about five to eight cases of CVT are identified among stroke patients of tertiary care hospitals [1]. Historically, CVT was considered a severe, almost inevitably fatal disease, as diagnosis in the pre-angiograph era was usually made post-mortem. However, modern neuroimaging techniques allow the diagnosis of CVT at an early stage and document that CVT is more frequent than was traditionally assumed, and that its prognosis is much better than is generally accepted, provided that the diagnosis is suspected, the respective neuroimaging examinations are performed in a timely manner, and therapy is initiated early, i.e. often with the diagnosis being clinically suspected only. The variety of clinical signs and symptoms renders the diagnosis of CVT a challenge to the physician. Diagnosis is still frequently overlooked or delayed due to the wide spectrum of clinical symptoms and the often subacute or lingering disease onset.

It is important to keep the diagnosis of CVT in mind in stroke cases that present with a fluctuating course, headache, epileptic seizures or disturbances of the level of consciousness. With timely therapeutic intervention, CVT has a favorable prognosis, with an overall mortality rate of about 8% in recent studies [2]. However, thrombosis of the inner cerebral veins as well as septic CVT remain severe diseases with high mortality rates.

Anatomy

The cerebral venous system consists of two distinct groups – the superficial and the deep cerebral veins –

which eventually drain into the cerebral sinuses. The superficial veins of the brain that drain the cortex and the underlying white matter form a network of anastomoses that drain into the cortical sinuses, but number, diameter and topography of these veins vary among individual patients. However, two major superficial veins can be identified in the majority of patients: the upper anastomotic vein of Trolard, which drains into the superior sagittal sinus, and the lower anastomotic vein of Labbé, which drains into the transverse sinus. Cerebral veins do not possess valves and therefore allow blood flow in both directions. This is the main reason why even larger thrombotic venous occlusions may remain clinically silent for a long time. In contrast, the deep veins that drain the basal ganglia and other deep subcortical structures do not possess the diversity of the superficial venous network. The basal veins of Rosenthal and the internal cerebral veins drain into the great cerebral vein of Galen and the straight sinus, and from there the transverse and sigmoid sinuses, finally reaching the vena cava via the jugular veins. Blood supply to the cerebellum and brainstem is drained from the posterior fossa by veins reaching the vein of Galen, the petrose or the lateral sinus. In contrast to veins, the cerebral sinuses are formed by duplication of the dura mater and are fixed to the osseous cranial structures. Thus, there is no possibility of influencing venous blood flow by means of vasoconstriction or vasodilatation.

> Cerebral veins have a peculiar anatomy, as they do not follow the arteries as in other parts of the body.

Etiology

CVT may be due to infectious and non-infectious causes. Septic CVT is observed as a complication of bacterial infections of the visceral cranium, namely otitis, sinusitis, mastoiditis and bacterial meningitis. The infectious agents reach the cerebral sinuses ascending

Table 11.1. Potential causes of and risk factors associated with cerebral venous thrombosis [3, 4, 14].

Genetic prothrombotic conditions

  Antithrombin III deficiency

  Protein C and protein S deficiency

  Factor V Leiden mutation

  Prothrombin AG20210 mutation

  Mutations in the methylenetetrahydrofolate reductase (MTHFR) gene

Acquired prothrombotic states

  Nephrotic syndrome

  Antiphospholipid antibodies

  Homocysteinemia

  Pregnancy

  Puerperium

Infections

  Otitis, mastoiditis, sinusitis

  Meningitis

  Systemic infectious disease

Inflammatory disease

  Systemic lupus erythematosus

  Wegener's granulomatosis

  Sarcoidosis

  Inflammatory bowel disease (Crohn's disease, colitis ulcerosa)

  Adamantiadis-Behçet syndrome

Hematological conditions

  Polycythemia, primary and secondary

  Thrombocythemia

  Leukemia

  Anemia, including paroxysmal nocturnal hemoglobinuria

Drugs

  Oral contraceptives

  Hormonal replacement therapy

  Steroids

  Cytotoxic drugs (e.g. asparaginase)

Mechanical causes, trauma

  Head injury

  Injury to sinuses or jugular vein, jugular catheterization

  Neurosurgical procedures

  Lumbar puncture

Miscellaneous

  Dehydration, especially in children

  Cancer

via the draining veins of the face, the sinuses or the ear, or following local inflammation that destroys osseous structures that separate the infectious focus from the brain. Clinical signs and symptoms of septic CVT comprise signs of systemic infection and of meningitis. Septic CVT remains a rare disease with high mortality in spite of modern therapeutic surgical and medical approaches (see below for details).

Aseptic CVT may stem from a variety of causes, all of them resembling those of extracranial thrombosis (Table 11.1). However, the cause of CVT remains unknown in approximately 15–20% of all patients, in spite of a thorough diagnostic workup [2–4].

> Septic CVT may be caused by bacterial infections of the visceral cranium, e.g. otitis, sinusitis, mastoiditis and bacterial meningitis. Aseptic CVT may be caused by the same causes as extracranial thrombosis (see Table 11.1).

Pathophysiology

Venous thrombosis of the CNS differs from arterial thromboses in many ways: venous thrombosis does not manifest acutely, as arterial thrombosis does, but is a subacute, often fluctuating process, in which endogenous pro-thrombotic and fibrinolytic processes occur concurrently. Regional cerebral blood flow (rCBF) is not significantly impaired, the auto-regulation of cerebral perfusion is nearly fully maintained, and administration of acetazolamide induces – in contrast to arterial thrombosis – a significant increase of rCBF [5]. In venous congestion, disturbances of neuronal functional metabolism are tolerated for a much longer time than in arterial occlusion, and full recovery from severe focal and generalized neurological signs and symptoms may be observed in CVT even after weeks.

Intracranial hemorrhage is often observed in CVT, and its incidence may reach 40–50% [3, 6], a percentage significantly higher than in cerebral arterial thrombosis or embolism. The most common form of intracranial hematoma in CVT is intracerebral bleeding, but subdural and – rarely – subarachnoid hemorrhage may be observed. In general, intracerebral hematoma in CVT is atypically localized in cortical and subcortical regions that do not correspond to territories of cerebral arteries. From a pathophysiological point of view, these bleedings are caused by the diapedesis of erythrocytes through the endothelial membrane, following the increase of the venous and capillary transmural pressure after venous thrombosis. The rationale for anticoagulant therapy with heparin or low-molecular-weight heparin (LMWH) is that preventing the re-occlusion of veins and sinuses re-opened by endogenous fibrinolysis will result in a lowering of venous and capillary pressure. Thus, even in the presence of hemorrhage due to CVT, immediate anticoagulation results in clinical amelioration without increase in hematoma volume.

Hemorrhages are frequent in CVT.

Clinical features

Abrupt occlusion of a cerebral artery results in the acute manifestation of focal neurological symptoms due to ischemia of the brain tissue perfused by this artery. In contrast, cerebral venous thrombosis may remain clinically silent, as long as venous drainage is maintained by collateral veins or sinuses. Eventually, failure of collateral venous drainage will result in the gradual, fluctuating or progressive clinical manifestation of focal or generalized brain dysfunction. An exception to this rule is CVT in pregnancy and puerperium, where signs and symptoms of venous thrombosis may present within minutes or hours [7].

Clinical features of CVT differ according to the venous structures involved. Cortical CVT will present with signs and symptoms different from that of deep CVT, and septic CVT will show findings other than aseptic thrombosis.

In most prospective clinical series [2, 3, 6, 8], intense and diffuse headache was either the first (>70%) or the most common (75–90%) symptom of cortical venous thrombosis. Headache, as well as nausea, papilledema, visual loss or sixth nerve palsy, is due to increased intracranial pressure. The onset of

headache in CVT is subacute over hours and may precede the manifestation of other symptoms and signs by days or even weeks. Acute appearance of epileptic seizures is observed in 40–50% of all cases of CVT [2, 3, 6, 8], a percentage much higher than in arterial thrombosis of the brain. Seizures in CVT may present as simple partial seizures with post-ictal limb paresis or as complex partial seizures, and in both cases secondary generalization is often observed. Focal neurological signs may be observed in 30–50% of CVT patients [2, 3, 6, 8], but their localizing value is limited, due to the excellent collateralization of cerebral veins and the lack of venous valves that allows inversion of venous drainage in the case of localized thrombotic occlusion. Furthermore, the intensity of focal signs and symptoms may fluctuate over time. Motor symptoms may initially present as a monoparesis that gradually develops into a full-blown hemiparesis. With cortical CVT, higher cortical functions may be impaired, and aphasia or apraxia may be observed. Impairment of the level of consciousness (any degree from somnolence to deep coma) may be present in 30–50% of patients, and acute delirium or psychotic symptoms are observed in 20–25% [2, 3, 6, 8]. As a rule, extended thrombosis of cortical sinuses will result in symptoms and signs of generalized brain dysfunction (headache and other signs of increased intracranial pressure, impairment of the level of consciousness, generalized seizures), while isolated cortical venous thrombosis will result in focal neurological signs or focal seizures.

The rare thromboses of the inner cerebral veins (veins of Rosenthal, great vein of Galen, straight sinus, etc.) will result in a severe dysfunction of the diencephalon, reflected by coma and disturbances of eye movements and pupillary reflexes, a condition usually associated with poor outcome [9].

Thrombosis of the cavernous sinus may present with the characteristic combination of ocular chemosis, eye protrusion, painful ophthalmoplegia, trigeminal dysfunction, and – occasionally – papilledema. Cavernous sinus thrombosis may be unilateral, but the good collateralization between the cavernous sinuses usually leads to bilateral symptoms, while extension of the thrombosis into the large sinuses is the exception. Most cases of cavernous sinus thrombosis are due to ascending infection from the orbita, the paranasal sinuses or other structures of the viscerocranium and are accompanied by signs of local or systemic infection.

Symptoms of CVT are manifold: they may remain clinically silent as long as venous drainage is still maintained. Headache is the most common and frequently the first symptom of CVT. Epileptic seizures, focal neurological signs, impairment of the level of consciousness and psychotic symptoms can occur.

Septic thrombosis of other sinuses is found as a complication of bacterial infection (e.g. otitis, mastoiditis, bacterial meningitis), and is always accompanied by symptoms and signs of systemic infection. Septic CVT accounts for about 5% of all cases of cerebral thrombosis, but its mortality remains extremely high.

Septic CVT is accompanied by symptoms of systemic infection.

Diagnostic workup

Owing to the multitude of clinical manifestations as well as etiologies, the diagnosis of CVT presents a challenge to the clinical physician. The less distinct the clinical presentation is, the more difficult is the diagnosis of CVT. CVT may be suspected in the presence of headache and other signs of intracranial hypertension, alone or in combination with epileptic seizures and fluctuating neurological signs, especially if conditions are present that may favor thrombogenesis (e.g. bacterial infection, pregnancy and puerperium, malignancies and known pro-thrombotic states; see Table 11.1). However, mono- or oligosymptomatic cases of CVT may be difficult to diagnose. In patients with signs and symptoms of systemic infection, CVT may be mistaken for meningo-encephalitis. The presence of CVT has to be suspected in young stroke patients, in painful stroke, in stroke with unusual presentation, and in patients with first-ever headache in combination with seizures of subtle focal signs.

The differential diagnosis of aseptic CVT comprises benign intracranial hypertension, but also all forms of intracranial hypertension due to neoplastic diseases. Aseptic thrombosis of the cavernous sinus leading to painful uni- or bilateral ophthalmoplegia has to be differentiated from the Tolosa-Hunt syndrome.

Computed tomography

Cerebral computed tomography (CCT) is widely available and is feasible in critically ill patients. Thus,

CCT is often the first neuroimaging technique applied to patients with CVT and should be performed before and after the intravenous application of iodinated contrast media. However, CCT findings in CVT are often nonspecific and may consist of one or more of the following: localized or diffuse brain edema, focal hypodensities that do not comply with the boundaries of cerebral arterial territories, atypical hemorrhagic infarctions or hematomas (Figure 11.1). Where available, CT venography may increase the diagnostic yield of CCT in CVT [9]. CCT may be entirely normal in up to 25% of patients with angiographically proven CVT. Thus, the main indication of CCT in CVT is to rule out other conditions that may mimic or be confounded with CVT.

However, there are two CCT findings that – if present – are highly suggestive of CVT (Figures 11.1 and 11.2). The thrombotic occlusion of an isolated cortical vein may present as a thread-like hyperdense structure on no-contrast CCT ("cord sign"). After

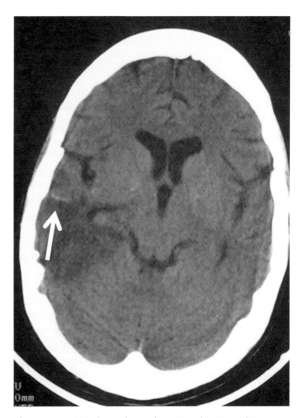

Figure 11.1. Unenhanced cranial computed tomography scan showing an atypical right temporal hemorrhagic venous infarction in a patient with isolated cortical venous thrombosis. Note the cord sign.

intravenous application of iodinated contrast media, the dura mater of the sinuses will show a distinct enhancement, and the non-enhancing intravenous thrombus may be discriminated as a triangle ("empty triangle" or "Delta-sign", in analogy to the design of the Greek capital letter Delta [Δ]). While the cord sign is found in up to 20% of CVT cases only, the Delta-sign has been described in 15–45% of CVT patients [10].

> A 'cord sign', a thread-like hyperdense structure on no-contrast CCT and a 'Delta-sign', a triangle-shaped non-enhanced structure showing after application of contrast media, are highly suggestive of CVT. Other findings are nonspecific, such as

brain edema. The main indication is to rule out other conditions.

Magnetic resonance imaging

Cerebral magnetic resonance imaging (MRI, Figure 11.3) and magnetic resonance venography (MRV) are extremely sensitive in detecting CVT as well as the underlying parenchymal alterations. The ability of MRI and MRV to obtain images in various planes facilitates the visualization of the different cerebral sinuses. It is important to obtain – at least initially – tri-planar MRI in sagittal, axial and coronal T1 and T2, T2* and FLAIR sequences in combination with

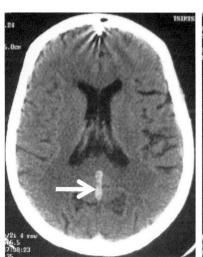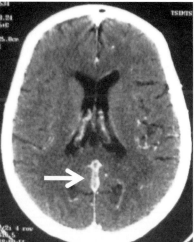

Figure 11.2. Cranial computed tomography in a patient with thrombosis of the straight sinus: the straight sinus presents as a hyperintense thread (cord sign) in non-enhanced CCT (left image), while after intravenous injection of iodinated contrast media the surrounding sinus structures show a distinct enhancement surrounding the thrombus (right image).

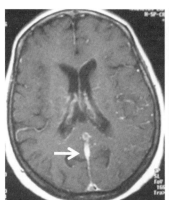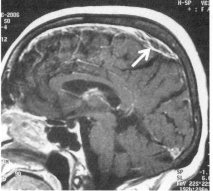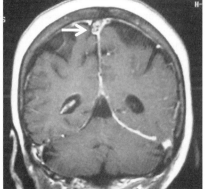

Figure 11.3. Magnetic resonance imaging (T1-weighted images after intravenous injection of paramagnetic contrast media) in a patient with thrombosis of the superior sagittal, straight and right transverse sinus.

MRV, in order to minimize confusion of CVT with sinus aplasia or hypoplasia and not to mistake the T2-weighted hypointense signal of deoxyhemoglobin and intracellular methemoglobin with flow voids [10, 11]. MRI and MRV allow direct imaging of the thrombus, whose signal intensity depends on clot age. Initially (days 1–5), thrombotic material gives an isointense signal on T1 images instead of the normal intraluminal flow void and a strongly hypointense signal on T2 images, indicating the presence of deoxyhemoglobin in erythrocytes of the thrombus. During the second week after clot formation, red blood cells are destroyed, and deoxyhemoglobin is metabolized into methemoglobin, and the thrombus yields a hyperintense signal on both T1- and T2-weighted images. After 2 weeks, the thrombus becomes hypointense on T1- and hyperintense on T2-weighted images, and recanalization may occur with the re-appearance of flow void signaling. Partial or total recanalization is observed within 4–5 months after thrombosis [10–12]. MRI and MRV are non-invasive neuroimaging techniques and may easily be repeated for follow-up and re-evaluation of the course of the disease. However, MRI and MRV are – in most cases – unable to detect isolated cortical venous thrombosis.

> MRI and MRV are highly sensitive in detecting CVT. They allow direct imaging of the thrombus; the signal intensity depends on clot age.

Digital subtraction angiography

Until recently, digital subtraction angiography (DSA) has been the gold standard for the diagnosis of CVT, documenting the partial filling of cerebral venous structures after intra-arterial injection of iodinated contrast media (Figure 11.4). However, DSA is an invasive diagnostic procedure, associated with a peri-procedural risk of death or stroke of about 1%. Furthermore, the interpretation of DSA (as of MRV or CT venography) may be complicated by the presence of anatomical variations, e.g. the hypoplasia of a transverse sinus [13]. Often, indirect signs of thrombosis, e.g. the dilatation of venous collaterals, or the regional prolongation of venous transition time are the only findings that indicate the presence of CVT. Thus, the role of DSA in the diagnosis of CVT remains restricted to those patients where the clinical suspicion cannot be corroborated by other neuroimaging techniques.

> Owing to the high peri-procedural risk, DSA is nowadays restricted to patients where other neuroimaging techniques are not feasible.

Other diagnostic findings

The diagnosis of CVT is based on the detection of venous thrombosis by the neuroimaging techniques described above. As differential diagnosis of CVT comprises a large number of diseases, diagnostic workup in patients with the final diagnosis of CVT requires extensive laboratory exams as well as other auxiliary testing: lumbar puncture, EEG and transcranial Doppler ultrasound are often performed, but most findings are nonspecific.

Most routine laboratory findings in the acute phase of aseptic CVT are nonspecific: mild leukocytosis, elevated erythrocyte sedimentation rate and CRP are the most common abnormalities. Acute thrombosis may be suspected if the D-dimers, a fibrinogen degradation product, are found to be elevated. However, elevated D-dimers just indicate active thrombosis (anywhere in the body), and normal values for D-dimers do not exclude acute CVT [14, 15].

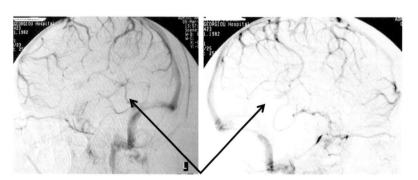

Figure 11.4. Digital subtraction angiography in a patient with isolated thrombosis of the right inferior anastomotic vein of Labbe (right), in contrast to physiological imaging of the cerebral vein findings of the contralateral hemisphere (left).

Table 11.2. Suggested thrombophilia screening in patients with cerebral venous thrombosis.

Genetic prothrombotic conditions

    Antithrombin III

    Protein S

    Protein C

    APC resistance

    Mutations in the MTHFR gene

    Prothrombin AG20210 mutation

    FV-Leiden mutation

    Factor VIII

Acquired prothrombotic conditions

    Homocysteine

    Vitamin B12

    Folic acid

Inflammatory diseases

    Lupus anticoagulant

    Anticardiolipin IgG and IgM antibodies

    Anti-beta2-GP IgG and IgM antibodies

    Anti-prothrombin IgG and IgM antibodies

Other laboratory markers for acute thrombosis include PAI-1, thrombin-antithrombin (TAT) and plasmin-antiplasmin (PAP) complexes. However, their diagnostic value in the acute phase of CVT is under debate, and testing is not widely available.

After the diagnosis of acute CVT, a thorough thrombophilia screening (Table 11.2) should be performed in all patients, but – if that is not feasible at a certain institution – at least patients with recurrent thromboembolic events or those with a positive family history of such disease should be referred to a specialized center for a hematological workup.

As the clinical features of CVT may be mistaken for those of meningo-encephalitis, lumbar puncture is often performed in these patients. CSF findings in acute CVT include increased CSF pressure, a mild pleocytosis and elevated CSF protein in about 50% of patients. However, these findings are nonspecific and do not allow the diagnosis of CVT. The diagnostic value of lumbar puncture in CVT patients is the exclusion of definite infectious meningo-encephalitis (or its diagnosis in septic CVT).

EEG in CVT patients may show focal or generalized slowing, or even focal or generalized epileptic discharges. However, EEG findings may be physiological in up to 25% of patients.

Transcranial duplex sonography may disclose an elevation in venous flow velocities in patients with severe CVT.

Laboratory parameters and CSF findings in aseptic CVT are nonspecific. Normal values for D-dimers do not exclude acute CVT.

Lumbar puncture is necessary to exclude or confirm infectious meningo-encephalitis in septic CVT. Thrombophilia screening should be performed especially in patients with recurrent thromboembolic events.

Therapy

Patients with acute CVT may present with signs and symptoms of acutely increased intracranial pressure or extended venous infarctions, and are in danger of dying within hours from cerebral herniation. Impaired consciousness and cerebral hemorrhage on admission are associated with a poor outcome. The treatment priority in the acute phase is to stabilize the patient and to prevent herniation, followed by the initiation of anticoagulant treatment and the treatment of underlying causes, especially bacterial infections.

In 2006, the European Federation of Neurological Societies published evidence-based guidelines on the treatment of CVT [1], which are outlined in the following sections. The question of anticoagulation therapy in acute CVT is also addressed in the recent guidelines issued by the Council on Stroke of the American Heart Association/American Stroke Association [16].

Acute management:
    stabilization of the patient
    prevention of herniation
    initiation of anticoagulant treatment
    treatment of underlying causes, especially bacterial infections.

Anticoagulation

The rationale for immediate anticoagulation therapy in patients with definite and acute CVT is to stop prothrombotic processes and allow endogenous fibrinolysis to recanalize the occluded veins and sinuses. However, concern has been raised about the possible dangers of anticoagulation in the presence of hemorrhagic venous infarction, found in up to 40% of all CVT patients [2]. The issue has been addressed in two small randomized controlled trials [6, 8] that compared anticoagulant treatment with dose-adjusted unfractionated heparin (UFH [8]) or weight-adjusted LMWH (nadroparin 90 anti-Xa units/kg BW bid) with placebo treatment [6]. The first study was terminated after inclusion of 10 patients in each group, as an interim analysis documented a beneficial effect of heparin treatment on morbidity and mortality. The second study documented a relative risk reduction for poor outcome of 38% with LMWH treatment, without reaching statistical significance. Both studies were criticized for inadequately small sample size [8] or baseline imbalance favoring the placebo group [6]. Patients with intracranial hemorrhage were included in both studies, and no new symptomatic cerebral hemorrhage occurred in either treatment group. A meta-analysis of the studies on immediate anticoagulation treatment for acute CVT showed a nonsignificant reduction in the pooled relative risk of death or dependency [17].

In the recently published ISCVT study [2], more than 80% of the enrolled patients with CVT were treated with anticoagulation (two-thirds of patients received dose-adjusted UFH, one-third were treated with LMWH). A minority of patients received either low-dose LMWH antiplatelet treatment or no anticoagulants at all. There was a non-significant trend towards favorable outcome in patients under anticoagulation treatment compared with those not receiving anticoagulation, but no differences in treatment safety or efficacy were observed between patients on UFH or LMWH.

Based on the results of these studies, meta-analyses and observational data, both UFH and LMWH are considered safe and probably effective in CVT, and immediate anticoagulation is recommended even in the presence of hemorrhagic venous infarcts [1, 16]. When using intravenous UFH, the therapeutic goal is the doubling of activated partial thromboplastin time (aPTT), while LMWH is administered subcutaneously twice daily in a body-weight-adjusted total dose of 180 (2×90) anti-Xa units per day. Whether treatment with full-dose UFH or subcutaneously applied LMWH is equally effective for CVT is not clear, as direct comparisons are lacking. A meta-analysis which compared the efficacy of fixed-dose subcutaneous LMWH versus adjusted-dose UFH for

extracerebral venous thromboembolism found a superiority for LMWH and significantly fewer major bleeding complications [18]. Other advantages of LMWH include the subcutaneous instead of intravenous route of administration, which increases the mobility of patients, and the lack of a need for laboratory monitoring and subsequent dose adjustments. The advantage of dose-adjusted intravenous heparin therapy, particularly in critical ill patients, may be the fact that the activated partial thromboplastin time normalizes within 1–2 h after discontinuation of the infusion, if complications occur or surgical intervention becomes necessary. In addition, the anticoagulatory effect of heparin may be immediately antagonized with protamin, while such an antidote is not available for LMWH. Following current guidelines, and for the reasons mentioned above, LMWH should be preferred over heparin in uncomplicated CVT cases [1].

> Immediate anticoagulation is recommended, even in the presence of hemorrhagic venous infarcts. In critically ill patients, dose-adjusted intravenous heparin therapy (therapeutic goal: doubling of activated partial thromboplastin time (aPTT)) has the advantage of a short half-life and the possibility of antagonization with protamin. In uncomplicated CVT cases, LMWH should be preferred over heparin (dose: body-weight-adjusted 90 anti-Xa units twice daily).

Long-term treatment of CVT – as of other forms of venous thrombosis – with intravenous UFH or subcutaneous LMWH poses the question of patient compliance. Therefore, a switch to oral anticoagulation with vitamin K antagonists aiming at an INR of 2.0–3.0 is recommended after the patient's condition has stabilized [1, 16]. There are insufficient data to determine the optimal duration of oral anticoagulation with vitamin K antagonists. As recanalization of occluded cerebral veins is observed until 5 months after diagnosis [12], it is suggested that effective anticoagulation should be performed for about 6 months after diagnosis of CVT. If no underlying disease is identified that justifies the continuation of oral anticoagulation, treatment with vitamin K antagonists should be stopped and antiplatelets (e.g. acetylsalicylic acid 100 mg qid) should be given for at least another 6 months [16]. Alternatively, and in analogy to patients with extracerebral venous thrombosis, oral anticoagulation may be given for 3 months if CVT was secondary to a transient risk factor, and for 6–12 months if it was idiopathic [19].

According to current guidelines [1], oral anti-coagulation is recommended for 6–12 months in patients with CVT and a "mild" hereditary thrombophilia such as protein C and S deficiency, heterozygous factor V Leiden or prothrombin G20210A mutations. Long-term treatment should be considered for patients with a "severe" hereditary thrombophilia which carries a high risk of recurrence, such as antithrombin-III deficiency, homozygous factor V Leiden mutation, or two or more thrombophilic conditions. "Indefinite" anticoagulation is recommended in patients with two or more episodes of idiopathic objectively documented extracerebral venous thrombosis [19]. In general, in the absence of controlled data, the decision on the duration of anticoagulant therapy must be based on individual hereditary and precipitating factors predisposing to CVT as well as on the potential bleeding risks of long-term oral anticoagulation. Regular follow-up visits should be performed after termination of anticoagulation and patients should be informed about early signs and symptoms (e.g. headache) indicating a possible relapse.

> For long-term treatment of CVT, a switch to oral anticoagulation with vitamin K antagonists (therapeutic goal: INR 2.0–3.0) is recommended.
> The duration of effective anticoagulation depends on CVT etiology.

Thrombolysis

Despite immediate anticoagulation, some patients show a distinct deterioration of their clinical condition, and this risk seems to be especially high in patients presenting with focal neurological signs and reduction of the level of consciousness. The recent ISCVT study identified coma on admission and thrombosis of the deep venous system apart from underlying causes as the most important predictors of a poor clinical outcome [2]. Thrombolytic therapy has the potential to provide faster restitution of venous outflow, and positive effects of both systemic and local thrombolytic treatment of CST have been reported from case reports and small uncontrolled series. However, systematic reviews of thrombolysis in CVT do not show sufficient evidence to support the use of either systemic or local thrombolysis in this disorder [20, 21]. A potential publication bias in the current published work has been assumed, with possible under-reporting of cases with poor outcome and complications. In addition, treatment and assessment were non-blind, leading to a possible bias in outcome assessment [14].

Current guidelines [1] state that there is insufficient evidence to support the use of either systemic or local thrombolysis in patients with CVT. If patients deteriorate despite adequate anticoagulation and other causes of deterioration have been ruled out, thrombolysis may be a therapeutic option in selected cases, possibly in those without hemorrhagic infarction or intracranial hemorrhage. However, optimal substance (urokinase or rt-PA), dosage, route (systemic or local), and method of administration (repeated bolus or bolus plus infusion) are not known.

> Thrombolysis is not recommended in current guidelines.

Symptomatic therapy

Symptomatic treatment of acute CVT comprises analgesia, sedation of agitated patients, management of epileptic seizures and treatment of elevated intracranial pressure.

Pain, nausea and agitation

Headache is the main symptom of CVT, may cause considerable agitation, and should be treated accordingly. Mild to moderate headache in CVT patients should be treated with paracetamol. Acetylsalicylic acid should be avoided, as the patients' bleeding risk may be increased due to the concomitant anticoagulation treatment. Severe headache may require treatment with opioids, but dose titration should be performed cautiously in order to avoid over-sedation.

Concomitant nausea requires parenteral anti-emetic treatment with metoclopramide, minor neuroleptics (e.g. levopromazine, chlorpromazine) or HT_3 antagonists (e.g. ondansetron, granisetron).

If sedation of agitated patients is required, first-choice drugs are major neuroleptics (e.g. haloperidine), because they do not have a relevant impact on the patient's level of consciousness. It has to be kept in mind that other sedative drugs (e.g. benzodiazepines) impair the evaluation of the course of the disease and therefore their use should be restricted to necessary diagnostic or therapeutic interventions.

> For the treatment of headaches, paracetamol should be preferred over acetylsalicylic acid because of the patients' bleeding risk.

Epileptic seizures

All CVT patients presenting with seizures should receive antiepileptic treatment, as the risk of seizure recurrence and status epilepticus is extremely high. For the same reason, effective drug plasma levels should be achieved as soon as possible. Therefore, first-line antiepileptic drugs (AEDs) in CVT patients are those that can be administered parenterally and allow a dosage that reaches therapeutic plasma drug levels within a short time, e.g. phenytoin, valproic acid and levetiracetam.

There are insufficient data regarding the effectiveness of a prophylactic use of AEDs in patients with CVT. One study identified focal sensory deficits and the presence of focal edema or infarcts on admission CT/MRI as significant predictors of early symptomatic seizures [22]. These findings suggest that prophylactic treatment with AED may be a therapeutic option for those patients, whereas treatment is not warranted when there are no focal neurological deficits and no focal parenchymal lesions on brain scan (e.g. patients with isolated intracranial hypertension).

In spite of the high incidence of epileptic seizures in the acute phase of CVT, the risk of residual epilepsy is low, with reported incidence rates between 5% and 10.6% [2, 22] and the vast majority of late seizures occurring within the first year. A hemorrhagic lesion in the acute brain scan was the strongest predictor of post-acute seizures [22]. Late seizures are more common in patients with early symptomatic seizures than in those patients with none. Thus, prolonged treatment with AED for 1 year may be reasonable for patients with early seizures and a hemorrhagic lesion on admission CCT or MRI, whereas in patients without these risk factors, antiepileptic therapy may be tapered off gradually after the acute stage.

Current guidelines [1] state that prophylactic antiepileptic therapy may be an option in patients with focal neurological deficits and focal parenchymal lesions on admission CT/MRI, but that the optimal duration of treatment for patients with seizures remains unclear.

> Epileptic seizures should be treated with parenterally administered antiepileptic drugs (phenytoin, valproic acid, levetiracetam). Prophylactic treatment with antiepileptic drugs may be an option in patients with focal sensory deficits and focal edema or infarcts on admission CT/MRI.

Elevated intracranial pressure

Localized or diffuse brain edema is observed in about 50% of all patients with CVT. However, minor brain swelling (e.g. not resulting in midline shift or uncal herniation) needs no other treatment than anticoagulation, as anticoagulation improves venous drainage to a degree that effectively reduces intracranial pressure.

In patients with the clinical signs of isolated intracranial hypertension only, but threatened vision due to papilledema, lumbar puncture with sufficient CSF removal should be performed. In these patients, anticoagulation may be started 24 hours after CSF removal. This intervention is usually followed by a rapid improvement of headache and visual function. Although controlled data are lacking, acetazolamide should be considered in patients not responding to lumbar puncture. If visual function continues to deteriorate despite CSF removal and acetazolamide therapy, shunting procedures (lumbo-peritoneal shunting, optic nerve fenestration) are recommended.

In the case of severe brain swelling, anti-edema treatment should follow the general rules for the treatment of raised intracranial pressure, i.e. head elevation to 30°, osmotic diuretics (e.g. glycerol or mannitol) and – after admission to an ICU – moderate controlled hyperventilation with a target pCO_2 of 30–35 mmHg. However, in CVT, osmodiuretic drugs are not as quickly eliminated from the intracerebral circulation as in other conditions of increased intracranial pressure. Osmodiuretics may thus reduce venous drainage and should therefore be used with caution only. Volume restriction should be avoided, as dehydration may further increase blood viscosity. Steroids cannot be generally recommended for treatment of elevated intracranial pressure, since their efficacy is unproven and their administration may be harmful, as steroids may promote the thrombotic process [1, 23]. In single patients with impending herniation due to unilateral hemispheric lesion, decompressive hemicraniectomy can be life-saving and even allow a good functional recovery, but evidence is anecdotal [24].

> Increased intracranial pressure in most cases responds to improved venous drainage after anticoagulation. In some patients with lumbar puncture with CSF removal, acetazolamide might be required.
>
> Steroids are not recommended, as they may promote the thrombotic process.

Infectious thrombosis

Infectious CVT requires immediate broad antibiotic treatment and – often – surgical treatment of the underlying disease (e.g. otitis, sinusitis, mastoiditis). Until the results of microbiological cultures are available, third-generation cephalosporins (e.g. cefaloxim 2 g tid or ceftriaxone 2 g bid i.v.) should be given. As in aseptic CVT, anticoagulation should be initiated immediately and symptomatic therapy of septic CVT should adhere to the principles outlined for aseptic CVT, although controlled studies on the efficacy of these measures in septic CVT are lacking.

> Infectious CVT requires immediate broad antibiotic treatment and often surgical treatment of the underlying disease.

Prognosis

The vital and functional prognosis of patients with acute CVT, as established in the ISCVT cohort, is astonishingly favorable, with an overall death or dependency rate of about 15% [2]. Long-term predictors of poor prognosis are the presence of CNS infection, malignancy, deep venous system thrombosis, intracranial hemorrhage, coma upon admission, age and male sex.

In the acute phase of CVT, the case fatality is around 4–8% [2, 14]. The main causes of acute death are transtentorial herniation secondary to a large hemorrhagic lesion, multiple brain lesions or diffuse brain edema. Other causes of acute death include status epilepticus, medical complications and pulmonary embolism. Deterioration after admission occurs in about 23% of patients, with worsening of mental status, headache or focal deficits, or with new symptoms such as seizures. A new parenchymal lesion is present in one-third of patients who deteriorate. Fatalities after the acute phase are predominantly associated with the underlying disorder. The individual prognosis is difficult to predict, but the overall vital and functional prognosis of CVT is much better than that of arterial stroke, with about two-thirds of CVT patients recovering without sequelae [14].

> The overall death or dependency rate is about 15%.

Recurrence of cerebral venous thrombosis

After the acute phase of CVT, anticoagulation is continued not only to facilitate the recanalization of the occluded cerebral veins, but also in order to prevent the recurrence of intra- or extracerebral thrombosis. Recurrent CVT may be difficult to diagnose, if follow-up MRI or MRV examinations are not available. Therefore, it seems feasible to repeat MR venography in CVT patients after 4–6 months, as further recanalization cannot be expected after this point. This follow-up venography may serve as a reference in those cases where recurrent CVT is suspected.

However, recurrence of CVT is rarely observed, and the manifestation of other (extracerebral) thrombotic events is observed in about 5% of CVT patients [2]. This should be pointed out to patients recovering from CVT, who may need reassuring of the very low risk of further thrombotic events.

As pregnancy and puerperium are conditions that favor the manifestation of CVT, concern has been raised about the risk of future pregnancies in women with CVT. On the basis of available evidence, CVT and even pregnancy- or puerperium-related CVT are no contraindication for future pregnancies. Antithrombotic prophylaxis during pregnancy is probably unnecessary, unless a prothrombotic disorder has been diagnosed. However, women on vitamin K antagonists should be advised not to become pregnant because of the teratogenic effects of these drugs [14].

Special aspects
CVT in neonates

While the symptomatology, etiology and therapy of CVT in older children resemble those of adult CVT in most respects, in neonates the causes, clinical presentation, outcome, and management are very different. Manifestation of CVT in neonates seems to be associated with maternal risk factors (hypertension, [pre-] eclampsia, gestational or chronic diabetes mellitus). The vast majority of neonates present with an acute illness at the time of diagnosis, most often dehydration, cardiac defects, sepsis or meningitis. Leading clinical symptoms are epileptic seizures in two-thirds and respiratory distress or apnea in one-third of the neonates. There is a high incidence of intracranial hemorrhages (40–60% hemorrhagic infarctions, 20% intraventricular bleedings). A significant number of children are left with a considerable impairment (motor or cognitive deficits, epilepsy). Treatment is mostly symptomatic and comprises rehydration, antibiotics in the case of sepsis, and antiepileptic therapy.

Heparin is rarely used in neonates, although a pilot study did not show any detrimental effect [25].

Taken together, the nonspecific presentation of neonatal CVT and its common association with an acute illness make the diagnosis even more difficult than in adults or older children. There is no consensus on heparin therapy in neonates, and the prognosis of CVT in neonates is more severe than in adults [14, 26].

CVT in elderly patients

Only recently, older patients were identified as a distinct subgroup of CVT patients. In ISCVT, about 8% of all patients were older than 65 years [27]. In general, these patients presented with clinical symptoms and signs different from those in younger patients: isolated intracranial hypertension was uncommon, whereas disturbances of mental status, alertness and the level of consciousness were common. Carcinoma was found more often in older patients with CVT. The prognosis was worse, with half of the patients being dead or dependent at the end of follow-up.

Future developments

Many issues in the etiology, diagnosis and management of CVT are still unresolved and controversially discussed. Epidemiological data on CVT are lacking from many parts of the planet. Open questions concern many of our current management decisions, such as the role of local or systemic thrombolysis, decompressive hemicraniectomy, initiation and duration of antiepileptic prophylaxis, and the duration of anticoagulation treatment. It is mandatory to increase the level of evidence supporting our diagnostic or therapeutic decisions through prospective registries, case–control studies, and, whenever possible, randomized controlled trials. As CVT is a rare disease with few cases diagnosed annually even at large tertiary health-care facilities, close cooperation between these centers is necessary to achieve progress in the diagnosis and treatment of CVT.

Chapter Summary

Clinical features
The most common and frequently the first symptom of CVT is headache. The onset of headache in CVT is subacute over hours and is due to the increased intracranial pressure.
Epileptic seizures, focal neurological signs, impairment of the level of consciousness and psychotic symptoms can occur.
Septic CVT is accompanied by symptoms of systemic infection.

Diagnostic workup
The main indication of CCT is to rule out other conditions.
MRI and MRV are highly sensitive in detecting CVT. They allow direct imaging of the thrombus; the signal intensity depends on clot age.
The diagnostic value of lumbar puncture in CVT patients is the exclusion or confirmation of infectious meningo-encephalitis in septic CVT.

Therapy
Stabilization of the patient.
Prevention of herniation.
Immediate initiation of anticoagulant treatment (LMWH with a body-weight-adjusted dose of 90 anti-Xa units twice daily or intravenous heparin with the therapeutic goal of doubling of aPTT).
Treatment of bacterial infections with broad antibiotics and surgery.
Switch to oral anticoagulation with vitamin K antagonists (therapeutic goal: INR 2.0–3.0) for long-term treatment.
Treatment of epileptic seizures with parenterally administered antiepileptic drugs (phenytoin, valproic acid, levetiracetam).

Acknowledgement

The author expresses his gratitude to Dr Ioannis Tsitouridis, Director of the Department of Diagnostic Radiology at the General Hospital "Papageorgiou" (Thessaloniki, Greece), in whose department the neuroimaging procedures shown in this article were performed.

References

1. Einhaupl K, Bousser MG, De Bruijn SFTM, et al. Guidelines on the treatment of cerebral venous and sinus thrombosis. *Eur J Neurol* 2006; **13**:553–9.

2. Ferro JM, Canhao P, Stam J, et al. Prognosis of cerebral vein and dural sinus thrombosis. Results of the International Study on Cerebral Vein and Dural Sinus Thrombosis (ISCVT). *Stroke* 2004; **35**:664–70.

3. Amery A, Bousser MG. Cerebral venous thrombosis. *Clin Neurol* 1992; **19**:87–111.

4. Stam J. Thrombosis of the cerebral veins and sinuses. *N Engl J Med* 2005; **352**:1791–8.

5. Schmiedek P, Einhaupl KM, Moser E. Cerebral blood flow in patients with sinus venous thrombosis. In: Einhaupl KM, Kempski O, Baethmann A, eds. *Cerebral Sinus Thrombosis: Experimental and Clinical Aspects.* New York: Plenum Press; 1990: 75–83.

6. De Bruijn SFTM, Stam J, for the Cerebral Venous Sinus Thrombosis Study Group. Randomized, placebo-controlled trial of anticoagulant treatment with low-molecular-weight heparin for cerebral sinus thrombosis. *Stroke* 1999; **30**:484–8.

7. Cantu C, Barinagarrementiera F. Cerebral venous thrombosis associated with pregnancy and puerperium: a review of 67 cases. *Stroke* 1993; **24**:1880–4.

8. Einhaupl K, Villringer A, Meister W, et al. Heparin treatment in sinus venous thrombosis. *Lancet* 1991; **338**:597–600.

9. Van den Bergh WM, van der Schaaf I, van Gijn J. The spectrum of presentations of deep venous infarction caused by deep cerebral vein thrombosis. *Neurology* 2005; **65**:192–6.

10. Renowden S. Cerebral venous sinus thrombosis. *Eur Radiol* 2004; **14**:215–26.

11. Tsitouridis I, Papapostolou P, Rudolf J, et al. Non-neoplastic dural sinus thrombosis: An MRI and MRV evaluation. *Riv Neuroradiologia* 2005; **18**:581–8.

12. Baumgartner RW, Studer A, Arnold M, et al. Recanalization of cerebral venous thrombosis. *J Neurol Neurosurgery Psychiatry* 2003; **74**:459–61.

13. Bono F, Lupo MR, Lavano A, et al. Cerebral MR venography of transverse sinuses in subjects with normal CSF pressure. *Neurology* 2003; **61**:1267–70.

14. Bousser MG, Ferro J. Cerebral venous thrombosis: an update. *Lancet Neurology* 2007; **6**:162–70.

15. Lalive PH, de Moerloose P, Lovblad K, et al. Is measurement of D-dimer useful in the diagnosis of cerebral venous thrombosis? *Neurology* 2003; **61**:1057–60.

16. Sacco RL, Adams R, Albers G, et al. Guidelines for the prevention of stroke in patients with ischemic stroke or transient ischemic attack. *Stroke* 2006; **37**:577–617.

17. Stam J, de Bruijn SFTM, de Veber G. Anticoagulation for cerebral sinus thrombosis. *Cochrane Database Syst Rev* 2002; **4**:CD002005.

18. Van Donden CJJ, van den Belt AGM, Prins HM, et al. Fixed dose subcutaneous low molecular weight heparins versus adjusted dose unfractionated heparin for venous thromboembolism. *Cochrane Database Syst Rev* 2004; **4**:CD001100.

19. Buller HR, Agnelli G, Hull RH, et al. Antithrombotic therapy for venous thromboembolic disease. The seventh ACCP conference on antithrombotic and thrombolytic therapy. *Chest* 2004; **126**:401–28.

20. Canhao P, Falcao F, Ferro JM. Thrombolytics for cerebral sinus thrombosis: a systematic review. *Cerebrovasc Dis* 2003; **15**:159–66.

21. Ciccone A, Canhao P, Falcao F, Ferro JM, Sterzi R. Thrombolysis for cerebral vein and dural sinus thrombosis. *Stroke* 2004; **35**:2428.

22. Ferro JM, Correia M, Rosas MJ, et al. Seizures in cerebral vein and dural sinus thrombosis. *Cerebrovasc Dis* 2003; **15**:78–83.

23. Canhao P, Cortesao A, Cabral M, et al. Are steroids useful for the treatment of cerebral venous thrombosis? ISCVT results. *Cerebrovasc Dis* 2004; **17**(Suppl. 5):16.

24. Rudolf J, Hilker R., Terstegge K, et al. Extended haemorrhagic infarction following isolated cortical venous thrombosis. *Eur Neurol* 1999; **41**:115–16.

25. deVeber G, Chan A, Monagle P, et al. Anticoagulation therapy in pediatric patients with sinovenous thrombosis: a cohort study. *Arch Neurol* 1998; **55**:1533–7.

26. Golomb MR. Sinovenous thrombosis in neonates. *Semin Cerebrovasc Dis Stroke* 2001; **1**:216–24.

27. Ferro JM, Canhao P, Bousser M-G, Barinagarrementeria F. Cerebral vein and dural sinus thrombosis in elderly patients. *Stroke* 2005; **36**:1927–32.

Chapter 12

Behavioral neurology of stroke

José M. Ferro, Isabel P. Martins and Lara Caeiro

Cognitive functions are related to our ability to build an internal representation of the world, the conceptual representation system, based on a large-scale neuronal network. This system is connected with more circumscribed and lateralized operational systems that allow us to translate thoughts into words (spoken, written or gestures), images, numbers or other symbols, to store and retrieve information when necessary and to make decisions or act upon them. Most of these operational abilities are subserved by distributed networks with areas of regional specialization, organized according to their specific processing capacities.

The pattern of cognitive/behavioral impairment observed after ischemic stroke is relatively stereotyped, since it follows the distribution of the vascular territories. However, in the hyperacute stage symptoms are likely to be amplified by additional regions of ischemic penumbra, mass effects and diaschisis (impairment of intact regions that are functionally connected with the damaged area), and, in the chronic stage, functional reorganization and brain plasticity mechanisms make neuroanatomical correlations loose and less predictable.

In hemorrhagic lesions, vasculitis, and cerebral venous thrombosis the pattern of cognitive defects is less stereotyped due to the variability of lesion localization, size and number, or particular pathogenic mechanisms that may cause diffuse impairment.

In this chapter we will present the most common cognitive and neurobehavioral deficits secondary to stroke, according to symptom presentation.

Language disorders

Language disorders, or aphasia, occur following peri-sylvian lesions (middle cerebral artery territory) of the left hemisphere and have a marked impact on the individual quality of life, autonomy and the ability to return to work or previous activities. Since these lesions are circumscribed, the conceptual representation system is not affected and these patients are not demented. This is an important distinction that should be explained to the family and caregivers.

> Language disorders occur following middle cerebral artery territory lesions of the left hemisphere.

A brief bedside evaluation of language comprises four cardinal tests that are useful in the taxonomic classification of aphasia and to localize lesions, since they have neuroanatomical correlates [1]. Although these tests are also included in brief exams of cognitive assessment, such as the Mini Mental State Examination (MMSE), they should be evaluated beforehand. In fact, language impairment will affect the majority of cognitive functions and needs to be ruled out before proceeding to the assessment of orientation, memory or executive functions.

The most sensitive task for the diagnosis of aphasia is confrontation naming, for it depends upon a large network around the Sylvian fissure and can be disrupted even by small lesions. It is also a rough measure of aphasia severity. The ability to retrieve a name is related to word frequency and the familiarity/imageability of stimuli. Presented objects should be common and easily recognized (spoon, comb, spectacles, pencil, wristwatch), to make the task specific for aphasia and not sensitive to cultural factors or aging. Patients' responses vary from pauses (word-finding difficulties), tip-of-the tongue phenomenon, paraphasias, the use of supraordinal responses (fruit for apple) and descriptions of use (circumlocutions). There are rare patients who suffer from a selective naming difficulty affecting a single category of names ("category-specific impairments"), such as living entities, actions but not objects, or proper names but not common names. These unusual cases demonstrate that the mental lexicon/semantic system is organized by the functional or physical properties of objects or living entities (see Martin [2] for review).

The analysis of speech is performed during spontaneous or induced conversation (asking patients to tell you an episode or to describe a picture). Speech is classified, dichotomically, as fluent (associated with temporo-parietal lesions) or nonfluent (pre-rolandic or subcortical lesions) [1] (Table 12.1). To make this classification easy the listener should try to ignore the content of speech (as if listening to a foreign language) and concentrate on the effort, speech rate and the number and duration of pauses. Fluent speech "sounds" normal as opposed to nonfluent speech.

Verbal auditory comprehension is tested through simple verbal commands ("close your eyes", "raise your arm", etc.). Poor comprehension of words/nouns (lexical comprehension) is usually associated with posterior temporal lesions, while inferior frontal/opercular lesions tend to impair the understanding of syntax and verbs but not the nouns.

Finally, one should ask the patient to repeat words, pseudowords (pronounceable strings of speech sounds that do not belong to the lexicon) and sentences, to evaluate the ability to decode, retain briefly in memory and reproduce phonemes (speech sounds). Transcortical aphasias are characterized by a disproportionate capacity to repeat, compared to other language abilities. Sometimes these patients repeat compulsively, a phenomenon called echolalia. In conduction aphasia, in contrast, patients have outstanding difficulty in repeating pseudowords or even words they can otherwise produce.

Difficulty in any of these four tasks may vary from mild (occasional difficulty) to severe, and the taxonomic classification of aphasia varies accordingly (Table 12.2).

Effective language recovery, in adults, depends mostly upon the reorganization of the intact areas of the left hemisphere in the neighborhood of the lesion [3].

> Four cardinal tests are useful for a bedside evaluation of aphasia and to localize lesions, since they have neuroanatomical correlates: (1) confrontation naming; (2) analysis of speech (fluent and nonfluent); (3) verbal auditory comprehension; (4) repetition of words, pseudowords and sentences. Language should be evaluated before cognitive assessment.

Certain brain lesions may impair the ability to read (alexia or acquired dyslexia) or to write (agraphia/dysgraphia). Both conditions are commonly

Table 12.1. Classification of speech fluency.

Speech fluency	
Fluent	**Non-fluent**
Normal output	Slow output
(words/minute)	Single words
Normal phrase length	Telegraphic sentences
Effortless	Effortful
No pauses	Hesitations, pauses, interruptions
Normal prosody	Loss of prosody
Sounds "normal"	Sounds "atypical"

Table 12.2. Classification of aphasic syndromes.

Taxonomic classification of aphasia			
Speech fluency	**Lexical comprehension**	**Word-pseudoword repetition**	**Aphasia type**
Non-fluent	Normal	Normal	Transcortical motor
Non-fluent	Normal	Poor	Broca's
Non-fluent	Poor	Normal	Isolation of speech areas
Non-fluent	Poor	Poor	Global
Fluent	Normal	Normal	Anomic
Fluent	Normal	Poor	Conduction
Fluent	Poor	Normal	Transcortical sensory
Fluent	Poor	Poor	Wernicke's

found in aphasia but may occur in isolation following lesions of the left hemisphere.

The study of patients with reading or writing disorders has contributed to the understanding of the cognitive processes subserving those abilities and to the building of theoretical models of them. They have shown that there are separate pathways to process particular categories of words (regular vs. irregular; meaningful words vs. functional words, such as "to", "if", "so") or specific tasks (copying vs. writing spontaneously). This information has been incorporated into the assessment and classification of these disorders (Figure 12.1) [4].

Alexia and agraphia can be classified as central or peripheral, depending on whether the impairment affects the central processing or the afferent or efferent pathways.

The best known peripheral alexia is "pure alexia" (alexia without agraphia or letter-by-letter reading). In this syndrome, patients can read through the tactile and auditory modalities (read a word that is spelled aloud to them), showing that the central processing is intact. They can also write to dictation or spontaneously. However, they cannot associate visually presented written words with their sound or meanings (cannot read). This syndrome results from a disconnection between the visual areas and the "word form area", due to left temporo-occipital infarcts involving the posterior splenium.

In central dyslexias, the impairment is independent of the presentation modality (visual, auditory or tactile) and therefore also involves writing and spelling. "Deep dyslexic" patients may reach the meaning of some written words, including irregular words (producing semantic paraphasias, *orange* for *lemon*),

but are unable to read function words or nonwords that are deprived of meaning. In contrast, in "surface dyslexia" patients can read aloud regular words and pseudowords (because they can convert letters, written graphemes, to their corresponding sound), but have difficulty reading irregular words or accessing their meaning. These opposite types of impairment have shown the existence of two pathways for reading, a fast whole-word recognition with access to meaning (used when one reads frequent meaningful words) and a step-by-step conversion that is useful for reading new or infrequent words.

Likewise, in central agraphias, the writing impairment is similar across different output modalities (handwriting, spelling or typing) and can be of a "deep type" (phonological dysgraphia) with preserved access to meaning, or a "surface type" (lexical agraphia, with preserved sound-to-grapheme conversion and particular difficulty writing irregular words). There are also cases whose defect involves the "graphemic buffer" (a short-term memory "device" that enables the writer to keep the word "on line" as it is being written in real time), which is characterized by a particular difficulty writing long words. In contrast, peripheral agraphia is a selective damage in the selection or the act of drawing letters (during handwriting) that can be overcome by typing or the use of anagrams and is associated with normal spelling.

Deep forms of dyslexia and dysgraphia are associated with large left hemisphere strokes [5], while surface types result from more limited lesions. It is possible that reading and writing/spelling rely on the same cognitive processes, but in reverse order (the "shared components hypothesis") and share the same neural network that includes the angular,

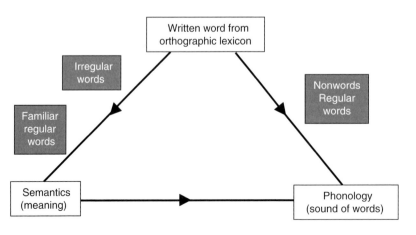

Figure 12.1. Cognitive models of reading. (After Plaut et al. [4].)

supramarginal and fusiform gyrus (BA 37) and BA 22 and 44/45, as suggested in a study performed in acute stroke patients [6].

> Alexia and agraphia are commonly found in aphasia, but may occur in isolation following lesions of the left hemisphere. Alexia can be classified as central and peripheral, and as 'deep' and 'surface' types.

Neglect

Neglect is an inability to attend to, orient or explore the hemispace contralateral to a brain lesion. Since the right hemisphere is dominant for selective attention, this syndrome is usually observed following right hemisphere stroke (affecting some 36–80% of acute stroke patients) [7] and affecting awareness of the left-hand side. Neglect has a negative impact on daily living activities and on functional recovery, because patients cannot be expected to focus on a symptom that consists exactly of lack of awareness.

Selective attention relies on a large network involving the anterior cingulate gyrus (responsible for its motivational aspects), frontal-parietal and superior temporal regions (afferent and intentional/exploratory aspects) as well as subcortical structures, such as the thalamus and the striatum. Lesions at any of these areas may produce neglect.

Neglect can produce different symptoms that must be looked for to be detected. It may be evident in different types of space: in the personal space (forgetting to dress, groom the left side of the body), the "hand reach" or peri-personal space (failing to detect or orient to surrounding objects or persons), the distant space ("at eye reach") leading to spatial disorientation, or in representational space (mental imagery). It may be present spontaneously or during competing sensory stimulation (extinction phenomena) and in any sensory modality (visual, tactile, auditory). In its most severe form it comprises anosognosia or denial of illness/impairment and a loss of identification of body parts as belonging to the self.

The most common tests used to diagnose neglect are performed in the peri-personal space and require the patient to draw, copy or cross out lines or other stimuli (cancellation tasks) or to read or write. A qualitative analysis of the defect allow us to further classify the defect as person-centered "egocentric neglect" (involving the angular gyrus) or object-centered or "alocentric neglect" (right superior temporal gyrus) [8].

Table 12.3. Memory systems.

| Primary (short term) |
| Declarative |
| Semantic |
| Episodic |
| Implicit |
| Procedural |
| Priming – facilitation from a previous exposure |
| Classic conditioning |
| Sensory recording systems |

> Neglect is an inability to attend to, orient or explore the hemispace contralateral to a brain lesion, usually of the right hemisphere.

Memory disturbances

Memory is not a unitary function. It consists of five independent systems and involves three processes (encoding, storing/consolidation and retrieval). Both depend on specific neural networks that may dissociate following a brain lesion.

Classification of memory systems (Table 12.3) [9] depends upon three main vectors: duration of memory traces (fractions of seconds, seconds or "for life"), content (explicit knowledge or motor routines) and access to consciousness (explicit or implicit). According to the processes affected amnesia is further subdivided in reference to a specific time event into anterograde (patients cannot encode/consolidate new information) and retrograde (the difficulty lies in retrieving information that was already stored).

Amnesic strokes, i.e. infarcts presenting amnesia for recent events as the main clinical feature, can result from posterior cerebral artery, posterior communicating artery, anterior and posterior choroidal artery, anterior cerebral and anterior communicating artery thrombosis or embolism. Infarcts in the territories of the two last arteries can also be secondary to subarachnoid hemorrhage and its complications and to the surgical and less often to the endovascular treatment of aneurysms located in these arteries. Single case reports or small case series of amnestic stroke have been reported following infarcts of the inferior genu of the internal capsule inferior, the

Table 12.4. Summary of main features of major amnestic stroke syndromes.

Characteristic stroke type	Hippocampal	Thalamic	Basal forebrain
	PCA infarct	anterior or mesial thalamic infarct	rupture of ACoA aneurysm
Anterograde amnesia	severe	severe	severe
Retrograde amnesia	none or mild	none or mild	moderate
Encoding defect	severe	severe	severe
Consolidation defect	severe	severe	severe
Retrieval defect	none or mild	severe	severe
Recognition defect	none or mild	none or mild	false recognitions
Working memory	normal	none or mild defect	normal
Procedural memory	normal	normal	normal
Meta-memory	normal or mild defect	normal or mild defect	impaired
Confabulations	occasional	frequent	very frequent

mammillothalamic tract, the fornix and the retrosplenium [10]. Anterolateral and medial thalamic hemorrhages, caudate and intraventricular hemorrhages and venous infarcts due to thrombosis of the deep venous system also produce memory defects.

A quarter of posterior cerebral artery infarcts result in memory defects [11] (Table 12.4). These amnestic strokes usually have mesial temporal involvement and the damage extends beyond the hippocampus to the entorhinal cortex, perirhinal cortex, collateral isthmus or parahippocampal gyrus. The memory defect is more frequent and severe after left-sided and especially after bilateral infarcts. Left posterior cerebral artery infarcts cause either a verbal amnesia or a global amnesia, while right lesions produce visuospatial memory defects, including deficits in the memory for familiar faces or locations and topographical amnesia. Confabulations appear to be more likely if there is a dual lesion (temporo-occipital and thalamic).

In thalamic infarcts [12], memory defects (Table 12.4) are also a distinct feature of anterior, dorsomedial and, in the variant types, anteromedian and central infarcts. Combined polar and paramedian infarcts also cause a severe and persistent amnesia. Left thalamic infarcts can produce "pure amnesia" in the form of a verbal or global amnesia. Memory disturbances are more frequent and severe after left than after right thalamic infarcts. Right thalamic infarcts cause visual and/or visuospatial amnesia.

Following unilateral infarcts (left or right) a complete or partial recovery of memory disturbances can be expected. Bilateral infarcts produce global and severe amnesia and a persistent deficit, with slow and limited improvement. In thalamic amnesia confabulations, intrusions and perseveration are frequent. Distractibility, alternating good and poor performance and better performance on first attempts are also characteristic.

Memory defects are a frequent clinical feature of subarachnoid hemorrhage due to ruptured anterior communicating artery aneurysms and may also follow posterior communicating aneurysm rupture. They are a frequent and disabling long-term sequela: the Australian Cooperative Research on Subarachnoid Haemorrhage Group (2000) [13] found problems with memory in 50% of survivors. Recently, hippocampal atrophy was found on neuroimaging studies in subarachnoid hemorrhage survivors [14].

Amnesia following rupture of anterior communicating aneurysms is characterized by a severe anterograde and a moderate retrograde amnesia (Table 12.4). There is a high susceptibility to interference, false recognitions, confabulations and anosognosia. Amnesia is related to damage to the anterior cingulum, subcalosal area and basal forebrain. Temporal error contexts are associated with ventromedial prefrontal cortex damage, but for spontaneous confabulations to occur there must be additional orbitofrontal deficit [15]. The brain has a mechanism to distinguish mental activity representing ongoing perception of reality from memories and ideas. Confabulations can be traced to fragments of previous actual experiences. Confabulators confuse ongoing reality with the past because they fail to suppress evoked memories that do not pertain to the current reality. The role of the anterior limbic system is the suppression of currently irrelevant mental associations. It represents "now" in human thinking.

> Classification of memory systems depends upon duration of memory traces, content, and access to consciousness.
> Amnesia can be further subdivided into anterograde and retrograde.
> Amnesia can result from lesions in hippocampus, thalamus or basal forebrain.

Executive deficits

Executive functions are classically assigned to the prefrontal lobes. Three types of prefrontal lobe functions are usually considered: (1) dorsolateral (executive/cognitive), including working memory, programming/planning, concept formation, monitoring of actions and external cues and metacognition; (2) orbital (emotional/self-regulatory), consisting of inhibition of impulses and of non-relevant sensorial information and motor activity; and (3) mesial (action regulation), including motivation. These functions are served by three prefrontal-subcortical loops: dorsolateral, lateral orbital and anterior cingulate, whose dysfunction produces three distinct clinical syndromes composed respectively of executive deficits, uninhibited behavior and apathy. Executive difficulties manifest as difficulty deciding, leaving decisions to proxy and being stubborn or rigid. Examples of uninhibited behavior include inappropriate familiarity, being distractible and shouting when constrained and manipulation or utilization behavior. Recent models propose four main executive functions: dual task coordination, switch retrieval, selective attention and holding and manipulation of information stored in long-term memory, so-called working memory; and three executive processes: updating, shifting and inhibition [16]. Table 12.5 lists instruments that can be used to evaluate executive functions.

There are few systematic studies of executive functioning and other "frontal" syndromes in stroke patients. About one-third of acute stroke patients show either disinhibition or indifference and 30–40%

Table 12.5. Neuropsychological evaluation of "frontal lobe" functions.

Interview

   Frontal Behavioral Inventory

   EXIT-25 – Executive Interview

   Neuropsychiatric Inventory (NPI)

Bedside evaluation

   Frontal Assessment Battery at bedside

Specific tests

   Speed and motor control – tapping test, reaction times, Pordue Pegboard

   Sustained attention – letter or other cancellation test, Trail Making A

   Speed and shifting – Digit-Symbol or Symbol-Digit, Trail Making B

   Inhibition – Stroop Test B

   Initiative – phonological and semantic verbal fluency tasks

   Concept formation and set shifting – Wisconsin Card Sorting Test, mazes

   Problem solving – mazes, Towers (Hanoi, London), gambling task

display executive deficits in formal testing [17, 18]. Among patients with subarachnoid hemorrhage one-half to two-thirds have executive deficits [19]. Stroke in some specific locations can cause executive deficits, disinhibition or apathy. Examples are middle cerebral artery infarcts with frontal lobe or striatocapsular involvement, uni- or bilateral anterior cerebral artery infarcts, anterior or paramedian thalamic infarcts, striatocapsular, thalamic, intraventricular or frontal intracerebral hemorrhages, subarachnoid hemorrhage due to rupture of anterior communicating artery aneurysms and thrombosis of the saggital sinus or of the deep venous system.

> Executive deficits due to lesions in the prefrontal lobe occur in about one-third of stroke patients and can be divided into three distinct clinical syndromes:
> - executive deficits – corresponding to the dorsolateral prefrontal lobe
> - uninhibited behavior – corresponding to the lateral orbital prefrontal lobe
> - apathy – corresponding to the anterior cingulate prefrontal lobe.

Visual agnosia

The human brain has two parallel visual systems: a ventral occipito-temporal stream, whose main function is the recognition of visual stimuli (the "what" system) and a dorsal occipito-parietal stream, whose main function is the spatial localization of visual stimuli (the "where" system) [20]. The paradigm of human dysfunction of the ventral system is visual agnosia while that of the dorsal system is Balint's syndrome.

Visual agnosias are disorders of visual recognition and are one of the clinical manifestations of posterior cerebral artery infarcts and occipito-temporal hemorrhages. Agnosias can be seen in patients improving from cortical blindness. Visual agnosias can be classified following the type of stimuli that is defectively recognized or following the impaired functional step in the processing of information from the visual system to the semantic and the language systems (Table 12.6).

Apperceptive visual object agnosia is characterized by the presence of perceptual defects in visuoperceptive tasks and a defective perception of elementary perceptual features (color, shape, contour, brightness). The most distinctive feature of patients with apperceptive visual agnosia is visual matching errors when trying to match identical visual stimuli. Their naming errors are morphological, based on visual similarity. They perform better with real objects than with drawings. There are two varieties of apperceptive visual agnosia: form and integrative agnosia. Patients with form agnosia cannot perceive contours, although they can perceive brightness, color or luster. They have a better recognition of moving than of static objects. In contrast, patients with integrative agnosia perceive single contours but cannot integrate them in a coherent structure of the object, and produce predominantly visual similarity errors. Apperceptive visual agnosia is due to bilateral occipital or occipito-temporal lesions.

In associative visual object agnosia the distinctive feature is the intact perception. Although minor errors can be detected in complex perceptual tasks, the perception of elementary perceptual features (color, shape, contour, brightness) is correct, as is the matching of visual stimuli. Naming errors are semantic-related, perseverations or confabulatory. A variety of associative visual agnosia is semantic access agnosia (visuo-verbal or visuo-semantic

Table 12.6. Classification of visual agnosias.

According to the type of visual stimuli
Visual agnosia for
Letters and words
Other symbols
Colors
Objects
Specific classes of objects
Faces
Locations
According to the functional processes involved
Apperceptive visual agnosia
Form agnosia
Integrative agnosia
Associative visual agnosia
Disconnection or loss of semantic access
Loss of semantic knowledge

disconnection). Patients with this type of agnosia show not only intact naming in other modalities (tactile, auditory) but also a correct use of objects. They may be able to select the correct name of an object in multiple-choice tasks and can sort objects by semantic categories. They may also be able to describe or pantomime the use of visually presented objects and have a superior naming of actions than of objects. Associative visual agnosia results from left or bilateral occipito-temporal lesions. In the literature the term optic aphasia is also found. It refers to a syndrome closely linked to visual agnosia and to transcortical sensory aphasia, and is often found during recovery from this. Patients have a disproportionate difficulty in naming stimuli presented visually, but otherwise do not display other features of visual agnosia (Figure 12.2).

Testing for color agnosia deserves a note. A careful check for achromatopsia in the whole or part of the visual field should precede other tasks. Color perception is checked by asking the patient to match identical colors. To test the visual–verbal connection we ask the patient to name colors and to point to named colors. To evaluate whether there is color anomia and to ensure that language is intact we ask

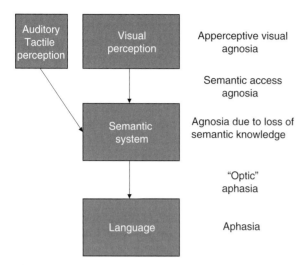

Figure 12.2. Processing of visual stimuli and visual agnosias.

for color names in responsive naming (e.g. "Tell me the names of the colors of the national flag"). Finally, we can test visual–semantic connections by showing the patient drawings of stimuli which are painted in the correct and the wrong colors (e.g. blue banana) and asking the patient whether the colors are correct. Functional and lesion localization studies found that the V4v, V8, V4a areas and the lingual gyrus are the human brain "color areas" [21]. Strokes causing color agnosia are left posterior cerebral infarcts with inferior temporal involvement. Color agnosia is more frequent than object agnosia.

Prosopagnosia is defined as an inability to recognize visually familiar faces, i.e. faces known by the patient, despite preserved visual perception. Recent studies using functional imaging indicate that the human brain areas activated by personally familiar faces (family, friends, etc.), famous familiar faces (media, politicians, sports people, etc.) and even of one's own child vs. familiar unrelated children are in part distinct. Current cognitive models consider a core system necessary for the recognition of visual appearance (the system which is disturbed in prosopagnosia), and an extended system relative to person knowledge and to emotion related to or triggered by the perception of a face [22]. Prosopagnosia should not be confused with visuo-perceptive deficits in tests using unknown faces, nor with the common complaint of prosopanomia (difficulty in recalling the names of known persons). Patients with prosopagnosia retain their ability to recognize people through

other cues, such as voice, gait, size and clothes. They may also be able to recognize faces by facial features, e.g. moustache, scar, or accessories, e.g. spectacles, rings. They may be able to identify gender, ethnicity, age and emotional expression. They have a normal semantic knowledge about people. Functional and anatomical studies identified the occipital face area, the fusiform face area and the superior temporal sulcus as the areas crucial in processing information relative to human faces [23]. Prosopagnosia can be found in 4–7% of posterior cerebral artery infarcts, either bilateral inferomedial or less commonly right inferomedial [24].

Hyperfamiliarity for unknown faces has also been reported.

> Visual agnosias are disorders of visual recognition and are one of the clinical manifestations of posterior cerebral artery infarcts and occipito-temporal hemorrhages. Special testing can identify apperceptive and associative visual object agnosia, color agnosia and prosopagnosia.

Delirium

Delirium is a disturbance of consciousness, with a change in cognition or development of a perceptual disturbance, which develops over a short period, fluctuates during the course of the day and cannot be explained by pre-existing dementia (Table 12.7). Stroke is a rare cause of delirium. On the other hand, delirium often (15–48%) complicates acute stroke [25–28]. Delirium must be differentiated clinically from disorientation in time, topographical disorientation, delusions and hallucinations, amnesia, fluent aphasia, mania, psychosis and even severe depression. Strokes in strategic locations (e.g. posterior cerebral artery, dorsomedial thalamic, caudate infarcts and hemorrhages, right middle cerebral artery, intraventricular hemorrhage, subarachnoid hemorrhage) [29] can cause acute agitated confusional states, with a variable combination of declarative episodic memory defect, hyperactive motor behavior, apathy and other personality changes, delusions or hallucinations and disturbed sleep cycle.

Delirium can be detected by the routine testing of mental status or with a specific simple instrument such as the Confusion Assessment Method. The severity of the delirium can be graded using scales such as the Delirium Rating Scale or the CIWA-Ar scale (if delirium is related to alcohol withdrawal).

Table 12.7. Main clinical features of delirium.

Acute onset

　Occurs abruptly, over a period of hours or days

Fluctuating course

　Symptoms came and go and fluctuate in severity over a 24-hour period

　Lucid intervals

Inattention

　Difficulty focusing, sustaining and shifting attention

　Difficulty maintaining conversation or following commands

Disorganized thinking

　Disorganized or incoherent speech

　Rambling or irrelevant conversation or an unclear or illogical flow of ideas

Altered level of consciousness

　Clouding of consciousness, with reduced clarity of awareness of environment

Cognitive deficits

　Global or multiple: orientation, memory, language

Perceptual disturbances

　Illusions, hallucinations

Psychomotor disturbances

　Hyperactive type: agitated, hyper-vigilant

　Hypoactive type: decreased motor activity, lethargy

Altered sleep–wake cycle

　Daytime drowsiness, night-time insomnia, fragmented sleep, reversed sleep cycle

Emotional disturbances

　Intermittent or labile fear, paranoia, anxiety, depression, apathy, irritability, anger or euphoria

Table 12.8. Check-list for precipitants of delirium in stroke patients.

- Previous dementia, MCI or cognitive decline
- Previous delirium
- Medication side-effect
- Medication with anticholinergic activity
- Medication intoxication or withdrawal
- Alcohol or illicit drug intoxication or withdrawal
- Fever; infection
- Pain: shoulder, bed sores, visceral, immobility
- Fall with bone fracture
- Subdural hematoma
- Full bladder
- Respiratory distress
- Metabolic disturbance
- Sleep apnea
- Nonconvulsive epileptic status
- Sensory deprivation

Predictors of the development of delirium in stroke patients can be grouped as (a) vulnerable patients, (b) stroke type and (c) precipitating factors. Older patients and those with previous dementia or cognitive decline, previous delirium or vision impairment are more prone to become delirious. Supratentorial strokes, total anterior circulation infarct (TACI) type, cardioembolic strokes, intracerebral hemorrhage as well as strokes causing severe paresis or neglect or a decrease in alertness are more likely to be complicated by delirium. Precipitating factors of delirium in stroke patients include intake of drugs with anticholinergic activity (even subtle anticholinergic activity, such as SSRIs, anti-emetics, baclofen or ipratropium bromide) before or during hospitalization, high blood urea nitrogen/creatinine, infections and metabolic complications. A check-list for the precipitants of delirium is given in Table 12.8.

The pathogenesis of delirium is incompletely understood (Figure 12.3). There is reduced oxidative metabolism and cerebral blood flow, mainly in the frontal lobes and parietal lobes. There is evidence of a cholinergic deficit and of increased serum anticholinergic activity. However, other neurotransmitters such as serotonin, GABA, dopamine and glutamate are probably also involved. A role of inflammation and of cytokines (interleukin-1,2,6, TNF-a) has been recently proposed. The stress-hypercortisolemia hypothesis of delirium is based on the finding of increased ACTH levels in the first hours of delirium and of higher post-dexamethasone cortisol levels in delirious patients.

Delirium is an ominous prognostic sign: acute stroke patients with delirium have a higher risk of

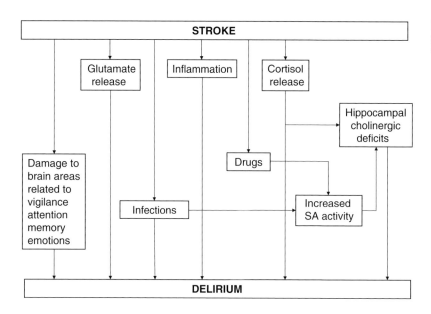

Figure 12.3. Proposed schematic pathophysiological model of post-stroke delirium.

longer hospital stay, in-hospital death, death and dependency at 6–12 months, being admitted to a nursing home or other long-term care facility, recurrent delirium and dementia.

> Delirium often complicates acute stroke and is a bad prognostic sign.
> Delirium is related to
> * vulnerable patients
> * stroke type and
> * precipitating factors.

Anger and aggressiveness

Anger and aggression are complex human emotions and behaviors depending on several anatomical structures, including the frontal lobes, the amygdala, the hypothalamus and the brainstem. Anger is a primary emotion with three components: the emotional (anger), the cognitive (hostility) and the behavioral (aggression).

A few studies [30–34] have evaluated anger and its components systematically in stroke patients and found a frequency ranging from 17% to 34%. In some studies, anger in stroke patients was associated with younger age, depression, anxiety, lower MMSE, and with hemorrhagic strokes with the proximity of the lesion to the frontal pole, while no such associations were found in other studies. Kim et al. [32] described an association with motor dysfunction, dysarthria, emotional incontinence and higher frequency of anger in strokes involving the frontal, lenticulocapsular and basal pontine areas, but three other studies found no association with a specific stroke localization.

An interesting aspect is the dissociations that were found in acute stroke patients between the emotional, cognitive and behavioral components of anger and between the subjective experience of anger and what could be observed [33]. Patients may behave aggressively without feeling angry or experience only hostility.

In acute stroke, aggressive behavior appears to be mainly due to a failure of regulatory inhibitory control. On the other hand the hospital environment may be or may be perceived as hostile or humiliating. The role of premorbid personality traits has not yet been investigated.

> In acute stroke, aggressive behavior appears to be mainly due to a failure of regulatory inhibitory control.

Psychotic disorders, hallucinations and delusions

Psychotic disorders due to stroke are rare. They are classified according to the predominant symptom, with prominent hallucinations or with delusions. Delusions are of two main types: delusional misidentification syndromes and delusional ideation. This can be observed in patients with Wernicke's aphasia and severe comprehension defect. Kumral and Oztürk [35] found that delusions started 0–3 days after stroke, and the predominant types were mixed, persecutory, jealousy and suspicion. Delusional ideation was transient, with a mean duration of 13 days. The prevalence of psychosis and of delusional ideation (1–5%) in stroke survivors is also low. It is predominantly associated with right hemispheric strokes. There is no association between delusion type and infarct site.

The delusional misidentification syndromes include Capgras syndrome, where the patient believes a familiar person is not the real person but has been replaced by a similar one; Fregoli syndrome, where the patient believes it is the same person but with different features; and intermetamorphosis, where the familiar person has been transformed into another one. Somatoparaphrenia is associated with hemiassomatognosia and denial of hemiplegia. In spatial delirium the patient believes he/she is in a different place than the actual one, even in the face of compelling counter-evidence. Spatial delirium can have three grades of severity or stages of evolution: (1) confabulatory mislocation: "I am not in hospital X but in hospital Y"; (2) reduplication: "I am not in the real hospital X but in an identical building"; (3) chimeric assimilation: "I am not in the real hospital X but in my house which was transformed into a hospital". Spatial delirium is in some cases associated with delirium, neglect, memory or visuospatial disturbances and is seen predominantly after right-hemispheric lesions.

Hallucinations in stroke patients are predominantly visual and can be due to: (1) sensory deprivation: poor vision (Charles Bonnet syndrome), darkness, deafness…; (2) delirium and substance withdrawal (alcohol, drugs); (3) rostral brainstem and thalamic lesions (peduncular hallucinosis) (subcortical hallucinations); (4) partial occipital lesions ("release" hallucinations) (cortical hallucinations). Functional imagery studies showed that in subjects with visual hallucinations there was activation of the ventral extrastriate visual cortex and that the type of hallucinations reflected the functional specialization of the activated region.

In rostral brainstem and thalamic strokes, hallucinations are vivid, complex, visual, naturalist and scenic. Less frequently they are auditory or combined. They appear during the day or night, and last for minutes. Patients have variable insight and reactive

behavior, but sometimes there is a strong emotional reaction of anxiety and fear. Peduncular hallucinosis can recur in a stereotyped manner over weeks. In posterior cerebral artery infarcts, hallucinations are more common after partial occipital lesions. Hallucinations are complex, colored, stereotyped, featuring animal or human figures. They are apparent in the abnormal visual field. They appear in general with a delay of days after the vascular event. The phenomenology of hallucinations does not always reflect the localization of the lesion, because the damaged area may serve as the focus of an abnormally activated neuronal network. Visual hallucinations can be associated with seizures and the EEG may show epileptiform activity. Visual hallucinations usually resolve spontaneously, but are resistant to treatment.

Auditory hallucinations are much rarer than visual hallucinations and have been reported following right temporal and left dorsomedial thalamic strokes. These auditory hallucinations are transient [36].

> Psychotic disorders due to stroke are rare. Most frequent are visual hallucinations related to rostral brainstem, thalamic and partial occipital lesions.

Disturbances of emotional expression control

The prevalence of crying in acute stroke patients has been estimated at between 12% and 27%, but disorders of emotional expression control are more frequent (11–40%) and often appear delayed after stroke onset [37]. This disorder consists of uncontrollable outbursts of laughing, crying or both, with paroxysmal onset, transient duration of seconds or minutes, stereotyped, precipitated by nonspecific or inappropriate stimuli but also by appropriate stimuli in an inappropriate context. Patients cannot control the extent or duration of the episode. The outbursts are incongruent or exaggerated in comparison with the emotional feelings. There is no mood change during the episode and no sense of relief when it ends. There are many crying situations and many content areas of crying situations. The crying frequency is very high. It is more frequent in men and in the presence of others.

Disorders of emotional expression control are sometimes associated with depression but more often they can be dissociated. Other behavioral and cognitive correlates include irritability and ideas of reference, decreased sexual activity and lower MMSE scores. Disorders of emotional expression control have an adverse impact on the quality of life of stroke survivors. They can disrupt communication, cause embarrassment and therefore curtail social activities.

Disorders of emotional expression control have been classically associated with bilateral subcortical strokes. More recent systematic studies have shown that they can follow not only bilateral subcortical strokes, but also bilateral pontine and unilateral strokes, including large anterior, cortico-subcortical lesions, lenticulocapsular or thalamocapsular lesions, and also basal pontine strokes.

The pathophysiology of the uncontrolled outbursts of laughing and crying is poorly understood. Wilson [38] proposed a patho-anatomical model consisting of a putative fasciorespiratory control center for emotional expression located in the brainstem with a dual route of control from the motor cortex: a voluntary pathway through the pyramidal and geniculate tracts, which initiates voluntary laughter and crying and inhibits involuntary initiated laughter or crying, and an involuntary pathway consisting of a frontal/temporal–basal ganglia–ventral brainstem circuitry, which initiates and also terminates involuntary laughter or crying. Uncontrolled laughing and crying could result from release of the fasciorespiratory control center from the motor cortex or from disruption of the involuntary pathway. Parvizi and the Damasios [39] proposed a modified version of Wilson's model, in which the cerebellar structures play a role in adjusting the execution of laughter and crying to the cognitive and situational context. There is recent evidence of disruption of ascending serotoninergic pathways in disorders of emotional expression control.

An uncontrollable prolonged burst of laughing, called after Féré *fou rire prodromique*, can exceptionally anticipate by seconds to days the onset of the focal deficit in acute stroke [40].

> Disorders of emotional expression control (outbursts of laughing, crying or both) are frequent and are often associated with bilateral subcortical strokes.

Anxiety disorders

Post-stroke anxiety disorders have received comparatively less attention than post-stroke depression. Anxiety in acute stroke can also be secondary to substance use or withdrawal (alcohol, benzodiazepines and illicit drugs).

The core symptoms of generalized anxiety disorder are being anxious or worried and having difficulty in controlling worries. Diagnostic and Statistical Manual (DSM) IV criteria require in addition three or more symptoms such as restlessness, decreased energy, poor concentration, irritation, nervous tension and insomnia.

In the acute stage restlessness, decreased energy, poor concentration, irritation, nervous tension and insomnia are more common in "anxious or worried" stroke patients, while during follow-up restlessness and nervous tension are more consistently associated with anxiety, while decreased energy is a nonspecific complaint.

The prevalence of post-stroke anxiety, with or without depression, is higher in hospital settings (acute stroke patients: 28, 15–17 and 3–13%, respectively; stroke survivors: 24, 6–17 and 3–11%, respectively) than in community studies (11, 8 and 1–2%, respectively). The prevalence of agoraphobia is estimated to be 17%. Anxiety disorders are often associated with major or minor depression. Besides depression, other consistent clinical and psychiatric correlates are previous psychiatric disorders, pre-stroke depression or anxiety and alcohol abuse. Less consistent correlates include younger age, female gender, aphasia, history of insomnia and cognitive impairment. Functional and social correlates of anxiety include impairment in activities of daily living, impairment in social functioning, being single, living alone or having no social contacts outside the family [41–43]. The most consistent anatomical association of post-stroke anxiety was with anterior circulation strokes.

Concerning the outcome of post-stroke anxiety, a sizeable proportion, ranging from one-quarter to one-half, do not recover: post-stroke anxiety with associated depression has an unfavorable prognosis and usually lasts longer. Post-stroke anxiety without depression does not influence functional or cognitive recovery but is associated with worse social functioning and quality of life.

> Post-stroke anxiety disorders are often associated with depression, previous psychiatric disorders and alcohol abuse.

Post-traumatic stress disorder

Stroke and TIA can be experienced as a traumatic event and it may be re-experienced as an unpleasant and uncontrollable intrusion. Post-traumatic stress disorder is estimated to affect 10% to 31% [44] of stroke survivors and is associated with depression and anxiety. Post-traumatic stress disorder after stroke is more common in women, in patients with low educational level, and in those with premorbid neuroticism or with a negative affect or appraisal of the stroke experience.

Post-stroke mania

Post-stroke mania is an infrequent complication of stroke (1–2%) [45]. It is a prominent and persistent disturbance in mood characterized by elevated, expansive or irritable mood. Clinical features of post-stroke mania also include increased rate or amount of speech, talkativeness, language thought and content disturbance, such as flights of ideas, racing thoughts, grandiose ideation and lack of insight, hyperactivity and social disinhibition and decreased need for sleep. In severe cases distractibility, confusion, delusions and hallucinations may be also present. To distinguish between true post-stroke mania and a reactivation of previous undiagnosed primary mania, it is crucial to obtain a careful history of previous manic or hypomanic episodes or symptoms.

Starkstein et al. [45] emphasized the relationship of post-stroke mania to predisposing genetic (family/ personal history of mood disorder) factors, subcortical brain atrophy and damage to the right corticolimbic (fronto-basal ganglia-thalamic-cortical) pathways. However, mania can also be detected in stroke patients without personal or familial predisposing factors, after lesions in both hemispheres and also after subarachnoid hemorrhage. Patients with post-stroke mania can experience recurrent episodes.

Post-stroke depression

Post-stroke depression is a prominent and persistent mood disturbance characterized by depressed mood or lack of interest or lack of pleasure (anhedonia) in all or almost all activities. Post-stroke depression has two subtypes: with depressive features and similar to a major depressive episode.

Figures related to the epidemiological features of post-stroke depression are highly variable, because they depend on the setting of the study, the time since stroke, the case mix and the criteria/method used to diagnose depression. The prevalence of post-stroke depression ranges from 5 to 67% among all types of stroke patients. Severe depression has a frequency ranging from 9 to 26%, while in the acute phase depression is present in 16–52% of the patients [46]. At two years, 18–55% of stroke survivors are depressed. A systematic review of 51 studies reported a mean prevalence of 33% (29–36%) [47].

The symptomatology of post-stroke depression is dominated by depressed mood, closely followed by anhedonia. Loss of energy, decreased concentration and psychomotor retardation are also frequent, as well as the somatic symptoms of decreased appetite and insomnia. Guilt and suicidal ideation are less common.

Concerning the features of stroke which increase the risk of post-stroke depression, all stroke types are similarly prone to depression. The hemispheric side is also not relevant [48], although in some studies the frequency and severity of depression were higher after left-sided lesions, in particular during the first months after stroke. Higher lesion volumes, cerebral atrophy, silent infarcts and white matter lesions are all associated with a higher risk of post-stroke depression.

The relationship between depression and disability depends on several factors: the personality of the patients, their subjectivity (i.e. the subjective experience of the stroke), their lifestyle, the severity of neurological impairment and social isolation. Acute depressive symptoms mainly have a biological determinism, while post-stroke depression at 1–2 years has an additional psycho-social determinism.

Post-stroke depression has a prevalence of about 30%.

Personality changes

Persistent personality disturbances, defined as a change from the previous characteristic personality, are one of the most annoying behavioral disturbances found after stroke. For the caregiver these changes are hard to cope with and they are difficult to control pharmacologically. There are several types of personality changes in stroke patients: aggressive, disinhibited, paranoid, labile and apathetic types. In the apathetic type the predominant feature is marked apathy and indifference. Apathy is a disorder of motivation. In severe forms, there is lack of feeling, emotion, interest and concern, flat affect, indifference, no initiative or decisions and little spontaneous speech or actions. Responses are either absent, delayed or slow. A key feature is the dissociation between impaired self-activation and preserved hetero-activation. Subtle symptoms of apathic personality change include lack of interest in previous activities and hobbies, preference for passive activities (sitting, watching TV), no "zapping" of TV channels, paucity in starting a conversation, speaking mainly in response to other people, and lack of complaining. Apathetic patients look depressed, but they deny "low" mood. Relatives are more worried than the patient. Stroke in anatomical locations that interrupt the cingulate-subcortical thalamo-striate loop can produce apathy. These include anterior thalamic, medial thalamic, caudate, inferior capsular genu, bilateral palidal, uni- or bilateral anterior cerebral artery and baso-frontal strokes.

In acute stroke, 17–71% of the patients present apathy, which is associated with older age, low educational level, cognitive impairment (mostly executive functions) and denial.

Systematic studies investigating apathy in stroke survivors detected apathy in 20–40% of the patients 1–6 months after stroke. Apathy was associated with cognitive impairment (defects in attention, concentration, working memory and reasoning) with deficits in activities of daily living. Apathy was associated with right-sided lesions involving subcortical circuits, which comprised the ipsilateral frontal white matter, anterior capsule, basal ganglia and thalamus. Apathy was independent of depression [49,50].

> Persistent personality changes (aggressive, disinhibited, paranoid, labile and apathetic) are frequent and for the caregiver one of the most annoying behavioral disturbances found after stroke.

Chapter Summary

- **Aphasia** occurs following middle cerebral artery territory lesions of the left hemisphere. Cardinal tests: (1) confrontation naming; (2) analysis of speech (fluent and nonfluent); (3) verbal auditory comprehension; (4) repetition of words, pseudo-words and sentences.
- **Alexia and agraphia** are commonly found in aphasia, but may occur in isolation following lesions of the left hemisphere. They can be classified as central and peripheral, and as 'deep' and 'surface' types.

- **Neglect** is an inability to attend to, orient or explore the hemispace contralateral to a brain lesion, usually of the right hemisphere.
- **Amnesia** can be classified according to the affection of the memory system (duration of memory traces, content, and access to consciousness) and further subdivided into anterograde and retrograde. Amnesia can result from thrombosis or embolism of the posterior cerebral artery, posterior communicating artery, anterior and posterior choroidal artery and anterior cerebral and anterior communicating arteries.
- Prefrontal lobe deficits:
  - executive deficits (showing difficulty deciding, leaving decisions to proxy and being stubborn or rigid), corresponding to the dorsolateral prefrontal lobe
  - uninhibited behavior (inappropriate familiarity, being distractible and manipulation or utilization behavior), corresponding to the lateral orbital prefrontal lobe
  - apathy, corresponding to the anterior cingulated prefrontal lobe.
- **Visual agnosias** are disorders of visual recognition (for classification see Table 12.6) and are one of the clinical manifestations of posterior cerebral artery infarcts and occipito-temporal hemorrhages.
- **Delirium** often complicates acute stroke and is a bad prognostic sign. Predictors are a vulnerable patient, the type of stroke and precipitating factors (e.g. drugs or infections).
- **Hallucinations** in stroke patients are predominantly visual. Lesion: rostral brainstem and thalamic and partial occipital. Other reasons: sensory deprivation or delirium or substance withdrawal.
- **Depression** has a prevalence of about 30%. All stroke types are similarly prone to depression, but higher lesion volumes, cerebral atrophy, silent infarcts and white matter lesions are associated with a higher risk.
- **Persistent personality changes** are most annoying for caregivers of patients after stroke.

References

1. Kreisler A, Godefroy O, Delmaire C, Debachy B, Leclercq M, Pruvo JP, et al. The anatomy of aphasia revisited. *Neurology* 2000; **4**:1117–23.

2. Martin A. The representation of object concepts in the brain. *Annu Rev Psychol* 2007; **58**:25–45.

3. Saur D, Lange R, Baumgaertner A, Schraknepper V, Willmes K, Rijntjes M, et al. Dynamics of language reorganization after stroke. *Brain* 2006; **129**:1371–1384.

4. Plaut D, McClelland J, Seidenberg M, Patterson K. Understanding normal and impaired word reading. *Psychol Rev* 1996; **103**:56–115.

5. Lambon Ralph MA, Graham NL. Acquired phonological and deep dyslexia. *Neurocase* 2000; **6**:141–3.

6. Philipose LE, Gottesman RF, Newhart M, Kleinman JT, Herskovits EH, Pawlak MA, et al. Neural regions essential for reading and spelling of words and pseudowords. *Ann Neurol* 2007; **62**:481–92.

7. Azouvi P, Samuel C, Louis-Dreyfus A, Bernati T, Bartolomeo P, Beis JM, et al. French Collaborative Study Group on Assessment of Unilateral Neglect (GEREN/GRECO). Sensitivity of clinical and behavioural tests of spatial neglect after right hemisphere stroke. *J Neurol Neurosurg Psychiatry* 2002; **73**:160–6.

8. Hillis AE, Newhart M, Heidler J, Barker PB, Herskovits EH, Degaonkar M. Anatomy of spatial attention: insights from perfusion imaging and hemispatial neglect in acute stroke. *J Neurosci* 2005; **25**:3161–7.

9. Tulving E. Organization of memory: Quo vadis? In: Gazzaniga M, ed. *The Cognitive Neurosciences*. Cambridge: MIT Press; 1995: 839–47.

10. Valenstein E, Bowers D, Verfaellie M, Heilman KM, Day A, Watson RT. Retrosplenial amnesia. *Brain* 1987; **110**:1631–46.

11. Victor M, Angevine JB Jr, Mancall EL, Fisher CM. Memory loss with lesions of hippocampal formation. Report of a case with some remarks on the anatomical basis of memory. *Arch Neurol* 1961; **5**:244–63.

12. Graff-Radford NR, Damasio H, Yamada T, Eslinger PJ, Damasio AR. Nonhaemorrhagic thalamic infarction. Clinical, neuropsychological and electrophysiological findings in four anatomical groups defined by computerized tomography. *Brain* 1985; **108**:485–516.

13. Hackett ML, Anderson CS. Health outcomes 1 year after subarachnoid hemorrhage: An international population-based study. The Australian Cooperative Research on Subarachnoid Hemorrhage Study Group. *Neurology* 2000; **55**:658–62.

14. Bendel P, Koivisto T, Hänninen T, Kolehmainen A, Könönen M, Hurskainen H, et al. Subarachnoid hemorrhage is followed by temporomesial volume loss: MRI volumetric study. *Neurology* 2006; **67**:575–82.

15. Gilboa A, Alain C, Stuss DT, Melo B, Miller S, Moscovitch M. Mechanisms of spontaneous confabulations: a strategic retrieval account. *Brain* 2006; **129**:1399–1414.

16. Collette F, Hogge M, Salmon E, Van der Linden M. Exploration of the neural substrates of executive functioning by functional neuroimaging. *Neuroscience* 2006; **139**:209–21.

17. Nys GM, van Zandvoort MJ, de Kort PL, Jansen BP, de Haan EH, Kapeplle LJ. Cognitive disorders in acute stroke: prevalence and clinical determinants. *Cerebrovasc Dis* 2007; **23**:408–16.

18. Zinn S, Bosworth HB, Hoenig HM, Swartzwelder HS. Executive function deficits in acute stroke. *Arch Phys Med Rehabil* 2007; **88**:173–80.

19. Keiter KT, Copeland D, Bernardini GL, Bates JE, Peery S, Claassen J, et al. Predictors of cognitive dysfunction after subarachnoid hemorrhage. *Stroke* 2002; **33**:200–8.

20. James TW, Culham J, Humphrey GK, Milner AD, Goodale MA. Ventral occipital lesions impair object recognition but not object-directed grasping: an fMRI study. *Brain* 2003; **126**:2463–75.

21. Bouvier SE, Engel SA. Behavioral deficits and cortical damage loci in cerebral achromatopsia. *Cereb Cortex* 2006; **16**:183–91.

22. Gobbini MI, Haxby JV. Neural systems for recognition of familiar faces. *Neuropsychologia* 2007; **45**:32–41.

23. Sorger B, Goebel R, Schiltz C, Rossion B. Understanding the functional neuroanatomy of acquired prosopagnosia. *Neuroimage* 2007; **35**:836–52.

24. Brandt T, Steinke W, Thie A, Pessin MS, Caplan LR. Posterior cerebral artery territory infarcts: clinical features, infarct topography, causes and outcome. Multicenter results and a review of the literature. *Cerebrovasc Dis* 2000; **10**:170–82.

25. Hénon H, Lebert F, Durieu I, Godefroy O, Lucas C, Pasquier F, Leys D. Confusional state in stroke: relation to preexisting dementia, patient characteristics, and outcome. *Stroke* 1999; **30**:773–9.

26. Caeiro L, Ferro JM, Albuquerque R, Figueira ML. Delirium in the first days of acute stroke. *J Neurol* 2004; **251**:171–8.

27. Gustafson Y, Olsson T, Eriksson S, Asplund K, Bucht G. Acute confusional states (delirium) in stroke patients. *Cerebrovasc Dis* 1991; **1**:257–64.

28. Sheng AZ, Shen Q, Cordato D, Zhang YY, Yin Chan DK. Delirium within three days of stroke in a cohort of elderly patients. *J Am Geriatr Soc* 2006; **54**:1192–8.

29. Caeiro L, Menger C, Ferro JM, Albuquerque R, Figueira ML. Delirium in acute subarachnoid haemorrhage. *Cerebrovasc Dis* 2005; **19**:31–38.

30. Ghika-Schmid F, van Melle G, Guex P, Bogousslavsky L. Subjective experience and behaviour in acute stroke: the Lausanne Emotion in Acute Stroke Study. *Neurology* 1999; **52**:22–8.

31. Paradiso S, Robinson RG, Arndt S. Self-reported aggressive behavior in patients with stroke. *J Nerv Ment Dis* 1996; **184**:746–53.

32. Kim JS, Choi S, Kwon SU, Seo YS. Inability to control anger or aggression after stroke. *Neurology* 2002; **58**:1106–8.

33. Santos CO, Caeiro L, Ferro JM, Albuquerque R, Luísa Figueira M. Anger, hostility and aggression in the first days of acute stroke. *Eur J Neurol* 2006; **13**:351–8.

34. Chan KL, Campayo A, Moser DJ, Arndt S, Robinson RG. Aggressive behavior in patients with stroke: association with psychopathology and results of antidepressant treatment on aggression. *Arch Phys Med Rehabil* 2006; **87**:793–8.

35. Kumral E, Oztürk O. Delusional state following acute stroke. *Neurology* 2004; **62**:110–13.

36. Lampl Y, Lorberboym M, Gilad R, Boaz M, Sadeh M. Auditory hallucinations in acute stroke. *Behav Neurol* 2005; **16**:211–16.

37. House A, Dennis M, Molyneux A, Warlow C, Hawton K. Emotionalism after stroke. *BMJ* 1989; **298**:991–4.

38. Wilson SAK. Some problems in neurology. II. Pathological laughing and crying. *J Neurol Psychopathol* 1923; **4**:299–333.

39. Parvizi J, Anderson SW, Martin CO, Damasio H, Damasio AR. Pathological laughter and crying: a link to the cerebellum. *Brain* 2001; **124**:1708–19.

40. Coelho M, Ferro JM. Fou rire prodromique. Case report and systematic review of literature. *Cerebrovasc Dis* 2003; **16**:101–4.

41. Burvill PW, Johnson GA, Jamrozik KD, Anderson CS, Stewart-Wynne EG, Chakera TM. Anxiety disorders after stroke: results from the Perth Community Stroke Study. *Br J Psychiatry* 1995; **166**:328–32.

42. Aström M. Generalized anxiety disorder in stroke patients. A 3-year longitudinal study. *Stroke* 1996; **27**:270–5.

43. Robinson RG. Poststroke anxiety disorders. Clinical and lesion correlates. In: Robinson RG, ed. *The Clinical Neuropsychiatry of Stroke. Cognitive, Behavioral, and Emotional Disorders Following Vascular Brain Injury*, 2nd ed. Cambridge: Cambridge University Press; 2006: 326–33.

44. Bruggimann L, Annoni JM, Staub F, von Steinbüchel N, Van der Linden M, Bogousslavsky J. Chronic posttraumatic stress symptoms after nonsevere stroke. *Neurology* 2006; **66**:513–16.

45. Starkstein SE, Pearlson GD, Boston JD, Robinson RG. Mania after brain injury. A controlled study of causative factors. *Arch Neurol* 1987; **44**:1069–73.

46. Caeiro L, Ferro JM, Santos CO, Figueira ML. Depression in acute stroke. *J Psychiatry Neurosci* 2006; **31**:377–83.

47. Hackett ML, Yapa C, Parag V, Anderson CS. Frequency of depression after stroke: a systematic review of observational studies. *Stroke* 2005; **36**:1330–40.

48. Carson AJ, MacHale S, Allen K, Lawrie SM, Dennis M, House A, et al. Depression after stroke and lesion location: a systematic review. *Lancet* 2000; **356**:122–6.

49. Hama S, Yamashita H, Shigenobu M, Watanabe A, Hiramoto K, Kurisu K, et al. Depression or apathy and functional recovery after stroke. *Int J Geriatr Psychiatry* 2007; **22**:1046–51.

50. Brodaty H, Sachdev PS, Withall A, Altendorf A, Valenzuela MJ, Lorentz L. Frequency and clinical, neuropsychological and neuroimaging correlates of apathy following stroke – the Sydney Stroke Study. *Psychol Med* 2005; **35**:1707–16.

Stroke and dementia

Didier Leys and Marta Altieri

For every three people currently living in Western countries, at least one will develop dementia, stroke or both [1, 2]. Stroke is the leading cause of physical disability in adults: of one million inhabitants, 2400 people have a stroke every year, of whom more than 50% will die or become dependent 1 year later [3]. Dependency after stroke is often due to dementia [4]. Even in stroke survivors who are independent, slight cognitive or behavioral changes may have consequences for familial and professional activities [5]. Dementia is also frequent in Western countries, especially after the age of 75 years, where its prevalence is close to 18% [6]. About 40% of demented people live in an institution, and among institutionalized residents two-thirds are demented [6]. Therefore, the economic burden of dementia is important.

Stroke and dementia are both frequent and their relationship is more complex than being just a coexistence of two frequent disorders. Besides being a potential cause of dementia, and a factor that negatively influences the time-course of Alzheimer's disease (AD), stroke also shares many risk factors with AD, such as increasing age, arterial hypertension and ApoE4 genotype [7]. The prevalence of stroke and of dementia is likely to increase in the coming years, because of the decline in mortality after stroke [8] and the aging of Western populations [9]. Therefore, the burden of stroke-related dementia is also likely to increase in the future [5].

Definitions

Post-stroke dementia (PSD) includes any dementia that occurs after a stroke, irrespective of its cause, i.e. vascular, degenerative or mixed [5]. The concept of PSD is useful for patients who are followed-up after a stroke, before an extensive diagnostic workup makes possible a classification into vascular dementia (VaD), degenerative dementia (especially AD) and mixed dementia (dementia due to the coexistence of vascular

lesions of the brain, and neurodegenerative lesions, usually of Alzheimer type, both types of lesions being not necessarily severe enough to induce dementia when isolated).

VaD is a dementia syndrome that is the direct consequence of cerebral infarcts, cerebral hemorrhages and white matter changes [10]. The term VaD cannot be used for all patients who have had a stroke and are demented, because many of them have AD.

> Post-stroke dementia (PSD) includes any dementia that occurs after a stroke, irrespective of its cause, i.e. vascular, degenerative or mixed.

This chapter will not cover: (i) cognitive impairment without dementia, but we should bear in mind that the cognitive burden of stroke is severely underestimated, cognitive impairment without dementia being three times more frequent in patients who have had a stroke than in stroke-free controls [11]; and (ii) dementia associated with apparently purely "silent" vascular lesions of the brain (silent infarcts, microbleeds and leukoaraiosis), i.e. brain lesions presumably of vascular origin that occur in the absence of clinical symptoms of stroke or transient ischemic attacks. Therefore, our review will focus only on dementia that occurs – or was already present – in patients who have had clinical symptoms of stroke.

Descriptive epidemiology of dementia occurring after stroke

Prevalence of dementia in stroke survivors

Prevalence studies include both dementia pre-existing to stroke and new-onset dementia occurring after stroke [5]. The prevalence of PSD ranges from 5.9% to 32%, depending on the mean age of the study population, exclusion or not of patients with aphasia or severe physical disability, mortality rates, delay between stroke onset and cognitive assessment, and criteria used for the diagnosis of dementia [5, 12]. Dementia is 3.5–5.8-fold more frequent in patients who have had a stroke than in stroke-free controls, after adjustment for age [13, 14]. Details of studies evaluating the prevalence of PSD are provided in Table 13.1.

> Dementia is 3.5–5.8-fold more frequent in patients who have had a stroke than in stroke-free controls.

Incidence of new-onset dementia in stroke survivors

Incidence studies are limited by similar methodological issues [5]. The incidence of dementia after stroke depends on whether the study excluded patients with pre-existing cognitive decline or dementia or not. Many so-called PSDs are not actually "new-onset" dementia, but pre-existing dementia revealed after stroke, pre-existing dementia being present in 7–16% of stroke patients, and often undiagnosed before stroke [15–21]. In a community-based study conducted over a 25-year period, the cumulative incidence of dementia after stroke was 7% after 1 year, 10% after 3 years, 15% after 5 years, 23% after 10 years and 48% after 25 years [22]. In hospital-based studies, the incidence of dementia after stroke ranged from 9% [23] to 16.8% [24] after 1 year, 24% to 28.5% [25] after 3 years, 21.5% [26] to 33.3% [27] after 4 years, and was 32% [27, 28] after 5 years. In the Lille Stroke/Dementia cohort after exclusion of patients who were demented at month 6, only 6% of survivors developed really "new-onset" dementia after 3 years [25].

> Incidence of dementia after stroke is 7% after 1 year, 10% after 3 years, 15% after 5 years, 23% after 10 years, and 48% after 25 years.

Relative risk of dementia after stroke

In the Rochester study, the relative risk of dementia (i.e. the risk of dementia in stroke survivors divided by the risk of dementia in stroke-free controls) was 8.8 one year after stroke, then declined progressively to 2.5 after 10 years, and 2.0 after 25 years [22]. The risk of AD was also doubled after 25 years [22]. In the Framingham study, the results were similar 10 years after stroke, after adjustment for age, gender, education level and exposure to individual risk factors for

stroke [29]. A study where stroke was not associated with an increased risk of dementia [30] was actually conducted in non-aphasic patients, with mild first-ever strokes, and only 1 year of follow-up, i.e. the best conditions to minimize the incidence of new-onset dementia. In hospital-based studies the risk of new-onset dementia within 4 years after ischemic stroke is 5–6-fold higher than in stroke-free controls [27, 31].

Finally, the results of hospital- and community-based studies can be summarized as follows: (i) stroke doubles the risk of dementia, (ii) the attributable risk is the highest within the first year after stroke, then declines, and the relative risk of dementia remains stable around 2, and (iii) the risk of delayed dementia (including AD) also remains doubled 10 years and more after stroke.

> Stroke doubles the risk of dementia; the attributable risk is the highest within the first year after stroke, and then declines.

Factors influencing the occurrence of dementia after stroke

Determinants of post-stroke dementia that have been found in at least two independent studies, or have been identified recently, are listed in Table 13.2.

Demographic and medical characteristics of the patient

The most important demographic predictors of dementia after stroke, in sufficiently powered studies, are increasing age and low education level, but not gender when the analysis is adjusted for age [5]. The risk of dementia after stroke is higher in patients who were already dependent before stroke [5]. Pre-stroke cognitive decline without dementia, assessed by standardized questionnaires, is also associated with a higher risk of dementia after stroke [5, 32].

Diabetes mellitus, atrial fibrillation and myocardial infarction were also independent risk factors for dementia after stroke in several studies [5]. Arterial hypertension, a risk factor for vascular dementia (VaD) and AD, has not been clearly identified as a risk factor for dementia after stroke.

Epileptic seizures [33], sepsis, cardiac arrhythmias and congestive heart failure are independently associated with an increased risk of dementia after stroke [5]. However, the statistical relationship found

Table 13.1. Prevalence of post-stroke dementia. Studies are classified by increasing duration of follow-up. The same study may appear several times if several assessments were performed at different time intervals after stroke. References of the studies cited in this table can be found in Leys et al. [5].

1st author, year	Follow-up (months)	Number of patients	Population characteristics	Criteria for dementia	Prevalence (%)
Tatemichi, 1990	7–10 days	726	Ischemic stroke, age ≥ 60 years	Clinician's opinion	16.3
Andersen, 1996	1	220	First-ever stroke, age: 60–80 years	Mattis Dementia Rating Scale	32.0
Tatemichi, 1992	3	251	Ischemic stroke, age ≥ 60 years	DSM III R	26.3
Censori, 1996	3	110	First-ever ischemic stroke	NINDS-AIREN	13.6
Pohjasvaara, 1998	3	337	Ischemic stroke, age: 55–85 years	DSM III	31.8
Desmond, 2000	3	453	Ischemic stroke, age ≥ 60 years	DSM III R	26.3
Barba, 2000	3	251	Stroke, age ≥ 18 years	DSM IV	22.1
Madureira, 2001	3	237	Stroke patients with no previous functional deficit	NINDS-AIREN	5.9
Lin, 2003	3	283	Ischemic stroke, no patient with previous TIA	ICD-10	9.2
Tang, 2004	3	280	Stroke, age ≥ 60 years	DSM IV	15.5
Mok, 2004	3	75	Ischemic stroke associated with small vessel disease	Clinical dementia rating scale ≥ 1	13.3
Zhou, 2004	3	434	Ischemic stroke, age ≥ 55 years	DSM IV	27.2
Rasquin, 2004	6	146	First-ever ischemic stroke, age ≥ 40 years MMS ≥ 15 (acute stage)	DSM IV	8.5
Andersen, 1996	6	220	First-ever stroke, age: 60–80 years	Mattis Dementia Rating Scale	26.0
Hénon, 2001	6	202	Stroke, age ≥ 40 years	ICD-10	22.8
Inzitari, 1998	12	339	Stroke	Proxy-informant interview based on ICD-10	16.8
Hénon, 2001	12	202	Stroke, age ≥ 40 years	ICD-10	21.4
Rasquin, 2004	12	196	First-ever ischemic stroke, age ≥ 40 years MMS ≥ 15 (acute stage)	DSM IV	10.0
Linden, 2004	18	149	Stroke, age ≥ 70 years	DSM III R	28.0
Hénon, 2001	24	202	Stroke, age ≥ 40 years	ICD-10	21.6
Hénon, 2001	36	202	Stroke, age ≥ 40 years	ICD-10	19.2

Table 13.2. Determinants of dementia after stroke. This table includes only determinants of dementia after stroke that have been found in at least two independent studies or identified recently. A few determinants may not have been confirmed in other studies, often because of lack of statistical power. References to the studies cited in this table and published before 30 April 2005 can be found in Leys et al. [5].

Demographic and medical characteristics of the patient

Demographic variables

    Increasing age

    Low education level

Pre-stroke dependency

    Dependency

Pre-stroke cognitive decline

    Pre-stroke cognitive decline without dementia [32, 50]

Vascular risk factors

    Diabetes mellitus

    Atrial fibrillation

    Myocardial infarction

    ApoE4 genotype [34]

Hypoxic-ischemic disorders

    Epileptic seizures [33]

    Sepsis

    Cardiac arrhythmias

    Congestive heart failure

Silent brain lesions

    Silent infarcts

    Global cerebral atrophy

    Medial temporal lobe atrophy [36]

    Leukoaraiosis

Stroke characteristics

Stroke severity

    More severe clinical deficit at onset

    Stroke recurrence

    Stroke volume [50]

Location of the cerebral lesions

    Supra-tentorial lesions

    Left hemispheric lesions

    Anterior and posterior cerebral artery territory infarcts

    Strategic infarcts

    Multiple lesions

between these disorders and dementia does not mean a causal relationship: it is also possible that dementia increases the risk of such events [5].

The influence of hyperlipidemia, hyperhomocysteinemia, alcohol consumption and cigarette smoking on dementia after stroke remains unproven [5]. The results concerning cigarette smoking should be interpreted with caution, because smoking influences mortality and stroke recurrence. ApoE4 genotype is associated with an increased risk of dementia after stroke [34].

> Risk factors for dementia after stroke include increasing age, low education level, diabetes mellitus, atrial fibrillation, myocardial infarction, epileptic seizures, sepsis, cardiac arrhythmias and congestive heart failure.

Pre-existing silent brain lesions in stroke patients

Silent infarcts, i.e. cerebral infarcts seen on CT or MRI scans that have never been associated with a relevant neurological deficit, are associated with an increased risk of dementia after stroke [5]. Their influence is more important when the follow-up is longer: in the Lille study, silent infarcts were associated with dementia after stroke at year 3 [25] but not at year 2 and in the Maastricht study silent infarcts were independently related to dementia after 12 months, but not after 1 or 6 months [35]. Stroke patients with associated silent infarcts seem to have a steeper decline in cognitive function than those without, but this decline might be confined to those with additional silent infarcts after base-line.

Global cerebral atrophy is associated with a higher risk of dementia after stroke [5]. Medial temporal lobe atrophy (MTLA) is more frequent in stroke patients who have pre-existing dementia but it may also be present in non-demented stroke patients. MTLA clearly differentiates demented from non-demented patients after a first-ever ischemic stroke, even after exclusion of patients who had pre-stroke cognitive impairment [5]. Stroke patients with MTLA may have pre-clinical AD that is clinically revealed by stroke [5, 7, 36]. However, MTLA is not specific for AD, as it has also been observed in VaD [5].

The presence and severity of leukoaraiosis are independent predictors of dementia after stroke [5], but there are many potential confounders, such as

(i) cerebral atrophy, more frequent in patients with leukoaraiosis, (ii) lacunar infarcts, which share a common pathogenesis with leukoaraiosis, and (iii) stroke recurrence, which is more frequent in stroke patients with leukoaraiosis [5].

Microbleeds are frequent in stroke patients and especially those with intracerebral arteriolopathies [37] and in patients with VaD, and to a lower degree AD [38]. However, the question of their influence on the risk of post-stroke dementia has never been systematically addressed.

> Pre-existing silent brain lesions in stroke patients, such as silent infarcts, global cerebral atrophy, medial temporal lobe atrophy and leukoaraiosis, are associated with a higher risk of dementia after stroke.

Stroke characteristics

Most studies found that a more severe clinical deficit at onset is associated with a higher risk of dementia after stroke [5]. The risk of dementia and its severity are not influenced by the type of stroke (ischemic or hemorrhagic) [5]. However, differences in survival rates between stroke subtypes make the results difficult to interpret. In the Framingham study large-artery infarcts, lacunar infarcts and infarcts of unknown origin were associated with a higher risk of dementia after stroke [29]. In other studies, the risk of dementia after stroke was lower in patients with small-vessel disease [5]. These results are influenced by the higher mortality rate in stroke subtypes associated with more severe deficits, i.e. in stroke patients who are the most likely to develop dementia after stroke when they survive [5]. A study where stroke volumes were evaluated showed a relationship between a higher stroke volume and the risk of dementia [39]. Previous stroke and stroke recurrence are also associated with a higher risk of dementia after stroke [5].

Supratentorial lesions, left hemispheric lesions, anterior and posterior cerebral artery territory infarcts, multiple infarcts and so-called "strategic infarcts", i.e. cerebral infarcts that may lead to dementia on their own in the absence of any other lesion, have been found to be associated with an increased risk of dementia after stroke in at least two independent studies [5]. However, strategic locations (left angular gyrus, inferomesial temporal and mesiofrontal locations, thalami, left capsular genu, caudate

nuclei) were described more than 20 years ago, in single case reports, or in small series, usually without MRI, and without follow-up [5]. Other vascular brain lesions and coexisting AD cannot be excluded in most cases [5]. Therefore, this concept should be revisited in large prospective studies, with MRI and a follow-up long enough to exclude associated AD [5].

> Stroke characteristics, such as severity of the clinical deficit or stroke localization, influence the risk of dementia after stroke. "Strategic infarcts" may lead to dementia on their own in the absence of any other lesion.

Causes of post-stroke dementia

The most frequent causes of dementia after stroke are VaD, AD and mixed AD-VaD [5]. AD and mixed AD-VaD account for 19% to 61% of patients with dementia after stroke (Table 13.3). Two Asian studies did not confirm this high proportion of AD patients, but in one [40] the study population was at least 10 years younger than in all other studies, and patients who were lost to follow-up at the 3-month evaluation were more cognitively impaired at the acute stage, and in the other [21] the diagnosis of VaD was based on the DSM IV criteria, which are the less specific [41].

In the following circumstances vascular lesions are the most prominent or only determinants of dementia after stroke: (i) in stroke patients who are too young to have Alzheimer lesions, and became demented just after stroke; (ii) when cognitive functions were normal before stroke, impaired immediately after, and did not worsen over time, or even slightly improved over time; (iii) when a specific vascular condition known to cause stroke and dementia (e.g. CADASIL) is proven by a specific marker; or (iv) when the lesion is located in a strategic area.

In many other circumstances dementia is the consequence of the coexistence of Alzheimer and vascular lesions.

Even when vascular lesions or Alzheimer pathology do not lead to dementia by themselves, their association may reach the threshold of brain lesions required to induce dementia [7]: when a stroke occurs in a patient with asymptomatic Alzheimer pathology, the period of pre-clinical AD may be shortened and the clinical onset of AD may therefore be anticipated [7]. Patients usually have a clinical presentation of AD that appears several months or years after stroke. These concepts of mixed dementia emphasize the fact

Table 13.3. Causes of new-onset dementia after stroke. Studies are classified by increasing duration of follow-up. The same study may appear several times in this table if several assessments were performed at different time intervals. References to the studies cited in this table can be found in Leys et al. [5].

Author, year	Follow-up after stroke*	Number of patients**	Study population	VaD (%)	AD (%)	AD + VaD (%)
Tatemichi, 1990	7–10 days	726	Hospital	39	36	25
Tatemichi, 1992	3	251	Hospital	56	36	–
Pohjasvaara, 1998	3	337	Hospital	81	19	–
Desmond, 2000	3	453	Hospital	57	39	–
Barba, 2000	3	251	Hospital	75	25	–
Tang, 2004	3	280	Hospital	98	–	2
Kokmen, 1996	12	–	Community	–	41	–
Hénon, 2001	36	202	Hospital	67	33	–
Zhu, 2000	36	–	Community	100	–	–
Ivan, 2004	120	–	Community	51	–	37

Notes: *In months unless specified; **available only for hospital-based studies. VaD, vascular dementia; AD, Alzheimer's disease.

that those patients have two disorders and should be treated for AD and receive appropriate stroke prevention. Considering those patients as having pure AD may lead to an underestimation of the need for secondary stroke prevention measures. The hypothesis of a possible summation of lesions is supported by the results of the Optima and the Nun studies, showing that amongst patients who met neuropathological criteria for AD, those with brain infarcts had poorer cognitive functions before death and a higher prevalence of dementia [42, 43]. This hypothesis was also supported by the results of the Syst-Eur dementia substudy showing that nitrendipine decreases the incidence rate of AD [44], suggesting that stroke prevention reduces the risk of new-onset AD.

> Frequently dementia is the consequence of the coexistence of Alzheimer and vascular lesions. Even when vascular lesions or Alzheimer pathology do not lead to dementia on their own, their summation might induce dementia.

Influence of dementia on stroke outcome

Mortality

Both population- and hospital-based studies have shown that stroke patients with dementia after stroke have higher mortality rates than non-demented stroke patients, independently of age and co-morbidities [45]. The long-term mortality rate after stroke is 2–6-fold higher in patients with dementia, after adjustment for demographic factors, associated cardiac diseases, stroke severity and stroke recurrence [27, 46–48]. This increase in mortality rate in stroke patients with dementia may be due to the increased overall mortality rate in patients with dementia, a more severe underlying vascular disease or a higher risk of any nonspecific complication in patients with dementia [5]. It is also possible that, in the presence of dementia, patients receive less appropriate stroke prevention [5]. Stroke patients with dementia may also be less compliant for stroke prevention.

Stroke recurrence

Dementia diagnosed 3 months after stroke is associated with a 3-fold increased risk of stroke recurrence [49]. Dementia may be a marker for a more severe vascular disease leading to an increased risk of recurrence [5]. Less intensive stroke prevention and lack of compliance may contribute to the increased risk of recurrence [49]. Leukoaraiosis could also be a confounding factor, as it is associated with an increased risk of stroke recurrence [25].

Functional outcome

The few available data on the influence of dementia on functional outcome after stroke suggest that stroke patients with dementia are more impaired and more dependent in daily living activities than stroke patients without dementia [5].

> Dementia after stroke is associated with a 3-fold increase in stroke recurrence and with higher mortality.

Treatments of stroke in patients with dementia

There are no data in randomized clinical trials that may help in determining how acute stroke therapy and stroke prevention should be conducted in patients who are demented before or develop dementia after stroke [5].

PSD is not a specific entity that requires a specific treatment. Patients with dementia after stroke are patients with dementia and they are also stroke patients. In the absence of studies specifically designed for stroke patients with dementia, current guidelines for stroke prevention should be applied, but we should bear in mind that the specific issue of secondary prevention of stroke in patients with dementia (either pre-existing or new-onset dementia) is not addressed in any guidelines. Accordingly, a symptomatic approach to the dementia syndrome is necessary, depending on the presumed cause (AD, VaD or mixed AD-VaD). Both AD and VaD share a cholinergic deficit, and both conditions show improvement under cholinesterase inhibitors [5].

> PSD does not require specific treatment, but pragmatic management of prevailing symptoms.

Conclusions

Recognition of dementia in stroke patients is important because it indicates a worse outcome with higher mortality rates, more recurrences and more functional impairment. Research should now focus on a delineation of the concept of post-stroke cognitive decline without dementia, which may be a preliminary stage of dementia after stroke, be much more frequent in practice, and be a better target for therapeutic approaches. Other epidemiological studies are also necessary to evaluate the evolution over time of the burden of dementia after stroke at the community level, in order to have better knowledge of the need in terms of resources and its evolution over time.

Chapter Summary

Dementia is one of the major causes of dependency in stroke patients. In community-based studies, the prevalence of dementia in stroke survivors is approximately 30% and the incidence of new-onset dementia after stroke increases from 7% after 1 year, up to almost 50% after 25 years. The risk of dementia is doubled after stroke. Patient-related variables associated with an increased risk of dementia after stroke are increasing age, low education level, dependency before stroke, pre-stroke cognitive decline without dementia, diabetes mellitus, atrial fibrillation, myocardial infarction, epileptic seizures, sepsis, cardiac arrhythmias, congestive heart failure, silent cerebral infarcts, global and medial temporal lobe atrophy and white matter changes. Stroke-related variables associated with an increased risk of dementia after stroke are severity, volume, location and recurrence. Dementia in stroke patients may be due to vascular lesions, Alzheimer pathology, white matter changes or a summation of these lesions. The proportion of patients with presumed Alzheimer's disease amongst those with dementia after stroke varies between 19% and 61%. Stroke patients with dementia have higher mortality rates, and are more often functionally impaired.

References

1. Hachinski V. The 2005 Thomas Willis Lecture: stroke and vascular cognitive impairment: a transdisciplinary, translational and transactional approach. *Stroke* 2007; **38**:1396.

2. Seshadri S, Wolf PA. Lifetime risk of stroke and dementia: current concepts, and estimates from the Framingham Study. *Lancet Neurol* 2007; **6**:1106–14.

3. Hankey GJ, Warlow CP. Treatment and secondary prevention of stroke: evidence, costs, and effects on individuals and populations. *Lancet* 1999; **354**:1457–63.

4. Pasquini M, Leys D, Rousseaux M, Pasquier F, Henon H. Influence of cognitive impairment on the institutionalisation rate 3 years after a stroke. *J Neurol Neurosurg Psychiatry* 2007; **78**:56–9.

5. Leys D, Henon H, Mackowiak-Cordoliani MA, Pasquier F. Poststroke dementia. *Lancet Neurol* 2005; **4**:752–9.

6. Helmer C, Peres K, Letenneur L, et al. Dementia in subjects aged 75 years or over within the PAQUID cohort: prevalence and burden by severity. *Dement Geriatr Cogn Disord* 2006; **22**:87–94.

7. Pasquier F, Leys D. Why are stroke patients prone to develop dementia? *J Neurol* 1997; **244**:135–42.

8. Ukraintseva S, Sloan F, Arbeev K, Yashin A. Increasing rates of dementia at time of declining mortality from stroke. *Stroke* 2006; **37**:1155–9.

9. Rothwell PM, Coull AJ, Giles MF, et al. Change in stroke incidence, mortality, case-fatality, severity, and risk factors in Oxfordshire, UK from 1981 to 2004 (Oxford Vascular Study). *Lancet* 2004; **363**:1925–33.

10. Roman GC, Tatemichi TK, Erkinjuntti T, et al. Vascular dementia: diagnostic criteria for research studies. Report of the NINDS-AIREN International Workshop. *Neurology* 1993; **43**:250–60.

11. Linden T, Skoog I, Fagerberg B, Steen B, Blomstrand C. Cognitive impairment and dementia 20 months after stroke. *Neuroepidemiology* 2004; **23**:45–52.

12. Erkinjuntti T, Ostbye T, Steenhuis R, Hachinski V. The effect of different diagnostic criteria on the prevalence of dementia. *N Engl J Med* 1997; **337**:1667–74.

13. Prencipe M, Ferretti C, Casini AR, Santini M, Giubilei F, Culasso F. Stroke, disability, and dementia: results of a population survey. *Stroke* 1997; **28**:531–6.

14. Zhu L, Fratiglioni L, Guo Z, Aguero-Torres H, Winblad B, Viitanen M. Association of stroke with dementia, cognitive impairment, and functional disability in the very old: a population-based study. *Stroke* 1998; **29**:2094–9.

15. Henon H, Pasquier F, Durieu I, et al. Preexisting dementia in stroke patients. Baseline frequency, associated factors, and outcome. *Stroke* 1997; **28**:2429–36.

16. Pohjasvaara T, Mantyla R, Aronen HJ, et al. Clinical and radiological determinants of prestroke cognitive decline in a stroke cohort. *J Neurol Neurosurg Psychiatry* 1999; **67**:742–8.

17. Barba R, Castro MD, del Mar Morin M, et al. Prestroke dementia. *Cerebrovasc Dis* 2001; **11**:216–24.

18. Klimkowicz A, Dziedzic T, Polczyk R, Pera J, Slowik A, Szczudlik A. Factors associated with pre-stroke dementia: the Cracow stroke database. *J Neurol* 2004; **251**:599–603.

19. Klimkowicz A, Dziedzic T, Slowik A, Szczudlik A. Incidence of pre- and poststroke dementia: Cracow stroke registry. *Dement Geriatr Cogn Disord* 2002; **14**:137–40.

20. Tang WK, Chan SS, Chiu HF, et al. Frequency and determinants of prestroke dementia in a Chinese cohort. *J Neurol* 2004; **251**:604–8.

21. Tang WK, Chan SS, Chiu HF, et al. Frequency and determinants of poststroke dementia in Chinese. *Stroke* 2004; **35**:930–5.

22. Kokmen E, Whisnant JP, O'Fallon WM, Chu CP, Beard CM. Dementia after ischemic stroke: a population-based study in Rochester, Minnesota (1960–1984). *Neurology* 1996; **46**:154–9.

23. Ballard C, Stephens S, Kenny R, Kalaria R, Tovee M, O'Brien J. Profile of neuropsychological deficits in older stroke survivors without dementia. *Dement Geriatr Cogn Disord* 2003; **16**:52–6.

24. Inzitari D, Di Carlo A, Pracucci G, et al. Incidence and determinants of poststroke dementia as defined by an informant interview method in a hospital-based stroke registry. *Stroke* 1998; **29**:2087–93.

25. Henon H, Durieu I, Guerouaou D, Lebert F, Pasquier F, Leys D. Poststroke dementia: incidence and relationship to prestroke cognitive decline. *Neurology* 2001; **57**:1216–22.

26. Altieri M, Di Piero V, Pasquini M, et al. Delayed poststroke dementia: a 4-year follow-up study. *Neurology* 2004; **62**:2193–7.

27. Tatemichi TK, Paik M, Bagiella E, et al. Risk of dementia after stroke in a hospitalized cohort: results of a longitudinal study. *Neurology* 1994; **44**:1885–91.

28. Bornstein NM, Gur AY, Treves TA, et al. Do silent brain infarctions predict the development of dementia after first ischemic stroke? *Stroke* 1996; **27**:904–5.

29. Ivan CS, Seshadri S, Beiser A, et al. Dementia after stroke: the Framingham Study. *Stroke* 2004; **35**:1264–8.

30. Srikanth VK, Anderson JF, Donnan GA, et al. Progressive dementia after first-ever stroke: a community-based follow-up study. *Neurology* 2004; **63**:785–92.

31. Desmond DW, Moroney JT, Sano M, Stern Y. Incidence of dementia after ischemic stroke: results of a longitudinal study. *Stroke* 2002; **33**:2254–60.

32. Gamaldo A, Moghekar A, Kilada S, Resnick SM, Zonderman AB, O'Brien R. Effect of a clinical stroke on the risk of dementia in a prospective cohort. *Neurology* 2006; **67**:1363–9.

33. Cordonnier C, Henon H, Derambure P, Pasquier F, Leys D. Early epileptic seizures after stroke are associated with increased risk of new-onset dementia. *J Neurol Neurosurg Psychiatry* 2007; **78**:514–6.

34. Jin YP, Ostbye T, Feightner JW, Di Legge S, Hachinski V. Joint effect of stroke and APOE 4 on dementia risk: the Canadian Study of Health and Aging. *Neurology* 2008; **70**:9–16.

35. Rasquin SM, Verhey FR, van Oostenbrugge RJ, Lousberg R, Lodder J. Demographic and CT scan features related to cognitive impairment in the first

year after stroke. *J Neurol Neurosurg Psychiatry* 2004; **75**:1562–7.

36. Firbank MJ, Burton EJ, Barber R, et al. Medial temporal atrophy rather than white matter hyperintensities predict cognitive decline in stroke survivors. *Neurobiol Aging* 2007; **28**:1664–9.

37. Cordonnier C, Al-Shahi Salman R, Wardlaw J. Spontaneous brain microbleeds: systematic review, subgroup analyses and standards for study design and reporting. *Brain* 2007; **130**:1988–2003.

38. Cordonnier C, van der Flier WM, Sluimer JD, Leys D, Barkhof F, Scheltens P. Prevalence and severity of microbleeds in a memory clinic setting. *Neurology* 2006; **66**:1356–60.

39. Sachdev P, Brodaty H. Vascular dementia: an Australian perspective. *Alzheimer Dis Assoc Disord* 1999; **13** Suppl 3:S206–12.

40. Lin JH, Lin RT, Tai CT, Hsieh CL, Hsiao SF, Liu CK. Prediction of poststroke dementia. *Neurology* 2003; **61**:343–8.

41. Gold G, Bouras C, Canuto A, et al. Clinicopathological validation study of four sets of clinical criteria for vascular dementia. *Am J Psychiatry* 2002; **159**:82–7.

42. Nagy Z, Esiri MM, Jobst KA, et al. The effects of additional pathology on the cognitive deficit in Alzheimer disease. *J Neuropathol Exp Neurol* 1997; **56**:165–70.

43. Snowdon DA, Greiner LH, Mortimer JA, Riley KP, Greiner PA, Markesbery WR. Brain infarction and the clinical expression of Alzheimer disease. The Nun Study. *JAMA* 1997; **277**:813–7.

44. Forette F, Seux ML, Staessen JA, et al. Prevention of dementia in randomised double-blind placebo-controlled Systolic Hypertension in Europe (Syst-Eur) trial. *Lancet* 1998; **352**:1347–51.

45. Aevarsson O, Svanborg A, Skoog I. Seven-year survival rate after age 85 years: relation to Alzheimer disease and vascular dementia. *Arch Neurol* 1998; **55**:1226–32.

46. Desmond DW, Moroney JT, Sano M, Stern Y. Mortality in patients with dementia after ischemic stroke. *Neurology* 2002; **59**:537–43.

47. Barba R, Morin MD, Cemillan C, Delgado C, Domingo J, Del Ser T. Previous and incident dementia as risk factors for mortality in stroke patients. *Stroke* 2002; **33**:1993–8.

48. Henon H, Vroylandt P, Durieu I, Pasquier F, Leys D. Leukoaraiosis more than dementia is a predictor of stroke recurrence. *Stroke* 2003; **34**:2935–40.

49. Moroney JT, Bagiella E, Tatemichi TK, Paik MC, Stern Y, Desmond DW. Dementia after stroke increases the risk of long-term stroke recurrence. *Neurology* 1997; **48**:1317–25.

50. Sachdev PS, Brodaty H, Valenzuela MJ, et al. Clinical determinants of dementia and mild cognitive impairment following ischaemic stroke: the Sydney Stroke Study. *Dement Geriatr Cogn Disord* 2006; **21**:275–83.

Ischemic stroke in the young and in children

Didier Leys and Valeria Caso

Introduction

Stroke is a major public health issue because of its high frequency, the risk of death and residual physical cognitive or behavioral impairments, and the risk of recurrent vascular events that may be cerebral or cardiac [1–3]. Although strokes occur at a mean age of 75 years in Western countries [4–6], they may also occur in younger patients, and even in children [4–7]. Most strokes occurring in young patients are ischemic in origin. They account for from 2 to 12% of all strokes, depending on whether figures are provided from community- or hospital-based data [8, 9].

The main specificities of ischemic strokes in young patients are their causes, their outcome and the possibility of occurring during pregnancy. These specificities may influence the management of patients. Therapeutic options should therefore take into account the presumed cause, the natural history of the disease and the long life expectancy. The clinical deficits and acute management have no specificity in young people, and will therefore not be addressed.

Epidemiology

Figures depend on the definition of "young". Three upper thresholds can be found in the literature, at 30, 45 and 55 years of age. The most frequently used upper age limit is 45 years. It constitutes a good compromise between an age category where common causes of cerebral ischemia, such as atheroma, atrial fibrillation and lipohyalinosis, are very rare, and on the other hand a disorder that is not too rare. The incidence of ischemic strokes increases with age even in young people: most young people with stroke are between 40 and 45 years of age [7]. The incidence of ischemic stroke in young people varies between 60 and 200 new cases per year per million inhabitants [10], depending on the characteristics of the population and the age limit. This incidence remains stable over time and does not decline, as does the incidence rate of ischemic stroke in other age categories. The incidence is higher in non-industrialized countries and in black populations [4]. In young women, the incidence of ischemic strokes during pregnancy is about 43 per million deliveries, i.e. similar to that observed in non-pregnant women of similar age [11]. Population-based estimates of the incidence of stroke in children, including hemorrhagic strokes, range from 2.3 to 13.0 per 100 000 children [12]. About 50% of incident strokes in children are ischemic, with a higher incidence in boys [12].

> The incidence of ischemic stroke in young people varies between 60 and 200 new cases per year per million inhabitants.

Diagnostic work-up

The diagnostic work-up should not differ from that of older patients except for the search for a cause. The same principles as those detailed in the recommendations of the European Stroke Organisation are also valid in young people, although they are not specific for this age category [13]. Cervical and transcranial ultrasounds, magnetic resonance angiography of cervical and intracranial arteries, continuous ECG monitoring, transthoracic and transesophageal echocardiography should be performed according to the same rules as in older patients, and will therefore not be detailed in this chapter.

Cerebral ischemia occurring during pregnancy requires the same diagnostic work-up as in non-pregnant women. However, MRI is the investigation of choice over CT and percutaneous angiography, although its safety profile for the fetus has never been evaluated. Gadolinium enhancement is, however, not recommended as its effects on the fetus remain unknown.

The patient interview

The patient interview can provide information on the potential cause of cerebral ischemia. It should be repeated, with the patient and close relatives. It should focus on the following features:

presence of cervical pain or headache that may have occurred before stroke (in favor of a dissection)

presence of pulsatile tinnitus (in favor of a dissection)

recent intake of illicit substances (in favor of toxic angiopathies)

recent intake of vasoconstrictive drugs (in favor of toxic angiopathies)

history of migraine with aura (in favor of migrainous infarct)

history of definite systemic inflammatory disorder, or suggestive clinical features such as photosensitivity, arthritis, pericarditis, pleuritis, repetitive spontaneous miscarriage, oral or genital aphthosis, unexplained fever, anemia, thrombopenia, proteinuria (in favor of cerebral vasculitis)

family history of ischemic stroke occurring in young patients (in favor of genetic causes, such as CADASIL)

family history of migraine with aura, severe depression or dementia occurring in young patients (in favor of CADASIL)

personal history of irradiation (in favor of post-irradiation arteriopathy)

any medical history that may orient towards a specific etiology of cerebral ischemia.

Skin examination

Skin examination is an important step in the search for a cause. It should be performed with the patient naked, and requires the advice of a dermatologist when necessary. The examination should focus on the search for:

features of abnormal skin elasticity, varicose veins, spontaneous ecchymosis, abnormal scars (in favor of Ehlers-Danlos disease)

papulosis (in favour of malignant atrophic papulosis, so-called Degos disease)

livedo racemosa (in favor of Sneddon disease)

neurofibromas and "*taches café-au-lait*" (in favor of von Recklinghausen disease)

angiokeratomas (in favor of Fabry disease)

facial lentiginosis (possibly associated with cardiac myxoma).

Fundoscopic examination

Fundoscopic examination is necessary, as it may identify signs of:

hypertensive retinopathy

cholesterol emboli

perivascular retinitis (in favor of Eales' syndrome)

multiple retinal ischemia (in favor of Susac's syndrome).

The biological work-up

The biological work-up should include:

in all patients, the same biological work-up as in older patients: blood cell count, glucose level, cholesterol and triglyceride levels, erythrocyte sedimentation rate, fibrinogen, and C-reactive protein

in selected patients in the absence of a clearly identified cause of cerebral ischemia:

- activated cephalin time (when increased, should lead to a search for lupus anticoagulant)
- serology for syphilis and human immunodeficiency virus
- electrophoresis of proteins
- dosage of antiphospholipid antibodies in the case of multiple spontaneous miscarriages, deep venous thrombosis, false positivity of syphilitic serology, or systemic disorder
- search for congenital thrombophilia in the presence of personal or family history of multiple venous thrombosis (proteins C and S, antithrombin III, resistance to activated protein C, mutation of factor V Leiden, mutation of thrombin gene), but these causes of thrombophilia are rarely causes of cerebral ischemia except in the case of cerebral venous thrombosis.

Diagnostic work-up must include a large variety of symptoms and careful examination of other systems (skin, retina) as well as a search for systemic diseases.

Causes of ischemic strokes in the young

There are huge differences in the breakdown of etiologies depending on the centers and countries where the data are collected [7, 8, 10, 14–23]. Despite an extensive diagnostic work-up, the cause of cerebral ischemia remains undetermined in up to 45% of patients [7, 8, 10, 14, 15, 19, 20, 23–25]. However, even in specialized centers it may happen that the diagnostic work-up is negative because it is not extensive enough or is performed too late after the onset [24]. The most frequent cause in Western countries is cervical artery dissection, and in non-industrialized countries valvulopathies. In this chapter we present the etiologies according to the TOAST classification [26] although the first three categories (large-vessel atherosclerosis, cardioembolism and small-vessel occlusion) are rare in young patients.

> The main differences between ischemic strokes occurring in young adults and children and those occurring later in life are the breakdown of causes, with a prominence of "unknown" and "other determined" causes, and an overall favorable outcome. Depending on how exhaustive the diagnostic work-up is, up to 50% of patients have no clearly identified cause.

Large-vessel atherosclerosis

Large-vessel atherosclerosis accounts for less than 10% of cerebral ischemia before the age of 45 years, and is found mainly in men between 40 and 45 years of age. Atherosclerosis has no specificity concerning the clinical presentation, diagnosis or predisposing factors. Smoking is a major risk factor in this age category, and a family history is frequent, suggesting a genetic predisposition [27].

Cardioembolism

The main causes of cardioembolism in young patients are listed in Table 14.1. A few of them deserve more detail.

Atrial fibrillation

Atrial fibrillation is associated with a very low risk of cerebral emboli in young people when occurring in the absence of underlying cardiopathy (lone atrial fibrillation) and of vascular risk factors. However, it confers a high risk of cerebral emboli when there are

Table 14.1. Main cardiac sources of cerebral ischemia in young adults.

High-risk cardiopathies
atrial fibrillation associated with cardiopathy, or vascular risk factors or previous systemic emboli
mitral stenosis
mechanical prosthetic valve
infectious endocarditis
marastic endocarditis
intracardiac thrombus
acute myocardial infarction
ventricular akinesia
dilated cardiomyopathy
intracardiac tumor (myxoma, papillary fibroelastoma)
paradoxical emboli through a PFO or interatrial communication
congenital cardiopathies with cyanosis
IASA plus PFO
complication of catheterism and cardiac surgery
Low-risk cardiopathies
lone atrial fibrillation
mitral valve prolapse
mitral calcification
bioprosthesis
aortic stenosis
bicuspid aortic valve
Lambl excrescence
isolated IASA
isolated PFO

risk factors for stroke, especially high blood pressure, or an underlying cardiopathy, such as mitral stenosis or cardiomyopathy. In the absence of evidence of atrial fibrillation on ECG, the search for paroxysmal atrial fibrillation by endovascular stimulation provided results that are difficult to interpret in the absence of reliable controls. Most studies were conducted in too small cohorts, and lack statistical power. The question of whether endovascular stimulation is useful remains unresolved, even in subgroups that may be at risk, such as patients with interatrioseptal abnormalities [28].

Infectious endocarditis

Infectious endocarditis is not always associated with fever. At an early stage, transthoracic echocardiography (TTE) and transesophageal echocardiography (TEE) may reveal vegetations. When negative, these investigations should be repeated.

Patent foramen ovale (PFO)

Patent foramen ovale is present in 10 to 20% of young patients with cerebral ischemia [29, 30]. It may be familial, especially in women [31]. PFO consists of a communication between right and left atrium which becomes functional when the pressure in the right atrium becomes higher than in the left one (e.g. pulmonary embolism, Valsalva maneuver). PFO may be diagnosed by TTE or TEE with contrast, or transcranial Doppler with contrast. When there is a causal relationship, possible mechanisms of cerebral ischemia are paradoxical emboli (requiring deep venous thrombosis, pulmonary embolism and cerebral ischemia without other potential cause), local thrombosis in the PFO (most likely hypothesis but almost never proven) or paroxysmal atrial fibrillation [28]. However, the presence of a PFO is frequent in practice and the causal relationship is unlikely in many patients. The risk of recurrence after a first ischemic stroke in the presence of an isolated PFO does not differ from that in ischemic stroke patients of similar age who have no PFO [32]. A causal relationship will be proven only if ongoing trials aiming at the closure of PFO show a clear reduction in the risk of recurrence after closure. Evidence of a right-to-left shunt by transcranial Doppler with contrast enhancement is, in most cases, a marker of the presence of a PFO. However, sometimes the cause of the right-to-left shunt is not a PFO but a pulmonary arteriovenous malformation, which is a rare disorder that occurs mainly in patients with Rendu-Osler-Weber disease. Evidence of a shunt without evidence of a PFO should therefore lead to a search for pulmonary arteriovenous malformation (see Chapter 9).

Interatrioseptal aneurysm (IASA)

Interatrioseptal aneurysm is a protrusion of the interatrial septum in either atrium. It is rare in the absence of PFO [32]. Diagnostic criteria are, on TEE, an excursion of 10 mm or more during cardiac contraction, and a base of at least 15 mm [32]. IASA is

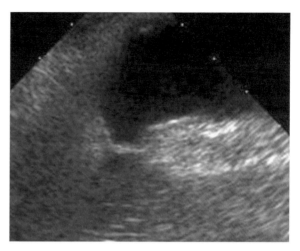

Figure 14.1. Transesophageal echography showing a patent foramen ovale and an interatrioseptal aneurysm.

more frequent in young patients who have had an ischemic stroke of unknown cause [30], but, in the absence of associated PFO, the presence of an IASA is not a marker of increased risk of recurrence [32]. Paroxysmal atrial fibrillation and local thrombosis in the IASA are the most likely mechanisms of cerebral ischemia when a causal relationship exists.

> The association of a patent foramen ovale and an interatrioseptal aneurysm is a marker of an increased risk of recurrence.

Associated PFO and IASA

The association of PFO and IASA (Figure 14.1) in patients aged 55 years or less who have had an ischemic stroke of unknown cause is a marker of increased risk of recurrence under aspirin [32]. In the FOP-ASIA study [32], after 4 years of follow-up, the rate of recurrent strokes was 15.2% (95% confidence interval [CI] 1.8–28.6%) in patients with PFO and IASA, whereas it was only 2.3% (95% CI 0.3–4.3%) in those with isolated PFO, 4.2% (95% CI 1.8–6.6%) in those without PFO and IASA, and 0.0% in those with isolated IASA. Therefore the coexistence of PFO and IASA is associated with a 4.2-fold increased risk of recurrence (95% CI 1.5–11.8). Ischemic stroke patients with coexistence of PFO and IASA have a higher risk of recurrence and are eligible for clinical randomized trials aiming at evaluating the safety and efficacy of closure of PFO compared with anticoagulant or antiplatelet therapy.

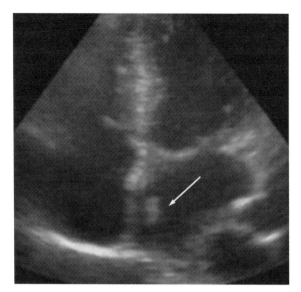

Figure 14.2. Transesophageal echography showing a left atrial myxoma (arrow).

Mitral valve prolapse

Mitral valve prolapse is a protrusion of one or two mitral valves in the left atrium, found in 2–6% of people in the community [33]. However, diagnostic criteria often lacked precision in studies and its role in cerebral ischemia remains very controversial. The risk of cerebral emboli in patients with mitral valve prolapse is very low except in the case of associated atrial fibrillation or endocarditis.

Intracardiac myxoma

Intracardiac myxoma (Figure 14.2) is the most frequent intracardiac tumour. Its prevalence is 10 per million inhabitants and it is usually located in the left atrium. In less than 50% of cases it leads to systemic emboli associated with fatigue, weight loss, fever, and sometimes cardiac signs such as dyspnea, murmur or variations in blood pressure. Most myxomas remain asymptomatic and are revealed by an ischemic stroke. The presence of facial lentiginosis (a rare autosomal dominant disorder) may be associated with a myxoma.

Papillary fibroelastoma

Papillary fibroelastoma is a benign tumor which is usually located on a cardiac valve and is difficult to distinguish from vegetations.

Peripartum cardiomyopathies

Peripartum cardiomyopathies are very rare in Western countries but are reported quite frequently in sub-Saharan countries during the last month of pregnancy and the post-partum period [34]. The clinical presentation is that of a cardiac failure [35], often associated with cerebral emboli [35]. This disorder is multifactorial and is associated with a high case-fatality rate.

Small-vessel occlusion

Lacunar infarcts are small infarcts of less than 15 mm located in the deep white matter, basal ganglia and brainstem. They are the consequence of the occlusion of a single deep perforating intracerebral artery of less than 400 μm in diameter. These perforators have no collaterals and their occlusion always leads to an infarct. The short-term outcome is usually good, but the risk is cognitive decline and dementia in the event of recurrences.

Lipohyalinosis of the deep perforators

Arterial hypertension is the most important risk factor for lipohyalinosis of the deep perforators, but such hypertensive arteriolopathies are very rare before the age of 45 years.

CADASIL

CADASIL (Cerebral Autosomal Dominant Arteriopathy with Subcortical Infarcts and Leukoencephalopathy) is a genetic disorder of small deep perforating arteries identified on the basis of clinical, MRI (Figure 14.3) and genetic criteria [36, 37]. CADASIL is due to a mutation of the *Notch3* gene on chromosome 19 [36], leading to an accumulation in the wall of small perforators leading to a progressive occlusion. CADASIL is associated with migraine with aura, depression, multiple subcortical infarcts and, at the end-stage, dementia with pseudobulbar palsy [36, 37]. White matter changes are always already severe on MRI when the first symptoms occur, usually during the third decade of life [37], leading to death within 20 years after the first symptoms (see Chapter 9) [37].

Other definite causes of cerebral ischemia

These are actually the most frequent causes of cerebral ischemia when a cause can be identified.

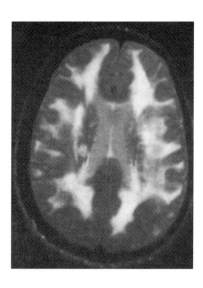

Figure 14.3. Brain MRI of a CADASIL patient showing severe white matter abnormalities and lacunas.

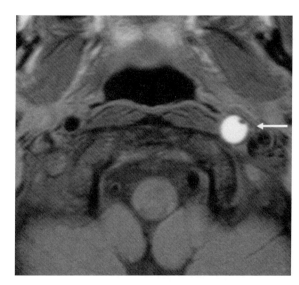

Figure 14.4. MRI of an internal carotid artery dissection, showing the mural hematoma (arrow).

Diseases of large arteries

- *Cervical artery dissections* are the leading cause of cerebral ischemia in the young in Western countries when a cause can be clearly identified [7, 38]. In most cases no trauma can be identified, or the trauma is mild and a causal relationship between a trivial trauma and dissection is even disputable [38, 39]. The most likely hypothesis to explain most cases is that of a trivial trauma of daily life [7] occurring on an artery prone to dissect for genetic [40, 41] or infectious reasons [42]. Inherited elastic tissue disorders, especially Ehler-Danlos type IV, predispose to dissections but they are rare and probably underdiagnosed in practice. The associations with intracranial aneurysms and cases occurring in the same family are rare but, when they occur, are in favor of elastic tissue disorder. Recurrences of stroke and of dissections are rare [38, 39], and the overall outcome can be considered excellent except when stroke was severe at the acute stage [38, 39]. Nowadays the diagnosis should be possible using exclusively non-invasive investigations, especially Doppler ultrasonography and MRI, both techniques being able to show the mural hematoma [38, 39] (see Chapter 9; Figure 14.4).

Cervical artery dissection is the leading cause of cerebral ischemia in young adults in Western countries and is usually associated with a good outcome in patients who survive the acute stage.

- *Post-irradiation cervical arteriopathies* in young persons are often due to irradiation for hematological disorders, and less frequently to throat cancers. Patients always have radiodermitis in the area of irradiation. The arterial lesion is atheroma, irradiation being a local factor in atheroma. The outcome is usually more dependent on the underlying disorder that led to irradiation, than on irradiation arteriopathy per se, especially in asymptomatic cases [43].
- *Cervical fibromuscular dysplasia of cervical arteries* is associated with a low risk of ischemic stroke except in the case of dissection. It can be isolated or associated with other locations such as renal arteries. It may be found in patients with von Recklinghausen disease or elastic tissue disorder.
- *Intracranial dissections* are very rare and difficult to diagnose. They may occur in children, are often revealed by cerebral ischemia, but may also lead to subarachnoid hemorrhage, especially when located in the vertebrobasilar territory. Their prognosis is usually poor but benign cases, if they exist, may remain undiagnosed.
- *Moyamoya disease* is a progressive intracranial vasculopathy that usually becomes symptomatic in children or young adults and may lead to ischemia, hemorrhage, or both. Angiography shows a tight stenosis or occlusion of the intracranial carotid arteries associated with

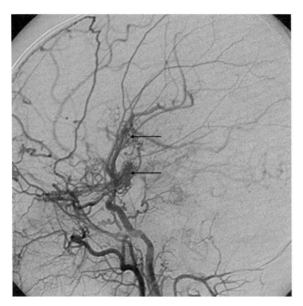

Figure 14.5. Conventional angiography of moyamoya (arrow) with distal occlusion of the internal carotid artery.

intracerebral neo-vessels (Figure 14.5). Any disorder that can lead to progressive stenosis or occlusion of intracranial carotid arteries in children or in young adults may be a cause of moyamoya.

- *Secondary vasculitis occurring in the context of systemic disorder.* Such vasculitis may occur in a patient whose systemic disorder is already known, or be the first manifestation.

  - Systemic disorders where cerebral vasculitis is usually not the most prominent feature (panarteritis nodosa, Churg-Strauss syndrome, systemic lupus erythematosus, Sjögren syndrome, Behcet syndrome, sarcoidosis, Crohn disease, ulcerative rectocolitis) are usually diagnosed on the basis of other manifestations of the disease and, depending on the type of systemic disorder, either a neuropathological proof (e.g. sarcoidosis) or association of diagnostic criteria (e.g. systemic lupus erythematosus).

  - Takayasu disease is a chronic inflammatory disease that progressively involves the aorta and the brachiocephalic arteries. It occurs predominantly in women before 45 years of age. Cerebral ischemia may be due to progressive stenosis or occlusion of the cervical arteries when they arise from the aortic arch.

  - Buerger disease, so-called thromboangiitis obliterans, is a segmental inflammatory vasculitis involving arteries of intermediate and small calibers and also superficial veins. This is usually a disorder involving peripheral arteries, which may exceptionally involve cerebral arteries.

  - Eales disease is an inflammatory vasculitis that involves predominantly retinal arteries and very rarely cerebral arteries. The causal relationship with cerebral ischemia is uncertain.

  - Acute multifocal placoid pigment epitheliopathy is a bilateral primary disorder that may rarely be associated with cerebral vasculitis and lead to permanent visual deficits [44]. The clinical picture is that of decreased visual acuity and fever. The diagnosis is based on evidence of specific lesions at fundoscopy and inflammatory CSF. Intravenous corticosteroids and immunosuppressant therapy are recommended [44].

  - Köhlmeier-Degos disease (or malignant atrophic papulosis) is a systemic vasculitis that predominantly involves the skin. The severity of the disease is due to the consequences of the vasculitis involving the brain or the bowel.

- *Secondary vasculitis occurring in a context of infectious disorder.* Such vasculitis may occur in patients with bacterial infections (syphilis, tuberculosis, Lyme disease, etc.), viral infections (ophthalmic herpes zoster, HIV, etc.), parasites (malaria, cysticercosis, etc.) or mycotic infections (aspergillosis, candidosis, cryptococcosis, etc.).

- *Primary vasculitis of the central nervous system* is granulomatous inflammatory non-sarcoidosic non-infectious vasculitis with giant cells, restricted to the leptomeningeal and cerebral arteries [45]. The incidence is approximately 2.4 new cases per year per million inhabitants [45]. They occur in both genders around 40 years of age. The first symptom is usually headache, followed by subacute focal neurological deficits, sometimes transient, and seizures [45]. Cerebral infarcts are usually multiple, cortical and sometimes associated with hemorrhages. Fever is possible. There is no systemic biological sign of inflammation. The CSF may be normal, but is usually characterized by an increased number of lymphocytes with or without oligoclonal bands. Brain imaging is suggestive when it shows (i) on CT or MRI scans multiple infarcts of small size in cortical areas, with or without associated hemorrhages, and (ii) on conventional angiography or MRA multiple beadings in intracranial arteries in various territories [45]. This finding is not specific and the proof of diagnosis is provided by a biopsy of leptomeningeal arteries. In the absence of treatment (corticosteroids sometimes associated with cyclophosphamide for at least 1 year) or, in the event of failure of treatment, the outcome is poor, with occurrence of cognitive decline, dementia and a high mortality rate [45]. It is possible that primary vasculitis of the central nervous system is a heterogeneous entity that actually consists of several subsets of diseases [45].

- *Sneddon syndrome* is a potential cause of recurrent cerebral ischemia. Each episode is usually of mild severity but their repetition may lead to dementia. This diagnosis should be discussed each time a young patient has recurrent episodes of cerebral ischemia of mild severity preceded by livedo racemosa, which is a purple livedo, involving the trunk and the most proximal part of the limbs that does not disappear with cutaneous warming, opposite to the more trivial livedo reticularis. Antiphospholipid antibodies are usually associated. Although there is not a high level of evidence, oral anticoagulation is recommended by experts.

- *Post-partum cerebral angiopathy* is a rare entity that occurs usually in the first 2 weeks after delivery. Despite a severe clinical presentation, the outcome is usually excellent [46, 47]. The clinical presentation consists of a combination of severe headache, vomiting, epileptic seizures and focal neurological deficits [46, 47]. Angiography (either conventional or preferably magnetic resonance angiography) shows multiple beadings in large intracranial arteries that disappear spontaneously within a few weeks [46, 47] (Figure 14.6). It might be a variety of toxic angiopathy favored by estrogen withdrawal, the use of vasoconstrictive drugs and possibly bromocriptine [46, 47].

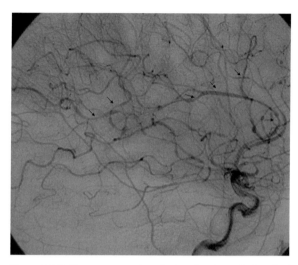

Figure 14.6. Post-partum angiopathy: beading (arrows) of cerebral arteries.

- *Other acute reversible cerebral angiopathies* have been reported. They have the same clinical presentation and outcome as the post-partum type. Possible etiologies are toxic (vasoconstrictive drugs, illicit substances such as cocaine or amphetamines), reversible hypertensive encephalopathies, pheochromocytoma, carcinoid tumors or vasospasm after subarachnoid hemorrhage.

- *Eclampsia* is the main cause of maternal mortality and preterm birth in Western countries [48]. The clinical presentation consists of headache, visual impairment, confusion or coma, epileptic seizures and focal neurological deficits [48, 49]. The HELLP syndrome (Hemolysis; Elevated Liver enzymes, Low Platelets) is a subtype of eclampsia [50]. MRI shows in FLAIR or T2 sequences multiple hyperintense signals, isolated or more frequently confluent, more prominent in posterior areas, frequently bilateral, located at the junction between the cortex and the subcortical white matter [51, 52]. These abnormalities completely disappear after a few days or weeks. Cerebral infarcts may lead to residual deficits, but in most patients who survive the acute stage the long-term outcome is favorable [11].

- *Unruptured aneurysms of intracranial arteries* may be a cause of cerebral ischemia secondary to a local intra-saccular thrombosis and subsequent distal emboli.

Hematological diseases

- *Thrombotic thrombocytopenic purpura (Moschcowitz syndrome)* is a systemic disorder characterized by fever, renal failure, thrombocytopenia and hemolytic anemia with a negative Coombs test [53]. Cerebral infarcts are present in most cases [53]. The neurological manifestations may be the first manifestations of the disease [53]. The diagnosis is made easy by the determination of platelet count and the search for schizocytes.
- Hemoglobinopathies:
  - Sickle-cell disease is a cause of ischemic stroke in children and young adults and during pregnancies [12]
  - Beta thalassemia is also a possible cause of cerebral ischemia.
- Nocturnal paroxysmal hemoglobinuria (Marchiafava-Micheli disease).
- *Congenital thrombophilia*: deficits in proteins C and S, or antithrombin III, resistance to activated protein C, mutation of factor V Leiden, and mutation of the thrombin gene are clearly proven causes of cerebral venous thrombosis, but their role in arterial ischemia remains disputable [54].
- *Acquired thrombophilia: antiphospholipid antibody syndrome.* This is a cause of arterial and venous occlusions, recurrent spontaneous miscarriages, and biological changes such as thrombocytopenia, false positivity of syphilis serology and activated cephalin time increase. It may be primary or associated with a clearly defined systemic disorder such as systemic lupus erythematosus. Cerebral ischemia may be due to various mechanisms: prothrombotic state, Libman-Sachs endocarditis or early atheroma.
- *Other hematological causes* of cerebral ischemia in young people are polycythemia, iron-deficiency anemia, leukemia, thrombocythemia, hypereosinophilic syndrome, endovascular lymphoma, disseminated intravascular coagulation, and hyperviscosity syndromes.

Metabolic disorders

- *Fabry disease* is an X-linked recessive lysosomal storage disease resulting from deficient alpha-galactosidase. It causes an endothelial vasculopathy followed by cerebral ischemia [55].

A few female cases have been reported [55]. Various types of mutation have been identified. The clinical picture associates episodes of unexplained fever, cutaneous angiokeratomas located in the trunk and proximal part of limbs, crisis of painful acroparesthesia of feet and hands, corneal opacities, hypohydrosis, and later in the time-course of the disease cardiac and renal failure. Ischemic strokes occur during the fourth decade and are often associated with headache. Strokes are more prominent in the vertebrobasilar territory. The possible mechanisms of ischemic stroke are dolichomega intracranial arteries, occlusions of the deep perforating arteries due to the accumulation of sphingolipids, cardiopathies and prothrombotic state. The frequency of the disorder has been found to be 1.2% in young ischemic stroke patients with a negative diagnostic work-up in a large German study [55], but this rate has never been confirmed thereafter. It is, however, important to recognize such cases because of possible therapeutic consequences with infusion of alpha-galactosidase [55]. The diagnosis is performed on the basis of a low plasma alpha-galactosidase activity or mutation in the alpha-GAL gene in men, and only by identification of the mutation in women (see Chapter 9) [55].

- *Homocystinuria* has a prevalence of three per million inhabitants. One-third of patients have a venous or arterial event during their life. A mutation in the gene for methyltetrahydrofolate reductase (MTHFR) can be found. It is more frequent to find a slight increase in plasma homocysteine ($>15 \mu mol/l$), which is more a factor than a cause. Folic acid supplementation reduces the serum level of homocysteine, but whether it also reduces the rate of vascular events remains to be proven.
- *MELAS syndrome (Mitochondrial Encephalopathy with Lactic Acidosis and Stroke-like episodes)* is a mitochondriopathy due to several types of mutation in the mitochondrial DNA. The major clinical features are, in a patient around 30 years of age, progressive deafness, stroke-like episodes, usually transient and located in posterior territories, seizures, cognitive impairment and recurrent episodes of headache and vomiting. Progressive external ophthalmoplegia with ptosis,

muscular pain at exercise, lactic acidosis after exercise, presence of ragged red fibers on muscle biopsy, cataract, hypogonadism, diabetes mellitus, hypothyroidism and cardiomyopathy are the other manifestations of the disease. The diagnosis needs evidence of the mitochondrial DNA mutation (see Chapter 9).

Non-cruoric emboli

- *Gas emboli* occur during cesarean sections, traumatic deliveries, subclavian catheter accidents, gynecological and cardiac surgery or diving accidents [56]. The clinical picture consists of acute respiratory failure and acute diffuse encephalopathy, preceded by severe anxiety and dyspnea [56]. In a few minutes the patient develops tachycardia, seizures and coma, leading to death [56]. As soon as the diagnosis is suspected the patient should be turned onto the left side.
- *Amniotic emboli* occur after difficult deliveries in the presence of a vaginal lesion. The patient develops acute pulmonary edema and seizures [11, 57].
- *Fat emboli* occur in long bone fractures or liposuction surgery [58].

Choriocarcinoma

Choriocarcinoma is a malignant trophoblastic tumor that occurs in one pregnancy in 40 000. Lesions of the arterial wall may occur and lead to cerebral ischemia in the absence of metastasis [59].

Rare causes of cerebral ischemia in young people of undetermined mechanism

- *Sweet syndrome (acute febrile neutrophilic dermatosis)* is a dermatological disorder characterized by multiple pustulae and painful purple skin lesions where a neutrophilic infiltration can be found [60]. This dermatological disorder has accompanying features of systemic inflammation such as fever, conjunctivitis or other types of ocular inflammation, and arthritis [60]. It occurs mainly around the age of 40 years and may be associated with cancer [60]. Cerebral ischemia may occur but a causal relationship is not proven.
- *Kawasaki syndrome* is a panarteritis of arteries of intermediate and small caliber that may lead to coronary or cerebral artery occlusions [61].

- *Susac syndrome (or Sicret syndrome)* is a rare disease occurring in young women of unknown pathogenesis consisting of a triad with retinal arterial occlusion, hearing loss by cochlear ischemia and diffuse vascular encephalopathy [62].
- *HERNS syndrome (Hereditary Endotheliopathy with Retinopathy and Stroke)* is an autosomal dominant hereditary syndrome consisting of retinopathy, nephropathy and ischemic stroke, leading to blindness. Fundoscopic examination reveals a typical vasculopathy [63].

Cerebral ischemia of undetermined and unknown causes

Before classifying a patient in this category it is important to be sure that the diagnostic work-up has been extensive enough and repeated over time. Sometimes the etiology is found during the follow-up.

Risk factors for stroke in the young
Classic risk factors

Classic risk factors for stroke (arterial hypertension, smoking and hypercholesterolemia) are also risk factors in the young, but the attributable risk is lower than in older patients. They are frequent in patients with a negative diagnostic work-up [7].

More specific risk factors in the young
Oral contraceptive therapy

Oral contraceptive therapy increases the risk of ischemic stroke even with compounds with low-dose estrogens: the relative risk of cerebral ischemia is 2.9 (95% CI 1.3–6.7) [64]. This relative risk increases in smokers. However, the absolute risk is low, and one case of cerebral ischemia can be attributed to oral contraceptive therapy for 5880 women without vascular risk factors treated during 1 year [64]. Therefore oral contraceptive therapy is contraindicated only in high-risk women, especially those who have already had a stroke or have other risk factors.

Migraine

Migraine is associated with a relative risk of ischemic stroke of 3.5, reaching 6 for migraine with aura [65] or even more in the presence of vascular risk factors.

Case–control studies conducted in several countries suggest that the association between migraine with aura and stroke is not an artifact, although none of these studies can be considered as providing a definite proof of association. It is less clear whether migraine without aura is associated with stroke or whether the association is restricted to migraine with aura. Similarly, there are few data examining the magnitude of the association among nonusers of oral contraceptives compared with those who use low-estrogen oral contraceptives. There is no convincing evidence on the mechanism that would be implicated. The concept of migrainous infarct is not proven: it requires exclusion of other causes and a typical temporal relationship, the neurological deficit being a prolongation of a typical aura.

HIV infection

HIV infection is also associated with an increased risk of ischemic stroke. The mechanisms of stroke are multiple in HIV-infected patients, with an important role of vasculitis and hypercoagulability state [66].

Pregnancy

Pregnancy is classically associated with an increased risk of ischemic stroke [6, 11, 67]. However, data supporting this classic statement are scarce. A study conducted in high-risk women, i.e. women who have already had an ischemic stroke, showed no significant increase in incidence of recurrent stroke during periods of subsequent pregnancy. The main difference during pregnancy is the breakdown of etiologies, with specific causes described that do not exist or are rare in non-pregnant women. Stroke occurring during pregnancy is one of the leading causes of maternal death [68–70].

> Classic risk factors for stroke: arterial hypertension, smoking, hypercholesterolemia.
> Migraine: the relative risk of ischemic stroke is 3.5, reaching 6 for migraine with aura or even more in the presence of vascular risk factors.

Outcome

Studies that evaluated the long-term outcome of young stroke patients are heterogeneous and can hardly be compared. Their findings are influenced by the inclusion or not of all types of stroke, including intracerebral ischemia [10, 19, 23, 71, 72],

subarachnoid hemorrhages [10, 19, 23, 71] and even sometimes TIA. Those studies used different age limits, and may have suffered recruitment bias in specialized centers [7, 10, 25, 73]. Moreover, most studies were conducted in small samples, were retrospective, had a partial follow-up [15, 19, 22, 23, 71, 73, 74], excluded recurrent cases [10, 19, 71, 75] or included only those who survived the acute stage, leading to a selection bias towards less severe cases and better outcomes.

Mortality

The mortality rate is low in the short and intermediate term [7, 8, 10, 15–23, 25, 73]. In the Lille cohort of 287 patients aged between 15 and 45 years, with a mean follow-up of 3 years and none lost to follow-up, the mortality rate was 4.5% after 1 year, 0.8% per year during the next 2 years [7].

Recurrent vascular events (stroke or coronary syndromes)

The risk of recurrent vascular events is low in this age category, but they depend on the presumed cause of cerebral ischemia. In the Lille cohort the risk of recurrent stroke was 1.4% during the first year then 1.0% per year during the next 2 years, and that of myocardial infarction 0.2% per year [7]. In cervical artery dissections the risk of recurrent stroke is very low [2, 38, 39, 76, 77]. A negative diagnostic work-up is also associated with a low risk of new events [7, 32]. In children the recurrence rate is higher than in young adults.

Epilepsy

Epilepsy is more frequent after an ischemic stroke in a young patient than stroke recurrence, with a risk at 3 years between 5 and 7% [7, 78]. Most patients had post-stroke epilepsy and the first seizure during the first year after stroke [7, 78].

Quality of life

Even if most patients remained independent, many of them lost their job or divorced during the 3 years after the ischemic stroke [7]. In the absence of a systematic evaluation it is difficult to identify the reason, but depression, fatigue, mild cognitive or behavioral changes or alteration in social cognition are likely explanations. Therefore ischemic strokes in young people are frequently associated with a decline in quality of life that is not explained by handicap [5, 7, 17].

Pregnancy after an ischemic stroke

A multicenter French study [79] conducted with 373 consecutive women who had an ischemic stroke between 15 and 40 years of age and followed-up over a 5-year period found an overall risk of recurrent stroke of 0.5% at year 5 (95% CI 0.3–0.95) in periods without pregnancy and 1.8% (95% CI 0.5–7.5) during pregnancies and puerperium, without significant difference. Therefore young women who have had an ischemic stroke have an overall low risk of recurrence during a subsequent pregnancy and do not significantly increase this risk during pregnancy [79].

Specificities for children

Besides a higher recurrence rate, children are also more prone to have seizures, altered mental status and also dystonia and dyskinesia than adults [12].

> The mortality rate (4.5% after 1 year) and the risk of recurrent stroke (1.4% during the first year) are low, especially in patients with a negative diagnostic work-up. Risk of epilepsy after an ischemic stroke is 5–7% at 3 years. Behavioral changes and dystonia in children are frequent sequelae.

Secondary prevention after ischemic stroke in young adults

The main characteristics of ischemic stroke occurring in young patients, i.e. their causes, the overall good outcome and interference with hormonal life in women (contraception, pregnancy and future menopause), influence secondary prevention after stroke. As for elderly subjects, secondary prevention measures mainly depend on the presumed cause. For this reason, an extensive and early diagnostic work-up is required, as well as an extensive evaluation of risk factors. The overall management of secondary prevention is based on principles similar to those in elderly subjects, i.e. an optimal management of vascular risk factors, an appropriate antithrombotic therapy (oral anticoagulation and antithrombotic agents depending on the cause) and removal of the source in specific cases (severe internal artery stenosis, cardiac

myxoma, etc.). Stroke prevention measures should take into account that short- and long-term mortality rates are low, and that the overall risk of new vascular events is also low.

The specificities of stroke prevention in young adults are the following: (i) oral contraceptive therapy should be avoided in most cases; (ii) in the absence of evidence-based data, cervical artery dissections may be treated either by antiplatelet therapy or by anticoagulation [80], but, because of the low rate of recurrence after the 4th week, there is no reason to give oral anticoagulation for more than a few weeks or in patients at increased risk of bleeding; (iii) patients who have a negative diagnostic work-up but a patent foramen ovale (PFO) at risk (large PFO, or PFO associated with an interatrioseptal aneurism) have a 4-fold increased risk of recurrence under aspirin, and should preferably be randomized in trials comparing oral anticoagulation and closure; (iv) aspirin plus dipyridamole is the standard therapy for patients who can tolerate aspirin, have no clear cardiac indication for clopidogrel and do not develop headache; (v) as randomized controlled trials suggest that estrogens increase the severity of ischemic strokes, patients should be informed that hormonal replacement therapy will not be recommended when the menopause occurs, if there are no new data showing that this attitude is inappropriate at that time; (vi) young women should be informed what to do in the event of pregnancy (continue aspirin except during the last 6 weeks, replace oral anticoagulation by subcutaneous heparin if pregnant).

An important question that remains unanswered is how long young patients should receive antiplatelet therapy after an ischemic stroke when the diagnostic work-up is negative. Due to the low risk of recurrence in patients without any risk factor, the reasons for continuing antiplatelet therapy for more than a few years are rather weak.

> Secondary prevention measures mainly depend on the presumed cause and consist of an optimal management of vascular risk factors, an appropriate antithrombotic therapy and removal of the source in specific cases.

Conclusion

The etiologies of ischemic stroke in the young are multiple and the outcome is good in most patients. New causes should now be identified.

Chapter Summary

Diagnostic work-up (additionally to the standard work-up as in older patients):

Intensive patient interview about the presence of headache, tinnitus, drug abuse, family history; careful skin examination; careful fundoscopic examination; and in selected patients serology for syphilis and HIV, electrophoresis of proteins, antiphospholipid antibodies and testing for thrombophilia.

Causes:
- Large-vessel atherosclerosis
- Cardioembolism (see Table 14.1)
- Small-vessel occlusion such as CADASIL
- Diseases of large arteries:
  - Cervical artery dissections
  - Post-irradiation cervical arteriopathies
  - Cervical fibromuscular dysplasia of cervical arteries in patients with von Recklinghausen disease or elastic tissue disorder
  - Intracranial dissections
  - Moyamoya
  - Secondary vasculitis in the context of a systemic disorder such as panarteritis nodosa, systemic lupus erythematodes, Takayasu disease or Buerger disease or the context of infectious disorder
  - Primary vasculitis of the central venous system
  - Sneddon syndrome
  - Post-partum cerebral angiopathy and eclampsia
  - Unruptured aneurysms of intracranial arteries
- Hematological disorders
- Metabolic disorders such as Fabry disease, homocystinuria and MELAS syndrome
- Gas emboli, amniotic emboli or fat emboli
- Choriocarcinoma

The most frequent cause in Western countries is cervical artery dissection, and in non-industrialized countries valvulopathies, but the cause of cerebral ischemia remains undetermined in up to 45% of patients.

Secondary prevention

Secondary prevention measures mainly depend on the presumed cause and consist of optimal management of vascular risk factors, an appropriate antithrombotic therapy (oral anticoagulation and antithrombotic agents, depending on the cause), and removal of the source in specific cases (severe internal artery stenosis, cardiac myxoma, etc.).

Specificities of stroke prevention in young adults: oral contraceptive therapy should be avoided in most cases; cervical artery dissections may be treated either by antiplatelet therapy or by anticoagulation (oral anticoagulation only for a few weeks); due to the low risk of recurrence in patients without any risk factor, the reasons for continuing antiplatelet therapy more than a few years are rather weak.

References

1. Bamford J, Sandercock P, Dennis M, Burn J, Warlow C. Classification and natural history of clinically identifiable subtypes of cerebral infarction. *Lancet* 1991; **337**:1521–6.

2. Hankey GJ, Warlow CP. Treatment and secondary prevention of stroke: evidence, costs, and effects on individuals and populations. *Lancet* 1999; **354**:1457–63.

3. Murray CJ, Lopez AD. Global mortality, disability, and the contribution of risk factors: Global Burden of Disease Study. *Lancet* 1997; **349**:1436–42.

4. Bonita R. Epidemiology of stroke. *Lancet* 1992; **339**:342–4.

5. Carolei A, Marini C, Di Napoli M, et al. High stroke incidence in the prospective community-based L'Aquila registry (1994–1998). First year's results. *Stroke* 1997; **28**:2500–6.

6. Giroud M, Milan C, Beuriat P, et al. Incidence and survival rates during a two-year period of intracerebral and subarachnoid haemorrhages, cortical infarcts, lacunes and transient ischaemic attacks. The Stroke Registry of Dijon: 1985–1989. *Int J Epidemiol* 1991; **20**:892–9.

7. Leys D, Bandu L, Henon H, et al. Clinical outcome in 287 consecutive young adults (15 to 45 years) with ischemic stroke. *Neurology* 2002; **59**:26–33.

8. Bogousslavsky J, Pierre P. Ischemic stroke in patients under age 45. *Neurol Clin* 1992; **10**:113–24.

9. Naess H, Nyland HI, Thomassen L, Aarseth J, Nyland G, Myhr KM. Incidence and short-term outcome of cerebral infarction in young adults in western Norway. *Stroke* 2002; **33**:2105–8.

10. Marini C, Totaro R, Carolei A. Long-term prognosis of cerebral ischemia in young adults. National Research Council Study Group on Stroke in the Young. *Stroke* 1999; **30**:2320–5.

11. Sharshar T, Lamy C, Mas JL. Incidence and causes of strokes associated with pregnancy and puerperium. A study in public hospitals of Ile de France. Stroke in Pregnancy Study Group. *Stroke* 1995; **26**:930–6.

12. Amlie-Lefond C, Sebire G, Fullerton HJ. Recent developments in childhood arterial ischaemic stroke. *Lancet Neurol* 2008; **7**:425–35.

13. Guidelines for management of ischaemic stroke and transient ischaemic attack 2008. *Cerebrovasc Dis* 2008; **25**:457–507.

14. Adams HP, Jr., Kappelle LJ, Biller J, et al. Ischemic stroke in young adults. Experience in 329 patients enrolled in the Iowa Registry of stroke in young adults. *Arch Neurol* 1995; **52**:491–5.

15. Bogousslavsky J, Regli F. Ischemic stroke in adults younger than 30 years of age. Cause and prognosis. *Arch Neurol* 1987; **44**:479–82.

16. Hoffmann M. Stroke in the young in South Africa – an analysis of 320 patients. *S Afr Med J* 2000; **90**:1226–37.

17. Kappelle LJ, Adams HP, Jr., Heffner ML, Torner JC, Gomez F, Biller J. Prognosis of young adults with ischemic stroke. A long-term follow-up study assessing recurrent vascular events and functional outcome in the Iowa Registry of Stroke in Young Adults. *Stroke* 1994; **25**:1360–5.

18. Kwon SU, Kim JS, Lee JH, Lee MC. Ischemic stroke in Korean young adults. *Acta Neurol Scand* 2000; **101**:19–24.

19. Leno C, Berciano J, Combarros O, et al. A prospective study of stroke in young adults in Cantabria, Spain. *Stroke* 1993; **24**:792–5.

20. Lisovoski F, Rousseaux P. Cerebral infarction in young people. A study of 148 patients with early cerebral angiography. *J Neurol Neurosurg Psychiatry* 1991; **54**:576–9.

21. Nayak SD, Nair M, Radhakrishnan K, Sarma PS. Ischaemic stroke in the young adult: clinical features, risk factors and outcome. *Natl Med J India* 1997; **10**:107–12.

22. Neau JP, Ingrand P, Mouille-Brachet C, et al. Functional recovery and social outcome after cerebral infarction in young adults. *Cerebrovasc Dis* 1998; **8**:296–302.

23. Nencini P, Inzitari D, Baruffi MC, et al. Incidence of stroke in young adults in Florence, Italy. *Stroke* 1988; **19**:977–81.

24. Chan MT, Nadareishvili ZG, Norris JW. Diagnostic strategies in young patients with ischemic stroke in Canada. *Can J Neurol Sci* 2000; **27**:120–4.

25. Ferro JM, Crespo M. Prognosis after transient ischemic attack and ischemic stroke in young adults. *Stroke* 1994; **25**:1611–16.

26. Adams HP, Jr., Bendixen BH, Kappelle LJ, et al. Classification of subtype of acute ischemic stroke. Definitions for use in a multicenter clinical trial. TOAST. Trial of Org 10172 in Acute Stroke Treatment. *Stroke* 1993; **24**:35–41.

27. Oliviero U, Orefice G, Coppola G, et al. Carotid atherosclerosis and ischemic stroke in young patients. *Int Angiol* 2002; **21**:117–22.

28. Berthet K, Lavergne T, Cohen A, et al. Significant association of atrial vulnerability with atrial septal abnormalities in young patients with ischemic stroke of unknown cause. *Stroke* 2000; **31**:398–403.

29. Lechat P, Mas JL, Lascault G, et al. Prevalence of patent foramen ovale in patients with stroke. *N Engl J Med* 1988; **318**:1148–52.

30. Lucas C, Goullard L, Marchau M Jr, et al. Higher prevalence of atrial septal aneurysms in patients with ischemic stroke of unknown cause. *Acta Neurol Scand* 1994; **89**:210–13.

31. Arquizan C, Coste J, Touboul PJ, Mas JL. Is patent foramen ovale a family trait? A transcranial Doppler sonographic study. *Stroke* 2001; **32**:1563–6.

32. Mas J, Arquizan C, Lamy C, et al. Recurrent cerebrovascular events in young adults with patent foramen ovale, atrial septal aneuvrysm or both. *N Engl J Med* 2001; **345**:1740–6.

33. Procacci PM, Savran SV, Schreiter SL, Bryson AL. Prevalence of clinical mitral-valve prolapse in 1169 young women. *N Engl J Med* 1976; **294**:1086–8.

34. Demakis JG, Rahimtoola SH, Sutton GC, et al. Natural course of peripartum cardiomyopathy. *Circulation* 1971; **44**:1053–61.

35. Homans DC. Peripartum cardiomyopathy. *N Engl J Med* 1985; **312**:1432–7.

36. Chabriat H, Vahedi K, Iba-Zizen MT, et al. Clinical spectrum of CADASIL: a study of 7 families. Cerebral autosomal dominant arteriopathy with subcortical infarcts and leukoencephalopathy. *Lancet* 1995; **346**:934–9.

37. Joutel A, Corpechot C, Ducros A, et al. Notch3 mutations in CADASIL, a hereditary adult-onset condition causing stroke and dementia. *Nature* 1996; **383**:707–10.

38. Leys D, Moulin T, Stojkovic T, Begey S, Chavot D. Follow-up of patients with history of cervical-artery dissection. *Cerebrovasc Dis* 1995; **5**:337–40.

39. Touze E, Gauvrit JY, Moulin T, Meder JF, Bracard S, Mas JL. Risk of stroke and recurrent dissection after a cervical artery dissection: a multicenter study. *Neurology* 2003; **61**:1347–51.

40. Gallai V, Caso V, Paciaroni M, et al. Mild hyperhomocyst(e)inemia: a possible risk factor for cervical artery dissection. *Stroke* 2001; **32**:714–18.

41. Pezzini A, Del Zotto E, Archetti S, et al. Plasma homocysteine concentration, C677T MTHFR genotype, and 844ins68bp CBS genotype in young adults with spontaneous cervical artery dissection and atherothrombotic stroke. *Stroke* 2002; **33**:664–9.

42. Guillon B, Berthet K, Benslamia L, Bertrand M, Bousser MG, Tzourio C. Infection and the risk of spontaneous cervical artery dissection: a case-control study. *Stroke* 2003; **34**:e79–81.

43. Marcel M, Leys D, Mounier-Vehier F, et al. Clinical outcome in patients with high-grade internal carotid artery stenosis after irradiation. *Neurology* 2005; **65**:959–61.

44. O'Halloran HS, Berger JR, Lee WB, et al. Acute multifocal placoid pigment epitheliopathy and central nervous system involvement: nine new cases and a review of the literature. *Ophthalmology* 2001; **108**:861–8.

45. Salvarani C, Brown RD Jr, Calamia KT, et al. Primary central nervous system vasculitis: analysis of 101 patients. *Ann Neurol* 2007; **62**:442–51.

46. Janssens E, Hommel M, Mounier-Vehier F, Leclerc X, Guerin du Masgenet B, Leys D. Postpartum cerebral angiopathy possibly due to bromocriptine therapy. *Stroke* 1995; **26**:128–30.

47. Rascol A, Guiraud B, Manelfe C, Clanet M. Accidents vasculaires cérébraux de la grossesse et du post-partum. In: Baillière JB, ed. *2o Conference de la Salpétrière sur les maladies vasculaires cérébrales*, Paris, 1979. 84–127.

48. Goldenberg RL, Culhane JF, Iams JD, Romero R. Epidemiology and causes of preterm birth. *Lancet* 2008; **371**:75–84.

49. Sibai B, Dekker G, Kupferminc M. Pre-eclampsia. *Lancet* 2005; **365**:785–99.

50. Barton JR, Sibai BM. Care of the pregnancy complicated by HELLP syndrome. *Obstet Gynecol Clin North Am* 1991; **18**:165–79.

51. Fredriksson K, Lindvall O, Ingemarsson I, Astedt B, Cronqvist S, Holtas S. Repeated cranial computed tomographic and magnetic resonance imaging scans in two cases of eclampsia. *Stroke* 1989; **20**:547–53.

52. Digre KB, Varner MW, Osborn AG, Crawford S. Cranial magnetic resonance imaging in severe preeclampsia vs eclampsia. *Arch Neurol* 1993; **50**:399–406.

53. Garg AX, Suri RS, Barrowman N, et al. Long-term renal prognosis of diarrhea-associated hemolytic uremic syndrome: a systematic review, meta-analysis, and meta-regression. *JAMA* 2003; **290**:1360–70.

54. Douay X, Lucas C, Caron C, Goudemand J, Leys D. Antithrombin, protein C and protein S levels in 127 consecutive young adults with ischemic stroke. *Acta Neurol Scand* 1998; **98**:124–7.

55. Rolfs A, Bottcher T, Zschiesche M, et al. Prevalence of Fabry disease in patients with cryptogenic stroke: a prospective study. *Lancet* 2005; **366**:1794–6.

56. Corson SL. Venous air and gas emboli in operative hysteroscopy. *J Am Assoc Gynecol Laparosc* 2002; **9**:106; author reply.

57. Levy R, Furman B, Hagay ZJ. Fetal bradycardia and disseminated coagulopathy: atypical presentation of amniotic fluid emboli. *Acta Anaesthesiol Scand* 2004; **48**:1214–15.

58. Mentz HA. Fat emboli syndromes following liposuction. *Aesthetic Plast Surg* 2008: **32**:737–8.

59. Weir B, MacDonald N, Mielke B. Intracranial vascular complications of choriocarcinoma. *Neurosurgery* 1978; **2**:138–42.

60. Cohen PR. Sweet's syndrome – a comprehensive review of an acute febrile neutrophilic dermatosis. *Orphanet J Rare Dis* 2007; **2**:34.

61. De Rosa G, Pardeo M, Rigante D. Current recommendations for the pharmacologic therapy in Kawasaki syndrome and management of its cardiovascular complications. *Eur Rev Med Pharmacol Sci* 2007; **11**:301–8.

62. Reiniger IW, Thurau S, Haritoglou C, et al. Susac-Syndrom: Fallberichte und Literaturübersicht. *Klin Monatsbl Augenheilkd* 2006; **223**:161–7.

63. Jen J, Cohen AH, Yue Q, et al. Hereditary endotheliopathy with retinopathy, nephropathy, and stroke (HERNS). *Neurology* 1997; **49**:1322–30.

64. Mant J, Painter R, Vessey M. Risk of myocardial infarction, angina and stroke in users of oral contraceptives: an updated analysis of a cohort study. *Br J Obstet Gynaecol* 1998; **105**:890–6.

65. Tzourio C, Kittner SJ, Bousser MG, Alperovitch A. Migraine and stroke in young women. *Cephalalgia* 2000; **20**:190–9.

66. Ortiz G, Koch S, Romano JG, Forteza AM, Rabinstein AA. Mechanisms of ischemic stroke in HIV-infected patients. *Neurology* 2007; **68**:1257–61.

67. Stirling Y, Woolf L, North WR, Seghatchian MJ, Meade TW. Haemostasis in normal pregnancy. *Thromb Haemost* 1984; **52**:176–82.

68. Bouvier-Colle MH, Varnoux N, Costes P, Hatton F, et le groupe d'experts sur la mortalité maternelle. Mortalité maternelle en France. Fréquence et raisons de sa sous-estimation dans la statistique des causes médicales de décès. *J Gynecol Obstet Biol Reprod (Paris)* 1991; **20**:885–91.

69. Gibbs CE. Maternal death due to stroke. *Am J Obstet Gynecol* 1974; **119**:69–75.

70. Kaunitz AM, Hughes JM, Grimes DA, Smith JC, Rochat RW, Kafrissen ME. Causes of maternal mortality in the United States. *Obstet Gynecol* 1985; **65**:605–12.

71. Marini C, Totaro R, De Santis F, Ciancarelli I, Baldassarre M, Carolei A. Stroke in young adults in the community-based L'Aquila registry: incidence and prognosis. *Stroke* 2001; **32**:52–6.

72. Qureshi AI, Safdar K, Patel M, Janssen RS, Frankel MR. Stroke in young black patients. Risk factors, subtypes, and prognosis. *Stroke* 1995; **26**:1995–8.

73. Chancellor AM, Glasgow GL, Ockelford PA, Johns A, Smith J. Etiology, prognosis, and hemostatic function after cerebral infarction in young adults. *Stroke* 1989; **20**:477–82.

74. Johnson DM, Kramer DC, Cohen E, Rochon M, Rosner M, Weinberger J. Thrombolytic therapy for acute stroke in late pregnancy with intra-arterial recombinant tissue plasminogen activator. *Stroke* 2005; **36**:e53–5.

75. Camerlingo M, Casto L, Censori B, et al. Recurrence after first cerebral infarction in young adults. *Acta Neurol Scand* 2000; **102**:87–93.

76. Pozzati E, Giuliani G, Acciarri N, Nuzzo G. Long-term follow-up of occlusive cervical carotid dissection. *Stroke* 1990; **21**:528–31.

77. Schievink WI, Mokri B, O'Fallon WM. Recurrent spontaneous cervical-artery dissection. *N Engl J Med* 1994; **330**:393–7.

78. Lamy C, Domigo V, Semah F, et al. Early and late seizures after cryptogenic ischemic stroke in young adults. *Neurology* 2003; **60**:400–4.

79. Lamy C, Hamon JB, Coste J, Mas JL. Ischemic stroke in young women: risk of recurrence during subsequent pregnancies. French Study Group on Stroke in Pregnancy. *Neurology* 2000; **55**:269–74.

80. Engelter ST, Brandt T, Debette S, et al. Antiplatelets versus anticoagulation in cervical artery dissection. *Stroke* 2007; **38**:2605–11.

Stroke units and clinical assessment

Risto O. Roine and Markku Kaste

Introduction

There is strong evidence that treatment of stroke patients in stroke units significantly reduces death, dependency and need for institutional care compared to treatment in general medical wards [1]. An acute stroke unit is one of the key elements in the critical pathway and the chain of recovery of acute stroke patients.

Only stroke unit care, thrombolytic therapy and hemicraniectomy have been shown to improve the outcome of stroke patients. The acute therapies and interventions in stroke are described in Chapter 16. The basic functions of the stroke unit, mainly covered in other chapters of this book, are etiological diagnostic work-up (Chapters 2–4 and 7–13), general management and proactive prevention of complications (Chapters 17 and 18), secondary prevention of stroke and other vascular endpoints (Chapter 19), and early rehabilitation (Chapter 20).

The purpose of this chapter is to characterize the chain of recovery of acute stroke patients from emergency phone call to acute stroke unit, including clinical evaluation of the patient and aspects of general stroke management that can be optimally delivered in stroke units, in light of current guidelines.

Prehospital care and referral

The essential building blocks for prehospital stroke care are the emergency medical service (EMS) organization consisting of an emergency response center (ERC), the EMS providers and the admitting stroke center, all of which should be involved in planning the prehospital critical pathway.

The general emergency phone number 112 (in Finland) (911 in the United States) is the first link in the chain of survival and recovery for acute stroke patients. National stroke-awareness campaigns always emphasize the importance of recognizing the symptoms of acute stroke and calling the emergency number immediately before doing anything else. This is usually done by a family member, since the stroke patient is not able to make the call himself/herself. There is class II level B evidence that educational programs to increase awareness of stroke at the population level are beneficial, and the same holds true for EMS professionals, both paramedics and physicians [2].

It does matter who is called and how the patient arrives: EMS transport to and arrival at the emergency department (ED) increase the likelihood of a patient presenting within the 3-hour time window allowing thrombolysis to be considered, compared to private physician referral and self-transport, and significantly reduce the time from symptom onset to CT evaluation [3, 4]. Failure to use the emergency number is the most common and most devastating error, with respect to the possibility of timely recanalization therapy [5, 6]. Delays during acute stroke management have been identified at three levels: at the population level (due to failure to recognize the symptoms of stroke and calling the emergency number), at the level of the emergency services and emergency physicians (due to a failure to implement stroke code) and at the hospital level (due to delays in in-hospital logistics and neuroimaging) [6].

To optimize stroke identification, prehospital professionals should use a prehospital stroke screening instrument that has been prospectively evaluated for sensitivity, specificity, reproducibility and validity. Such instruments include the Los Angeles Prehospital Stroke Screen (LAPSS), the Cincinnati Prehospital Stroke Scale (CPSS, or Face-Arm-Speech-Test [FAST]) and the Melbourne Ambulance Stroke Screen (MASS), which all have been reported to have a sensitivity exceeding 90% [7, 8, 9, 10, 11]. The electronic validated algorithm of questions should be used during the emergency phone call.

The stroke code is activated immediately when stroke is suspected [12, 13]. Using a predefined protocol, the patient will be transported to the stroke center, which will be notified in advance. Prehospital notification of an inbound stroke patient has been demonstrated to shorten the delay from ED arrival to initial neurological assessment and initial brain imaging, and to increase the proportion of patients treated with rtPA. Physicians, nurses, CT/MR technologists and pharmacists are able to utilize early notification to mobilize necessary resources for the patient. This is called the Stroke Alarm at the ED. Stroke alarm also means that the patient has a priority for CT and emergency laboratory evaluation. The ESO Guidelines include a class II level B recommendation for immediate EMS contact, priority EMS dispatch and priority transport with prenotification of the receiving hospital, and a class III level B recommendation that suspected stroke victims should be transported without delay to the nearest medical center with a stroke unit that can provide ultra-early treatment [2]. In current guidelines, there is also a class III level B recommendation for immediate ED triage, clinical, laboratory and imaging evaluation, accurate diagnosis, therapeutic decision and administration of appropriate treatments at the receiving hospital [2].

In-hospital delay may account for at least 16% of total time lost between stroke onset and recanalization therapy. Reasons for in-hospital delays are a failure to identify stroke as emergency, inefficient in-hospital transport, delayed medical assessment and imaging and uncertainty in administering thrombolysis [14–16]. In Helsinki, the ED reorganization of acute stroke care has been shown to result in reduced delays in acute stroke treatment, i.e. shorter door-to-rtPA times. The present mean door-to-needle time is 25 minutes, which is based on over 200 patients treated. The main components of the reorganization were:

- Triage
- neuro-ED with written protocols
- ED prenotification by the EMS
- ED rebuild with easy-access CT
- digital patient records, including digital imaging system (PACS) [16].

In remote and rural areas helicopter transfer should be considered to improve access to treatment (class III level C) [2]. Telemedicine is also a feasible, valid and reliable means of facilitating thrombolysis for patients in distant or rural hospitals, where timely air or ground transportation is not feasible (class II level B). The quality of treatment, complication rates and short- and long-term outcomes are similar for acute stroke patients treated with rtPA via a telemedicine consultation at local hospitals and those treated in academic centers [17, 18].

To ensure that a stroke patient presents within the time window allowing thrombolysis to be considered, several pre-admission conditions have to be guaranteed:
- awareness of stroke at the population level
- emergency medical service transport to the emergency department
- prehospital notification of the stroke patient
- emergency department reorganization with easy-access CT.

Stroke unit care

A stroke unit is defined as an organized inpatient area that exclusively or nearly exclusively takes care of stroke patients and is managed by a multidisciplinary team of specialists who are knowledgeable about stroke care. The most distinctive features are a multidisciplinary team specialized in the care of stroke patients (i.e. medical staff, nursing staff and therapists with expertise in stroke and rehabilitation), educational programs for the staff, involvement of caregivers, written care protocols and, more recently, an integrated emergency response system, availability of computed tomography scans 24 hours every day, rapid laboratory testing and experience in stroke thrombolysis [2, 19–22]. Acute stroke patients are more likely to survive, return home and regain independence if they receive stroke unit care [1]. Stroke unit care is effective for all age groups and for any stroke type or severity. Elderly patients and those with severe stroke benefit the most [23]. In spite of such strong scientific evidence, the majority of stroke patients in Europe are treated in general medicine, geriatric and neurology wards by non-specialized staff and only about 14% receive stroke unit care [24]. There have been concerns that the benefits revealed in randomized clinical trials (RCT) including Cochrane systematic reviews may not be possible to achieve in routine practice. A recent systematic review of observational studies verified that the benefits associated with stroke unit care in routine practice are comparable to those of RCTs [1].

There are many types of stroke units, including acute stroke units, combined acute and rehabilitation stroke units, and rehabilitation stroke units admitting patients after a delay of 1–2 weeks, all of which have been shown to improve the outcome of stroke patients, while mobile stroke teams have no major impact on death, dependency or need for institutional care [1, 25–27]. The first generation of stroke intensive care units failed to improve the outcome of stroke patients and there are no RCTs comparing modern stroke intensive care unit care with ordinary acute stroke unit care.

Five principles are relevant for the beneficial effect of stroke units [23–32]:

- a dedicated stroke unit confined only to acute stroke patients
- a multidisciplinary team approach including physicians, nurses, physiotherapists, occupational therapists, speech therapists, neuropsychologists and social workers, all specialized in the care of stroke patients
- a comprehensive stroke unit concept delivering both hyper-acute treatment and early mobilization and rehabilitation by the same multidisciplinary team, including diagnostics and secondary prevention
- automated monitoring of vital functions within the first 72 hours
- thrombolysis for selected patients.

The European Stroke Initiative (EUSI) recently performed a survey among 83 European stroke specialists to learn which in their opinion are the essential components and facilities for good stroke care at three levels: any hospital treating stroke patients (AHW), primary stroke centers (PSC) and comprehensive stroke centers (CSC) [28]. The results needed for AHW are shown in Table 15.1, those needed for PSC in Table 15.2 and those for CSC in Table 15.3. Definitions are in line with the American recommendations of Primary Stroke Centers [33]. The criteria were clearly too demanding for many hospitals, as was detected in the second random survey, which investigated whether European hospitals treating acute stroke patients were able to provide appropriate care as evaluated by these criteria. A questionnaire was sent to 4261 randomly selected hospitals, 1688 of which admitted acute stroke patients. Of these 886 agreed to participate and returned the questionnaire. These 886 hospitals treated over 330 000 acute stroke patients, i.e. approximately one-third of all stroke patients supposed to

Table 15.1. Infrastructure components considered as absolutely necessary (in bold) or as important in AHW treating acute stroke patients on a regular basis by more than 50% of the experts (centers had to meet only 50% of these requirements within each category to qualify as suboptimal minimal standard) [28].

Personnel
Emergency department staff
Multidisciplinary team
Stroke-trained nurses
Neurologists on call
Stroke-trained physician on call
Diagnostic radiologist on call
Internist on staff
Cardiologist on staff
Social worker
Speech therapy start within 2 days
Physiotherapy start within 2 days
Diagnostic procedures
Brain CT scan 24/7
CT priority for stroke patients
Extracranial Doppler sonography
Extracranial duplex sonography
Transthoracic echocardiography
Transesophageal echocardiography
Monitoring
Automated ECG monitoring at bedside
Automated monitoring of pulsoximetry
Automated monitoring of blood pressure
Monitoring of temperature
Infrastructures
Emergency department (in-house)
Collaboration with outside rehabilitation center
Stroke outpatient clinic
Multidisciplinary ICU
Respiratory support
Outpatient rehabilitation available
Treatment, procedures and protocols
Stroke pathways
Stroke care map for patient admission
Prevention program
Intravenous rt-PA protocols 24/7
Community stroke-awareness program

Table 15.2. Infrastructural components considered as absolutely necessary or as important in the PSC by more than 75% of the experts (in bold) or by more than 50% of the experts (normal print) [28].

Personnel
Multidisciplinary team
Stroke-trained nurses
Neurologists on call
Neurologists on staff
Stroke-trained physician (24/7)
Diagnostic radiologist on call
Emergency department staff
Physician expert in carotid ultrasonography
Social worker
Speech therapy start within 2 days
Physiotherapy start within 2 days
Diagnostic procedures
Brain CT scan 24/7
CT priority for stroke patients
Extracranial Doppler sonography
Extracranial duplex sonography
Transthoracic echocardiography
Transesophageal echocardiography
Monitoring
Automated ECG monitoring at bedside
Automated monitoring of pulsoximetry
Automated monitoring of blood pressure
Automated monitoring of breathing
Monitoring of temperature
Infrastructures
Emergency department (in-house)
Stroke outpatient clinic
Multidisciplinary ICU
Inpatient rehabilitation (in-house)
Outpatient rehabilitation available
Collaboration with outside rehabilitation center
Treatment, procedures and protocols
Intravenous rt-PA protocols 24/7
Stroke care map for patient admission
Community stroke-awareness program
Prevention program
Stroke pathways

have suffered stroke in 2005, of whom 8489 received thrombolysis, constituting 3.3% of ischemic strokes. Of 886 hospitals 43 (4.9%) met the criteria for CSC, 32 (3.6%) for PSC and 356 (40.2%) for AHW, while 455 (51.4%) did not meet even the lowest level of care as defined by the European stroke specialists. Of all stroke patients 8.3% were treated in CSC, 5.5% in PSC and 44.1% in AHW, while 42.3% were treated in hospitals meeting none of the accepted levels [24].

Both the First and Second Helsingborg Declarations recommend that all stroke patients should have access to care in specialized stroke units [29, 30]. The recent guidelines by the European Stroke Organisation (ESO) recommends the same thing although the EUSI survey revealed that only one out of seven acute stroke patients are treated in an acute stroke unit and only a minority of European hospitals can provide an optimal level of care for stroke patients. There were huge disparities between countries. According to the survey, only in Finland, Sweden, the Netherlands and Luxemburg were the criteria for decent care met [1, 24]. The Second Helsingborg Declaration listed the minimum criteria for stroke units (Table 15.4) and accepted that these criteria may not be met in all stroke units in all EU member states owing to economic constraints [30].

> Acute stroke patients are more likely to survive, return home and regain independence if they receive stroke unit care.

Early activities at a stroke unit

The time window for treatment of patients with acute stroke is narrow and requires well-organized services at the ED and acute stroke unit. The points which must be kept in mind include:

- acute emergency management of stroke requires parallel processes at different levels of patient management
- acute assessment of neurological and vital functions parallels treatment of acutely life-threatening conditions

Table 15.3. Components considered as absolutely necessary for a CSC by 75% (in bold) or 50% of the experts (normal print) [28].

Personnel
Multidisciplinary team
Stroke-trained nurses
Physiotherapy start within 2 days
Neurologists (24/7)
Stroke-trained physician (24/7)
Interventional neuroradiologist on call
Neurosurgeon on call
CEA vascular surgeon
Emergency department staff
Physician expert in carotid ultrasonography
Physician expert in echocardiography
Speech therapy start within 2 days
Physiotherapy start within 2 days

Diagnostic procedures
Brain CT scan 24/7
CT priority for stroke patients
Extracranial Doppler sonography
Extracranial duplex sonography
Transthoracic echocardiography
MRI (T1, T2, T2*, FLAIR) 24/7
Diffusion-weighted MRI
Extracranial Doppler sonography 24/7
Extracranial duplex sonography 24/7
Transcranial Doppler 24/7
CT angiography 24/7
Magnetic resonance angiography 24/7
Transfemoral cerebral angio 24/7
Transesophageal echo

Monitoring
Automated ECG monitoring at bedside
Automated monitoring of pulsoximetry
Automated monitoring of blood pressure
Automated monitoring of breathing
Monitoring of temperature

Invasive treatments provided
Intravenous rtPA protocols 24/7
Carotid surgery
Angioplasty and stenting
Intra-arterial thrombolysis 24/7
Respiratory support
Surgery for aneurysms
Hemicraniectomy
Ventricular drainage

Table 15.4. Helsingborg Declaration 2006: minimum criteria for a stroke unit [30].

- Dedicated beds for stroke patients
- Dedicated team: stroke physician, trained nurses and rehabilitation staff (e.g. physical therapy, speech therapy, occupational therapy)
- Immediate imaging 24 hours (CT or MRI). It is realized that this criterion may not be met in all stroke units in all EU member states due to economic constraints
- Written protocols and pathways for diagnostic procedures, acute treatment, monitoring to prevent complications and secondary prevention
- Availability of neurosurgery, vascular surgery, interventional neuroradiology, cardiology is preferable but not an absolute requirement for a stroke unit
- Immediate start of mobilization and access to early rehabilitation
- Continuing staff education

- the selection of special treatment strategies may already be ongoing before the final decision on the subtype of acute stroke has been made.

Time is the most important factor, especially the first minutes and hours after stroke onset. During those hours the following tasks need to be performed:
- differentiate between different types of stroke
- assess the underlying cause of brain ischemia
- provide a basis for physiological monitoring of the stroke patient

223

- identify concurrent diseases or complications associated with stroke
- rule out other brain diseases
- assess prognosis.

Stroke unit care reduces the risk of death after stroke but it is not entirely clear how that is achieved. Further analysis of systemic reviews revealed that organized stroke unit care appears to reduce the risk of death after stroke through prevention and treatment of complications, in particular infections [2].

Clinical assessment

There is general agreement that stroke severity should be assessed by trained staff using the National Institutes of Health Stroke Scale (NIHSS). In addition, the initial examination should include:

- observation of breathing and pulmonary function
- early signs of dysphagia, preferably using a validated scale
- evaluation of concomitant heart disease
- assessment of blood pressure (BP) and heart rate
- determination of arterial oxygen saturation using infrared pulse oximetry.

Close monitoring is essential (see Chapter 17) to ascertain stable vital functions (airway, breathing and cardiovascular function). If they are compromised, intensive care may be necessary until the clinical situation is stable.

Diagnostic work-up

Table 15.5 lists the recommended diagnostic procedures as advocated by the ESO. Although not yet clearly stated in the guidelines, the exact neurovascular diagnosis based on predominantly non-invasive angiographic tests is soon likely to be the standard, and is already applied in the majority of stroke centers [2, 24]. In-depth discussion of diagnostic work-up can be found in Chapters 2–4.

In addition to imaging, early evaluation of physiological parameters, routine blood tests and 12-channel electrocardiography (ECG) followed by continuous ECG recording should be performed according to the ESO class I level A recommendation. When arrhythmias are suspected and no other cause of stroke is found, a 24-hour Holter ECG monitoring should also be performed, although modern patient-monitoring systems may have the same functionality

Table 15.5. Diagnostic tests at the acute stroke unit recommended by ESO [2].

In all patients	
1	Brain imaging: CT or MRI
2	ECG
3	Laboratory tests Complete blood count and platelet count, prothrombin time or INR, PTT, serum electrolytes, blood glucose, CRP or sedimentation rate Hepatic and renal chemical analysis
When indicated	
4	Extracranial and transcranial duplex/Doppler ultrasound
5	MRA or CTA
6	Diffusion and perfusion MR or perfusion CT
7	Echocardiography (transthoracic and/or transesophageal)
8	Chest X-ray
9	Pulse oximetry and arterial blood gas analysis
10	Lumbar puncture
11	EEG
12	Toxicology screen

built in. Diagnostic cardiac ultrasound is recommended in selected patients (class III level B). Systematic use of these methods may result in an increased proportion of cardioembolic stroke [2, 34].

General management, monitoring and complications

The success of stroke unit care is believed to depend on general management, careful monitoring and normalization of physiological parameters, as well as proactive prevention and treatment of medical complications. No RCTs address this, therefore level I class A recommendations do not exist. The recommendations are based on consensus statements of experts such as Guidelines for Management of Ischaemic Stroke and Transient Ischaemic Attack by the ESO and Recommendations for the Establishment of Primary Stroke Centers by the Brain Attack Coalition [33]. The cornerstones of this approach, as recommended by the ESO, are summarized in Tables 15.6 and 15.7 and will be discussed in more detail in Chapter 17 [2].

Table 15.6. ESO Guidelines for general monitoring and treatment [2].

- Intermittent monitoring of neurological status, pulse, blood pressure, temperature and oxygen saturation is recommended for 72 hours in patients with significant persisting neurological deficits

- It is recommended that oxygen should be administered if the oxygen saturation falls below 95%

- Regular monitoring of fluid balance and electrolytes is recommended in patients with severe stroke or swallowing problems (class IV, GCP)

- Normal saline (0.9%) is recommended for fluid replacement during the first 24 hours after stroke

- Routine blood pressure lowering is not recommended following acute stroke

- Cautious blood pressure lowering is recommended in patients with extremely high blood pressures (>220/120 mmHg) on repeated measurements, or with severe cardiac failure, aortic dissection or hypertensive encephalopathy

- It is recommended that abrupt blood pressure lowering be avoided. It is recommended that low blood pressure secondary to hypovolemia or associated with neurological deterioration in acute stroke should be treated with volume expanders

- Monitoring serum glucose levels is recommended

- Treatment of serum glucose levels >180 mg/dl (>10 mmol/l) with insulin titration is recommended

- It is recommended that severe hypoglycemia (<50 mg/dl [<2.8 mmol/l]) should be treated with intravenous dextrose or infusion of 10–20% glucose

- It is recommended that the presence of pyrexia (temperature > 37.5°C) should prompt a search for concurrent infection. Treatment of pyrexia (temperature > 37.5°C) with paracetamol and fanning is recommended

- Antibiotic prophylaxis is not recommended in immunocompetent patients

- Swallowing assessment is recommended but there are insufficient data to recommend a specific approach for treatment

- Oral dietary supplements are only recommended for non-dysphagic stroke patients who are malnourished

- Early commencement of nasogastric (NG) feeding (within 48 hours) is recommended in stroke patients with impaired swallowing

- It is recommended that percutaneous enteral gastrostomy (PEG) feeding should not be considered in stroke patients in the first 2 weeks

Table 15.7. ESO Guidelines for management of complications [2].

- It is recommended that infections after stroke should be treated with appropriate antibiotics

- Prophylactic administration of antibiotics is not recommended, and levofloxacin can be detrimental in acute stroke patients

- Early rehydration and graded compression stockings are recommended to reduce the incidence of venous thromboembolism

- Early mobilization is recommended to prevent complications such as aspiration pneumonia, DVT and pressure ulcers

- It is recommended that low-dose subcutaneous heparin or low molecular weight heparins should be considered for patients at high risk of DVT or pulmonary embolism

Acute treatment

Acute treatments and interventions for stroke including thrombolytic therapy and endovascular procedures are discussed in Chapter 16. From the organizational point of view, intravenous thrombolytic therapy is most often administered in the ED instead of the stroke unit, where rescue therapies after unsuccessful intravenous thrombolysis may still be considered, provided that the time window is still open and depending on the indications and possible contraindications for the therapy. Stroke unit administration of i.v. rtPA requires immediate transfer of the patient, bypassing the ED. The specific treatments at a stroke unit are shown in Table 15.8 [2].

Elevated intracranial pressure

The most common cause of death in the acute stage of a major stroke is increased intracranial pressure and herniation due to brain edema. Decompressive craniectomy has now a class I level A recommendation in malignant ischemic MCA stroke patients younger than

225

Table 15.8. ESO Guidelines for specific treatments [2].

- Intravenous rtPA (0.9 mg/kg body weight, maximum 90 mg), with 10% of the dose given as a bolus followed by a 60-minute infusion, is recommended within 3 hours of onset of ischemic stroke

- Intravenous rtPA may be of benefit also for acute ischemic stroke beyond 3 hours after onset but is not recommended for routine clinical practice

- The use of multimodal imaging criteria may be useful for patient selection for thrombolysis but is not recommended for routine clinical practice

- It is recommended that blood pressures of 185/110 mmHg or higher are lowered before thrombolysis

- It is recommended that intravenous rtPA may be used in patients with seizures at stroke onset, if the neurological deficit is related to acute cerebral ischemia

- It is recommended that intravenous rtPA may also be administered in selected patients under 18 years and over 80 years of age, although this is outside the current European labeling

- Intra-arterial treatment of acute MCA occlusion within a 6-hour time window is recommended as an option

- Intra-arterial thrombolysis is recommended for acute basilar occlusion in selected patients. Intravenous thrombolysis for basilar occlusion is an acceptable alternative even after 3 hours

- It is recommended that aspirin (160–325 mg loading dose) be given within 48 hours after ischemic stroke

Table 15.9. ESO Guidelines for elevated intracranial pressure [2].

- Surgical decompressive therapy within 48 hours after symptom onset is recommended in patients up to 60 years of age with evolving malignant MCA infarcts

- It is recommended that osmotherapy can be used to treat elevated intracranial pressure prior to surgery if this is considered

- No recommendation can be given regarding hypothermic therapy in patients with space-occupying infarctions

- It is recommended that ventriculostomy or surgical decompression be considered for treatment of large cerebellar infarctions that compress the brainstem

of treatment is based on the most likely etiology of the stroke and all the patient's risk factors. Secondary prevention strategies should be planned and initiated at the stroke unit and continued in community health care by a general practitioner or family doctor as soon as the patient has been discharged from the hospital [2].

Early rehabilitation

Rehabilitation of stroke patients will be discussed in Chapter 19. All patients need to be assessed at the stroke unit by a physiotherapist, occupational therapist, speech therapist and neurophysiologist of the multidisciplinary stroke team within the first week after the onset of stroke. There is great variability in rehabilitation resources and staff between geographical regions and hospitals, but in general all available therapists should be involved in the early assessment and design of the rehabilitation plan of every acute stroke patient. The rehabilitation plan is much like a tailor-made suit, which is started at the stroke unit and continued and modified based on the progress of the patient at a rehabilitation hospital, outpatient clinic and at home. For all stroke patients follow-up by community health care is crucial to ensure that the functional outcome reached during rehabilitation will endure. Many patients need the rehabilitation services of the community from time to time to be able to keep their independence in daily life and to be able to live in their own homes, knowing that such late rehabilitation is not supported by RCTs [2].

60–65 years of age, and it is currently the only treatment shown in RCTs to be able to reduce mortality in this patient group [32]. Except for craniectomy for selected patients, recommendations are based on a lower level of evidence. The recent ESO Guidelines give practical advice on how to treat stroke patients with increased intracranial pressure (Table 15.9) [2, 20–22].

Secondary prevention

Secondary prevention, discussed in detail in Chapter 19, should start as early as possible, i.e. at the ED or in the stroke unit at the latest. It is recommended that aspirin (160–325 mg loading dose) should be given within 48 hours after ischemic stroke if thrombolysis is not administered, or 24 hours after thrombolysis. Selection

Advantages of centralized stroke management organization

In Finland, as in most Scandinavian countries, stroke care is organized in a more straightforward and centralized manner if compared to most EU countries and the USA. The EMS organization consists of a national ERC administration providing emergency response services for the entire country. There are no overlapping EMS services, and in many areas only one EMS provider, supervised by an EMS physician at the university hospital or regional hospital. Furthermore, only one hospital is in charge for acute stroke care of the municipality. Tertiary referral is rare because even comprehensive stroke centers take primary responsibility for stroke care, i.e. are the first admitting hospitals for most stroke patients. The Nordic type of centralized care also means easier administration, so that all involved in the chain of recovery, from EMS to rehabilitation and community health care, can be instantly instructed in new paradigms.

A stroke unit oversees:
- emergency management
- clinical assessment of vital functions
- diagnostic work-up, including stroke type, cause of brain ischemia and other brain diseases
- management of complications
- acute treatment, including thrombolytic therapy and endovascular procedures
- implementation of secondary prevention and rehabilitation.

Conclusions

According to the frequently cited ESO 2008 Guidelines, it is now recommended (class I level A) that all stroke patients irrespective of age, sex, gender or severity of stroke should be treated in a stroke unit in a primary (or comprehensive) stroke center. The healthcare system should ensure that acute stroke patients can access high-technology medical and surgical stroke care when required (class III level B). The development of clinical networks, including telemedicine, is recommended to expand the access to high-technology specialist stroke care (class II level B) [2].

Is this the recipe for the future? It is easy to predict that among the key elements for future success in acute stroke care will be centralized acute care, shortening delays at every step, increasing stroke awareness, identification of barriers that may prevent direct and immediate access to a stroke center, ERC, EMS and ED involvement in prehospital management, in-hospital pathways and protocols as well as well-organized systematic routines for fast implementation of evidence-based medicine, including telestroke in selected hospitals.

Chapter Summary

Emergency medical service (EMS) transport of a stroke patient to the emergency department (ED) increases the likelihood of a patient presenting within the 3-hour time-window allowing thrombolysis to be considered. To reduce delays, awareness of stroke at the population level is pivotal. Prehospital professionals should use a prehospital stroke screening instrument that has been prospectively evaluated for sensitivity, specificity, reproducibility and validity. Prehospital notification of inbound stroke patients has been demonstrated to shorten the delay from ED arrival to initial neurological assessment and initial brain imaging, and to increase the proportion of patients treated with rtPA. Reorganization of acute stroke care has been shown to result in reduced delays in acute stroke treatment, i.e. shorter door-to-rtPA times.

A stroke unit is defined as an organized inpatient area that exclusively or nearly exclusively takes care of stroke patients and is managed by a multidisciplinary team of specialists who are knowledgeable about stroke care. Acute stroke patients are more likely to survive, return home and regain independence if they receive stroke unit care. Five principles are relevant for the beneficial effect of stroke units:
- a dedicated stroke unit confined only to acute stroke patients
- a multidisciplinary team approach
- a stroke unit concept delivering both hyperacute treatment and early mobilization and rehabilitation by the same multidisciplinary team, including diagnostics and secondary prevention
- automated monitoring of vital functions within the first 72 hours
- thrombolysis for selected patients.

Activities at a stroke unit:
- early assessment, including type of stroke, the underlying cause of brain ischemia and other brain diseases
- clinical assessment of stroke severity, breathing and pulmonary function, dysphagia, concomitant

heart disease, blood pressure, heart rate and arterial oxygen saturation
- diagnostic work-up
- general management, careful monitoring and normalization of physiological parameters, as well as proactive prevention and treatment of medical complications
- acute treatments and interventions of stroke, including thrombolytic therapy and endovascular procedures (see Table 15.8)
- management of elevated intracranial pressure (e.g. decompressive craniectomy)
- start of secondary prevention measures, e.g. aspirin
- design of the rehabilitation plan.

References

1. Stroke Unit Trialists' Collaboration: Organised inpatient (stroke unit) care for stroke. *Cochrane Database Syst Rev* 2007; CD000197.

2. European Stroke Organisation (ESO) Executive Committee; ESO Writing Committee. Guidelines for management of ischaemic stroke and transient ischaemic attack 2008. *Cerebrovasc Dis* 2008; 25(5):457–507.

3. Kothari R, Jauch E, Broderick J, et al. Acute stroke: delays to presentation and emergency department evaluation. *Ann Emerg Med* 1999; 33(1):3–8.

4. Schroeder EB, Rosamond WD, Morris DL, et al. Determinants of use of emergency medical services in a population with stroke symptoms: the second delay in accessing stroke healthcare (dash ii) study. *Stroke* 2000; 31:2591–6.

5. Morris DL, Rosamond W, Madden K, et al. Prehospital and emergency department delays after acute stroke: the Genentech Stroke Presentation Survey. *Stroke* 2000; 31 (11):2585–90.

6. Kwan J, Hand P, Sandercock P. A systematic review of barriers to delivery of thrombolysis for acute stroke. *Age Ageing* 2004; 33:116–21.

7. Kothari R, Barsan W, Brott T, et al. Frequency and accuracy of prehospital diagnosis of acute stroke. *Stroke* 1995; 26(6):937–41.

8. Kothari RU, Pancioli A, Liu T, et al. Cincinnati prehospital stroke scale: reproducibility and validity. *Ann Emerg Med* 1999; 33(4):373–8.

9. Nor A, Mc Allister C, Louw S, et al. Agreement between ambulance paramedic – and physician – recorded neurological signs using the Face Arm Speech Test (FAST) in acute stroke patients. *Stroke* 2004; 35:1355–9.

10. Kidwell CS, Starkman S, Eckstein M, et al. Identifying stroke in the field. Prospective validation of the Los Angeles prehospital stroke screen (LAPSS). *Stroke* 2000; 31(1):71–6.

11. Bray JE, Martin J, Cooper G, et al. Paramedic identification of stroke: community validation of the Melbourne ambulance stroke screen. *Cerebrovasc Dis* 2005; 20(1):28–33.

12. Belvis R, Cocho D, Martí-Fàbregas J, et al. Benefits of a prehospital stroke code system. *Cerebrovasc Dis* 2005; 19(2):96–101.

13. Gomez CR, Malkoff MD, Sauer CM, et al. Code stroke. An attempt to shorten inhospital therapeutic delays. *Stroke* 1994; 25(10):1920–3.

14. Nor AM, Davis J, Sen B, et al. The Recognition of Stroke in the Emergency Room (ROSIER) scale: development and validation of a stroke recognition instrument. *Lancet Neurol* 2005; 4(11):727–34.

15. Morgenstern LB, et al. Improving delivery of acute stroke therapy: The TLL Temple Foundation Stroke Project. *Stroke* 2002; 33(1):160–6.

16. Lindsberg PJ, Häppölä O, Kallela M, et al. Door to thrombolysis: ER reorganization and reduced delays to acute stroke treatment. *Neurology* 2006; 67(2):334–6.

17. Audebert H, Schenkel J, Heuschmann P, et al. Effects of the implementation of a telemedical stroke network: the Telemedic Pilot Project for Integrative Stroke Care (TEMPiS) in Bavaria, Germany. *Lancet Neurol* 2006; 5:742–8.

18. Hess DC, Wang S, Gross H, et al. Telestroke: extending stroke expertise into underserved areas. *Lancet Neurol* 2006; 5(3):275–8.

19. Alberts MJ, Hademenos G, Latchaw RE, et al. Recommendations for the establishment of primary stroke centers. Brain Attack Coalition. *JAMA* 2000; 283(23):3102–9.

20. Acker JE 3rd, Pancioli AM, Crocco TJ, et al. American Heart Association; American Stroke Association Expert Panel on Emergency Medical Services Systems, Stroke Council. Implementation strategies for emergency medical services within stroke systems of care: a policy statement from the American Heart Association/American Stroke Association Expert Panel on Emergency Medical Services Systems and the Stroke Council. *Stroke* 2007; 38(11):3097–115.

21. Adams HP Jr, del Zoppo G, Alberts MJ, et al. Guidelines for the early management of adults with ischemic stroke: a guideline from the American Heart Association/American Stroke Association Stroke

Council, Clinical Cardiology Council, Cardiovascular Radiology and Intervention Council, and the Atherosclerotic Peripheral Vascular Disease and Quality of Care Outcomes in Research Interdisciplinary Working Groups. *Stroke* 2007; **38**(5):1655–711.

22. Broderick J, Connolly S, Feldmann E, et al. Guidelines for the management of spontaneous intracerebral hemorrhage in adults: 2007 update: a guideline from the American Heart Association/American Stroke Association Stroke Council, High Blood Pressure Research Council, and the Quality of Care and Outcomes in Research Interdisciplinary Working Group. *Stroke* 2007; **38**(6):2001–23.

23. Langhorne P, Dennis M. *Stroke Units: an evidence based approach*. London: BMJ Books; 1999.

24. Leys D, Ringelstein E, Kaste M, Hacke W, and the Executive Committee of the European Stroke Initiative. Facilities Available in European Hospitals Treating Stroke Patients. *Stroke* 2007; **38** (11):2985–91.

25. Seenan P, Long M, Langhorne P. Stroke units in their natural habitat. Systematic review of observational studies. *Stroke* 2007; **38**(6):1886–92.

26. Langhorne P, Dey P, Woodman M, et al. Is stroke unit care portable? A systematic review of the clinical trials. *Age Aging* 2005; **34**(4):324–30.

27. Asplund K, Indredavik B. Stroke units and stroke teams: evidence-based management of stroke. In: Castillo J, Davalos A, Toni D, eds. *Management of Acute Ischemic Stroke*. Barcelona: Springer Verlag Iberica; 1997: 3–15.

28. Leys D, Ringelstein EB, Kaste M, et al. for the European Stroke Initiative executive committee. The main components of stroke unit care: results of a European Expert survey. *Cerebrovasc Dis* 2007; **23**(5–6):344–52.

29. Aboderin I, Venables G, for the Pan European Consensus Meeting. Stroke management in Europe. *J Intern Med* 1996; **240**(4):173–80.

30. Kjellström T, Norrving B, Shatchkute A. Helsingborg Declaration 2006 on European stroke strategies. *Cerebrovasc Dis* 2007; **23**(2–3):231–41.

31. Govan L, Langhorne P, Weir CJ, for the Stroke Unit Trialists' Collaboration. Does the prevention of complications explain the survival benefit of organized inpatient (Stroke Unit) care? Further analysis of a systematic review. *Stroke* 2007; **38** (9):2536–40.

32. Vahedi K, Hofmeijer J, Juettler E, et al. for DECIMAL, DESTINY, and HAMLET investigators. Early decompressive surgery in malignant infarction of the middle cerebral artery: a pooled analysis of three randomised controlled trials. *Lancet Neurol* 2007; **6**(3):215–22.

33. Alberts MJ, Latchaw RE, Selman WR, et al. Recommendations for comprehensive stroke centers: a consensus statement of the Brain Attack Coalition. *Stroke* 2005; **36**(7):1597–616.

34. Sulter G, Elting JW, Langedijk M, et al. Admitting acute ischemic stroke patients to a stroke care monitoring unit versus a conventional stroke unit: a randomized pilot study. *Stroke* 2003; **34**:101–4.

Chapter 16

Acute therapies and interventions

Richard O'Brien, Thorsten Steiner and Kennedy R. Lees

Introduction

Over recent decades the early management of acute stroke has changed dramatically and the early post-stroke period has been the focus of much research. With advances in pharmacotherapeutics, and on the basis of many randomized controlled trials, the potential interventions now available within the first 24–48 hours following acute stroke are numerous.

This chapter will present the evidence and best practice guidance for interventions during the first 24–48 hours following stroke, based upon the European Stroke Organisation Guidelines 2008 and the European Stroke Initiative recommendations for the management of intracranial hemorrhage [1, 2]. For the purposes of this chapter, the interventions discussed will generally be limited to the initial 48 hours following ictus. Access to some of these therapies may not be universal and may be dictated by local availability at individual stroke units. As with other aspects of stroke care, however, close cooperation and inter-disciplinary communication are essential.

Thrombolysis

In respect of acute interventions, one of the most significant advances during the last two decades has been the introduction of intravenous thrombolysis as a standard therapy for a well-selected population of patients with acute ischemic stroke. At present, the only thrombolytic agent licensed in Europe for the treatment of ischemic stroke is recombinant-tissue plasminogen activator (rtPA), alteplase. The evidence for its use comes from six landmark clinical trials: the Alteplase Thrombolysis for Acute Noninterventional Therapy in Ischaemic Stroke (ATLANTIS) trials A and B; the European Cooperative Stroke Study (ECASS) and ECASS II; and the two-part National Institute of Neurological Disorders and Stroke

(NINDS) rtPA study [1, 3–6]. These studies varied in timing and dose of rtPA, which may account for some of the differences in outcomes reported in each of the trials. The NINDS rtPA study demonstrated an odds ratio of 1.7 (95% confidence interval 1.2 to 2.6) for a favorable outcome at 3 months with rtPA treatment when administered within 3 hours of ischemic stroke onset, with the number needed to treat to achieve a favorable outcome of 7 [4]. In contrast, the ECASS studies (I and II) did not confirm significant benefit of rtPA although this was when administration occurred within 6 hours of ictus [3, 5]. However, analysis of the pooled data from the ATLANTIS, ECASS and NINDS rtPA trials has confirmed the beneficial effect of timely intervention with intravenous thrombolysis [7]. This analysis included 2775 patients in whom thrombolysis was initiated within 6 hours of ischemic stroke onset. The odds of a favorable outcome were inversely associated with delay from stroke onset to treatment, with those patients treated earliest following their stroke having the most favorable outcome. Favorable outcome at 3 months was defined as a modified Rankin Score of 0 or 1, a Barthel Index between 95 and 100, and National Institutes of Health Stroke Scale score of 0 or 1. More specifically, the analysis identified an adjusted odds ratio for favorable outcome at 3 months of 2.81 (95% confidence interval 1.75–4.50) for patients treated within the first 90 minutes of stroke, 1.55 (1.12–2.15) when treatment was commenced 91–180 minutes following onset, falling to 1.40 (1.05–1.85) and 1.15 (0.90–1.47) when thrombolytic treatment was commenced within 181–270 and 271–360 minutes from stroke onset respectively [7]. These benefits have been demonstrated without a significantly increased risk of death, but the proportion of patients with significant parenchymal hemorrhage, defined as blood clot exceeding 30% infarct volume with significant space-occupying effect, was larger in rtPA-treated patients (5.6% versus 1.0% in those who received treatment between 91 and 180 minutes following stroke onset). Of clinical importance, the proportion of patients suffering secondary parenchymal hemorrhage was associated with increasing age, but not with time from onset to treatment or baseline NIHSS score.

> Intravenous thrombolysis is a standard therapy for a well-selected population of patients with acute ischemic stroke. Within the 3-hour window the number needed to treat to achieve one favorable outcome is 7.

The benefits of intravenous thrombolysis are therefore greatest when treatment is initiated early following stroke. Until now, regulatory authorities have placed an upper limit of 3 hours for routine use of alteplase after stroke. The benefits extend beyond 3 hours, however. The SITS register has shown that treatment at an average of 3 hours 15 minutes and out until 4.5 hours after stroke onset remains as safe as earlier treatment in routine clinical practice [54]. This suggests that whilst early treatment remains desirable, patients in whom treatment cannot start within 3 hours should not be deprived of therapy for the sake of a few minutes delay. More compelling are the results of the third ECASS trial, which found an odds ratio for achieving favorable outcome of 1.34 (95% confidence interval 1.02–1.76) with treatment in the 3.0–4.5-hour window [55], effectively confirming the estimate of 1.4 that derives from meta-analysis [7]. There is thus good reason for clinicians and regulatory authorities to consider relaxation of the strict 3-hour window for alteplase treatment in favor of a 4.5-hour limit, provided that all unnecessary delays are avoided. Patients who receive timely treatment with intravenous rtPA have better odds of minimizing disability following their stroke, and although the risks of parenchymal hemorrhage are slightly greater in patients who receive thrombolysis, the odds of death are not significantly increased. The benefits of thrombolysis are not necessarily seen immediately but are present after 3 months following stroke [7]. It is good practice to discuss the risks and benefits of treatment with patients or their family before treatment is commenced and to emphasize that the aim of thrombolytic treatment is to improve the chances of the patients being independent several months after their stroke.

Post hoc analyses of thrombolysis data have identified factors associated with a poor outcome following intravenous thrombolysis, and these results have helped to inform clinical practice. Elevated serum glucose, increasing age and increasing stroke severity are among the poor prognostic factors which have been identified [8]. Appropriate patient selection is therefore important when considering whether a patient may be suitable for thrombolysis treatment. At present European regulatory agencies do not support the routine use of intravenous rtPA in patients beyond 3 hours, or in those with severe stroke (NIHSS > 24), extended early ischemic changes on CT or in those over the age of 80 years [1]. There is some evidence that thrombolysis is safe in elderly patients and therefore most clinicians will base their decision to offer thrombolysis upon the patient's 'physiological age' rather than their 'chronological age' [9]. The European license for alteplase does, however, exclude its use in those over the age of 80 years. Thrombolysis is contraindicated in patients with seizure at stroke onset due to the possibility of confusion with Todd's paresis, which may be present as a stroke mimic. Patients with severe hypertension at the time of admission were excluded from the trials of thrombolysis and therefore blood pressure is recommended to be below 185/110 mmHg before, and for the first 24 hours after, thrombolytic therapy. Severe hypertension increases the risks of hemorrhagic transformation following thrombolysis [8]. Indications and contraindications for thrombolysis are listed in Table 16.1. The dose of alteplase is weight-dependent at 0.9 mg/kg up to a maximum dose of 90 mg. Ten percent of the total dose is administered as an intravenous bolus with the remaining 90% delivered over 1 hour. Aspirin and other antiplatelets or anticoagulants should be avoided for 24 hours following thrombolysis, as should arterial puncture at a non-compressible site.

Various techniques have been employed to help facilitate effective thrombolysis and vessel recanalization, including transcranial Doppler "sonothrombolysis" and microbubble administration, but these are not currently in routine clinical use [1, 10]. Multimodal imaging technologies, such as perfusion CT and diffusion-weighted MRI, are being studied in the hope of improving patient selection for thrombolysis and extending the time window for intervention, but such procedures are not currently in routine use and are beyond the scope of this chapter.

Table 16.1. Indications and contraindications for intravenous thrombolysis in acute ischemic stroke.

Indication	Contraindication
Stroke onset within 3 hours	Previous intracranial hemorrhage
CT/MRI exclusion of hemorrhage and extensive infarct (>1/3 of MCA territory)	Ischemic stroke within 3 months
Serum glucose >2.7 and <22.2 mmol/l	Seizure at stroke onset
BP <185 mmHg systolic and/or 110 mmHg diastolic	Recent major surgery
NIHSS >3 and <25	Unexplained hemorrhage
Age 18–80 years	INR > 1.4
	Platelets < 150 × 10^9/l
	Rapid neurological recovery

The approved agent is recombinant tissue plasminogen activator (rtPA), alteplase, in a dose of 0.9 mg/kg up to a maximum dose of 90 mg (10% administered as a bolus, 90% over 1 hour). Patients with a delay > 3 hours, age > 80 years, blood pressure > 185/110 mmHg, severe stroke (NIHSS > 24) or seizure at stroke onset should be excluded.

Having identified patients who are potential candidates for intravenous thrombolysis, systems must be in place to ensure their timely transfer to an appropriate medical facility and rapid access to assessment and imaging once admitted. The exact structure of a stroke service will vary depending on local factors. Structuring thrombolysis services in places where patient populations are spread over large rural areas can be particularly challenging. The structure of such a service will differ depending on local needs and no single model can be claimed to be superior to another. Novel technologies such as telemedicine have been employed in some rural areas. The important common factors which ensure a safe and effective service are that patients should be assessed and diagnosed by physicians experienced in stroke care [1, 11]. Brain imaging should also be reviewed by a physician with the appropriate experience and training, although this does not necessarily need to be a radiologist.

In practice, due to the time constraint of initiating therapy within 3 hours of stroke onset, consideration needs to be given to the geographical location of the acute stroke unit in comparison to radiology and other acute services.

A request associated with the European license for alteplase was that outcome data should be collected prospectively for the first 3 years or 1000 patients on patients in whom alteplase was used for acute ischemic stroke thrombolysis. The Safe Implementation of Thrombolysis in Stroke – Monitoring Study (SITS-MOST) collected data on 6483 patients [11]. Reassuringly, it provided evidence that the use of intravenous thrombolysis in routine clinical practice results in outcomes comparable to those observed in clinical trials. The proportions of patients achieving independence (modified Rankin Score, mRS < 3) at 3 months were similar in the SITS-MOST group compared to the pooled randomized controlled trials, with lower rates of symptomatic intracerebral hemorrhage and mortality observed in the SITS-MOST data. This confirms the safety and efficacy of using rtPA for acute ischemic stroke in well-selected patients with acute ischemic stroke.

Although some evidence exists to support the use of intra-arterial thrombolysis for proximal occlusions of the middle cerebral artery (MCA) within 6 hours of onset, it is not currently established as a routine treatment option in the majority of centers [1]. The studies investigating intra-arterial thrombolysis have used pro-urokinase, which is currently not available in Europe, and large-scale studies using rtPA as an intra-arterial agent are lacking. A clinical trial investigating the efficacy of the combination of intravenous and intra-arterial rtPA compared to intravenous thrombolysis alone is currently under way [1]. No significant difference between intravenous and intra-arterial thrombolysis has been demonstrated for patients with basilar artery occlusion in non-randomized comparisons [1].

Intra-arterial thrombolysis is used in selected cases up to 6 hours after MCA occlusion, but is not established as a routine treatment option.

Patients who meet the criteria for intravenous thrombolysis remain in the minority, with rates for intravenous thrombolysis varying, but relatively low, throughout Europe. Whilst strategies are being developed to improve the rapid recognition and assessment of patients who may be suitable for intravenous thrombolysis, the majority of patients remain ineligible. For those who are ineligible for intravenous thrombolysis as part of routine clinical care, and in whom participating in a clinical research trial is either inappropriate or impossible, best supportive care is offered and other alternative interventions should be considered.

Mechanical embolus removal

The Mechanical Embolectomy Removal in Cerebral Ischemia (MERCI) trial, published in 2005, reported vessel re-canalization in 68 of the 141 (48%) patients ineligible for conventional intravenous thrombolysis and in whom the embolectomy device was deployed within 8 hours of stroke onset [12]. This exceeds the proportion expected from a historical control population (18%) and favorable neurological outcomes were observed in those patients who achieved successful re-canalization. To date there are no randomized controlled trial data available for embolectomy devices and consequently their use is not currently part of routine clinical practice.

> Mechanical embolus removal achieves recanalization in a high proportion, but controlled trial data are not yet available.

Aspirin

The benefits of low-dose aspirin in preventing recurrent serious vascular events in patients with transient ischemic attack, ischemic stroke or myocardial infarction have been established for more than 10 years [13]. The potential benefits of commencing aspirin therapy in patients early after the onset of ischemic stroke were not realized until the publication of two large randomized controlled trials, the Chinese Acute Stroke Trial (CAST) and the International Stroke Trial (IST) [14, 15]. With a combined study population of more than 40 000 patients, these two landmark studies provide strong evidence supporting the early introduction of aspirin following ischemic stroke. Aspirin was commenced within 48 hours of stroke onset in both studies, and continued for up to 14 days in IST and up to 4 weeks in CAST. In the CAST aspirin treatment was associated with a slight increase in hemorrhagic stroke (1.1% vs. 0.9%), offset by a significant 14% reduction in mortality (3.3% vs. 3.9%) and early recurrent ischemic stroke (1.6% vs. 2.1%). This corresponded to 11 fewer patients per 1000 treated with aspirin who were dead

or dependent at the time of discharge [15]. Similar results were observed in the IST with a significant reduction in early recurrent ischemic stroke observed in the aspirin-treated group (2.8% vs. 3.9%) without an associated excess of intracerebral hemorrhage, although the number of early deaths was similar between groups [14]. Early aspirin use (within 48 hours of stroke onset) was associated with a significant reduction in death or non-fatal recurrent stroke. In absolute terms, 13 fewer patients per 1000 treated with aspirin were dead or dependent at 6 months following their stroke. In both studies, a computed tomography (CT) scan to exclude intracerebral hemorrhage was mandatory only in comatose patients, although it was considered preferable prior to randomization. Given that access to brain imaging, either by CT or MRI, is now generally universally available within the first 24 hours of admission to an acute stroke unit, aspirin can justifiably be withheld until intracerebral bleeding has been excluded. CT readily distinguishes between ischemic and hemorrhagic stroke within the first 5–7 days and is most cost-effective when performed immediately [1, 16]. The dose of aspirin prescribed varied between the CAST and IST (160 mg daily and 300 mg daily respectively) and other doses have been used in other studies. Once intracranial hemorrhage has been excluded aspirin should be administered at the earliest opportunity at a dose of 300 mg either orally or rectally depending on the patient's ability to swallow safely. Subsequent doses can be lower (75–300 mg), with the evidence suggesting that the same benefit can be conferred with 75 mg daily whilst avoiding the potential side-effects which are more commonly observed at higher doses [17]. Although the absolute benefits provided by early aspirin use are small, this intervention is available to the majority of patients who have suffered ischemic strokes. Therefore, on a population level, initiating early aspirin treatment has the potential to reduce the number of recurrent vascular events by several thousand worldwide.

> A dose of 300 mg aspirin should be administered within 48 hours of stroke onset after exclusion of intracerebral hemorrhage through a CT scan. Subsequent doses can be lower (75–300 mg).

Other antiplatelets

Whether or not other antiplatelet agents, with or without aspirin, confer additional vascular risk reduction has been extensively investigated. Evidence exists

233

to support the use of the combination of aspirin and dipyridamole in secondary prevention [18], and also that the antiplatelet agent clopidogrel is at least equivalent to aspirin and dipyridamole combined [19]. The combination of aspirin and clopidogrel has been shown to be of some value in patients with significant internal carotid artery stenosis with distal emboli [20], although the same combination has also been shown to be associated with increased hemorrhagic risk in patients with completed stroke [21]. However, the efficacy of either dipyridamole, clopidogrel, or a combination of antiplatelet agents has not been investigated in the context of acute stroke and therefore there is no evidence to support their routine use in the acute setting. It is, however, good practice to commence appropriate secondary prevention antiplatelet therapy at the earliest opportunity in appropriate patients with a safe swallow. The glycoprotein-IIa-IIIb inhibitor abciximab has been studied in acute stroke patients but showed an increased risk of symptomatic or fatal intracranial hemorrhage without an associated benefit and therefore its use is not advised [1].

> There is no evidence of the efficacy of either dipyridamole, clopidogrel, or a combination of antiplatelet agents in the context of acute stroke.

Heparin for cardioembolic stroke

The International Stroke Trial investigated the use of aspirin and subcutaneous unfractionated heparin in a two-by-two factorial design. The beneficial effects of aspirin have already been discussed but the study also identified three fewer deaths within 14 days per 1000 patients treated with heparin (non-significant) and significantly fewer early recurrent strokes (2.9% vs. 3.8%) and pulmonary emboli (0.5% vs. 0.8%) [14]. After 6 months, however, the mortality rate was identical in those patients treated with heparin compared to those who were not. Unfortunately, heparin use was associated with more hemorrhagic strokes (1.2% vs. 0.4%) and resulted in a significant excess of nine transfused or fatal extracranial hemorrhages per 1000 patients treated. The risk of hemorrhagic complications was greater in the group which received a higher dose of subcutaneous heparin. Studies of other unfractionated heparin preparations have also failed to show significant benefit when commenced early following ischemic stroke, with the increased risk of hemorrhagic complications outweighing any potential benefit [1]. In a meta-analysis of early anticoagulant

therapy, the reduction in recurrent ischemic stroke observed was almost identical to the risk excess for symptomatic intracranial hemorrhage [22]. There is therefore currently no evidence to support the routine use of anticoagulants in all patients in the early aftermath of ischemic stroke.

For patients in whom stroke is due to a cardioembolic etiology, in a meta-analysis of seven trials involving 4624 patients within 48 hours of stroke onset, anticoagulation was associated with a non-significant reduction in early recurrent ischemic stroke (odds ratio 0.68, 95% confidence interval 0.44–1.06) without any significant change in death or disability at final follow-up (odds ratio 1.01, 95% confidence interval 0.82–1.24) [23]. A significant and almost 3-fold risk (odds ratio 2.89, 95% confidence interval 1.19–7.01) of symptomatic intracranial hemorrhage was identified with number needed to harm being 55. Despite the lack of supporting evidence, some authorities would advocate early anticoagulation with full-dose heparin in selected patients at high risk of re-embolization [1]. Evidence of a large infarction on brain imaging (e.g. >50% of the middle cerebral artery territory) or extensive microvascular disease and uncontrolled arterial hypertension are contraindications to full anticoagulation in the early post-stroke period.

> There is currently no evidence to support the routine use of anticoagulants in all patients in the early aftermath of ischemic stroke.

Neuroprotection

Neuronal injury progresses rapidly following the onset of cerebral ischemia and therefore a substance which attenuates this process may potentially reduce the extent of cerebral damage. The free-radical-trapping agent NXY-059 showed initial promise as a potential neuroprotective agent when introduced within 6 hours of ischemic stroke onset, but a larger randomized controlled trial involving more than 3000 patients did not demonstrate any benefit of NXY-059 over placebo [24]. The agent was also ineffective in those patients who had been treated with intravenous thrombolysis. Furthermore there was also no effect in patients with primary intracerebral hemorrhage. Whilst other studies of novel neuroprotective agents are ongoing, there is currently no evidence to support their routine clinical use at present.

Up to now all neuroprotective therapies have been without clinical efficacy.

Blood pressure – see Chapter 17

Hypertension is a well-recognized risk factor for first ever and recurrent stroke [25, 26] and is commonly observed in the immediate post-stroke period. In the International Stroke Trial, 82% of patients had systolic blood pressures measured in excess of 140 mmHg during the first 48 hours following admission, with 28% having a systolic BP $\geq$ 180 mmHg [27]. Similarly, in the Chinese Acute Stroke Trial three-quarters had systolic BP $\geq$ 140 mmHg, with one-quarter of patients having systolic BP $\geq$ 180 mmHg within 48 hours of admission [15]. Of the 624 patients who were included in the NINDS rtPA Stroke Trial, 19% had admission systolic BP > 185 mmHg and diastolic BP > 110 mmHg. Within the first 24 hours of randomization, 60% had blood pressure in excess of 180 mmHg systolic or 105 mmHg diastolic [28]. Despite high blood pressure being very common following stroke, the early management of blood pressure following ischemic stroke remains controversial and is the subject of ongoing research.

Although hypertension in the immediate post-stroke period is frequently observed, blood pressure tends to spontaneously fall within the first hours and days following the acute event, with the pattern of blood pressure change varying with stroke subtype [26, 29]. Precipitous falls in blood pressure have, however, been associated with poor outcome and should be avoided [30, 31]. A 'U-shaped' association between admission BP and stroke outcome has been identified, with very high and very low blood pressure being associated with poor post-stroke outcome. Analysis of the IST revealed a 3.8% increased risk of death and 4.2% increased risk of early recurrent stroke within 14 days with each 10 mmHg rise in systolic BP above 150 mmHg. For every 10 mmHg admission systolic BP was below 150 mmHg, the risk of early death rose by 17.9%, and the risk of death or dependency was increased by 3.6% at 6 months [27]. Further analyses have confirmed the association between elevated systolic, diastolic and mean arterial BP in the acute stroke period and poor outcome following ischemic stroke. Early recurrent stroke has been suggested as one possible mechanism by which elevated BP may be associated with poor outcome [32]. Cerebral perfusion becomes dependent upon systemic arterial BP following stroke due to impairment of cerebral autoregulation, and therefore changes in systemic BP can directly influence cerebral perfusion [26, 33]. Hypertension may sustain cerebral perfusion to the ischemic penumbra [34], with BP having been shown to fall spontaneously in response to successful re-canalization of cerebral vessels following thrombolytic treatment, perhaps suggesting the restoration of cerebral autoregulation [35]. High pre-thrombolysis BP has also been shown to be associated with poor re-canalization [36] and sustained hypertension may contribute to worsening cerebral edema and hemorrhagic transformation following acute ischemic stroke. Cardiovascular complications as well as early stroke recurrence in patients with elevated post-stroke blood pressures have been proposed as possible mechanisms for poor outcome [32].

There is therefore evidence that high (and low) post-stroke BP is associated with a poor outcome, although the relationship is not a straightforward one. The true relationship may depend on a combination of absolute BP level and the variability in BP following stroke and also upon stroke sub-type and co-morbidities. The optimum post-stroke BP, and how to achieve it, is therefore yet to be identified. Indeed, it is also unclear as to whether pre-existing antihypertensive medication should be continued or withdrawn following stroke and this is the focus of current research [37].

> A U-shaped relationship between baseline systolic blood pressure and both early and late death or dependency after ischemic stroke has been demonstrated in clinical trials.

A Cochrane systematic review of published and unpublished studies examining various interventions aimed at deliberately altering blood pressure within 2 weeks of acute stroke concluded that there was insufficient evidence to evaluate the effects of altering BP on outcome during the acute phase of stroke [38]. Numerous clinical trials are currently ongoing and each hopes to provide valuable knowledge and insight into how this common clinical situation is best managed.

This lack of certainty is reflected in clinical guidance, with clinicians avoiding the active reduction of blood pressure in the early post-stroke period [39]. Until evidence is available to the contrary, current clinical guidelines do not advocate the active reduction of hypertension in the immediate post-stroke period unless there is a concurrent indication to do so [1]. Such indications include hypertensive encephalopathy, myocardial infarction, aortic dissection and pre-eclampsia. Similarly, there is no conclusive evidence that low BP should be actively elevated following acute ischemic stroke [1]. Until strong evidence becomes available, some centers have developed local protocols for cautiously lowering BP when systolic BP exceeds the threshold required for thrombolysis (185/110 mmHg), although these are based on clinical experience rather than specific evidence [1]. If elevated BP is to be lowered in the acute post-stroke period, the reduction should be cautious (North American guidelines suggest a maximum reduction of 15–25% in the first 24 hours) [40], and by means of a short-acting agent. A short-acting intravenous beta-blocker such as labetolol or intravenous nitrates may be useful in this situation as the effects are readily reversed on withdrawal of the agent. Sub-lingual calcium-channel blockers should be avoided.

> The optimum post-stroke BP, and how to achieve it, is yet to be identified. Current clinical guidelines do not advocate the active reduction of hypertension in the immediate post-stroke period unless there is a concurrent indication to do so. If elevated BP is to be lowered in the acute post-stroke period, the reduction should be cautious.

Blood glucose – see Chapter 17

Measurement of blood glucose is mandatory for all patients with suspected stroke. Hypoglycemia (serum glucose < 2.8 mmol/l) with consequent neuroglycopenia is an important stroke mimic and is readily corrected by the intravenous infusion of 10–20% dextrose [1]. Hyperglycemia has a reported prevalence of up to 68% of acute stroke admission, and is not restricted to those patients with previously diagnosed diabetes mellitus [41]. The prevalence of previously unrecognized diabetes mellitus or impaired glucose tolerance may be between 20% and 30% [42]. There is evidence of a positive association between elevated admission plasma glucose and poor post-stroke outcome, with increasing stroke severity, higher mortality and reduced functional recovery observed in those with hyperglycemia [41, 43]. Tight control of hyperglycemia following myocardial infarction and in critically ill patients being managed in intensive care units appears to confer a beneficial outcome, and so it has been suggested that the same may be true in the context of acute stroke [44, 45]. Currently, however,

there is no evidence to support the routine active lowering of hyperglycemia following acute stroke. The largest randomized controlled trial of an active intervention aimed at achieving and maintaining euglycemia following stroke (ischemic and hemorrhagic) recruited 933 patients and randomized them to glucose-potassium-insulin (GKI) infusion versus 0.9% saline (control group) [46]. Only small reductions in plasma glucose were achieved, with the mean difference between the active treatment and control groups being 0.57 mmol/l, which probably reflects the median glucose at admission, which was only modestly elevated at 7.8 mmol/l and 7.6 mmol/l in the active treatment and control groups respectively. The 90-day mortality did not differ significantly between the groups although this study was limited by slow recruitment and therefore underpowered. A post hoc analysis identified an increase in the proportion of patients with a poor outcome where a reduction in glucose of ≥2 mmol/l was achieved using GKI, which raises the possibility that large reductions in post-stroke hyperglycemia may not be well tolerated. Until additional evidence becomes available, the routine use of insulin infusion regimes to control moderate post-stroke hyperglycemia cannot be recommended. Based upon clinical opinion, some acute stroke units may intervene to control post-stroke hyperglycemia in patients with blood glucose >10 mmol/l, although this decision must be made on an individual patient basis [1]. Further research is required in order to determine the optimum method of achieving and maintaining post-stroke euglycemia.

> Measurement of blood glucose is mandatory for all patients with suspected stroke. Hypoglycemia should be corrected by an intravenous dextrose infusion. The routine use of insulin regimes to control post-stroke hyperglycemia cannot be recommended.

Body temperature – see Chapter 17

Increased body temperature following stroke has been shown to be associated with poor outcome. Studies of anti-pyretic medication and thermal cooling devices have not provided conclusive evidence of efficacy but it is good practice to monitor and treat pyrexia in the immediate post-stroke period. A rise in body temperature can be centrally mediated following stroke, but more commonly it suggests the presence of intercurrent infection. Its occurrence should alert the clinician to this possibility and, if clinically appropriate, such infections should be treated. Raised body temperature following stroke is commonly treated with antipyretic medication [1]. Paracetamol 1 g can be administered every 4–6 hours, to a total dose of 4 g/24 h in adult patients, via the oral, rectal or intravenous routes. For patients who have suffered severe middle cerebral artery infarction, induced mild hypothermia (brain temperature 32–33°C) reduces mortality, but increases the risks of severe side-effects during re-warming, including recurrent intracranial pressure crisis [1]. Mild hypothermia in combination with decompressive surgery may be of benefit in patients with severe MCA infarction, although the evidence for temperature reduction is limited [1].

> Raised body temperature following stroke is commonly treated with antipyretic medication.

Brain edema and surgical intervention

For patients suffering from large middle cerebral artery (MCA) territory infarctions mortality is as high as 80% [47]. Early deterioration and death are often due to cerebral edema and rising intracranial pressure, which can occur within 24 hours of stroke, but usually becomes evident between days 2 and 5 following stroke onset [1]. Medical therapy includes airway management, oxygenation, pain control and control of body temperature [1]. Intracranial pressure should be maintained at ~70 mmHg and can be lowered by using intravenous mannitol (25–50 g every 3–6 hours), glycerol (4 × 250 ml 10% glycerol over 30–60 minutes) or hypertonic saline, although the evidence for such interventions comes from mainly observational data [1]. Dexamethasone and corticosteroids are not indicated and hypotonic and dextrose-containing solutions should be avoided [1].

Surgical decompression of evolving malignant MCA infarction should be considered in certain selected patients. Evidence for this comes from the pooled analysis of three European studies of decompressive craniotomy: the DECIMAL (decompressive surgery in malignant middle cerebral artery infarcts) study; the DESTINY (decompressive surgery for the treatment of malignant infarction of the middle cerebral artery) study; and the HAMLET trial (hemicraniectomy after middle cerebral artery infarction with life-threatening edema trial) [47]. The effects of surgery in the three trials were consistent and, based upon the 93 patients included in the pooled analysis, showed a significant improvement in the proportion

of patients with mRS ≤ 4 at one year, mRS ≤ 3 at 1 year and survivors at 1 year irrespective of function. The numbers needed to treat were 2, 4 and 2 respectively [47]. Importantly, there was no increase in the numbers of survivors left with severe disability (mRS 5). Patients who should be considered for decompressive hemicraniectomy are those up to 60 years old with evolving MCA infarction and NIHSS > 15 in whom consciousness is impaired (score of 1 or greater on item 1a of the NIHSS) and who have evidence of infarct in >50% of the MCA territory on CT [1]. Neurosurgical opinion should be sought at an early opportunity, with the aim of performing surgery within 48 hours of stroke onset.

> Intracranial pressure should be maintained at ~70 mmHg and can be lowered by using intravenous mannitol (25–50 g every 3–6 hours), glycerol (4 × 250 ml 10% glycerol over 30–60 minutes) or hypertonic saline. Surgical decompression of evolving malignant MCA infarction should be considered in certain selected patients.

Cerebellar infarction

Neurosurgical opinion should also be sought in patients with space-occupying posterior fossa infarctions. Although randomized controlled trial evidence is not available, expert opinion advises that decompressive surgery and ventriculostomy can be considered in cases of cerebellar infarction as prognosis can be favorable [1].

Intracerebral hemorrhage

Intracerebral hemorrhage (ICH) is not an isolated clinical entity, but a term used to describe the consequences of a variety of pathologies. It accounts for around 20% of strokes and includes primary ICH, secondary ICH and subarachnoid hemorrhage (SAH) [2]. Primary ICH is commonly associated with hypertension or cerebral amyloid angiopathy, while secondary ICH results from a number of pathologies including, but not limited to, aneurysms, arteriovenous malformation (AVM), neoplastic disease, cerebral vasculitis and venous sinus thrombosis [2]. Whilst a detailed description of the management of all ICH is beyond the scope of this chapter, an outline of the principles of the initial management of ICH will be discussed here.

Once ICH has been confirmed on brain imaging, some aspects of the patients' immediate management differ from that following ischemic stroke. Clearly, thrombolysis is contraindicated! Coagulopathy should be identified and treated as quickly as possible, although ICH associated with oral anticoagulation will be discussed separately.

Early blood pressure manipulation is also controversial in patients with ICH. Patients with ICH are frequently chronically hypertensive and may therefore tolerate, and perhaps require, higher cerebral perfusion pressures in order to maintain adequate cerebral perfusion. Conversely, hypertension may be associated with hematoma expansion [2]. Limited data are available to guide clinical practice, but the current European Stroke Initiative recommendations advise that in patients following ICH in whom there is a history of chronic hypertension, BP should be gradually lowered to below a mean arterial pressure (MAP) of 120 mmHg, whilst avoiding reductions of >20%, and MAP should not be lowered below 84 mmHg. A target BP of 160/100 mmHg is used for such patients. In patients without a history or clinical evidence of previously sustained hypertension, upper limits of 160/95 mmHg are accepted before BP lowering is advocated, with a target BP of 150/90 mmHg (MAP 110 mmHg) [2]. In support of active blood pressure reduction following ICH, the Intensive Blood Pressure Reduction in Acute Cerebral Haemorrhage Trial (INTERACT) reported reductions in mean hematoma growth in patients following ICH without intraventricular hemorrhage who had intensive blood pressure lowering (target systolic blood pressure of 140 mmHg) compared to those patients who received standard-guideline-based blood pressure control (target systolic blood pressure of 180 mmHg) commenced within 6 hours of onset and continued for 7 days (13.7% vs. 36.3% proportional increase, $p = 0.04$) [48]. Although the difference in proportional mean hematoma growth within 6 hours was no longer significant ($p = 0.06$) after adjustment for initial hematoma volume and time from onset to CT, the data would suggest that intensive lowering of blood pressure appears to reduce hematoma expansion. No difference in death, neurological deterioration or disability was identified between the groups at 90-day follow-up in this study of 404 patients, although a larger study to determine the effects on clinical outcomes is under way. Furthermore, results from the Antihypertensive Treatment of Acute Cerebral Haemorrhage (ATACH) study provide additional data to support the association between active blood

pressure lowering and reduced hematoma expansion [49]. A number of oral and intravenous agents have been studied and no single agent has been shown to be superior. Titration and revision of these thresholds may be required in order to maintain an adequate cerebral perfusion pressure.

Avoiding venous thromboembolism is as important in patients following ICH as it is in post-ischemic stroke patients. Graduated compression stockings have not yet been confirmed to be effective in patients following ICH, although their use is widespread [2]. Anticoagulants in the form of subcutaneous heparins may cause hematoma expansion and are therefore best avoided within the initial days following ICH [2]. The advice of the Seventh ACCP Conference on Antithrombotic and Thrombolytic Therapy recommends that low doses of unfractionated or low molecular weight heparin can be started on the second day following ICH in patients who are neurologically stable, although evidence of the efficacy of doing so is not available [50].

Raised intracranial pressure can be lowered if necessary by using medical methods previously discussed. Where this is unsuccessful, therapeutic hyperventilation can be utilized in order that adequate cerebral perfusion pressures are achieved [2]. Seizure is more commonly encountered in patients with ICH compared to ischemic stroke and non-convulsive status has been described, which will require anticonvulsant therapy [2].

Surgical intervention for ICH depends on a number of factors, including size, location, and the presence of intraventricular expansion of the hemorrhage (IVH). In the Surgical Trial in Intracerebral Haemorrhage (STICH) study, there was no difference in outcome between those patients who received early surgical intervention (<24 hours) and those who were managed conservatively [51]. However, a trend towards a significant benefit was observed in patients who suffered a deterioration in conscious level, from a Glasgow Coma Score of between 9 and 12, and in whom the ICH was superficial (≤1 cm from the surface) and no IVH compared to patients with deep hematomas who do not benefit from surgical intervention. This particular subset of patients warrants further investigation, which is currently ongoing. Although not confirmed by randomized controlled trials, surgical intervention for cerebellar hematoma should be considered, as outcomes are favorable [2]. In particular, ventricular drainage for subsequent hydrocephalus should be considered depending on the individual patient. For patients with intraventricular hemorrhage, there is some evidence to support the use of intraventricular drainage with thrombolytic agents administered via the catheter to prevent catheter obstruction, though trials on this continue [2].

The use of recombinant factor VIIa (rFVIIa) has been studied in patients with spontaneous ICH [2]. Recombinant factor VIIa initiates coagulation and therefore may be associated with increased thrombotic tendency. Consequently, trials of its use have been limited to patients without a history of previous ischemic events. In the first clinical trial with rFVIIa, the use of recombinant factor VIIa within 4 hours of ICH limited hematoma expansion, decreased mortality and improved 3-month outcome, although arterial thromboembolic events were significantly increased in the highest-dose group (160 μg/kg). A further trial involving more than 800 patients also found reduced hematoma expansion and significantly improved NIHSS scores compared to placebo when rFVIIa was used within 4 hours of ICH at a dose of 80 μg/kg, but no sustained advantage in terms of functional outcome was identified [52, 53]. Until more data are available, use of rFVIIa cannot be regarded as part of standard clinical care.

ICH whilst anticoagulated is associated with more severe hemorrhage, larger re-bleeds and a worse outcome, with an increased risk of death [2]. For patients who suffer ICH whilst anticoagulated, the priority is to reverse the anticoagulation. This can usually be effectively achieved by using a combination of intravenous vitamin K and prothrombin complex concentrate, or fresh frozen plasma.

> With intracerebral hemorrhage, thrombolysis is contraindicated. Hypertension should be gradually lowered. Raised intracranial pressure can be lowered if necessary. Surgical intervention for ICH depends on a number of factors, including size, location, and the presence of intraventricular expansion of the hemorrhage.

Summary

In order that patients obtain the full potential benefit of acute stroke therapies, significant changes in the way stroke services are configured have been required. Patient education and early recognition of symptoms and an appreciation that patients with suspected stroke should be transported to an appropriate medical facility in a time-efficient manner have been essential. Additionally, the recognition by medical and nursing staff of stroke as a medical emergency necessitating rapid clinical assessment, diagnosis and treatment has been essential in maximizing the potential benefit from the array of established and evolving acute stroke interventions.

Chapter Summary

Intravenous thrombolysis is a standard therapy for a well-selected population of patients with acute ischemic stroke. The only thrombolytic agent licensed in Europe for the treatment of ischemic stroke is recombinant tissue plasminogen activator (rtPA), alteplase. For routine use of alteplase after stroke there is an upper limit of 3 hours after the onset of stroke, but an extension of this time limit to 4.5 hours can be discussed.

At present European regulatory agencies do not support the routine use of intravenous rtPA in patients beyond 3 hours, or in those with severe stroke (NIHSS > 24), extended early ischemic changes on CT or in those over the age of 80 years. Factors associated with a poor outcome following intravenous thrombolysis are elevated serum glucose, increasing age and increasing stroke severity. Thrombolysis is contraindicated in patients with seizure at stroke onset. Blood pressure is recommended to be below 185/110 mmHg.

The dose of alteplase is weight-dependent at 0.9 mg/kg up to a maximum dose of 90 mg. Ten percent of the total dose is administered as an intravenous bolus with the remaining 90% delivered over 1 hour. Aspirin and other antiplatelets or anticoagulants should be avoided for 24 hours following thrombolysis.

Transcranial Doppler 'sonothrombolysis', microbubble and intra-arterial thrombolysis administration are currently not in routine clinical use.

Strong evidence supports the early introduction of **aspirin** following ischemic stroke. A dose of 300 mg (orally or rectally) should be administered within 48 hours of stroke onset, but after exclusion of intracerebral hemorrhage through a CT scan. Subsequent doses can be lower (75–300 mg).

The efficacy of either dipyridamole, clopidogrel, or a combination of antiplatelet agents has not been investigated in the context of acute stroke and therefore there is no evidence to support their routine use in the acute setting. It is, however, good practice to commence appropriate secondary prevention antiplatelet therapy at the earliest opportunity in appropriate patients.

There is currently no evidence to support the routine use of **anticoagulants** in all patients in the early aftermath of cardio-embolic ischemic stroke. Despite the lack of supporting evidence, some authorities would advocate early anticoagulation with full-dose heparin in selected patients at high risk of re-embolization. Evidence of a large infarction on brain imaging (e.g. >50% of the middle cerebral artery territory) or extensive microvascular disease and uncontrolled arterial hypertension are contraindications to full anticoagulation in the early post-stroke period.

Despite **high blood pressure** being very common following stroke, the early management of blood pressure following ischemic stroke remains controversial. A 'U-shaped' association between admission BP and stroke outcome has been identified, with very high and very low blood pressure being associated with poor post-stroke outcome. Hypertension may sustain cerebral perfusion to the ischemic penumbra, but sustained hypertension may contribute to worsening cerebral edema and hemorrhagic transformation, as well as leading to cardiovascular complications. The optimum post-stroke BP, and how to achieve it, is therefore yet to be identified. Current clinical guidelines do not advocate the active reduction of hypertension in the immediate post-stroke period unless there is a concurrent indication to do so. If elevated BP is to be lowered in the acute post-stroke period, the reduction should be cautious (North American guidelines suggest a maximum reduction of 15–25% in the first 24 hours), and by means of a short-acting agent.

Measurement of **blood glucose** is mandatory for all patients with suspected stroke. Hypoglycemia should be corrected by an intravenous dextrose infusion. There is evidence of a positive association between elevated admission plasma glucose and poor post-stroke outcome, with increasing stroke severity, higher mortality and reduced functional recovery observed in those with hyperglycemia. Currently, however, there is no evidence to support the routine active lowering of hyperglycemia following acute stroke. The routine use of insulin infusion regimens to control moderate post-stroke hyperglycemia cannot be recommended. On an individual patient basis, extreme hyperglycemia can be corrected.

Raised body temperature following stroke is commonly treated with antipyretic medication. Induced mild hypothermia (brain temperature 32–33°C) reduces mortality, but increases the risk of severe side-effects.

Intracranial pressure should be maintained at ~70 mmHg and can be lowered by using intravenous mannitol (25–50 g every 3–6 hours), glycerol (4 × 250 ml 10% glycerol over 30–60 minutes) or hypertonic saline. Surgical decompression of evolving malignant MCA infarction should be considered in certain selected patients.

With **intracerebral hemorrhage**, thrombolysis is contraindicated. Hypertension should be gradually lowered (target blood pressure 160/100 mmHg in patients with, and 150/100 mmHg in patients without chronic hypertension). No single antihypertensive agent has been shown to be superior. Low doses of unfractionated or low molecular weight heparin may be started on the second day following ICH in patients who are neurologically stable. Raised intracranial pressure can be lowered if necessary. Surgical intervention for ICH depends on a number of factors, including size, location, and the presence of intraventricular expansion of the hemorrhage. The use of recombinant factor VIIa (rFVIIa) cannot be recommended.

References

1. The European Stroke Organisation (ESO) Executive Committee and the ESO Writing Committee. Guidelines for the management of ischaemic stroke and transient ischaemic attack 2008. *Cerebrovasc Dis* 2008; **25**:457–507.

2. The European Stroke Initiative Writing Committee and the Writing Committee for the EUSI Executive Committee. Recommendations for the Management of Intracranial Haemorrhage – Part 1: Spontaneous Intracerebral Haemorrhage. *Cerebrovasc Dis* 2006; **22**:294–316.

3. Hacke W, et al. Intravenous thrombolysis with recombinant tissue plasminogen activator for acute hemispheric stroke. The European Cooperative Acute Stroke Study (ECASS). *JAMA* 1995; **274**(13): 1017–25.

4. The National Institute of Neurological Disorders and Stroke rt-PA stroke study group. Tissue plasminogen activator for acute ischaemic stroke. *N Engl J Med* 1995; **333**:1581–8.

5. Hacke W, et al. Randomised double-blind placebo controlled trial of thrombolytic therapy with intravenous Alteplase in acute ischaemic stroke (ECASS II). *Lancet* 1998; **352**:1245–51.

6. Clark WM, et al. Recombinant tissue-type plasminogen activator (alteplase) for ischemic stroke 3 to 5 hours after symptom onset: the ATLANTIS Study:

a Randomized Controlled Trial. *JAMA* 1999; **282** (21):2019–26.

7. Hacke W, et al. Association of outcome with early stroke treatment: pooled analysis of ATLANTIS, ECASS and NINDS rt-PA stroke trials. *Lancet* 2004; **363**:768–74.

8. Lansberg MG, et al. Risk factors of symptomatic intracerebral hemorrhage after tPA therapy for acute stroke. *Stroke* 2007; **38**(8):2275–8.

9. Sylaja PN, et al. Thrombolysis in patients older than 80 years with acute ischaemic stroke: Canadian Alteplase for Stroke Effectiveness Study. *J Neurol Neurosurg Psychiatry* 2006; **77**(7):826–9.

10. Molina CA, et al. Microbubble administration accelerates clot lysis during continuous 2-MHz ultrasound monitoring in stroke patients treated with intravenous tissue plasminogen activator. *Stroke* 2006; **37**(2):425–9.

11. Wahlgren N, et al. Thrombolysis with Alteplase for acute ischaemic stroke in the Safe Implementation of Thrombolysis in Stroke-Monitoring Study (SITS-MOST): an observational study. *Lancet* 2007; **369**:275–82.

12. Smith WS, et al. Safety and efficacy of mechanical embolectomy in acute ischemic stroke: results of the MERCI Trial. *Stroke* 2005; **36**(7):1432–8.

13. Collaborative overview of randomised trials of antiplatelet therapy. Prevention of death, myocardial infarction, and stroke by prolonged antiplatelet therapy in various categories of patients. *BMJ* 1994; **308**(6921):81–106.

14. International Stroke Trial Collaborative Group. The International Stroke Trial (IST): a randomised trial of aspirin, subcutaneous heparin, both, or neither among 19,435 patients with acute ischaemic stroke. *Lancet* 1997; **349**:1569–81.

15. CAST (Chinese Acute Stroke Trial) Collaborative Group. CAST: randomised placebo-controlled trial of early aspirin use in 20 000 patients with acute ischaemic stroke. *Lancet* 1997; **349**:1641–9.

16. Wardlaw JM, et al. What is the best imaging strategy for acute stroke? *Health Technol Assess* 2004; **8**:1–180.

17. Antithrombotic Trialists' Collaboration. Collaborative meta-analysis of randomised trials of antiplatelet therapy for prevention of death, myocardial infarction, and stroke in high risk patients. *BMJ* 2002; **324** (7329):71–86.

18. The ESPRIT Study Group. Aspirin plus dipyridamole versus aspirin alone after cerebral ischaemia of arterial origin (ESPRIT): randomised controlled trial. *Lancet* 2006; **367**:1665–73.

19. Sacco RL, et al. Aspirin and extended-release dipyridamole versus clopidogrel for recurrent stroke. *N Engl J Med* 2008; **359**(12):1238–51.

20. Markus HS, et al. Dual antiplatelet therapy with clopidogrel and aspirin in symptomatic carotid stenosis evaluated using Doppler embolic signal detection: the Clopidogrel and Aspirin for Reduction of Emboli in Symptomatic Carotid Stenosis (CARESS) Trial. *Circulation* 2005; **111**(17):2233–40.

21. Diener H-C, et al. Aspirin and clopidogrel compared with clopidogrel alone after recent ischaemic stroke or transient ischaemic attack in high-risk patients (MATCH): randomised, double-blind, placebo-controlled trial. *Lancet* 2004; **364**:331–37.

22. Gubitz G, Sandercock P, Counsell C. Anticoagulants for acute ischaemic stroke. *Cochrane Database of Systematic Reviews* 2004; CD000024.

23. Paciaroni M, et al. Efficacy and safety of anticoagulant treatment in acute cardioembolic stroke: a meta-analysis of randomized controlled trials. *Stroke* 2007; **38**(2):423–30.

24. Ashfaq Shuaib, et al. NXY-059 for the treatment of acute ischaemic stroke. *N Engl J Med* 2007; **357**:562–71.

25. Friday G, Alter M, Lai S-M. Control of hypertension and risk of stroke recurrence. *Stroke* 2002; **33** (11):2652–7.

26. Robinson TG, Potter JF. Blood pressure in acute stroke. *Age Ageing* 2004; **33**:6–12.

27. Leonardi-Bee J, et al. Blood pressure and clinical outcomes in the International Stroke Trial. *Stroke* 2002; **33**:1315–20.

28. Brott T, et al. Hypertension and its treatment in the NINDS rt-PA stroke trial. *Stroke* 1998; **29**:1504–9.

29. Bath P, et al. International Society of Hypertension (ISH): statement on the management of blood pressure in acute stroke. *J Hypertens* 2003; **21**:665–72.

30. Castillo J, et al. Blood pressure decrease during the acute phase of ischaemic stroke is associated with brain injury and poor stroke outcome. *Stroke* 2004; **35**:520–7.

31. Oliveira-Filho J, et al. Detrimental effect of blood pressure reduction in the first 24 hours of acute stroke onset. *Neurology* 2003; **61**:1047–51.

32. Willmot M, Leonardi-Bee J, Bath PM. High blood pressure in acute stroke and subsequent outcome. A systemic review. *Hypertension* 2004; **43**:18–24.

33. Eames P, et al. Dynamic cerebral autoregulation and beat to beat blood pressure control are impaired in acute ischaemic stroke. *J Neurol Neurosurg Psychiatry* 2002; **72**:467–72.

34. Powers W. Acute hypertension after stroke: the scientific basis for treatment decisions. *Neurology* 1993; **43**:461–7.

35. Mattle HP, et al. Blood pressure and vessel recanalization in the first hours after ischemic stroke. *Stroke* 2005; **36**:264–9.

36. Tsivgoulis G, et al. Association of pretreatment blood pressure with tissue plasminogen activator-induced arterial recanalization in acute ischemic stroke. *Stroke* 2007; **38**:961–6.

37. Continue or Stop Antihypertensives Collaboration Study. 2005. http://www.le.ac.uk/cv/research/COSSACS/COSSACShome.html [cited 18 June 2005].

38. Blood Pressure in Acute Stroke Collaboration (BASC). Interventions for deliberately altering blood pressure in acute stroke. *Cochrane Database of Systematic Reviews*, 2001; Issue 3. CD000039. DOI 10.1002/114651858.CD000039.

39. O'Connell J, Gray C. Treatment of post-stroke hypertension. A practical guide. *Drugs Aging* 1996; **8**(6):408–15.

40. Adams HP Jr, et al. Guidelines for the early management of adults with ischemic stroke: a guideline from the American Heart Association/American Stroke Association Stroke Council, Clinical Cardiology Council, Cardiovascular Radiology and Intervention Council, and the Atherosclerotic Peripheral Vascular Disease and Quality of Care Outcomes in Research Interdisciplinary Working Groups: The American Academy of Neurology affirms the value of this guideline as an educational tool for neurologists. *Stroke* 2007; **38**(5):1655–711.

41. Capes SE, et al. Stress hyperglycaemia and prognosis of stroke in nondiabetic and diabetic patients: a systematic overview. *Stroke* 2001; **32**:2426–32.

42. Scott J, et al. Glucose and insulin therapy in acute stroke; why delay further? *Q J Med* 1998; **91**:511–15.

43. Weir CJ, et al. Is hyperglycaemia an independent predictor of poor outcome after acute stroke? Results of a long term follow up study. *BMJ* 1997; **314**:1303–6.

44. Malmberg K, et al. Randomised trial of insulin glucose infusion followed by subcutaneous insulin treatment in diabetic patients with acute myocardial infarction. The DIGAMI Study. *J Am Coll Cardiol* 1995; **26**:57–65.

45. Van den Berghe G, et al. Intensive insulin therapy in critically ill patients. *N Engl J Med* 2001; **345**:1359–67.

46. Gray CS, et al. Glucose-potassium-insulin infusions in the management of post-stroke hyperglycaemia: the UK Glucose Insulin in Stroke Trial (GIST-UK). *Lancet Neurol* 2007; **6**:397–406.

47. Vahedi K, et al. Early decompressive surgery in malignant infarction of the middle cerebral artery: a pooled analysis of three randomised controlled trials. *Lancet Neurol* 2007; **6**:215–22.

48. Anderson CS, et al. Intensive blood pressure reduction in acute cerebral haemorrhage trial (INTERACT): a randomised pilot trial. *Lancet Neurol* 2008; 7(5):391–9.

49. Quresh, AI. Antihypertensive treatment of acute cerebral haemorrhage (ATACH). In *International Stroke Conference*, New Orleans, LA, USA. 2008.

50. Albers GW, et al. Antithrombotic and antithrombolytic therapy for ischaemic stroke: the Seventh ACCP Conference on Antithrombotic and Thrombolytic Therapy. *Chest* 2004; **126**:483S–512S.

51. Mendelow AD, et al. Early surgery versus initial conservative treatment in patients with spontaneous supratentorial intracerebral haematomas in the International Surgical Trial in Intracerebral Haemorrhage (STICH): a randomised trial. *Lancet* 2005; **365**(9457):387–97.

52. Mayer SA, et al. Recombinant activated Factor VII for acute intracerebral hemorrhage. *N Engl J Med* 2005; **352**(8):777–85.

53. Mayer SA, et al. Efficacy and safety of recombinant activated Factor VII for acute intracerebral hemorrhage. *N Engl J Med* 2008; **358**(20):2127–37.

54. Wahlgren N, et al. for the SITS investigators. Thrombolysis with alteplase 3 to 4.5 h after acute ischaemic stroke in the Safe Implementation of Treatments in Stroke Register (SITS-ISTR): an observational study. *Lancet* 2008; 372(9646):1303–9.

55. Hacke W, et al. for the European Cooperative Acute Stroke Study (ECASS) investigators. Alteplase compared with placebo within 3 to 4.5 hours for acute ischemic stroke. *N Engl J Med* 2008; 359:1317–29.

Management of acute ischemic stroke and its complications

Natan M. Bornstein and Eitan Auriel

General management of elevated blood pressure, blood glucose and body temperature

Monitoring the blood pressure (BP), glucose levels and temperature in acute stroke patients is an often neglected matter although it may have an important impact upon the patients' outcome. In the Tel Aviv stroke register, recorded between the years 2001 and 2003, 32% of acute stroke patients in the emergency room had glucose levels higher than 150 mg/dl, higher systolic BP than 140 mmHg was found in 77% of the patients and 17% of patients had temperatures above 37°C on admission. These numbers are representative of other centers as well. This chapter will summarize the current knowledge regarding the management of the above.

Hypertensive blood pressure values in acute ischemic stroke

Several observations have demonstrated spontaneous elevation of blood pressure in the first 24–48 hrs after stroke onset with a significant spontaneous decline after a few days [1–3]. Several mechanisms may be responsible for the increased blood pressure, including stress, pain, urinary retention, Cushing effect due to increased intracranial pressure and the activation of the sympathetic, renin–angiotensin and ACTH–cortisol pathways. Despite the increased prevalence of hypertension following stroke, optimal management has not been yet established. Several arguments speak for lowering the elevated BP: risks of hemorrhagic transformation, cerebral edema, recurrence of stroke and hypertensive encephalopathy. On the other hand, it may be important to maintain the hypertensive state due to the damaged autoregulation in the ischemic brain and the risk of cerebral hypoperfusion exacerbated by the lowered systemic blood pressure.

Blood pressure and outcome

Analysis of 17 398 patients in the International Stroke Trial [4] demonstrated a U-shaped relationship between baseline systolic blood pressure and both early death and late death or dependency. Both high blood pressure and low blood pressure were independent prognostic factors for poor outcome. Early death increased by 17.9% for every 10 mmHg below 150 mmHg ($P < 0.0001$) and by 3.8% for every 10 mmHg above 150 mmHg ($P = 0.016$). A prospective study among 1121 patients admitted within 24 hours from stroke onset and followed up for 12 months demonstrated similar findings of the "U shape" phenomenon [5]. It should be taken into consideration that prolongation of the elevated blood pressure may be caused by more severe stroke as compensation for the persistent vessel occlusion.

On the other hand, the GAIN study [6], done among 1455 patients with ischemic stroke, demonstrated that baseline mean arterial pressure was not associated with poor outcome. However, variables describing the course of BP over the first days have a marked and independent relationship with 1- and 3-month outcomes.

In a Cochrane systematic review of 32 studies involving 10 892 patients [7] after ischemic and hemorrhagic stroke, death was found to be significantly associated with elevated mean arterial BP (OR, 1.61; 95% CI 1.12–2.31) and high diastolic BP (OR, 1.71; 95% CI 1.33–2.48).

> A U-shaped relationship between baseline systolic blood pressure and both early and late death or dependency after ischemic stroke has been demonstrated in clinical trials.

BP and outcome in thrombolysed patients

Several observations, including the NINDS-tPA trial [8, 9], found an association between high blood pressure on admission, and its prolongation, with poor outcome and mortality. Although in one study no such association was found in alert patients, stroke patients with impaired consciousness showed higher mortality rates with increasing blood pressure [10]. The association between elevated blood pressure and recanalization was evaluated in 149 patients after intra-arterial thrombolysis using angiography [11]. The study demonstrated that the course of elevated systolic blood pressure, but not diastolic blood pressure, after acute ischemic stroke was inversely associated with the degree of vessel recanalization. When recanalization failed, systolic BP remained elevated longer than when it succeeded.

Controlling BP in the acute stroke phase

The theory that elevated systemic BP may compensate for the decreased cerebral blood flow in the ischemic region led to attempts to elevate blood pressure as a treatment for acute ischemic stroke. The hemodynamic and metabolic impact of pharmacologically increased systemic blood pressure on the ischemic core and penumbra was evaluated in rats. The mild induced hypertension was found to increase collateral flow and oxygenation and to improve cerebral metabolic rate of oxygen in the core and penumbra [12]. Several small studies in humans have addressed this question and administered vasopressors, including phenylephrine and norepinephrine, to patients with acute stroke [13–15]. Despite a documented improvement in CBF [16], the concept was abandoned because of the increased risk of hemorrhage and brain edema. In a systemic review of 12 relevant publications including 319 subjects, the small size of the trials and the inconclusive results limit conclusion as to the effects on outcomes, both benefits and harms. A randomized controlled trial is needed to determine the role of pressors in acute ischemic stroke [17].

> Elevated systemic BP may compensate for the decrease of cerebral blood flow in the ischemic region, but raises the risks of hemorrhagic transformation, cerebral edema, recurrence of stroke and hypertensive encephalopathy.

According to a systematic review of the literature [3] no conclusive evidence to support the lowering of blood pressure in the acute phase of ischemic stroke was found and more research is needed to identify the effective strategies for blood pressure management in

that phase [3]. Despite the controversy over the management of BP in the acute phase, the benefit of blood pressure reduction as a secondary prevention of stroke is well established and has been demonstrated in many studies. However, in most of these studies antihypertensive agents were administrated several weeks after stroke onset. Only a few trials were performed in the acute stage. The ACCESS trial [18] was a prospective, double-blind, placebo-controlled, randomized study evaluating the angiotensin receptor blocker candesartan vs. placebo for 342 hypertensive patients in the first week following stroke. Treatment was started with 4 mg candesartan or placebo on day 1 and dosage was increased to 8 or 16 mg candesartan or placebo on day 2, depending the blood pressure values. Treatment was aimed at a 10–15% blood pressure reduction within 24 hours. Although no difference was found in stroke outcome at 3 months, a significantly lower recurrent cardiovascular event rate and lower mortality after 1 year were documented in the treatment group. The authors concluded that when there is need for or no contraindication against early antihypertensive therapy, candesartan is a safe therapeutic option.

In the UK's Control of Hypertension and Hypotension Immediately Post-Stroke (CHHIPS) pilot trial [19], researchers randomized 179 patients who had suffered ischemic or hemorrhagic strokes within the previous 36 hours and who also had hypertension defined as systolic blood pressure greater than 160 mmHg. Patients received doses of either the antihypertensive drugs lisinopril at a dosage of 5 mg or labetalol at a dosage of 50 mg or a placebo at increasing doses for 14 days. Three months after treatment began, the active treatment group had a significantly lower mortality compared to the placebo group.

Despite the somewhat confusing and unclear data the current European Stroke Organisation (ESO) 2008 Guidelines [20] recommend that blood pressure up to 220 mmHg systolic or 120 diastolic may be tolerated in the acute phase without intervention unless there are cardiac complications. According to the American guidelines [21] it is generally agreed that patients with markedly elevated blood pressure may have their blood pressure lowered by not more than 15% during the first 24 hours after the onset of stroke. There is an indication to treat blood pressure only if it is above 220 mmHg systolic or if the mean blood pressure is higher than 120 mmHg. No data are available to guide selection of medication for the lowering of blood pressure in the setting of acute ischemic stroke. The recommended medication and doses are based on general consensus. More studies are needed to identify the optimal strategy for BP management. Several ongoing clinical trials such as the Efficacy of Nitric Oxide in Stroke (ENOS) trial may help answer the remaining questions.

> Guidelines recommend blood pressure lowering therapy above 220 mmHg (European Stroke Organisation (ESO) 2008 Guidelines and American Guidelines) systolic blood pressure.

Hyperglycemia

It has been well established that elevated glucose levels play a major role in microvascular and macrovascular morbidity and in hematological abnormalities as well. Several processes were found to be associated with these conditions, including impaired vascular tone and flow, disruption to endothelial function, changes at the cellular level, intracellular acidosis and increased aggregation and coagulability. Some animal studies [22, 23] have demonstrated the relations between acute ischemic stroke and hyperglycemia. In these models the administration of glucose to animals resulted in worsened brain ischemia. Those findings were attributed to the accumulation of lactate, decreased intracellular pH, increase in free radicals and excitatory amino acids, damage to the blood–brain barrier (BBB), formation of edema and elevated risk of hemorrhagic transformation. Pretreatment with insulin was found to limit the ischemia.

As mentioned, 30–40% of acute stroke patients are found to have elevated glucose levels on admission, about half of them have known diabetes, while the others are newly diagnosed or suffer from stress-induced hyperglycemia [24].

In one systematic study [24b] it was shown that glucose pathology is seen in up to 80% of acute patients, many of them showing a high probability of previously unrecognized diabetes. Out of 238 consecutive acute stroke patients, 20.2% had previously known diabetes; 16.4% were classified as having newly diagnosed diabetes, 23.1% as having impaired glucose tolerance (IGT), and 0.8% as having impaired fasting glucose; and only 19.7% showed normal glucose levels. Another 47 patients (19.7%) had hyperglycemic values only in the first week (transient hyperglycemia) or could not be fully classified due to missing data in the oral glucose tolerance test.

Increased mortality [25] was found in both diabetic and stress-induced hyperglycemia groups, independent of age, stroke type and stroke size. Stress hyperglycemia was associated with a 3-fold risk of fatal 30-day outcome and 1.4-fold risk of poor functional outcome in non-diabetic patients with acute ischemic stroke. Similar findings were also demonstrated in the NINDS tPA stroke trial. Hyperglycemia on admission [26] was correlated with decreased neurological improvement and the risk of hemorrhagic transformation in reperfused thrombolysed patients but not in non-reperfused tPA-treated patients. On the other hand, in the NINDS study, glucose level on admission was not associated with altered effectiveness of thrombolysis. All of these findings suggest that glucose level is an important risk factor for morbidity and mortality after stroke. However, it is not clear whether hyperglycemia itself affects stroke outcome or reflects, as a marker, the severity of the event due to the activation of stress hormones such as cortisol or norepinephrine. Diffusion–perfusion MRI analysis supports the first hypothesis. Hyperglycemia greater than 12.1 mmol/l in patients with perfusion–diffusion mismatch, shown on diffusion-weighted imaging–perfusion-weighted imaging (DWI–PWI) MRI, was associated with higher lactate production and with reduced salvage of mismatch tissue and increased conversion of tissue "at risk" of infarcted tissue compared with patients who arrived with the value of 5.2 mmol/l [27].

Among the factors found to contribute to the post-acute-stroke hyperglycemia [28] are the involvement of the insular cortex, which is known to play a role in sympathetic activation, involvement of the internal capsule, pre-existing diabetes, elevated systolic BP and NIHSS higher than 14 points.

> Glucose level is an important risk factor for morbidity and mortality after stroke, but it is unclear whether hyperglycemia itself affects stroke outcomes or reflects the severity of the event as a marker.

The previous data raise the question how, and especially to what extent, should post-acute-stroke hyperglycemia be treated. Intensive insulin therapy administered i.v. and aimed at maintaining blood glucose levels at 4.5–6.1 mmol/l in the surgical intensive care set-up was found to reduce mortality by more than 40% [29]. Similar results were documented among patients after myocardial infarction [30]. The question remains regarding the application in acute stroke patients. The GIST-UK trial [31] addressed this question. The study was conducted among 933 hyperglycemic acute stroke patients who received glucose-potassium-insulin infusion versus placebo. In the treatment group significantly lowered glucose and blood pressure values were documented; however, no clinical benefit was found among the treated patients. The time window for treating post-stroke hyperglycemia still remains uncertain. There are a variety of methods of insulin administration, including continuous intravenous (i.v.) infusion, repeated subcutaneous dosing and i.v. infusion containing insulin and dextrose with potassium supplementation [32]. Ongoing trials address the role of i.v. insulin for hyperglycemic stroke patients. The Glucose Regulation in Acute Stroke Patients Trial (GRASP) is continuing recruitment. Patients with hyperglycemia (glucose > 6.1 mmol/l) within 24 hours of symptom onset are randomized to tight glucose control (3.9 to 6.1 mmol/l), loose glucose control (6.1 to 11.1 mmol/l), or normal care. The insulin is delivered as a GKI infusion. The primary outcome of the GRASP trial is the rate of hypoglycemic events, and definitive information on clinical endpoints is not expected [33].

A randomized, multicenter, blinded pilot trial, Treatment of Hyperglycemia in Ischemic Stroke (THIS) [34], compared the use of aggressive treatment with continuous intravenous insulin, with no glucose or potassium in the insulin solution, with insulin administered subcutaneously in acute stroke patients. The aggressive-treatment group was associated with somewhat better clinical outcomes, which were not statistically significant. According to the ESO 2008 recommendations [20], a blood glucose of 180 mg/dl (10 mmol/l) or higher is an indication for treatment with i.v. insulin. According to the American guidelines [21], even lower serum glucose levels, possibly between 140 and 185 mg/dl, should trigger administration of insulin. Despite the current recommendation, a more aggressive approach is advised, especially in pre-thrombolysis patients. Many questions surrounding the role of glucose lowering therapy remain unanswered [32]. What level of blood glucose is best for intervention? What is the therapeutic time window? Will identification of the penumbra with CT and MR imaging help in selecting appropriate patients? How long should the insulin infusion last? What level of monitoring is required? All these questions are still to be answered.

> Guidelines recommend i.v. insulin therapy for blood glucose levels of 180 mg/dl (10 mmol/l). In pre-thrombolysis patients, an even more aggressive approach may be advisable.

Hyperthermia

Several animal studies [35, 36] demonstrated the correlation of elevated temperature and poor outcome in ischemic stroke models. Similar results were found in human observations. In the Copenhagen stroke study [37] stroke severity was correlated with hyperthermia higher than 37.5°C, while a temperature lower than 36.5°C was associated with a favorable outcome.

Other studies limited the correlation between stroke severity and hyperthermia to only the first 24 hours following stroke onset. In a prospective study temperature was recorded every 2 hours for 72 hours in 260 patients with a hemispheric ischemic stroke. Hyperthermia initiated only within the first 24 hours from stroke onset, but not afterward, was associated with larger infarct volume and worse outcome [38].

These animal studies and human observations raised the question regarding the role of hypothermia as a treatment for acute stroke. Hypothermia was introduced more than 50 years ago as a protective measure for the brain [39]. Mild induced hypothermia was found to improve neurological outcomes and reduce mortality following cardiac arrest due to ventricular fibrillation [40]; on the other hand, treatment with hypothermia aiming at 33°C within the first 8 hours after brain injury was not found to be effective [41]. Other applications for which therapeutic hypothermia was suggested include acute encephalitis, neonatal hypoxia and near drowning [39].

The use of antipyretics, such as acetaminophen, in high doses ranging between 3900 and 6000 mg daily [42,43], caused only very mild reduction in body temperature, ranging from 0.2 to 0.4°C respectively. The clinical benefit of this reduction is not well established. The use of external cooling aids [44], such as cooling blankets, cold infusions and cold washing, aiming at a body temperature of 33°C for 48 to 72 hours in patients with severe middle cerebral artery (MCA) infarction, was not associated with severe side-effects and was found to help control elevated ICP values in cases of severe space-occupying edema. Similar results, of decreasing acute post-ischemic cerebral edema, were found in a small pilot study of endovascular induced hypothermia [45]. The use of an endovascular cooling device which was inserted into the inferior vena cave was evaluated among patients with moderate to severe anterior circulation territory ischemic stroke in a randomized trial. Although no difference was found in the clinical outcome between the treatment group and the group randomized to standard medical management, the results suggest that this approach is feasible and that moderate hypothermia can be induced in patients with ischemic stroke quickly and effectively and is generally safe and well tolerated in most patients [46]. However, the current data do not support the use of induced hypothermia for treatment of patients with acute stroke. In conclusion, despite its therapeutic potential, hypothermia as a treatment for acute stroke has been investigated in only a few very small studies. Therapeutic hypothermia is feasible in acute stroke but owing to side-effects such as hypotension, cardiac arrhythmia, and pneumonia it is still thought of as experimental, and evidence of efficacy from clinical trials is needed [47]. According to the 2008 ESO recommendations [20], at a temperature of 37.5°C or above reducing the body temperature should be advised. The American Heart and Stroke Association [21] recommend that antipyretic agents should be administered in post-stroke febrile patients but the effectiveness of treating either febrile or non-febrile patients with antipyretics is not proven.

> Hyperthermia within the first 24 hours from stroke onset was associated with larger infarct volume and worse outcome, but the current data do not support the use of induced hypothermia aiming at a body temperature of 33°C for treatment of patients with acute stroke. The 2008 ESO guidelines recommend reducing body temperature only if above 37°C.

In summary, hypertension, hyperglycemia and hyperthermia are common conditions following acute stroke. All three have a major and independent impact on the severity of outcome. Occasionally, the benefit of this impact is no less than that of more "heroic" strategies such as intravenous and intra-arterial thrombolysis. Despite the lack of consensus on the data and optimal management, one should carefully monitor these three "hyper links" and treat them appropriately.

Summary

Optimal management of hypertension following stroke has not been yet established. A U-shaped relationship between baseline systolic blood pressure and both early death and late death or dependency has been demonstrated in clinical trials: early death increased by 17.9% for every 10 mmHg below 150 mmHg and by 3.8% for every 10 mmHg above 150 mmHg. Stroke patients with impaired consciousness showed higher mortality rates with increasing blood pressure. On the other hand, elevated systemic BP may compensate for the decrease in cerebral blood flow in the ischemic region. The benefit of blood pressure reduction as a secondary prevention of stroke is well established, but only a few trials have been performed in the acute stage. However, these few trials demonstrate a beneficial effect of lowering blood pressure. The current European Stroke Organisation (ESO) 2008 guidelines recommend that blood pressure up to 200 mmHg systolic or 120 diastolic may be tolerated in the acute phase. According to the American guidelines, indication to treat blood pressure starts with a systolic blood pressure of 220 mmHg, and lowering of blood pressure should not exceed 15% during the first 24 hours after the onset of stroke (Table 17.1).

Increased mortality was found in both diabetic and stress-induced hyperglycemia groups, independent of age, stroke type and stroke size. Glucose level is an important risk factor for morbidity and mortality after stroke, but it is unclear whether hyperglycemia itself affects stroke outcomes or reflects the severity of the event as a marker. According to the ESO 2008 recommendations (Table 17.2) a blood glucose of 180 mg/dl (10 mmol/l) or higher is an indication for treatment with i.v. insulin. According to the American guidelines even lower serum glucose levels, possibly between 140 and 185 mg/dl, should trigger administration of insulin. In pre-thrombolysis patients, an even more aggressive approach may be advisable.

Hyperthermia within the first 24 hours from stroke onset was associated with larger infarct volume and worse outcome. Mild induced hypothermia was found to improve neurological outcome and reduce mortality following cardiac arrest due to ventricular fibrillation, but the current data (few very small studies) do not support the use of induced hypothermia for treatment of patients with acute

Table 17.1. ESO 2008 and American Heart and Stroke Association recommendations in the acute stroke phase.

	European Stroke Organisation (ESO) 2008	American Heart Association/ American Stroke Association 2008
Blood pressure	Treat only if higher than 220/120 unless there are cardiac complications	Treat only if higher than 220/120. Not to lower BP by more than 15% in the first 24 hrs
Hyperglycemia	Treat with i.v. insulin if glucose levels are higher than 180 mg/dl	Insulin should be administered even at glucose levels between 140 and 185 mg/dl
Hyperthermia	Antipyretics should be administered if body temperature higher than 37.5°C	Antipyretics should be administered in febrile post-stroke patients

stroke. Because of side-effects such as hypotension, cardiac arrhythmia and pneumonia, therapeutic hypothermia aiming at a body temperature of 33°C is feasible in acute stroke, but is still thought of as experimental. The 2008 ESO recommendations are to reduce body temperature at temperatures of 37.5°C or above.

Management of post-stroke complications

Stroke is a major cause of long-term physical, cognitive, emotional and social disability. In addition to the neurological impairment appearing in the acute phase, there are infrequently late complications which are often neglected. These complications have a great impact on the quality of life, outcome and chances of rehabilitation and may include post-stroke epilepsy, dementia, depression and fatigue. Other complications, such as infections, are dealt with in the

Table 17.2. General stroke treatment recommendations according to current European Guidelines of the European Stroke Organisation [20].

Recommendations

- Intermittent monitoring of neurological status, pulse, blood pressure, temperature and oxygen saturation is recommended for 72 hours in patients with significant persisting neurological deficits (Class IV, GCP)

- It is recommended that oxygen should be administered if the oxygen saturation falls below 95% (Class IV, GCP)

- Regular monitoring of fluid balance and electrolytes is recommended in patients with severe stroke or swallowing problems (Class IV, GCP)

- Normal saline (0.9%) is recommended for fluid replacement during the first 24 hours after stroke (Class IV, GCP)

- Routine blood pressure lowering is not recommended following acute stroke (Class IV, GCP)

- Cautious blood pressure lowering is recommended in patients with extremely high blood pressures (>220/ 120 mmHg) on repeated measurements, with severe cardiac failure, aortic dissection, or hypertensive encephalopathy (Class IV, GCP)

- It is recommended that abrupt blood pressure lowering be avoided (Class II, Level C)

- It is recommended that low blood pressure secondary to hypovolemia or associated with neurological deterioration in acute stroke should be treated with volume expanders (Class IV, GCP)

- Monitoring serum glucose levels is recommended (Class IV, GCP)

- Treatment of serum glucose levels >180 mg/dl (>10 mmol/l) with insulin titration is recommended (Class IV, GCP)

- It is recommended that severe hypoglycemia (<50 mg/dl [<2.8 mmol/l]) should be treated with intravenous dextrose or infusion of 10–20% glucose (Class IV, GCP points)

- It is recommended that the presence of pyrexia (temperature >37.5°C) should prompt a search for concurrent infection (Class IV, GCP)

- Treatment of pyrexia (temperature >37.5°C) with paracetamol and fanning is recommended (Class III, Level C)

- Antibiotic prophylaxis is not recommended in immunocompetent patients (Class II, Level B) following chapter. Table 17.3 gives an overview of the recommendations of the ESO for the prevention and management of complications [20].

Post-stroke seizures

Epilepsy is one of the most common serious neurological disorders and is associated with numerous social and psychological consequences. Stroke is the most commonly identified etiology of secondary epilepsy and accounts for 30% of newly diagnosed seizures in patients older than 60 years [48]. Although recognized as a major cause of epilepsy in the elderly, many questions still arise regarding the epidemiology, treatment and outcome of post-stroke seizures.

The common definition of epilepsy includes at least two seizures with a time interval of at least 24 hours between the episodes. The current clinical classification of post-stroke seizures is made according to the period between the stroke and the first epileptic episode. A post-stroke seizure is defined as early if it occurs in the first 2 weeks after the stroke. A seizure occurring later is defined as late [49].

The estimated rate of early post-ischemic stroke seizures ranges from 2 to 33% and that of late seizures varies from 3 to 67% [50–58]. The wide range is due to the different methodologies, terminologies and sizes of the populations in the different studies. The overall rate of post-stroke epilepsy, as previously defined as at least two episodes, is 3–4% and is higher in patients who have had a late seizure [58].

In an observational study among 1428 patients after stroke [58], 51 patients (3.6%) developed epilepsy. Post-stroke epilepsy was found to be more common among patients with hemorrhagic strokes, venous infarctions and localization in the right hemisphere and MCA territory. The SASS (Seizures After Stroke Study) was a prospective multicenter study held among 1897 patients after an ischemic or hemorrhagic stroke [49]. In that study 14% of the patients with ischemic stroke and 20% of patients with hemorrhagic stroke had seizures during the first year; a second episode, required to establish epilepsy, was found in 2.5% of the patients. Most of the patients with post-stroke epilepsy have simple partial seizures, while complex partial seizures are relatively rare. The risk of status epilepticus varies from 0.14 to 13%. It should be emphasized that it is not always clear whether the patient has had a seizure; seizures in the elderly are sometimes difficult to diagnose and may

Table 17.3. Prevention and management of complications according to current European Guidelines of the European Stroke Organisation [20].

Recommendations
• It is recommended that infections after stroke should be treated with appropriate antibiotics (**Class IV, GCP**)
• Prophylactic administration of antibiotics is not recommended, and levofloxacin can be detrimental in acute stroke patients (**Class II, Level B**)
• Early rehydration and graded compression stockings are recommended to reduce the incidence of venous thromboembolism (**Class IV, GCP**)
• Early mobilization is recommended to prevent complications such as aspiration pneumonia, DVT and pressure ulcers (**Class IV, GCP**)
• It is recommended that low-dose subcutaneous heparin or low molecular weight heparins should be considered for patients at high risk of DVT or pulmonary embolism (**Class I, Level A**)
• Administration of anticonvulsants is recommended to prevent recurrent post-stroke seizures (**Class I, Level A**). Prophylactic administration of anticonvulsants to patients with recent stroke who have not had seizures is not recommended (**Class IV, GCP**)
• An assessment of risk of falls is recommended for every stroke patient (**Class IV, GCP**)
• Calcium/vitamin D supplements are recommended in stroke patients at risk of falls (**Class II, Level B**)
• Bisphosphonates (alendronate, etidronate and risedronate) are recommended in women with previous fractures (**Class II, Level B**)
• In stroke patients with urinary incontinence, specialist assessment and management are recommended (**Class III, Level C**)
• Swallowing assessment is recommended but there are insufficient data to recommend a specific approach for treatment (**Class III, GCP**)
• Oral dietary supplements are only recommended for non-dysphagic stroke patients who are malnourished (**Class II, Level B**)
• Early commencement of nasogastric (NG) feeding (within 48 hours) is recommended in stroke patients with impaired swallowing (**Class II, Level B**)
• It is recommended that percutaneous enteral gastrostomy (PEG) feeding should not be considered in stroke patients in the first 2 weeks (**Class II, Level B**)

present as acute confusion, behavioral changes or syncope of unknown origin [59].

> Post-stroke epilepsy is defined as at least two episodes of seizures. The overall rate is 3–4% of stroke patients.

Other predictors for post-stroke seizures found in various studies are cortical location, large infarct, evaluated clinically or radiologically, intracerebral hemorrhage and cardiac emboli, most probably due to the tendency of the latter to involve the cortex [54–57]. Post-stroke seizures are also more common among patients with pre-existing dementia evaluated using the validated IQCODE questionnaire (risk ratio of 4.66, CI 1.34–16.21). Patients in this population should be advised to avoid factors increasing the risk of seizures, such as certain drugs [60]. In a retrospective study the presence of chronic obstructive pulmonary disease (COPD) was found to be an independent risk factor for the development of seizures in stroke patients [61].

The pathophysiology of early seizures is thought to be due to the increased excitatory activity mediated by the release of glutamate from the hypoxic tissue [62]. Late seizures are due to the development of tissue gliosis and neuronal damage in the infarct area [63]. An interesting question is whether post-stroke seizures worsen the outcome of patients after stroke. A cortical cerebral infarction disability was found to be greater in patients with seizures; on the other hand, in patients with cortical hemorrhage disability was found to be less [49].

The attending physician is required to deal with two important questions, the first being whether to start treatment after the first episode and the second being which anti-epileptic drug to prefer. According to the common clinical approach, treatment should be initiated only after the second episode. Observational studies suggest that isolated early seizures after stroke do not require treatment [52, 53]. Beginning treatment after early-onset seizures has not been associated with reduction of recurrent seizures after discontinuing the medication [64].

At this stage there are no evidence-based studies to recommend one drug over the others. It is best to avoid the old drugs, especially phenytoin, because of their pharmacokinetic profile and interactions with anticoagulants and salicylates [65]. A single study has found neurontine to be a safe and effective treatment; however, this recommendation should be taken with caution since the study had no control group [66]. In a prospective study comparing lamotrigine versus carbamazepine in 64 patients with post-stroke epilepsy, lamotrigine was found to be significantly tolerated and with a trend to be also more efficacious ($p = 0.06$) [67].

> There is no evidence to prefer one antiepileptic drug over the others, but it is advised to avoid phenytoin because of interactions with anticoagulants and salicylates.

Post-stroke depression

Post-stroke depression (PSD) is considered to be the most frequent and important neuropsychiatric consequence of stroke and has a major impact on functional recovery, cognition and even survival.

The incidence of PSD ranges in various studies between 18 and 61%. Once again, the large variation in frequencies is due to methodological differences, including the point in time at which patients were assessed relative to the stroke onset and the different instruments and criteria for diagnosing depression that were used in the different studies.

A systematic review [68] of collected data from 51 observational studies conducted between 1977 and 2002 found that the frequency of post-stroke depression is 33% (95% CI, 29–36) and that the depression resolves spontaneously within several months of onset in most of the patients. The Italian multicenter observational study of post-stroke depression (DESTRO) [69] assessed 1064 patients with ischemic or hemorrhagic stroke in the first 9 months after the event. Patients with depression were followed for 2 years. PSD was detected in 36% of the patients, most of whom had minor depression with dysthymia, rather than major depression, and adaptation disorder. Although no correlation between PSD and mortality was found in the DESTRO study, an Australian study [70] found that among stroke patients in rehabilitation the depressed ones were eight times more likely to have died by 15-month follow-up than the non-depressed.

The potential etiology for PSD [71] includes neuroanatomic mechanisms such as disruption of monoaminergic pathways and depletion of cortical biogenic amines, especially in the case of lesions in the left frontal and left basal ganglia territories [72], and psychological mechanisms such as the difficulty in adjusting to the new limitations and requirements of the disease. In a systematic review [73] of 26 studies regarding the correlation of left hemispheric stroke and the risk of PSD no significant correlation was found. Differences in the measurement of depression, study design, and presentations of results may also have contributed to the heterogeneity of the findings. Other risk factors for PSD include female gender, severe physical disability, previous depression and history of psychiatric and emotional liability during the first days after stroke. Some studies have found aphasia as a risk factor, while others have not obtained similar results [74]. Dementia was also found to be an important predictor for the development of PSD [75].

> The frequency of post-stroke depression is 33% and it resolves spontaneously within several months of onset in most patients.

The treating physician should be aware of the diagnosis of depression in stroke survivors since it may be hindered by a number of conditions, including aphasia, agnosia, apraxia and memory disturbances. The differential diagnosis of PSD includes anosognosia, apathy, fatigue and disprosody [74]. Despite some encouraging data regarding the prophylactic use of antidepressants in post-stroke patients there is still insufficient randomized evidence to support this approach in routine post-stroke management [68]. A single recent double-blind placebo-controlled study evaluated the administration of escitalopram in a population of non-depressed patients following stroke [76]. Patients who received placebo were significantly more likely to develop depression than ones who received escitalopram after 12 months follow-up. Problem-solving therapy did not achieve significant results over placebo.

According to the ESO 2008 recommendations [20] antidepressant drugs such as selective serotonin reuptake inhibitors (SSRIs) and heterocyclics can improve mood after stroke, but there is less evidence that these agents can effect full remission of a major depressive episode or prevent depression. SSRIs are better tolerated than heterocyclics. There is no good evidence to recommend psychotherapy for treatment or prevention of post-stroke depression, although such therapy can elevate mood.

In spite of growing information, many questions still surround various aspects of PSD, including the development of standardized measure of depression, the optimal time after stroke onset to screen for PSD,

the creation of predictors for PSD and identifying the appropriate management.

> Antidepressant drugs can improve mood after stroke, but there is less evidence that these agents can be effective in a major depressive episode or prevention.

Post-stroke dementia

Stroke is an important risk factor for dementia and cognitive decline. According to the NINDAS-AIREN criteria, in order to make the diagnosis of post-stroke dementia (PSD) the patient has to be demented, with either historical, clinical or radiological evidence of cerebrovascular disease and the two disorders must be reasonably related [77]. On the other hand, according to the Diagnostic and Statistical Manual of Mental Disorders, fourth edition (DSM-4) [78], vascular dementia is diagnosed by the development of multiple cognitive deficits manifested by memory impairment and at least one of the following cognitive disturbances: aphasia, apraxia, agnosia and disturbance in executive functioning with the presence of focal neurological signs and symptoms or laboratory evidence indicative of cerebrovascular disease that is judged to be etiologically related to the disturbance. The deficits should not occur exclusively during the course of an episode of delirium.

Despite the lack of accurate data due to poor definition of the disorder, the use of different tools and diagnostic difficulties in distinguishing between PSD and other types of dementia, PSD is considered to be the second most common type of dementia. Since several studies used different tools for the diagnosis of PSD and there were also differences in the methodologies and study populations, the incidence varies in the different studies from 8 to 30%. One study, done among a population of elderly demented patients, demonstrated that the frequency of dementia was found to depend upon the diagnostic criteria used [79]. For instance, using the NINDAS-AIREN criteria only 14% of the patients were diagnosed with PSD, compared to 76% using the DSM-4 as a diagnostic tool. Interestingly there are also noticeable differences in the incidence rates between countries; an almost 3-fold difference in the age-standardized incidence ratios (SIR) of PSD rates between Germany and the Netherlands was demonstrated (1.23 and 0.42 respectively) [80], indicating that geographical variation is still present after taking into account the countries' differential age distributions. It is unclear whether these differences are due to genetic or environmental factors since, as in the previous trials mentioned, there were methodological differences between the studies.

Despite the conflicting data the overall estimated frequency of dementia in post-stroke patients is about 28% and the fact that stroke is a major risk factor for dementia is well established [81]. The mechanisms of PSD [82, 83] consist of large-vessel disease, including multi-infarcts or single infarcts in a strategic area such as the thalamus, hippocampus, basal forebrain or the angular gyrus, or small-vessel disease such as lacunes or leukoaraiosis. Other mechanisms include hypoperfusion, hypoxic-ischemic disorders and shared pathogenic pathways with degenerative dementia, especially Alzheimer type.

Risk factors for PSD include large and left-sided infarcts, bilateral infarcts, frontal lobe infarcts, large MCA infarcts and previous strokes. Diabetes, hyperlipidemia and atrial fibrillation were also found as predictors for the development of PSD [82–84]. Silent brain infarcts demonstrated on CT, however, were not found to predict the development of PSD in one prospective study [85], while in another higher grades of white matter findings on MRI were associated with impaired cognitive function [86]. Since it has also been shown in that study that the extent of white matter lesions is related to the blood pressure level, even in normotensive patients, and since these lesions are correlated with the risk of PSD, it would be reasonable to assume that lowering blood pressure would lower the risk of PSD. Abnormal EEG performed close to the ischemic stroke appears to be an indicator of subsequent PSD in a prospective study done among 199 patients, probably because it indicates cortical involvement [87].

The borders between dementia of the neurodegenerative type and vascular dementia are nowadays less visible and both types of dementia include many similar risk factors and clinical and pathological characteristics. It is suggested that cerebrovascular disease may play an important role in the presence and severity of AD [88].

There is no evidence-based treatment for PSD. In a meta-analysis of randomized controlled trials cholinesterase inhibitors, which are administered for the treatment of degenerative-type dementia, were found to produce only small benefits in cognition of uncertain clinical significance in patients with mild to moderate vascular dementia. There are insufficient data to recommend the use of these agents in PSD [89].

> The frequency of dementia (PSD) in post-stroke patients is about 28%. There is no evidence-based treatment for PSD.

Post-stroke fatigue

Another common and disabling late sequel of stroke is general fatigue [90, 91]. It is important to distinguish between "normal" fatigue, which is a state of general tiredness that is a result of overexertion and can be ameliorated by rest, and "pathological" fatigue, which is a more chronic condition, not related to previous exertion and not ameliorated by rest. Many other central and peripheral neurological conditions, beside stroke, are known to be a cause of fatigue, including multiple sclerosis, amyotrophic lateral sclerosis, Parkinson's disease, post-polio syndrome, HIV, collagen diseases and others [92–95]. It is important to emphasize that post-stroke fatigue is not always a part of post-stroke depression and can occur in the absence of depressive features [90, 96]. It is estimated that about 70% of post-stroke patients experience "pathological" fatigue. Fatigue was also rated by 40% of stroke patients as either their worst symptom or among their worst symptoms. Fatigue was found to be an independent predictor of functional disability and mortality [97]. Risk factors for post-stroke fatigue include older age and female sex, ADL impairment, living alone or in an institution, poor general health, anxiety, pain and depression. Some studies suggest the involvement of the brainstem and thalamus [91].

The caring physician should be alert to identify possible predisposing factors and to diagnose "pathological" fatigue. The initial treatment should focus on optimizing the management of potential factors, exercise, sleep hygiene, stress reduction and cognitive behavior therapy. The pharmacological therapy includes the stimulant agents amantadine and modafinil.

> It is estimated that about 70% of post-stroke patients experience fatigue and 40% of patients rate it among their worst symptoms. Pharmacological treatment includes the stimulating agents amantadine and modafinil.

Appropriate diagnosis and treatment of the late complications of stroke, which are often underdiagnosed and undertreated, are a crucial component in the management of stroke and should always be taken into consideration when dealing with stroke patients.

Chapter Summary

The overall rate of **post-stroke epilepsy**, defined as at least two episodes, is 3–4%. It is higher in patients who have a late seizure (early post-stroke seizures occur within the first 2 weeks after a stroke, late post-stroke seizures occur later). Predictors for post-stroke seizures are cortical location, large infarct, intracerebral hemorrhage and the presence of cardiac emboli and pre-existing dementia. Treatment should be initiated only after the second episode. There is no evidence to recommend one drug over the others but it is advised to avoid phenytoin because of interactions with anticoagulants and salicylates.

The frequency of **post-stroke depression** is 33% and it resolves spontaneously within several months of onset in most patients. Risk factors for post-stroke depression are female gender, severe physical disability, previous depression and dementia. According to the ESO 2008 recommendations antidepressant drugs such as selective serotonin reuptake inhibitors (SSRIs) and heterocyclics can improve mood after stroke.

For the diagnosis of **post-stroke dementia** (PSD) the patient has to be demented, with either historical, clinical or radiological evidence of cerebrovascular disease, and the two disorders must be reasonably related. PSD is the second most common type of dementia. The frequency of dementia in post-stroke patients is about 28%. Risk factors for PSD are large and left-sided infarcts, bilateral infarcts, frontal lobe infarcts, large MCA infarcts, previous strokes, diabetes, hyperlipidemia, and atrial fibrillation. There is no evidence-based treatment for PSD. Cholinesterase inhibitors were found to produce only small benefits in patients with mild to moderate vascular dementia.

Post-stroke fatigue is not related to previous exertion and is not ameliorated by rest and can occur in the absence of depressive features. It is estimated that about 70% of post-stroke patients experience fatigue and 40% of the patients rate it among their worst symptoms. The initial treatment should focus on the management of potential risk factors; pharmacological therapy includes the stimulant agents amantadine and modafinil.

References

1. Wallace JD, Levy LL. Blood pressure after stroke. *JAMA* 1981; 13; **246**(19):2177–80.

2. Carlberg B, Asplund K, Hägg E. Factors influencing admission blood pressure levels in patients with acute stroke. *Stroke* 1991; **22**:527–30.

3. Urrutia VC, Wityk RJ. Blood pressure management in acute stroke. *Crit Care Clin* 2006; **22**(4):695–711.

4. Leonardi-Bee J, Bath PM, Phillips SJ, Sandercock PA. IST Collaborative Group. Blood pressure and clinical outcomes in the International Stroke Trial. *Stroke* 2002; **33**:1315–20.

5. Vemmos KN, Tsivgoulis G, Spengos K, Zakopoulos N, Synetos A, Manios E, et al. U-shaped relationship between mortality and admission blood pressure in patients with acute stroke. *J Intern Med* 2004; **255**:257–65.

6. Aslanyan S, Fazekas F, Weir CJ, Horner S, Lees KR; GAIN International Steering Committee and Investigators. Effect of blood pressure during the acute period of ischemic stroke on stroke outcome: a tertiary analysis of the GAIN International Trial. *Stroke* 2003; **34**:2420–5.

7. Willmot M, Leonardi-Bee J, Bath PM. High blood pressure in acute stroke and subsequent outcome: a systematic review. *Hypertension* 2004; **43**(1):18–24.

8. Brott T, Lu M, Kothari R, Fagan SC, Frankel M, Grotta JC, et al. Hypertension and its treatment in the NINDS rt-PA Stroke Trial. *Stroke* 1998; **29**:1504–9.

9. Chamorro A, Vila N, Ascaso C, Elices E, Schonewille W, Blanc R. Blood pressure and functional recovery in acute ischemic stroke. *Stroke* 1998; **29**:1850–3.

10. Carlberg B, Asplund K, Hägg E. The prognostic value of admission blood pressure in patients with acute stroke. *Stroke* 1993; **24**:1372–5.

11. Mattle HP, Kappeler L, Arnold M, Fischer U, Nedeltchev K, Remonda L, et al. Blood pressure and vessel recanalization in the first hours after ischemic stroke. *Stroke* 2005; **36**:264–8.

12. Shin HK, Nishimura M, Jones PB, Ay H, Boas DA, Moskowitz MA, et al. Mild induced hypertension improves blood flow and oxygen metabolism in transient focal cerebral ischemia. *Stroke* 2008; **39**:1548–55.

13. Rordorf G, Koroshetz WJ, Ezzeddine MA, Segal AZ, Buonanno FS. A pilot study of drug-induced hypertension for treatment of acute stroke. *Neurology* 2001; **56**:1210–3.

14. Marzan AS, Hungerbühler HJ, Studer A, Baumgartner RW, Georgiadis D. Feasibility and safety of norepinephrine-induced arterial hypertension in acute ischemic stroke. *Neurology* 2004; **62**:1193–5.

15. Hillis AE, Ulatowski JA, Barker PB, Torbey M, Ziai W, Beauchamp NJ, et al. A pilot randomized trial of induced blood pressure elevation: effects on function and focal perfusion in acute and subacute stroke. *Cerebrovasc Dis* 2003; **16**:236–46.

16. Olsen TS, Larsen B, Herning M, Skriver EB, Lassen NA. Blood flow and vascular reactivity in collaterally perfused brain tissue. Evidence of an ischemic penumbra in patients with acute stroke. *Stroke* 1983; **14**:332–41.

17. Mistri AK, Robinson TG, Potter JF. Pressor therapy in acute ischemic stroke: systematic review. *Stroke* 2006; **37**(6):1565–71.

18. Schrader J, Lüders S, Kulschewski A, Berger J, Zidek W, Treib J, et al. Acute Candesartan Cilexetil Therapy in Stroke Survivors Study Group. The ACCESS Study: evaluation of Acute Candesartan Cilexetil Therapy in Stroke Survivors. *Stroke* 2003; **34**:1699–703.

19. Potter JF, Robinson TG, Ford GA, James M, Chernova J, Jagger C. Controlling hypertension and hypotension immediately post-stroke (CHHIPS): a randomised, placebo-controlled, double-blind pilot trial. *Lancet Neurol* 2009; **8**:48–56.

20. The European Stroke Organisation (ESO) Executive Committee and the ESO Writing Committee. Guidelines for Management of Ischaemic Stroke and Transient Ischaemic Attack 2008. *Cerebrovasc Dis* 2008; **25**:457–507.

21. Adams HP Jr, del Zoppo G, Alberts MJ, Bhatt DL, Brass L, Furlan A, et al. American Heart Association; American Stroke Association Stroke Council; Clinical Cardiology Council; Cardiovascular Radiology and Intervention Council; Atherosclerotic Peripheral Vascular Disease and Quality of Care Outcomes in Research Interdisciplinary Working Groups. Guidelines for the early management of adults with ischemic stroke: a guideline from the American Heart Association/American Stroke Association Stroke Council, Clinical Cardiology Council, Cardiovascular Radiology and Intervention Council, and the Atherosclerotic Peripheral Vascular Disease and Quality of Care Outcomes in Research Interdisciplinary Working Groups: the American Academy of Neurology affirms the value of this guideline as an educational tool for neurologists. *Stroke* 2007; **38**:1655–711.

22. Vázquez-Cruz J, Martí-Vilalta JL, Ferrer I, Pérez-Gallofré A, Folch J. Progressing cerebral infarction in relation to plasma glucose in gerbils. *Stroke* 1990; **21**(11):1621–4.

23. Martín A, Rojas S, Chamorro A, Falcón C, Bargalló N, Planas AM. Why does acute hyperglycemia worsen the outcome of transient focal cerebral ischemia? Role of corticosteroids, inflammation, and protein O-glycosylation. *Stroke* 2006; **37**(5):1288–95. Epub 2006 Apr 6.

24. Kiers L, Davis SM, Larkins R, Hopper J, Tress B, Rossiter SC, et al. Stroke topography and outcome in relation to hyperglycaemia and diabetes. *J Neurol Neurosurg Psychiatry* 1992; **55**:263–70.

24b. Matz K, Keresztes K, Tatschl C, Nowotny M, Dachenhausen A, Brainin M, et al. Disorders of glucose metabolism in acute stroke patients: an underrecognized problem. *Diabetes Care* 2006; **29**:792–7.

25. Capes SE, Hunt D, Malmberg K, Pathak P, Gerstein HC. Stress hyperglycemia and prognosis of stroke in nondiabetic and diabetic patients: a systematic overview. *Stroke* 2001; **32**:2426–32.

26. Alvarez-Sabín J, Molina CA, Montaner J, Arenillas JF, Huertas R, Ribo M, et al. Effects of admission hyperglycemia on stroke outcome in reperfused tissue plasminogen activator-treated patients. *Stroke* 2003; **34**:1235–41.

27. Parsons MW, Barber PA, Desmond PM, Baird TA, Darby DG, Byrnes G, et al. Acute hyperglycemia adversely affects stroke outcome: a magnetic resonance imaging and spectroscopy study. *Ann Neurol* 2002; **52**(1):20–8.

28. Allport LE, Butcher KS, Baird TA, MacGregor L, Desmond PM, Tress BM, et al. Insular cortical ischemia is independently associated with acute stress hyperglycemia. *Stroke* 2004; **35**:1886–91.

29. van den Berghe G, Wouters P, Weekers F, Verwaest C, Bruyninckx F, Schetz M, et al. Intensive insulin therapy in critically ill patients. *N Engl J Med* 2001; **345**(19):1359–67.

30. Malmberg K. Prospective randomized study of intensive insulin treatment on long term survival after acute myocardial infarction in patients with diabetes mellitus. DIGAMI (Diabetes Mellitus, Insulin Glucose Infusion in Acute Myocardial Infarction) Study Group. *BMJ* 1997; **24**; **314**:1512–5.

31. Gray CS, Hildreth AJ, Sandercock PA, O'Connell JE, Johnston DE, Cartlidge NE, et al. GIST Trialists Collaboration. Glucose-potassium-insulin infusions in the management of post-stroke hyperglycaemia: the UK Glucose Insulin in Stroke Trial (GIST-UK). *Lancet Neurol* 2007; **6**:397–406.

32. McCormick MT, Muir KW, Gray C, Walters MR. Management of hyperglycemia in acute stroke: how, when, and for whom? *Stroke* 2008; **39**(7):2177–85.

33. Glucose Regulation in Acute Stroke Patients Trial (GRASP). The internet stroke center. American Stroke Association. 2008.

34. Bruno A, Kent TA, Coull BM, Shankar RR, Saha C, Becker KJ, et al. Treatment of hyperglycemia in ischemic stroke (THIS): a randomized pilot trial. *Stroke* 2008; **39**(2):384–9. Epub 2007 Dec 20.

35. Memezawa H, Zhao Q, Smith ML, Siesjö BK. Hyperthermia nullifies the ameliorating effect of dizocilpine maleate (MK-801) in focal cerebral ischemia. *Brain Res* 1995; **670**(1):48–52.

36. Wass CT, Lanier WL, Hofer RE, Scheithauer BW, Andrews AG. Temperature changes of > or = 1 degree C alter functional neurologic outcome and histopathology in a canine model of complete cerebral ischemia. *Anesthesiology* 1995; **83**:325–35.

37. Reith J, Jørgensen HS, Pedersen PM, Nakayama H, Raaschou HO, Jeppesen LL, et al. Body temperature in acute stroke: relation to stroke severity, infarct size, mortality, and outcome. *Lancet* 1996; **347**:422–5.

38. Castillo J, Dávalos A, Marrugat J, Noya M. Timing for fever-related brain damage in acute ischemic stroke. *Stroke* 1998; **29**(12):2455–60.

39. Varon J, Acosta P. Therapeutic hypothermia: past, present, and future. *Chest* 2008; **133**:1267–74.

40. Hypothermia After Cardiac Arrest Study Group. Mild therapeutic hypothermia to improve the neurological outcome after cardiac arrest. *N Engl J Med* 2002; 346:549–56.

41. Clifton GL, Miller ER, Choi SC, Levin HS, McCauley S, Smith KR Jr, et al. Lack of effect of induction of hypothermia after acute brain injury. *N Engl J Med* 2001; **344**:556–63.

42. Kasner SE, Wein T, Piriyawat P, Villar-Cordova CE, Chalela JA, Krieger DW, et al. Acetaminophen for altering body temperature in acute stroke: a randomized clinical trial. *Stroke* 2002; **33**:130–4.

43. Dippel DW, van Breda EJ, van Gemert HM, van der Worp HB, Meijer RJ, Kappelle LJ, et al. Effect of paracetamol (acetaminophen) on body temperature in acute ischemic stroke: a double-blind, randomized phase II clinical trial. *Stroke* 2001; **32**:1607–12.

44. Schwab S, Schwarz S, Spranger M, Keller E, Bertram M, Hacke W. Moderate hypothermia in the treatment of patients with severe middle cerebral artery infarction. *Stroke* 1998; **29**:2461–6.

45. Guluma KZ, Oh H, Yu SW, Meyer BC, Rapp K, Lyden PD. Effect of endovascular hypothermia on acute ischemic edema: morphometric analysis of the ICTuS trial. *Neurocrit Care* 2008; **8**(1):42–7.

46. Olsen TS, Weber UJ, Kammersgaard LP, et al. Therapeutic hypothermia for acute stroke. *Lancet Neurol* 2003; **2**:410–6.

47. De Georgia MA, Krieger DW, Abou-Chebl A, Devlin TG, Jauss M, Davis SM, et al. Cooling for Acute Ischemic Brain Damage (COOL AID): a feasibility trial of endovascular cooling. *Neurology*. 2004; **63**(2):312–7.

48. Forsgren L, Bucht G, Eriksson S, Bergmark L. Incidence and clinical characterization of unprovoked seizures in adults: a prospective population-based study. *Epilepsia* 1996; **37**:224–9.

49. Bladin CF, Alexandrov AV, Bellavance A, Bornstein N, Chambers B, Coté R, et al. Seizures after stroke: a prospective multicenter study. *Arch Neurol* 2000; **57**:1617–22.

50. Lesser RP, Luders H, Dinner DS, Morris HH. Epileptic seizures due to thrombotic and embolic cerebrovascular disease in older patients. *Epilepsia* 1985; **26**:622–30.

51. So EL, Annegers JF, Hauser WA, O'Brien PC, Whisnant JP. Population-based study of seizure disorders after cerebral infarction. *Neurology* 1996; **46**:350–5.

52. Kilpatrick CJ, Davis SM, Tress BM, Rossiter SC, Hopper JL, Vandendriesen ML. Epileptic seizures in acute stroke. *Arch Neurol* 1990; **47**:157–60.

53. Shinton RA, Gill JS, Melnick AK. The frequency, characteristics, and prognosis of epileptic seizures at the onset of stroke. *J Neurol Neurosurg Psychiatry* 1988; **51**:273–276.

54. Arboix A, Garcia-Eroles L, Massons JB, Oliveres M, Comes E. Predictive factors of early seizures after acute cerebrovascular disease. *Stroke* 1997; **28**:1590–4.

55. Reith J, Jørgensen HS, Nakayama H, Raaschou HO, Olsen TS. Seizures in acute stroke: the Copenhagen Stroke Study. *Stroke* 1997; **28**:1585–9.

56. Giroud M, Gras P, Fayolle H, André N, Soichot P, Dumas R. Early seizures after stroke: a study of 1,640 cases. *Epilepsia* 1994; **35**:959–64.

57. Olsen TS. Post-stroke epilepsy. *Curr Atheroscler Rep* 2001; **3**(4):340–4. Review.

58. Benbir G, Ince B, Bozluolcay M. The epidemiology of post-stroke epilepsy according to stroke sub types. *Acta Neurol Scand* 2006; **114**:8–12.

59. Myint PK, Staufenberg EF, Sabanathan K. Post-stroke seizure and post-stroke epilepsy. *Postgrad Med J* 2006; **82**:568–72.

60. Cordonnier C, Hénon H, Derambure P, Pasquier F, Leys D. Influence of pre-existing dementia on the risk of post-stroke epileptic seizures. *J Neurol Neurosurg Psychiatry* 2005; **76**:1649–53.

61. De Reuck J, Proot P, Van Maele G. Chronic obstructive pulmonary disease as a risk factor for stroke-related seizures. *Eur J Neurol* 2007; **14**:989–92.

62. Sun DA, Sombati S, DeLorenzo RJ. Glutamate injury-induced epileptogenesis in hippocampal neurons: an in vitro model of stroke-induced "epilepsy". *Stroke* 2001; **32**:2344–50.

63. Stroemer RP, Kent TA, Hulsebosch CE. Neocortical neural sprouting, synaptogenesis, and behavioral

recovery after neocortical infarction in rats. *Stroke* 1995; **26**:2135–44.

64. Gilad R, Lampl Y, Eschel Y, Sadeh M. Antiepileptic treatment in patients with early postischemic stroke seizures: a retrospective study. *Cerebrovas Dis* 2001; **12**:39–43.

65. Ryvlin P, Montavont A, Nighoghossian N. Optimizing therapy of seizures in stroke patients. *Neurology* 2006 26; **67**(12 Suppl 4):S3–9.

66. Alvarez-Sabín J, Montaner J, Padró L, Molina CA, Rovira R, Codina A. Gabapentin in late-onset poststroke seizures. *Neurology* 2002; **59**(12):1991–3.

67. Gilad R, Sadeh M, Rapoport A, Dabby R, Boaz M, Lampl Y. Monotherapy of lamotrigine versus carbamazepine in patients with poststroke seizure. *Clin Neuropharmacol* 2007; **30**:189–95.

68. Hackett ML, Yapa C, Parag V, Anderson CS. Frequency of depression after stroke: a systematic review of observational studies. *Stroke* 2005; **36**:1330–4.

69. Paolucci S, Gandolfo C, Provinciali L, Torta R, Toso V. DESTRO Study Group. The Italian multicenter observational study on post-stroke depression (DESTRO). *J Neurol* 2006; **253**:556–62.

70. Morris PL, Robinson RG, Samuels J. Depression, introversion and mortality following stroke. *Aust N Z J Psychiatry* 1993; **27**:443–9.

71. Gainotti G, Marra C. Determinants and consequences of post-stroke depression. *Curr Opin Neurol* 2002; **15**(1):85–9.

72. Narushima K, Kosier JT, Robinson RG. A reappraisal of poststroke depression, intra- and inter-hemispheric lesion location using meta-analysis. *J Neuropsychiatry Clin Neurosci* 2003; **15**:422–30.

73. Bhogal SK, Teasell R, Foley N, Speechley M. Lesion location and poststroke depression: systematic review of the methodological limitations in the literature. *Stroke* 2004; **35**:794–802.

74. Gaete JM, Bogousslavsky J. Post-stroke depression. *Expert Rev Neurother* 2008; **8**:75–92.

75. Brodaty H, Withball A, Sachdev PS. Rates of depression at 3 and 15 months poststroke and their relationship with cognitive decline: the Sydney Stroke Study. *Am J Geriatr Psychiatry* 2007; **15**:477–486.

76. Robinson RG, Jorge RE, Moser DJ, Acion L, Solodkin A, Small SL, et al. Escitalopram and problem-solving therapy for prevention of poststroke depression: a randomized controlled trial. *JAMA* 2008; **299**:2391–400.

77. Román GC, Tatemichi TK, Erkinjuntti T, Cummings JL, Masdeu JC, Garcia JH, et al. Vascular dementia: diagnostic criteria for research studies. Report of the NINDS-AIREN International Workshop. *Neurology* 1993; **43**(2):250–60.

78. *Diagnostic and Statistical Manual of mental disorders (DSM-4)*, 4th ed. Washington DC: American Psychiatric Association; 1994.

79. Wetterling T, Kanitz RD, Borgis KJ. Comparison of different diagnostic criteria for vascular dementia (ADDTC, DSM-IV, ICD-10, NINDS-AIREN). *Stroke* 1996; **27**:30–6.

80. Dubois MF, Hébert R. The incidence of vascular dementia in Canada: a comparison with Europe and East Asia. *Neuroepidemiology* 2001; **20**(3):179–87.

81. Hénon H, Durieu I, Guerouaou D, Lebert F, Pasquier F, Leys D. Poststroke dementia: incidence and relationship to prestroke cognitive decline. *Neurology* 2001; **57**:1216–22.

82. Ince PG, Fernando MS. Neuropathology of vascular cognitive impairment and vascular dementia. *Int Psychogeriatr* 2003; **15** Suppl 1:71–5.

83. Jellinger KA. Pathology and pathophysiology of vascular cognitive impairment. A critical update. *Panminerva Med* 2004; **46**(4):217–21.

84. Skoog I. Status of risk factors for vascular dementia. *Neuroepidemiology* 1998; **17**(1):2–9.

85. Bornstein NM, Gur AY, Treves TA, Reider-Groswasser I, Aronovich BD, Klimovitzky SS, et al. Do silent brain infarctions predict the development of dementia after first ischemic stroke? *Stroke* 1996; **27**:904–5.

86. Longstreth WT Jr, Manolio TA, Arnold A, Burke GL, Bryan N, Jungreis CA, et al. Clinical correlates of white matter findings on cranial magnetic resonance imaging of 3301 elderly people. The Cardiovascular Health Study. *Stroke* 1996; **27**:1274–82.

87. Gur AY, Neufeld MY, Treves TA, Aronovich BD, Bornstein NM, Korczyn AD. EEG as predictor of dementia following first ischemic stroke. *Acta Neurol Scand* 1994; **90**(4):263–5.

88. Snowdon DA, Greiner LH, Mortimer JA, Riley KP, Greiner PA, Markesbery WR. Brain infarction and the clinical expression of Alzheimer disease. The Nun Study. *JAMA* 1997; **277**:813–7.

89. Kavirajan H, Schneider LS. Efficacy and adverse effects of cholinesterase inhibitors and memantine in vascular dementia: a meta-analysis of randomised controlled trials. *Lancet Neurol* 2007; **6**:782–92.

90. Ingles JL, Eskes GA, Phillips SJ. Fatigue after stroke. *Arch Phys Med Rehabil* 1999; **80**(2):173–8.

91. Staub F, Bogousslavsky J. Fatigue after stroke: a major but neglected issue. *Cerebrovasc Dis* 2001; **12**:75–81.

92. Fisk JD, Pontefract A, Ritvo PG, Archibald CJ, Murray TJ. The impact of fatigue on patients with multiple sclerosis. *Can J Neurol Sci* 1994; **21**:9–14.

93. Rose L, Pugh LC, Lears K, Gordon DL. The fatigue experience: persons with HIV infection. *J Adv Nurs* 1998; **28**:295–304.

94. Riemsma RP, Rasker JJ, Taal E, Griep EN, Wouters JM, Wiegman O. Fatigue in rheumatoid arthritis: the role of self-efficacy and problematic social support. *Br J Rheumatol* 1998; **37**:1042–6.

95. Zwarts MJ, Bleijenberg G, van Engelen BG. Clinical neurophysiology of fatigue. *Clin Neurophysiol* 2008; **119**:2–10.

96. van der Werf SP, van den Broek HL, Anten HW, Bleijenberg G. Experience of severe fatigue long after stroke and its relation to depressive symptoms and disease characteristics. *Eur Neurol* 2001; **45**:28–33.

97. Glader EL, Stegmayr B, Asplund K. Poststroke fatigue: a 2-year follow-up study of stroke patients in Sweden. *Stroke* 2002; **33**:1327–33.

Chapter 18

Infections in stroke

Achim Kaasch and Harald Seifert

Introduction

Bacterial, viral and parasitic infections are associated with stroke in several ways. First, at least 20% of strokes are preceded by a bacterial infection in the month prior to stroke. Second, many pathogens that affect the central nervous system are able to directly cause stroke. Third, patients who suffer a stroke are prone to develop infectious complications due to post-stroke immunodepression and impaired swallow and cough reflexes.

In this chapter, we will briefly summarize available evidence on how bacterial infections can trigger stroke. Then, specific infectious diseases are reviewed that are a direct cause of stroke, such as endocarditis, vasculitis and chronic meningitis. Furthermore, aspiration pneumonia is discussed, as an example of an early infectious complication that arises within the first week after stroke. Late infectious complications, occurring later than a week after stroke, such as ventilator-associated pneumonia or catheter-related infections, will not be covered since they are common infections in the hospital with no specific link to stroke.

Infections preceding stroke

Recent infection and stroke

Several studies have supplied evidence that acute infection in the week preceding stroke is an independent risk factor for cerebral infarction (odds ratio 3.4–14.5) [1–3]. Especially bacterial respiratory and urinary tract infections can trigger ischemic stroke [4]. Since a heterogeneous group of microbial pathogens is involved, the systemic inflammatory response is probably more important than microbial invasion per se. However, a detailed molecular understanding of events that lead to a higher susceptibility to cerebral infarction is lacking. Numerous mechanisms have been discussed. For example, inflammation has been implicated in atheroma instability and subsequent plaque rupture, alteration of the coagulation system, platelet aggregation, adhesion and lysis. Furthermore, alteration of the lipid metabolism, spasms in vascular smooth muscle, anti-phospholipid antibody formation, and impairment of endothelial function by endotoxin and bacterial toxins have been reported. Apart from these factors, dehydration, bed rest and mechanical factors such as sneezing may play a role.

Aside from bacterial infections, common viral diseases such as seasonal flu may trigger stroke. Several observational studies suggest that influenza vaccination lowers the risk of cerebral infarction (for review see Lichy and Grau [4]). However, conclusive evidence for a protective effect is still lacking.

Chronic infections and stroke

Atherosclerosis is a common disease and a major risk factor for stroke. Its etiology can largely be explained by the classic risk factors (age, gender, genetic predisposition, hypertension, diabetes, hypercholesterolemia, diet, smoking, low physical activity, etc.). Additionally, pathogens such as *Helicobacter pylori*, cytomegalovirus, herpes simplex virus and *Chlamydia pneumoniae* have been proposed to be associated with atherosclerosis.

Most studies on the infectious etiology of atherosclerosis have been focused on *Chlamydia pneumoniae* (for review see Watson and Alp [5]). *C. pneumoniae* is an obligate intracellular bacterium and usually causes mild upper respiratory tract infections, and occasionally pneumonia. Exposure to this agent is common and by the age of 20 years 50% of individuals are seropositive.

Animal models support a role of *C. pneumoniae* in the initiation, maintenance and rupture of atherosclerotic lesions, but clinical and epidemiological studies have not come to conclusive results. This shortcoming might be explained by the difficulty in attributing causality to a common pathogen and a multifactorial disease.

As with atherosclerosis, the contribution of chronic bacterial infections to the etiology of stroke is unclear. Some studies found an increased risk of stroke in patients with elevated antibody titers suggesting previous *C. pneumoniae* infection, *H. pylori* gastritis, and periodontal disease (caused by a great variety of bacteria). For these pathogens conflicting information has been published [6, 7] and randomized interventional trials, for example, aiming at the eradication of *C. pneumonia* by macrolide therapy, failed to reduce the incidence of vascular events [8, 9].

Since an association between a single pathogen and an increased risk of stroke has so far not been proven, the "infectious burden concept" was developed. It states that the aggregate burden of microbial antigens determines stroke risk rather than the occurrence of a single pathogen [10]. However, which bacteria should be included in a stroke-risk panel and how the microbial burden is measured remains an open question, as does, even more so, whether and when antimicrobial intervention may be appropriate.

Acute and chronic infections can raise the risk of cerebral infarction.

Infectious diseases that cause stroke

Multiple pathophysiological mechanisms can lead to stroke in bacterial, viral and parasitic diseases. An overview of organisms implicated in infectious diseases that may lead to stroke and their associated pathophysiology is presented in Table 18.1. For example, (i) emboli from infected heart valves may obstruct cerebral arteries in bacterial or fungal endocarditis; (ii) direct microbial invasion and inflammation of the vessel wall can lead to wall destruction and obliteration of the lumen, as in obliterative vasculitis or necrotizing panarteritis; (iii) chronic inflammation of the meninges leads to stroke through several mechanisms; (iv) mycotic aneurysms can rupture and cause hemorrhagic stroke. In the following section we will review some of these diseases and associated pathogenic principles.

Embolic stroke

Infective endocarditis

Infective endocarditis (IE) is an infection of the endocardium, a thin tissue layer that lines heart valves and mural myocardium (Figure 18.1). The incidence of IE

Table 18.1. Infectious causes of stroke and associated mechanisms.

Embolism	
Bacteria and fungi	
Infective endocarditis	*Staphylococcus aureus, Streptococcus* spp., *Enterococcus* spp., *Aspergillus* spp., and others
Protozoa	
Chagas disease	*Trypanosoma cruzi*
Meningitis	
Bacteria	
Acute meningitis	*Neisseria meningitidis, Haemophilus influenzae, Streptococcus pneumoniae,* and others
Chronic meningitis	*Mycobacterium tuberculosis, Borrelia burgdorferi, Treponema pallidum*
Fungi	
Chronic meningitis	*Cryptococcus neoformans, Coccidioides immitis*
Helminths	
Chronic meningitis	*Taenia solium*
Vasculitis	
Virus	
Vasculopathy	Varicella zoster virus, HIV
Mycotic aneurysm	
Bacteria	*Staphylococcus aureus, Salmonella enteritidis,* and others
Fungi	*Aspergillus, Candida* spp.

is about 5–10 cases per 100 000 person-years and it is a serious disease with about 20% mortality. The main risk factors for endocarditis are injection drug use, an underlying structural heart disease (such as congenital heart defects or degenerative valvular lesions), hemodialysis and invasive intravascular procedures. Carriers of a prosthetic heart valve are especially at risk, with a 1–4% chance of developing IE within the first year following surgery [11].

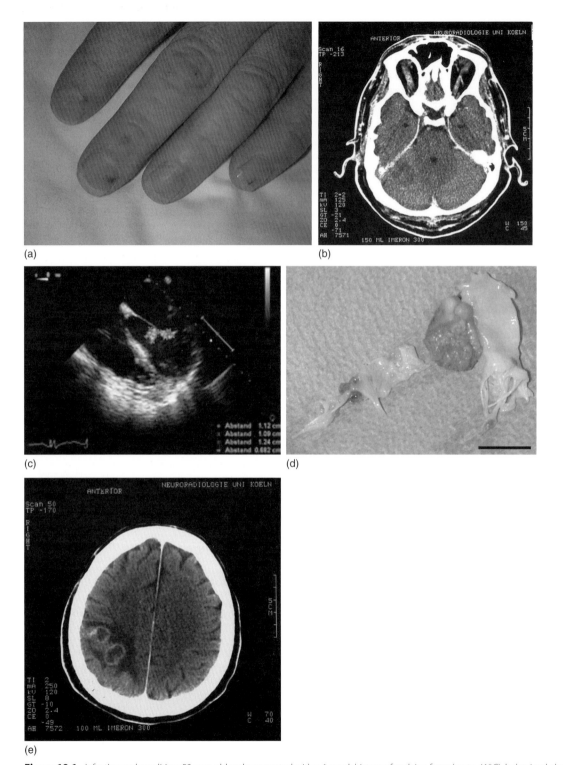

(a)

(b)

(c)

(d)

(e)

Figure 18.1. Infective endocarditis: a 53-year-old male presented with a 1-week history of malaise, fever (up to 41°C), behavioral changes and headache. On clinical examination mild meningeal signs, left-sided ataxia, and splinter hemorrhages (a) were noted. Computed tomography (CT) of the brain showed several ischemic lesions in both hemispheres and right cerebellum (b). *Staphylococcus aureus* was cultured from blood and cerebrospinal fluid. Transesophageal echocardiography revealed a large mitral valve lesion (c) which was subsequently removed surgically (d, bar = 1 cm). A CT scan 3 weeks after initial symptoms showed abscess formation with contrast enhancement and marked edema (e). (Courtesy of K. Lackner, Department of Radiology, F. Dodos, Department of Cardiology, and J. Wippermann, Department of Cardiac Surgery, University Hospital of Cologne).

Table 18.2. Distribution of etiological agents in patients with endocarditis (adapted from Wisplinghoff and Seifert [50]).

Pathogen	Mean	Range
Streptococci	50%	35–53
Viridans group streptococci	33%	17–48
Other streptococci	17%	5–33
Enterococci	8%	6–10
Staphylococci	30%	29–38
Staphylococcus aureus	23%	22–31
Coagulase-negative staphylococci	7%	6–8
Gram-negative aerobic bacilli (e.g. HACEK group*)	3%	1–3
Fungi (e.g. *Candida* spp., *Aspergillus* spp.)	1%	0–1
Other bacteria	2%	1–4
Polymicrobial infections	3%	3–4
Culture negative	8%	6–12

Notes: *Haemophilus aphrophilus, Aggregatibacter actinomycetemcomitans, Cardiobacterium hominis, Eikenella corrodens,* and *Kingella kingae.*

IE is caused by bacteria or fungi that attach to and damage the endocardium or the prosthetic valve and grow into vegetations measuring up to several centimeters in size. If left untreated, destruction of the heart valve ultimately leads to heart failure and death. Complications, e.g. stroke, can arise when emboli break off from the vegetation and occlude blood vessels, leading to infarction of the supplied tissues.

Microbiology of IE

Many bacteria and fungi can cause IE, some of which are listed with their overall frequency of isolation in Table 18.2. Different clinical conditions favor certain microbes, e.g. right-sided endocarditis in injection drug abusers is commonly caused by *Staphylococcus aureus* (>80%). In patients with prosthetic heart valves, late IE (i.e. more than 2 months after surgery) is less often caused by *S. aureus* than by coagulase-negative staphylococci (about 30% of all cases). Although fungal pathogens are rarely a cause of IE, *Candida* or *Aspergillus* spp. may occur in immunocompromised patients.

Depending on the causative organisms different clinical courses can be observed. *Staphylococcus*

aureus and Enterobacteriaceae such as *Escherichia coli* or *Klebsiella pneumoniae* are associated with an acute course and high mortality. Patients with IE due to enterococci or viridans group streptococci usually report several weeks of symptoms before a clinical diagnosis is made.

Clinical presentation and diagnostic criteria in IE

Clinical signs and symptoms for IE are highly variable and often misleading. Fever, heart murmur, malaise, anorexia, weight loss, night sweats and myalgia may or may not occur. The clinical course can be acute or subacute. Therefore IE is often recognized late, e.g. when complications have occurred.

To facilitate diagnosis of IE, diagnostic criteria have been developed. From the results of the clinical examination, blood cultures and ultrasound imaging (preferably transesophageal echocardiography, TEE) a clinical score is derived that describes the likelihood of IE in a specific patient (e.g. Duke criteria, see Table 18.3).

Neurological complications of IE are common (about 20–40%) and are associated with a worse outcome. They include stroke, intracranial or subarachnoidal hemorrhage, meningitis, seizures, encephalopathy, brain abscess, and mycotic aneurysm (frequencies in Table 18.4). Most neurological complications may go unnoticed. In a recent study cerebrovascular events were detected by MRI in 65% of patients with left-sided IE, but clinical symptoms were observed in only 35% of patients [12].

Pathogenesis of IE

IE is the result of a complex interaction between microorganism, matrix molecules and platelets at the site of endocardial cell damage. The pathophysiological process can be divided into several stages: formation of nonbacterial thrombotic endocarditis (NBTE), bacterial colonization of the lesion and growth into vegetations [13].

Endocardial damage is the starting point of IE pathogenesis. It is caused by congenital or acquired heart diseases that are associated with a turbulent blood flow. Then, fibrin and platelets are deposited on traumatized endothelium, which results in NBTE. Microorganisms that have gained access to the bloodstream (bacteremia) and possess the necessary virulence factors may now colonize the lesion and lead to IE.

Table 18.3. Modified Duke Criteria for the diagnosis of infective endocarditis [51, 52]. The diagnosis of IE is *definite* when (i) pathological/microbiological examination of vegetation shows active endocarditis, or (ii) two major criteria, (iii) one major and three minor, or (iv) five minor criteria are met. IE is *possible* when (i) one major and one minor, or (ii) three minor criteria are met. It is *rejected* when (i) a firm alternative diagnosis explaining evidence of IE or (ii) resolution of IE syndrome with ≤ 4 days of antimicrobial treatment, or (iii) no pathological evidence of IE at surgery or autopsy with ≤ 4 days of antimicrobial treatment, or criteria for possible or (iv) definite IE are not met.

Major criteria

Blood culture positive for IE

Typical microorganism consistent with IE isolated from two separate blood cultures

(viridans group streptococci, *Streptococcus bovis*, HACEK group, *Staphylococcus aureus*; or community-acquired enterococci, in the absence of a primary focus)

or Microorganism consistent with IE from persistently positive blood cultures (defined as at least two positive cultures of blood samples drawn >12 h apart; *or* all of three or a majority of four or more separate cultures of blood, with first and last sample drawn at least 1 h apart)

Evidence of endocardial involvement

Echocardiogram positive for IE* as follows: oscillating intracardiac mass on valve or supporting structures, in the path of regurgitant jets, or on implanted material in the absence of an alternative anatomic explanation; *or* abscess; *or* new partial dehiscence of prosthetic valve

or New valvular regurgitation (worsening or changing of pre-existing murmur not sufficient)

Minor criteria

Predisposition (predisposing heart condition or injection drug use)

Fever (temperature >38°C)

Vascular phenomena

major arterial emboli, septic pulmonary infarcts, mycotic aneurysm, intracranial hemorrhage, conjunctival hemorrhage, and Janeway's lesions

Immunological phenomena

glomerulonephritis, Osler's nodes, Roth's spots, and rheumatoid factor

Suggestive microbiological findings

positive blood culture not meeting major criterion or serological evidence of active infection with organism consistent with IE

Notes: *Transesophageal echocardiography (TEE) recommended in patients with prosthetic valves, rated at least 'possible IE' by clinical criteria, or complicated IE (paravalvular abscess). TTE as first test in other patients.

Table 18.4. Frequencies of neurological complications in infective endocarditis based on 1365 cases from seven studies (adapted from Cavassini et al. [53]).

Complication	Frequency
Emboli	20–57%
Intra- or subarachnoidal hemorrhage	7–25%
Mycotic aneurysm	3–16%
Meningitis	6–39%
Abscess	2–16%
Encephalopathy	17–33%
Seizure	2–29%
Headache	9–25%

A frequent cause of bacteremia is damage of a mucosal surface. All mucosal surfaces, such as oral cavity, nasopharynx, GI tract, urethra or vagina, are populated by a dense endogenous flora with many diverse bacterial species. Even a minor trauma such as tooth brushing or tooth extraction may lead to a temporary occurrence of bacteria in the bloodstream (transient bacteremia).

After having gained access to the bloodstream, IE-causing pathogens adhere to the NBTE. Adhesion to fibrin and platelets or to the surface of medical devices, such as artificial heart valves, is facilitated by virulence factors, many of which have been identified in staphylococci, streptococci, and enterococci.

Following adhesion, bacteria stimulate the deposition of further fibrin and platelets and a secluded compartment is formed, which hides bacteria from the host immunological defense. The microorganisms proliferate and produce a mucilaginous polysaccharide matrix which is called biofilm. In a biofilm less than 10% of bacteria divide actively and responsiveness to antimicrobial treatment is decreased. Additionally, antimicrobials need to penetrate the biofilm to reach the bacterial targets. Therefore, optimal antimicrobial treatment is crucial for a successful therapy of IE.

Pathogenic mechanisms leading to stroke in IE

Occlusion of cerebral arteries by septic or sterile emboli that originate from the vegetations is a common cause of stroke in IE. Impairment of the cerebral blood flow can lead to transient ischemia (TIA) or manifest stroke. Depending on the localization and duration of reduced blood flow, focal clinical signs occur. When multiple emboli occlude several independent vessels, multifocal clinical signs may become apparent.

The source of emboli to the central nervous system is usually the left heart, from vegetations on the mitral or aortic valve. Emboli from the right heart are filtered by intrapulmonary arteries and cause pulmonary embolism. Therefore, tricuspid valve endocarditis, which is common among intravenous drug users, rarely leads to stroke. However, in rare cases paradoxical embolism has been reported.

Other complications of IE, such as brain abscesses and meningitis, can also lead to stroke. A brain abscess occurs after hematogenous seeding of bacteria to the brain parenchyma. It is a rare complication of IE, but in 2–4% of patients with brain abscesses IE is the source of bacteria.

A brain abscess typically develops over 2–3 weeks. Initial imaging studies show a poorly demarcated lesion with localized edema. Over the weeks a clearly defined lesion develops, often accompanied by an extensive edema. The early stage is called cerebritis and is histologically defined by acute inflammation without tissue necrosis.

During abscess development tissue necrosis, liquefaction, and a fibrotic capsule become more prominent. A typical histological finding is a central necrotic area containing bacteria and debris and a hyperemic margin with bacteria and immune cells. In many cases antimicrobial therapy of a brain abscess alone is unsuccessful and has to be backed by surgical drainage.

Hematogenous seeding of microorganisms to the meninges causes bacterial meningitis. The resulting inflammation can damage arterial vessel walls and cause mycotic aneurysms (see below). Ischemic stroke occurs through obstruction of inflamed vessels, hemorrhagic stroke through rupture of a mycotic aneurysm. The significance of immune-mediated injury in pathogenicity, e.g. by immune-complex deposition, is unknown.

Therapy of IE

Before the advent of antimicrobials, IE has inadvertently led to death. Selection of the appropriate antimicrobial depends strongly on the isolation of the causative organism and its antimicrobial susceptibility. Therefore enough blood needs to be cultured. With the use of current technology, culturing about 40–60 ml of blood is considered sufficient. The chances of a successful isolation are higher when blood cultures are drawn at the beginning of a fever slope, and before antimicrobial drugs are administered.

Antimicrobial therapy should be carefully selected according to the results of antimicrobial susceptibility testing. Many scientific societies have issued guidelines that recommend specific drug treatment schemes for certain organisms [14, 15]. The standard duration of antimicrobial therapy is at least 4–6 weeks. If possible, a combination therapy of two antimicrobials with different modes of action is advised.

In addition to antimicrobial drug treatment, surgical therapy needs to be considered in the case of relapse or treatment failure, especially when a prosthetic heart valve is involved. Furthermore, surgical therapy needs to be considered in the case of severe heart failure, persistently positive blood cultures, local extension of infection (e.g. paravalvular abscess), and fungal or highly resistant organisms.

Patients who have suffered a recent stroke are considered to be at a high risk during cardiac surgery. The anticoagulation necessary for the cardiopulmonary bypass will greatly augment the risk of hemorrhagic transformation of a non-hemorrhagic infarct. Therefore, it has been suggested that heart valve replacement surgery should be performed later than two weeks after stroke. Successful surgery has been performed at earlier time points, but available data are scarce and thus careful judgement is required in each individual case.

> Occlusion of cerebral arteries by septic or sterile emboli that originate from the vegetations is a common cause for stroke in infective endocarditis (IE). IE is often diagnosed late and should be treated with a carefully selected antimicrobial therapy for at least 4–6 weeks. Additionally, surgical therapy needs to be considered.

Embolic stroke due to Chagas disease

Chagas disease is an infection with the protozoan parasite *Trypanosoma cruzi* which is most prevalent in South and Central America. It is transmitted by an insect vector (*Triatoma* and other assassin bug species) and can lead to a persistent chronic infection. Parasitic invasion of the heart muscle leads to cardiomyopathy, probably through chronic inflammation. Cardiomyopathy develops in about 10–30% of patients with long-lasting parasitemia and manifests itself years or even decades after initial infection [16].

Embolic stroke may be the first sign of cardiac Chagas disease. Conditions that predispose to cardiac emboli in Chagas disease are cardiac arrhythmias, congestive heart failure, apical aneurysms and mural thrombus formation. By the time stroke occurs, the damage to the heart is irreversible and thus effort needs to be directed towards prevention of *Trypanosoma* infection by vector control and improvement of basic housing conditions, as well as early diagnosis and treatment.

Meningitis as a cause of stroke

Meningitis denotes the inflammation of the leptomeninges, which consist of the pia mater and arachnoid mater. These layers ensheath the spinal cord and brain and confine the subarachnoidal space, which contains cerebrospinal fluid (CSF). Infection of the meninges by bacteria or fungi leads to an inflammatory response which causes the typical clinical symptoms, headache and nuchal rigidity. Depending on the time course, meningitis can be classified as acute or chronic.

Acute bacterial meningitis is prevalent worldwide and accounts for an estimated 1.2 million cases with 185 000 deaths per year. Patients present with fever, nuchal rigidity, and lethargy or confusion. Other less frequent symptoms are photophobia, seizures, petechial bleeding, and arthritis. The disease occurs in all age groups, but the causative organisms vary depending on age (Table 18.5). If left untreated, the disease is fatal.

Diagnosis is based on clinical symptoms, CSF analysis and microbiological testing. Empiric antimicrobial treatment needs to be initiated as early as possible with antimicrobials that reach adequate bactericidal concentrations in the CSF. The choice of antimicrobial therapy needs to be reconsidered when the causative organism is identified and susceptibility testing results become available.

Table 18.5. Acute bacterial meningitis: age groups and most common causative organisms.

Age group	Main pathogens
Neonates (≤1 month)	Enterobacteriaceae, Streptococcus agalactiae (group B streptococcus), coagulase-negative staphylococci (in preterm infants)
Children (1 month to 15 years)	*Haemophilus influenzae, Neisseria meningitidis, Streptococcus pneumoniae*
Adults (>15 years)	*Streptococcus pneumoniae, Neisseria meningitides*

Common complications of acute bacterial meningitis include raised intracranial pressure, seizures, and hyponatremia. Stroke is most prevalent in infants (less than 1 year of age) with an incidence of up to 10%, which is attributed to a more susceptible brain tissue.

Research into the molecular pathogenesis of stroke in meningitis has been scarce. Most likely, the spreading inflammation involves intracranial vessels and leads to thrombosis and subsequent ischemia or hemorrhage [17].

Chronic meningitis lasts for more than 4 weeks, has a subacute onset, and is often accompanied by fever, headache, and vomiting. There are many infectious and non-infectious causes of chronic meningitis and despite advances in diagnostic techniques, such as PCR, about 30% of cases are idiopathic. In the following sections we will discuss several organisms that cause chronic meningitis with a high incidence of stroke.

Tuberculous meningitis

Tuberculous meningitis is caused by *Mycobacterium tuberculosis*, a hardy slow-growing bacterium whose only natural reservoir is the human. It is taken up by inhalation, phagocytosed by alveolar macrophages and transported to the lung tissue, where an exudative inflammation is initiated. During the first couple of weeks, mycobacteria are undetected by the cellular immune system and spread to the draining hilar lymph nodes. There they slowly proliferate and the host immune system finally mounts a T-cell response. Depending on the capacity of the host immune system the infection can be cleared or mycobacteria survive within granulomata.

Granulomata are caseous foci with a fibrotic capsule that enwraps viable mycobacteria. They are formed by the host immune system to keep the bacteria contained and prevent further spread of infection. However, they allow the pathogen to persist within its host for decades, until the conditions for growth become more favorable, e.g. when the host immune system is impaired.

The granuloma at the site of initial infection and the swollen hilar lymph nodes together are called the primary complex, a typical feature of early tuberculosis. From there lymphogenous and hematogenous spread may occur to various distant organs, e.g. the meninges, where further granulomata are formed.

When reactivation of the disease occurs, the center of a granuloma liquefies, mycobacteria proliferate and the granuloma ruptures. Bacteria are released into the surrounding tissue, which leads, in the case of a meningeal granuloma, to tuberculous meningitis.

In tuberculous meningitis, the meningeal inflammation produces a basilar, gelatinous inflammatory exudate in the subarachnoid space. The walls of small and medium-sized arteries that traverse the exudate are invaded by inflammatory cells. Furthermore, disturbance of CSF circulation leads to an increased intracranial pressure.

Ischemic stroke is a relatively frequent complication of tuberculous meningitis and occurs in about 30% of cases [18]. Most cerebral infarcts occur in the anterior circulation. Strangulation and spasm of blood vessels by an intense inflammatory exudate, periarteriitis or necrotizing panarteritis, and stretching of blood vessels by increased intracranial pressure are pathogenic mechanisms. Compression of the M1 or M2 segment of the middle cerebral artery by the exudate causes large artery infarctions, whereas multiple infarcts are most likely due to secondary thrombosis.

When tuberculous meningitis is suspected in a patient, the diagnosis needs to be confirmed by microbiological techniques, i.e. direct microscopic examination, culture, or PCR-based techniques, before a long-lasting drug therapy is initiated.

Cryptococcal meningitis

The fungus *Cryptococcus neoformans* is a soil pathogen with a high potential to invade the central nervous system. It causes an often fatal disease, despite antimycotic therapy. Especially immunocompromised individuals with a defect in cellular immunity (e.g. AIDS patients) are at risk of developing cryptococcal disease. The frequency of ischemic complications is unknown, but stroke is associated with a worse outcome [19, 20].

Coccidioidomycosis

Coccidioides immitis is a fungal pathogen restricted to the deserts of south-western USA and Central and South America. Inhalation of contaminated soil normally leads to asymptomatic infection or mild pulmonary symptoms. Fewer than 2% of patients develop a disseminated disease within weeks to months after exposure. Most common extrapulmonary sites of infection are skin and subcutaneous soft tissue, the meninges and the skeleton.

Patients with basilar, coccidioidal meningitis have a 40% risk of developing cerebral infarcts and they often develop communicating hydrocephalus. A long course of antifungal drug treatment is required and there is a significant risk of relapse [21].

Neurosyphilis and neuroborreliosis

Other bacterial infections that have been implicated in stroke are the spirochetes *Treponema pallidum* and *Borrelia burgdorferi*. Meningovascular syphilis, caused by *T. pallidum*, is now a rare complication, since syphilis is most often recognized and treated at an earlier stage.

Stroke in syphilis develops as a result of inflammatory infiltration of medium to large arteries. Most often the middle cerebral artery and to a lesser extent basilar arteries are involved [22]. Typically, the onset of stroke is subacute. A diagnosis is based on serological testing of cerebrospinal fluid. Additionally, syphilis can cause stroke by other mechanisms, e.g. compression of the left carotid artery by a large aneurysm of the thoracic aorta has been reported [23].

Chronic meningitis in neuroborreliosis, an infection with *B. burgdorferi*, rarely causes stroke [24].

Neurocysticercosis

Neurocysticercosis is the most common parasitic central nervous system infection. The pork tapeworm *Taenia solium* is prevalent worldwide, especially in developing countries. In the human, the definite host, *Taenia solium* lives as a tapeworm in the small intestine and sheds eggs with the feces. The cystic larval form (termed cysticercus) is usually found in the pig. However, when humans ingest shed tapeworm eggs invasive larvae may develop in the intestines, penetrate the mucosa, enter the bloodstream, migrate to the tissues and mature into cysticerci.

Cysticerci have a predilection for neural tissue and can settle in the brain, subarachnoid space, and ventricle. Symptoms depend on localization and size of the larvae and include seizures, headache, visual problems, confusion, and hydrocephalus. About 50% of patients develop arteriitis with associated lacunar infarcts. Erosion of large vessels can occasionally lead to a large artery stroke, preferentially in the territory of the middle cerebral artery.

The diagnosis in non-endemic areas can be difficult and is generally made by a combination of clinical, radiographic, and serological criteria. Cysticerci normally die within 5–7 years after arrival in the brain, a process which can be accelerated by antiparasitic drug treatment. In many cases of symptomatic disease, drug treatment is not sufficient and neurosurgical procedures are required.

> Chronic meningitis, caused by, for example, tuberculosis, neurosyphilis or neuroborreliosis, can lead to stroke when the spreading inflammation involves intracranial vessels and leads to thrombosis.

Infectious diseases causing vasculitis
Varicella zoster virus vasculopathy

Varicella zoster virus (VZV) can lead to stroke due to viral infection of the cerebral artery walls (for review see Nagel et al. [25]). Two different types of infection can be differentiated depending on the immune status of the patient. Immunocompromised individuals, e.g. organ transplant or AIDS patients, show a diffuse inflammation of cerebral blood vessels of all sizes. Immunocompetent patients may develop herpes zoster associated cerebral angiitis, a granulomatous angiitis that usually affects larger arteries. In both cases, histopathological features include multinucleated giant cells, Cowdry A inclusion bodies, and VZV particles.

Diagnosis of VZV vasculopathy can be difficult, and is based on patient history, imaging studies, and analysis of the cerebrospinal fluid (CSF). It should be suspected in patients with ischemic lesions in MRI or CT, combined with a positive VZV PCR or serological detection of VZV IgG. Patient history often reveals a typical herpetiform rash. The rash can precede the manifestation of stroke by up to several months. When cerebral angiography is performed, unifocal or multifocal vascular lesions with corresponding lesions in CT or MRI imaging studies can be found.

Randomized clinical trials for standard treatment are lacking. Based on expert opinion, current treatment includes intravenous acyclovir in combination with steroids. A vaccination for VZV is available and has significantly diminished VZV-related morbidity and mortality in children. Prevention of herpes zoster by this vaccine has so far not been demonstrated [26].

HIV-associated vasculopathy and vasculitis

Several cohort studies around the world have shown that stroke in patients with acquired immunodeficiency syndrome (AIDS) is more frequent than in an age-adjusted HIV-negative population. However, a firm causal relationship between HIV infection and stroke has yet to be proven. A recent cohort study on young patients with stroke in South Africa suggests that the mechanisms leading to stroke in HIV-positive patients are largely similar to those in HIV-negative controls [27]. In this study, frequent causes were opportunistic infections (tuberculosis, neurosyphilis, varicella zoster vasculopathy, cryptococcal meningitis), coagulopathy, and cardioembolism. In 10–20% of the cases, HIV-associated vasculitis was suspected as a cause of stroke.

In the early stages of HIV infection an intracranial vasculopathy of small arteries can be found [28]. Histological features are thickening of the vessel wall, perivascular space dilatation, rarefaction, pigment deposition, and occasional perivascular inflammatory cell infiltrates. This condition is associated with asymptomatic microinfarcts and may predispose to ischemic stroke.

In later stages of AIDS, HIV-associated vasculitis can be found, a poorly characterized entity that involves large or medium sized intra- or extracranial arteries. It results in fusiform aneurysms, stenosis or thrombosis and can lead to ischemic or hemorrhagic stroke. Whether HIV-associated vasculitis is directly caused by HIV infection or is due to an undetected opportunistic infection is still under debate [29].

> Vasculitis from infectious diseases, e.g. varicella zoster virus and HIV, can result in ischemic stroke.

Mycotic aneurysms as cause of stroke

Mycotic aneurysms are caused by bacteria or fungi and account for a minority (about 3%) of all intracranial aneurysms. They develop in a significant fraction of patients with infective endocarditis (3–16%), due to microemboli that congest the vasa vasorum of the cerebral arteries. In these patients, rupture of a mycotic aneurysm without adequate antimicrobial therapy is frequent (57%) but the risk after a full course of antimicrobial treatment is very low, although it is a potentially devastating event [30].

Different mechanisms have been implicated in aneurysm formation; (1) septic microemboli to the vasa vasorum; (2) hematogenous seeding of bacteria to atherosclerotic vessels; (3) extension from a contiguous infected focus; and (4) direct contamination through trauma of the arterial wall. Infection of the vessel wall leads to necrosis, local hemorrhage, and abscess formation. The muscularis and elastica layers are destroyed, but the intima often remains intact. Bacterial aneurysms are usually small, saccular, and localized at multiple sites, whereas fungal aneurysms are long, large, and fusiform.

The causative organisms of intracerebral aneurysms are the same as for infective endocarditis, mainly viridans group streptococci, *S. aureus*, enterococci, and other *Streptococcus* spp. Enterobacteriaceae, in particular non-typhi *Salmonella* spp., play an important role in extracranial aneurysms but rarely cause intracranial aneurysms.

Among the fungi, *Aspergillus* spp. are a well described cause of true fungal mycotic aneurysms. An important virulence factor of *Aspergillus* spp. is the enzyme elastase, which degrades elastic fibers of the vessel wall [31].

Central nervous system aspergillosis usually occurs in immunocompromised patients and manifests as a triad: mycotic aneurysm, stroke, and granuloma formation. The mortality associated with intracranial aspergillosis is at least 85% and patients with mycotic aneurysms who survived have not been reported. Aside from aneurysm rupture, *Aspergillus* spp. can lead to stroke by thrombotic occlusion due to vascular extension of hyphae.

> In patients with infective endocarditis and in immunocompromised patients, rupture of mycotic aneurysms can be the cause of stroke.

Infectious diseases with similarities to stroke – toxoplasmosis and malaria encephalitis

Cerebral toxoplasmosis, an infection with the protozoan parasite *Toxoplasma gondii*, mainly occurs in immunocompromised individuals, especially in AIDS patients. The parasite is transmitted by undercooked meat or cat feces and taken up by the oral route.

During often asymptomatic initial infection, the parasite disseminates into various tissues and forms dormant tissue cysts, especially in the brain and muscle tissue. Reactivation of the dormant parasites during an impaired immune response leads to lesions with a necrotic central area, hyperemic border and sometimes a thin fibrotic capsule. A feature that distinguishes these lesions from an abscess is a hypertrophic arteriitis with or without thrombotic arterial occlusion that causes discrete infarcts. Thus cerebral toxoplasmosis results in a slowly expanding ischemic lesion [32].

Clinical signs depend on the localization of the lesions and, in contrast to acute ischemic stroke, onset is often subacute. MR and CT imaging studies often show multiple ring enhancing lesions that can occur anywhere in the brain or spinal cord, but are most often localized in the basal ganglia. Definite diagnosis requires histological demonstration of the organism or PCR-based methods. To prevent the occurrence of toxoplasmosis in immunocompromised patients, primary antimicrobial prophylaxis is initiated depending on $CD4^+$ T-cell counts.

The pathogenesis of cerebral malaria shares some similarity with stroke (for review see Idro et al. [33]). The causative organism of malaria tropica is the protozoan *Plasmodium falciparum*, which is transmitted by mosquitoes (*Anopheles* spp.). Common clinical manifestations of cerebral malaria are seizures, respiratory distress, and impaired consciousness.

During infection *P. falciparum* invades red blood cells and alters their surface properties. As a result, erythrocytes stick to the endothelium of the cerebral blood vessels and reduce the microvascular flow. Additionally, the membrane of infected erythrocytes becomes less deformable and thus travelling through narrow capillaries is more difficult.

As in stroke, the reduced blood flow impairs the delivery of substrates, which causes hypoxia, reduction of the blood–brain barrier, and ultimately brain swelling. At autopsy petechial hemorrhages are regularly observed, but infarction, necrosis, and large hemorrhages are rare.

In the course of malaria and toxoplasmosis, ischemic lesions mimicking stroke can occur.

Infectious diseases as complication of stroke
Early-onset infectious complications

Infectious complications after acute stroke are common. In a prospective study of 3866 patients with ischemic stroke hospitalized in neurological stroke units in Germany, 7.4% developed pneumonia and 6.3% urinary tract infections within 7 days after cerebral infarction [34]. Other studies report an even higher incidence of urinary tract infections and pneumonia, 24% and 22% respectively [35]. Stroke-associated pneumonia is associated with a higher fatality and worse long-term clinical outcome [34, 36].

Diagnostic work-up of infections post-stroke

When clinical signs or laboratory testing results (e.g. fever or hypothermia, leukocytosis, elevated CRP serum levels) point towards an infection, diagnostic specimens should be obtained for micro-biological testing. A diagnostic work-up is guided by the clinical signs and symptoms and should include blood cultures, urine culture, and a chest X-ray. If pneumonia is suspected, sputum or tracheal aspirate should be sampled. Microbiological specimens should be obtained before antimicrobial therapy is initiated.

Aspiration pneumonia

Pneumonia in stroke patients is most often caused by dysphagia and secondary aspiration. In up to 70% of stroke patients the cough and swallow reflexes are impaired and oropharyngeal or gastric content may gain access to the lungs [37]. In the lungs, bacteria can initiate an infectious process. Major risk factors for aspiration pneumonia are older age, stroke, altered mental state, poor oral hygiene, and gastroesophageal reflux disease (for review see Shige-mitsu and Afshar [38]).

The high frequency of aspiration pneumonia in stroke patients has led to the search for other mechanisms that may facilitate pneumonia [39], especially since aspiration of nasopharyngeal secretions regularly occurs in healthy individuals during sleep, at an estimated volume of 0.01–0.2 ml [40].

In a murine model, stroke induces a severe immunodepression through over-activation of the sympathetic nervous system. Dampening of the sympathetic activation by propranolol prevented pneumonia and bacteremia in 80% of the mice and improved 7-day survival by 50% [41, 42]. Downregulation of the immune system during a life-threatening condition seems paradoxical but it may serve to prevent damage to the brain by immune cells [43].

To prevent aspiration pneumonia, post-stroke patients need to be screened for potential aspiration of fluids or semi-solids and the diet should be adapted accordingly [44]. Other measures (positioning, oral hygiene, tube feeding) have been proposed for the prevention of aspiration pneumonia. However, controlled clinical trials in stroke patients are lacking.

Preventive antimicrobial therapy is effective in a mouse model [45], and a few small clinical trials have been carried out to assess its usefulness. In the ESPIAS trial, a 3-day regimen of levofloxacin vs. placebo started within 24 hours of stroke onset did not improve outcome or reduce the frequency of aspiration pneumonia [46]. The PANTHERIS trial, a 5-day regimen of moxifloxacin vs. placebo started within 36 hours of stroke onset, was not sufficiently powered to show significant differences between the groups [47]. To assess the usefulness of preventive antibiotic therapy further trials are needed.

Therapy of aspiration pneumonia is largely dependent on antibiotic treatment. Empiric regimens should cover *S. pneumoniae*, *S. aureus*, *Haemophilus influenzae*, Gram-negative enteric bacilli and anaerobic bacteria and should follow current treatment guidelines [48]. To guide further treatment, proper specimens for microbiological analysis, preferably bronchoalveolar lavage and blood cultures, should be obtained.

Urinary tract infections

Urinary tract infections (UTI) are common infections post-stroke, since many patients have indwelling catheters in place, which convey a significant risk of infection. Asymptomatic occurrence of bacteria in the urine (bacteriuria) needs to be distinguished from a true infection. Signs of UTI include mild irritative symptoms, such as frequency and urgency, dysuria, fever, and severe systemic manifestations, such as bacteremia and sepsis.

Microbiological examination of a urine specimen confirms the diagnosis, identifies the causative organism, and provides susceptibility testing results. Since antimicrobial treatment is initiated only in symptomatic infections, routine culture is not recommended.

Initial treatment is strongly dependent on local resistance patterns and should follow current guidelines (e.g. [49]). Urine cultures should be obtained prior to the start of antimicrobial therapy.

Infectious complications after acute stroke are common, mostly pneumonia and urinary tract infections.

Chapter Summary

Acute infection in the week preceding stroke is an independent risk factor for cerebral infarction; the "infectious burden concept" states that the aggregate burden of microbial antigens determines stroke risk rather than the occurrence of a single pathogen.

Embolic stroke can be caused by infective endocarditis (IE). The main risk factors for endocarditis are injection drug use, an underlying structural heart disease (especially prosthetic valves), hemodialysis and invasive intravascular procedures. Clinical signs and symptoms of IE are highly variable and often misleading, therefore IE is often diagnosed late.

Occlusion of cerebral arteries by septic or sterile emboli that originate from vegetations, usually in the left heart, is a common cause of stroke in IE. To isolate the causative organism, enough blood needs to be cultured (40–60 ml). Antimicrobial therapy should be carefully selected according to the results of antimicrobial susceptibility testing and be given for at least 4–6 weeks. In addition, surgical therapy needs to be considered. Embolic stroke may also be the first sign of cardiac Chagas disease.

Meningitis can lead to stroke. Most likely the spreading inflammation involves intracranial vessels and leads to thrombosis and subsequent ischemia or hemorrhage. Organisms that cause chronic meningitis with a high incidence of stroke are:

- Tuberculosis. Ischemic stroke is a relatively frequent complication of tuberculous meningitis and occurs in about 30% of cases.
- Coccidioidomycosis. Patients with basilar, coccidioidal meningitis have a 40% risk of developing cerebral infarcts and they often develop communicating hydrocephalus.
- Neurosyphilis and neuroborreliosis.
- Neurocysticercosis.

Vasculitis from infectious diseases, e.g. varicella zoster virus and HIV, can result in ischemic stroke.

Mycotic aneurysms account for about 3% of all intracranial aneurysms. Rupture of a mycotic aneurysm without adequate antimicrobial therapy is frequent.

Cerebral toxoplasmosis results in a slowly expanding ischemic lesion because it leads to a hypertrophic arteritis with or without thrombotic arterial occlusion that causes discrete infarcts. In **cerebral malaria** the infected erythrocytes stick to the endothelium of the cerebral blood vessels and reduce the microvascular flow.

Infectious complications after acute stroke are common, mostly pneumonia and urinary tract infections. Pneumonia in stroke patients is most often caused by dysphagia and secondary aspiration. To prevent aspiration pneumonia, post-stroke patients need to be screened for potential aspiration of fluids or semi-solids and the diet should be adapted accordingly.

References

1. Grau AJ, Buggle F, Heindl S, et al. Recent infection as a risk factor for cerebrovascular ischemia. *Stroke* 1995; **26**:373–9.

2. Paganini-Hill A, Lozano E, Fischberg G, et al. Infection and risk of ischemic stroke: differences among stroke subtypes. *Stroke* 2003; **34**:452–7.

3. Smeeth L, Thomas SL, Hall AJ, et al. Risk of myocardial infarction and stroke after acute infection or vaccination. *N Engl J Med* 2004; **351**:2611–8.

4. Lichy C, Grau AJ. Investigating the association between influenza vaccination and reduced stroke risk. *Expert Rev Vaccines* 2006; **5**:535–40.

5. Watson C, Alp NJ. Role of Chlamydia pneumoniae in atherosclerosis. *Clin Sci (Lond)* 2008; **114**:509–31.

6. Elkind MS, Cole JW. Do common infections cause stroke? *Semin Neurol* 2006; **26**:88–99.

7. Grau AJ, Marquardt L, Lichy C. The effect of infections and vaccinations on stroke risk. *Expert Rev Neurother* 2006; **6**:175–83.

8. Grayston JT, Kronmal RA, Jackson LA, et al. Azithromycin for the secondary prevention of coronary events. *N Engl J Med* 2005; **352**:1637–45.

9. O'Connor CM, Dunne MW, Pfeffer MA, et al. Azithromycin for the secondary prevention of coronary heart disease events: the WIZARD study: a randomized controlled trial. *JAMA* 2003; **290**:1459–66.

10. Ngeh J, Goodbourn C. Chlamydia pneumoniae, Mycoplasma pneumoniae, and Legionella pneumophila in elderly patients with stroke (C-PEPS, M-PEPS, L-PEPS): a case-control study on the infectious burden of atypical respiratory pathogens in elderly patients with acute cerebrovascular disease. *Stroke* 2005; **36**:259–65.

11. Bayer AS. Infective endocarditis. *Clin Infect Dis* 1993; **17**:313–20.

12. Snygg-Martin U, Gustafsson L, Rosengren L, et al. Cerebrovascular complications in patients with left-sided infective endocarditis are common: a prospective study using magnetic resonance imaging and neurochemical brain damage markers. *Clin Infect Dis* 2008; **47**:23–30.

13. Garrison PK, Freedman LR. Experimental endocarditis I. Staphylococcal endocarditis in rabbits resulting from placement of a polyethylene catheter in the right side of the heart. *Yale J Biol Med* 1970; **42**:394–410.

14. Baddour LM, Wilson WR, Bayer AS, et al. Infective endocarditis: diagnosis, antimicrobial therapy, and management of complications: a statement for healthcare professionals from the Committee on Rheumatic Fever, Endocarditis, and Kawasaki Disease, Council on Cardiovascular Disease in the Young, and the Councils on Clinical Cardiology, Stroke, and Cardiovascular Surgery and Anesthesia, American Heart Association: endorsed by the Infectious Diseases Society of America. *Circulation* 2005; **111**:e394–434.

15. Horstkotte D, Follath F, Gutschik E, et al. Guidelines on prevention, diagnosis and treatment of infective endocarditis executive summary; the task force on infective endocarditis of the European Society of Cardiology. *Eur Heart J* 2004; **25**:267–76.

16. Carod-Artal FJ. Chagas cardiomyopathy and ischemic stroke. *Expert Rev Cardiovasc Ther* 2006; **4**:119–30.

17. Takeoka M, Takahashi T. Infectious and inflammatory disorders of the circulatory system and stroke in childhood. *Curr Opin Neurol* 2002; **15**:159–64.

18. Chan KH, Cheung RT, Lee R, et al. Cerebral infarcts complicating tuberculous meningitis. *Cerebrovasc Dis* 2005; **19**:391–5.

19. Ecevit IZ, Clancy CJ, Schmalfuss IM, et al. The poor prognosis of central nervous system cryptococcosis among nonimmunosuppressed patients: a call for better disease recognition and evaluation of adjuncts to antifungal therapy. *Clin Infect Dis* 2006; **42**:1443–7.

20. Leite AG, Vidal JE, Bonasser Filho F, et al. Cerebral infarction related to cryptococcal meningitis in an HIV-infected patient: case report and literature review. *Braz J Infect Dis* 2004; **8**:175–9.

21. Williams PL, Johnson R, Pappagianis D, et al. Vasculitic and encephalitic complications associated with Coccidioides immitis infection of the central nervous system in humans: report of 10 cases and review. *Clin Infect Dis* 1992; **14**:673–82.

22. Flint AC, Liberato BB, Anziska Y, et al. Meningovascular syphilis as a cause of basilar artery stenosis. *Neurology* 2005; **64**:391–2.

23. Nakane H, Okada Y, Ibayashi S, et al. Brain infarction caused by syphilitic aortic aneurysm. A case report. *Angiology* 1996; **47**:911–7.

24. Scheid R, Hund-Georgiadis M, von Cramon DY. Intracerebral haemorrhage as a manifestation of Lyme neuroborreliosis? *Eur J Neurol* 2003; **10**:99–101.

25. Nagel MA, Cohrs RJ, Mahalingam R, et al. The varicella zoster virus vasculopathies: clinical, CSF, imaging, and virologic features. *Neurology* 2008; **70**:853–60.

26. Reynolds MA, Chaves SS, Harpaz R, et al. The impact of the varicella vaccination program on herpes zoster epidemiology in the United States: a review. *J Infect Dis* 2008; **197** Suppl 2:S224–7.

27. Tipping B, de Villiers L, Wainwright H, et al. Stroke in patients with human immunodeficiency virus infection. *J Neurol Neurosurg Psychiatry* 2007; **78**:1320–4.

28. Connor MD, Lammie GA, Bell JE, et al. Cerebral infarction in adult AIDS patients: observations from the Edinburgh HIV Autopsy Cohort. *Stroke* 2000; **31**:2117–26.

29. Ortiz G, Koch S, Romano JG, et al. Mechanisms of ischemic stroke in HIV-infected patients. *Neurology* 2007; **68**:1257–61.

30. Salgado AV, Furlan AJ, Keys TF. Mycotic aneurysm, subarachnoid hemorrhage, and indications for cerebral angiography in infective endocarditis. *Stroke* 1987; **18**:1057–60.

31. Ho CL, Deruytter MJ. CNS aspergillosis with mycotic aneurysm, cerebral granuloma and infarction. *Acta Neurochir (Wien)* 2004; **146**:851–6.

32. Huang TE, Chou SM. Occlusive hypertrophic arteritis as the cause of discrete necrosis in CNS toxoplasmosis in the acquired immunodeficiency syndrome. *Hum Pathol* 1988; **19**:1210–4.

33. Idro R, Jenkins NE, Newton CR. Pathogenesis, clinical features, and neurological outcome of cerebral malaria. *Lancet Neurol* 2005; 4:827–40.

34. Weimar C, Roth MP, Zillessen G, et al. Complications following acute ischemic stroke. *Eur Neurol* 2002; 48:133–40.

35. Langhorne P, Stott DJ, Robertson L, et al. Medical complications after stroke: a multicenter study. *Stroke* 2000; 31:1223–9.

36. Hilker R, Poetter C, Findeisen N, et al. Nosocomial pneumonia after acute stroke: implications for neurological intensive care medicine. *Stroke* 2003; 34:975–81.

37. Martino R, Foley N, Bhogal S, et al. Dysphagia after stroke: incidence, diagnosis, and pulmonary complications. *Stroke* 2005; 36:2756–63.

38. Shigemitsu H, Afshar K. Aspiration pneumonias: under-diagnosed and under-treated. *Curr Opin Pulm Med* 2007; 13:192–8.

39. Perry L, Love CP. Screening for dysphagia and aspiration in acute stroke: a systematic review. *Dysphagia* 2001; 16:7–18.

40. Gleeson K, Eggli DF, Maxwell SL. Quantitative aspiration during sleep in normal subjects. *Chest* 1997; 111:1266–72.

41. Prass K, Braun JS, Dirnagl U, et al. Stroke propagates bacterial aspiration to pneumonia in a model of cerebral ischemia. *Stroke* 2006; 37:2607–12.

42. Prass K, Meisel C, Hoflich C, et al. Stroke-induced immunodeficiency promotes spontaneous bacterial infections and is mediated by sympathetic activation reversal by poststroke T helper cell type 1-like immunostimulation. *J Exp Med* 2003; 198:725–36.

43. Dirnagl U, Klehmet J, Braun JS, et al. Stroke-induced immunodepression: experimental evidence and clinical relevance. *Stroke* 2007; 38:770–3.

44. Trapl M, Enderle P, Nowotny M, et al. Dysphagia bedside screening for acute-stroke patients: the Gugging Swallowing Screen. *Stroke* 2007; 38:2948–52.

45. Meisel C, Prass K, Braun J, et al. Preventive antibacterial treatment improves the general medical and neurological outcome in a mouse model of stroke. *Stroke* 2004; 35:2–6.

46. Chamorro A, Horcajada JP, Obach V, et al. The Early Systemic Prophylaxis of Infection After Stroke study: a randomized clinical trial. *Stroke* 2005; 36:1495–500.

47. Harms H, Prass K, Meisel C, et al. Preventive antibacterial therapy in acute ischemic stroke: a randomized controlled trial. *PLoS ONE* 2008; 3:e2158.

48. Guidelines for the Management of Adults with Hospital-acquired, Ventilator-associated, and Healthcare-associated Pneumonia. *Am J Respir Crit Care Med* 2005; 171:388–416.

49. Naber KG, Bergman B, Bishop MC, et al. EAU guidelines for the management of urinary and male genital tract infections. Urinary Tract Infection (UTI) Working Group of the Health Care Office (HCO) of the European Association of Urology (EAU). *Eur Urol* 2001; 40:576–88.

50. Wisplinghoff H, Seifert H. Bloodstream infection and endocarditis. In Borriello SP, Murray PR, Funke G, eds. *Bacteriology*. London: Hodder Arnold; 2005: 509–54.

51. Durack DT, Lukes AS, Bright DK. New criteria for diagnosis of infective endocarditis: utilization of specific echocardiographic findings. Duke Endocarditis Service. *Am J Med* 1994; 96:200–9.

52. Li JS, Sexton DJ, Mick N, et al. Proposed modifications to the Duke criteria for the diagnosis of infective endocarditis. *Clin Infect Dis* 2000; 30:633–8.

53. Cavassini M, Meuli R, Francioli P. Complications of infective endocarditis. In Scheld WM, Whitley RJ, Marra CM, eds. *Infections of the central nervous system*, 3rd ed. Philadelphia: Lippincott Williams and Wilkins; 2004: 537–68.

Hans-Christoph Diener and Greg W. Albers

Introduction

Secondary prevention aims at preventing a stroke after a transient ischemic attack (TIA) or a recurrent stroke after a first stroke. About 80–85% of patients survive a first ischemic stroke [1, 2]. Of those between 8% and 15% suffer a recurrent stroke in the first year. Risk of stroke recurrence is highest in the first few weeks and declines over time [3–5]. The risk of recurrence depends on concomitant vascular diseases (CHD, PAD) and vascular risk factors and can be estimated by risk models [6, 7]. Stroke risk after a TIA is highest in the first 3 days [8]. Therefore immediate evaluation of patients with stroke or TIA, identification of the pathophysiology and initiation of pathophysiology based treatment is of major importance [9]. In the following sections, we will deal with the treatment of risk factors, antithrombotic therapy and surgery or stenting of significant stenosis of extra- or intracranial arteries. Each paragraph will be introduced by recommendations, followed by the scientific justification.

Treatment of risk factors

Hypertension

- Antihypertensive therapy reduces the risk of stroke. The combination of an ACE inhibitor (perindopril) with a diuretic (indapamide) was significantly more effective than placebo, and an angiotensin-receptor blocker (ARB, eprosartan) was more effective than a calcium-channel blocker (nitrendipin). Ramipril reduces vascular events in patients with vascular risk factors.
- Early initiation of antihypertensive therapy with telmisartan on top of the usual antihypertensive therapy is not more effective than placebo.
- Most likely all antihypertensive drugs are effective in secondary stroke prevention. Beta-blockers (atenolol) show the lowest efficacy. More

important than the choice of a class of antihypertensives is to achieve the systolic and diastolic blood pressure targets (<140/90 mmHg in non-diabetics and <130/80 in diabetics). In many cases this requires combination therapy. Concomitant diseases (kidney failure, congestive heart failure) have to be considered.
- Lifestyle modification will lower blood pressure and should be recommended in addition to drug treatment.

There are very few studies investigating the efficacy of classes of antihypertensive drugs in secondary stroke prevention. One has to remember that two concepts exist in this field. Placebo-controlled trials may try to achieve a maximum of blood pressure lowering in patients with high blood pressure. Vascular protectives such as HOPE [10] include patients with vascular risk factors even with normal blood pressure under the assumption that end organs such as the brain will be protected. A meta-analysis comprised seven studies of 15 527 patients with TIA, ischemic or hemorrhagic stroke who were followed for 2–5 years. Treatment with antihypertensives reduced the risk of stroke by 24%, non-fatal stroke by 21%, risk of myocardial infarction (MI) by 21% and the risk of all vascular events by 21% [11]. For the endpoint stroke the combination of an ACE inhibitor with a diuretic was more effective (45% risk reduction) than a diuretic as monotherapy (32%), monotherapy with an ACE inhibitor (7% N.S.) or a beta-blocker (7%).

ACE inhibitors and ARBs were thought to have pleiotropic and protective vascular effects beyond lowering high blood pressure. Therefore the HOPE study compared ramipril with placebo. In the subgroup of patients with TIA or stroke as the qualifying event, ramipril resulted in a relative reduction of the combined endpoint of stroke, MI or vascular death by 24% and an absolute risk reduction of 6.3% in 5 years [12].

PROGRESS was the first large-scale trial specifically performed in patients after stroke. Patients ($n = 6105$) were treated with perindopril as monotherapy or in combination with indapamide or placebo. Across the 4-year observation time blood pressure was lowered on average by 9/4 mmHg. The absolute risk reduction for recurrent stroke was 4% and the relative risk reduction was 28%. Monotherapy with the ACE inhibitor was not superior to placebo, but also did not achieve the same level of blood pressure lowering as the combination therapy. The relative risk reduction for combination therapy was 43% [13].

ACCESS was a small phase II safety study in stroke patients with high blood pressure (>200/110 mmHg) in the early phase after an acute stroke. Patients were randomized to receive either candesartan or placebo in the first 7 days after stroke and continued with candesartan [14]. In the 12-month observation period the rate of vascular events was significantly lower in the candesartan group (9.8% vs. 18.7%, relative risk reduction RRR = 52%).

MOSES included 1352 patients with hypertension who had suffered a stroke in the previous 24 months. Patients were treated either with eprosartan (600 mg) or with nitrendipin (10 mg) on top of additional antihypertensive therapy when appropriate. For an identical drop in blood pressure, eprosartan was superior to nitrendipin in preventing recurrent vascular events (21% relative risk reduction). Optimal systolic blood pressure in the MOSES trial was 120–140 mmHg.

PRoFESS randomized 20 332 patients with a recent ischemic stroke to receive telmisartan at 80 mg/day or placebo in addition to other therapies, for a median duration of 2.4 years. Mean blood pressure over the trial period was lower in the telmisartan group by 3.8/2.0 mmHg. Recurrent strokes occurred in 8.7% in the telmisartan group compared to 9.2% in the placebo group, which was not significant. Therefore initiation of telmisartan early after a stroke, and continuation for a median of 2.4 years, did not significantly lower the rate of recurrent strokes, other major vascular events or new diabetes [15].

> Antihypertensive therapy reduces the risk of stroke. Most likely all antihypertensive drugs are effective in secondary stroke prevention.

High cholesterol

- Patients with TIA or ischemic stroke and coronary heart disease (CHD) should be treated with a statin irrespective of the initial LDL cholesterol level. The target range of LDL is 70–100 mg/dl. Patients with atherosclerotic ischemic stroke or TIA without CHD and LDL cholesterol levels between 100 and 190 mg/dl will benefit from a treatment with 80 mg atorvastatin. Statin therapy reduces the rate of recurrent stroke and vascular events.
- Lowering high LDL is more important than the use of a particular statin. Therefore lowering LDL cholesterol <100 mg/dl or ≥50% of the initial LDL cholesterol level is recommended.

The association of cholesterol levels and the risk of recurrent stroke is lower than the association with the risk of MI. Statins will, however, lower the risk of stroke in patients with CHD [16]. The relative risk reduction calculated from a meta-analysis is 21% [17]. NCEP ATP III guidelines recommend treating stroke patients with CHD with a statin. The LDL cholesterol level should be <100 mg/dl and <70 mg/dl in high-risk patients [18].

Patients with stroke without CHD were investigated in a subgroup of the Heart Protection Study (HPS) and the SPARCL trial. Within the HPS patient population of 20 536 high-risk patients, 3280 patients had TIA or stroke, 1820 of them without concomitant CHD. The relative risk reduction achieved by simvastatin given for 5 years for vascular events was 20% and the absolute risk reduction 5.1% [19]. In the overall population the RRR for stroke was 25%, whereas there was no significant reduction in the stroke rate in the subgroup of patients with TIA or stroke as the qualifying event [20]. The Stroke Prevention by Aggressive Reduction in Cholesterol Levels (SPARCL) study was performed in 4731 patients with TIA or stroke without CHD and LDL cholesterol levels between 100 and 190 mg/dl. Patients received either 80 mg atorvastatin or placebo. After an average of 4.9 years the primary endpoint (stroke) was reduced by 16% relative and 2.2% absolute [21]. The discrepancy with the HPS trial might be explained by the fact that HPS recruited patients on average 4.3 years after the initial vascular event whereas this time interval was only 6 months in SPARCL. The RRR for the combined endpoint of stroke, MI and vascular death was 20% and the ARR 3.5%. The rate of ischemic stroke was reduced (218 vs. 274) whereas hemorrhagic strokes were more frequent with atorvastatin (55 vs. 33).

Therapy with a statin should be initiated early after an ischemic stroke or TIA. The sudden

273

discontinuation of a statin in patients with a stroke or acute coronary syndrome might be associated with higher morbidity and mortality [22, 23]. Therefore, patients on a statin should continue treatment following an acute ischemic event.

> Patients with TIA or ischemic stroke and coronary heart disease (CHD) should be treated with a statin irrespective of the initial LDL cholesterol level.

Diabetes mellitus

Randomized controlled studies were unable to show an effect of glitazones on vascular events in stroke patients with diabetes mellitus [24]. Aggressive lowering of blood glucose does not reduce the risk of stroke and might even increase mortality [25, 26]. Therefore, treatment of diabetes mellitus should not be restricted to drug treatment but should also include diet, weight loss and regular exercise.

Supplementation of vitamins

- Treatment of increased plasma levels of homocysteine with vitamin B6, B12 and folic acid is not effective in secondary stroke prevention.

The VISP study was unable to show a benefit of the treatment of high homocysteine in stroke patients with B-vitamins and folic acid [27]. The HOPE-2 study also failed to demonstrate benefit [28]; the study included 5522 patients aged >55 years and a vascular event or diabetes mellitus and treated them for 5 years with either placebo or 2.5 mg folic acid, 50 mg vitamin B6 and 1 mg vitamin B12. This resulted in a significant reduction in homocysteine levels but not in a reduction of vascular events.

Hormone replacement therapy after menopause

- Hormone replacement after menopause is not effective in the secondary prevention of stroke and may even increase the risk of fatal strokes.

A randomized, placebo-controlled study in women who suffered a stroke receiving hormone replacement therapy after menopause found an increase in stroke mortality and a poorer prognosis in non-fatal strokes [29]. Therefore, in general, hormone replacement should be avoided following a stroke.

Antiplatelet therapy

- Patients with TIA or ischemic stroke should receive antiplatelet drugs. The choices are acetylsalicylic acid (ASA 50–150 mg), the combination of ASA (2 × 25 mg) and extended release dipyridamole (ER-DP 2 × 200 mg) or clopidogrel (75 mg).
- ASA is recommended in patients with a low risk of recurrence (<4%/year). Patients with a higher risk of recurrent stroke should be treated with ASA + ER-DP or clopidogrel. ASA + ER-DP and clopidogrel appear to be equally effective. ASA + ER-DP has more side-effects.
- Doses of ASA >150 mg/day result in an increased risk of bleeding complications.
- The combination of clopidogrel plus ASA is not more effective than either ASA or clopidogrel monotherapy, and carries a higher bleeding risk.
- The efficacy of antiplatelet therapy beyond 4 years after the initial event has not been studied in randomized trials. Theoretically, treatment should continue beyond that period.
- In the case of a recurrent ischemic event the pathophysiology of the ischemic event should be evaluated. When there is an indication for antiplatelet therapy the recurrence risk should be evaluated and the antiplatelet therapy adapted to the new risk. There is no evidence that changing antiplatelet therapy from ASA plus ER-DP to clopidogrel or vice versa provides greater protection.
- Patients with a history of TIA or ischemic stroke and an acute coronary syndrome should receive the combination of clopidogrel and ASA for at least 3 months. The same is true for patients with a coronary stent. This therapy is also typically extrapolated to patients with carotid stents.

Antiplatelet drugs are effective in secondary stroke prevention after TIA or ischemic stroke. This has been shown in many placebo-controlled trials and in several meta-analyses [30–32]. The RRR for non-fatal stroke achieved by antiplatelet therapy in patients with TIA or stroke is 23% (reduced from 10.8% to 8.3% in 3 years) [31]. The combined endpoint of stroke, MI and vascular death is reduced by 17% (from 21.4% to 17% in 29 months).

A meta-analysis of eleven randomized and placebo-controlled trials investigating ASA monotherapy in secondary stroke prevention found a RRR of 13% (95% CI 6–19) for the combined endpoint of stroke, MI and vascular death [33]. There is no relationship between the dose of ASA and its efficacy in secondary stroke prevention [31, 33, 34]. Therefore, the recommended dose of ASA is 75–150 mg/day. Gastrointestinal adverse events (AEs) and bleeding complications are, however, dose-dependent and bleeding rates increase significantly beyond a daily ASA dose of 150 mg [35, 36].

Clopidogrel monotherapy (75 mg/day) was compared to ASA (325 mg/day) in almost 20 000 patients with stroke, MI or peripheral arterial disease (PAD). The combined endpoint of stroke, MI and vascular death showed a relative risk reduction of 8.7% in favor of clopidogrel. The ARR was 0.51% [37]. The highest benefit of clopidogrel was seen in patients with PAD. The risk of GI bleeds (1.99% versus 2.66%) and gastrointestinal side-effects (15% versus 17.6%) was smaller with clopidogrel than with ASA.

The MATCH study compared the combination of clopidogrel 75 mg and ASA 75 mg with clopidogrel monotherapy in high-risk patients with TIA or ischemic stroke [38] and failed to show the superiority of combination antiplatelet therapy for the combined endpoint of stroke, MI, vascular death and hospitalization due to a vascular event. The combination resulted in a significant increase in bleeding complications, and therefore is not recommended.

The CHARISMA trial (Clopidogrel for High Atherothrombotic Risk and Ischemic Stabilization, Management, and Avoidance) was a combined primary and secondary prevention study in 15 603 patients and compared the combination of clopidogrel and ASA with ASA monotherapy [39]. Similarly to MATCH, the study failed to show a benefit of combination therapy and displayed a higher bleeding rate with the combination. Symptomatic patients, however, showed a trend towards a benefit for combination antiplatelet therapy [40].

The combination of low-dose ASA and extended-release dipyridamole (ER-DP) was investigated in the second European Stroke Prevention Study (ESPS2) with 6602 patients with TIA or stroke [41]. Patients were randomized to ASA (25 mg bid), ER-DP (200 mg bid), the combination of ASA and ER-DP or placebo. For the primary endpoint stroke, the combination was superior to ASA monotherapy (RRR 23%, ARR 3%) and placebo (RRR 37%, AAR 5.8%). ASA monotherapy lowered the risk of stroke by 18% (AAR 2.9%) and dipyridamole monotherapy

by 16% (AAR 2.6%) compared to placebo. Major bleeding complications were seen more frequently with ASA and the ASA + ER-DP combination, whereas DP monotherapy had a similar bleeding rate to placebo. Cardiac events occurred at similar frequency in the groups treated with dipyridamole compared to ASA [42]. The industry-independent ESPRIT study [43] randomized 2739 patients with presumed atherothrombotic TIA or minor stroke to ASA (30 to 325 mg) or the combination of ASA with DP and followed them for a mean period of 3.5 years. The primary endpoint was the combination of vascular death, stroke, MI and major bleeding complications. The event rate for the primary endpoint was 16% with ASA monotherapy and 13% with ASA + DP, resulting in a RRR of 20% (ARR 1%). In the combination arm 34% of patients terminated the trial prematurely, mostly because of AEs such as headache (13% in the ASA arm of the study). A meta-analysis of all stroke prevention trials testing ASA monotherapy versus ASA + DP showed a relative risk reduction in favor of the combination for the combined vascular endpoint of 18% (95% CI 9–26) [43].

A head-to-head comparison of clopidogrel and ASA + ER-DP was performed in the PRoFESS study [44]. The study randomized 20 332 patients with ischemic stroke and followed them for a mean period of 2.4 years. There was no difference in efficacy across all endpoints and no subgroup of patients. ASA + ER-DP resulted in more intracranial bleeds and a higher drop-out rate due to headache compared with clopidogrel (5.9% vs. 0.9%).

Table 19.1 gives an overview of absolute and relative risk reductions for different approaches in secondary stroke prevention. The calculation of the Essen risk score is shown in Table 19.2 [7, 45, 46].

Glycoprotein-IIb/IIIa-receptor antagonists are effective in the acute coronary syndrome [47]. Oral GP-IIb-IIIa-antagonists are not superior to ASA and carry a higher bleeding risk as shown in the BRAVO trial [35].

Patients with TIA or ischemic stroke should receive antiplatelet drugs.

Anticoagulation in cerebral ischemia due to cardiac embolism

- Patients with a cardiac source of embolism, in particular atrial fibrillation (AF), should be treated with oral anticoagulation (INR 2.0 to 3.0).

Table 19.1. Strategies for prevention of recurrent stroke after an initial TIA or ischemic stroke.

Intervention	Relative RR	Absolute RR/year	NNT/ year	Comments
Antihypertensive therapy	24%	0.46%	217	Proven for perindopril + indapamide and eprosartan
Statins	16%	0.4%	250	Proven for atorvastatin and simvastatin
ASA 50–150 mg after TIA or ischemic stroke	18–22%	1.3%	77	ASA doses >150 mg = higher bleeding risk
ASA 50 mg + dipyridamole 400 mg versus ASA	23%	1.0–1.5%	33–100	Combination also superior to placebo
Clopidogrel versus ASA	8%	0.5%	200	Based on a subgroup analysis from CAPRIE
Surgery of a high-degree carotid stenosis*	65%	3.1%	32	Efficacy declines with time interval from event
ASA in high-degree intracranial stenosis	?	?	?	In comparison to warfarin there was no significant benefit
Oral anticoagulation in cardiac source of embolism (AF) INR 3.0	68%	8%	12	Only one placebo-controlled study available (EAFT)
ASA in AF	19%	2.5%	40	In patients with contraindications for warfarin

Notes: *Outcome stroke and death.
NNT = number needed to treat/year; RR = risk reduction; AF = atrial fibrillation.

Table 19.2. Essen risk score for the calculation of the risk of a recurrent stroke after an initial ischemic stroke of atherothrombotic origin. A score of ≥3 points indicates a recurrence risk of ≥4%/year.

Risk factor	Points
Age <65 years	0
Age 65–75 years	1
Age >75 years	2
Hypertension	1
Diabetes mellitus	1
Myocardial infarction	1
Other cardiovascular events	1
Peripheral arterial disease	1
Smoking	1
Additional TIA or ischemic stroke	1

- Patients with contraindications or unwilling to use oral anticoagulation should receive ASA 100–300 mg/day.

- Patients with mechanical heart valves should be anticoagulated with an INR between 2.0 and 3.5.
- Patients with biological heart valves are anticoagulated for 3 months.
- In patients with TIA or minor stroke, oral anticoagulation can be initiated immediately after the exclusion of cerebral hemorrhage.
- The combination of ASA plus clopidogrel is inferior to oral anticoagulation with warfarin and carries a similar bleeding risk.

The evidence that oral anticoagulation prevents recurrent strokes in patients with atrial fibrillation results from the European Atrial Fibrillation Trial [48]. This randomized placebo-controlled trial showed a 68% relative risk reduction for a recurrent stroke for patients treated with warfarin compared to only 19% for patients receiving 300 mg ASA. Numbers needed to treat (NNT) are 12/year [48]. Therefore, oral anticoagulation in patients with AF is by far the most effective treatment for secondary stroke prevention. A Cochrane analysis concluded that oral anticoagulation is more effective than ASA for the prevention of vascular events (OR 0.67; 95% CI 0.50–0.91) or recurrent stroke (OR 0.49; 95% CI 0.33–0.72) [49]. The risk of major bleeding complications is significantly increased but not the risk of intracranial bleeds. Patients with intermittent AF have a similar stroke risk to patients with permanent AF [50, 51]. The optimal INR range for oral anticoagulation is between 2.0 and 3.0 [52]. INR values >3.0 lead to an increased risk of major bleeding complications in particular in the elderly [53].

The ACTIVE study [54] compared the combination of ASA and clopidogrel versus oral anticoagulation with warfarin in patients with AF: the study was terminated prematurely due to a significant reduction of stroke and systemic embolism in favor of warfarin. The rate of major bleeding complications was not different between the two regimens.

> Patients with a cardiac source of embolism, in particular atrial fibrillation (AF), should be treated with oral anticoagulation (INR 2.0 to 3.0).

Anticoagulation in cerebral ischemia of non-cardiac origin

- Oral anticoagulation is not superior to ASA and is not recommended.
- The benefit of anticoagulation for patients with arterial dissection of the vertebral or carotid arteries versus antiplatelet drugs has not been studied in head-to-head trials.
- Patients with cryptogenic stroke and coagulation disorders, e.g. protein C or S deficiency or factor V (Leiden) mutation, may benefit from oral anticoagulation. The optimal treatment duration and specific coagulation disorders that warrant anticoagulation are not clear.

The Stroke Prevention in Reversible Ischemia Trial (SPIRIT) studied oral anticoagulation with an INR between 3.0 and 4.5 versus ASA 30 mg in patients with TIA or minor stroke without a cardiac source of embolism [55]. The study was terminated due to a significantly increased bleeding risk with anticoagulation. The risk of bleeding was increased by a factor of 1.43 (95% CI 0.96–2.13) for an increase of the INR by 0.5. The Warfarin Aspirin Recurrent Stroke Study (WARSS) had a similar rate of ischemic events and bleeding complications comparing

warfarin (INR 1.4–2.8) and ASA in stroke patients without a cardiac source of embolism [56]. This result was replicated in the ESPRIT study [57]. ESPRIT found a lower rate of ischemic events with anticoagulation counterbalanced by an increased risk of intracranial bleeds.

A Cochrane analysis of five trials, with 4076 patients, was unable to show that anticoagulants are more or less efficacious in the prevention of vascular events than antiplatelet therapy (medium-intensity anticoagulation relative risk (RR) 0.96, 95% CI 0.38–2.42; high-intensity anticoagulation RR 1.02, 95% CI 0.49–2.13). The relative risk of major bleeding complications for low-intensity anticoagulation was 1.27 (95% CI 0.79–2.03) and for medium-intensity anticoagulation 1.19 (95% CI 0.59–2.41). High-intensity oral anticoagulants with INR 3.0 to 4.5 resulted in a higher risk of major bleeding complications (RR 9.0, 95% CI 3.9–21) [58].

The Antiphospholipid Antibodies and Stroke Study (APASS) found no difference in stroke, MI or vascular death in patients with antiphospholipid antibodies (aPL) treated with warfarin (INR 1.4–2.8) compared to 325 mg ASA [59]. There was in addition no difference in event rates between patients positive or negative for aPL. The evidence for anticoagulation in patients with protein C, protein S or antithrombin deficiency is derived from patients with deep vein thrombosis and not from patients with stroke.

The possible benefit of oral anticoagulation for the long-term treatment of dissections has never been studied in a randomized trial compared to antiplatelet drugs. An observational study from Canada in 116 patients with angiographically proven dissection of the vertebral or carotid arteries found a rate of TIA, stroke or death in the first year of 15%. The event rate in patients with anticoagulation was 8.3% and in patients receiving ASA 12.4%; the difference was not statistically significant [60]. A Cochrane review of 26 observational studies in 327 patients found no difference between anticoagulation and antiplatelet drugs for the endpoints death and severe disability [61]. A more recent review came to a similar conclusion [62].

Carotid endarterectomy and stenting with balloon angioplasty

- Symptomatic patients with significant stenosis of the internal carotid artery (ICA) should undergo carotid endarterectomy. The benefit of surgery increases with the degree of stenosis between 70% and 95%. The benefit of surgery is highest in the first 2 to 4 weeks after the initial TIA or minor stroke.

- The benefit of surgery is lower in patients with a stenosis between 50 and 70%, in high-degree stenosis (pseudo-occlusion), in women and in cases when surgery is performed 12 weeks or later after the initial event.
- The benefit of surgery is no longer present when the complication rate exceeds 6%.
- Patients should receive ASA prior to, during and after endarterectomy. Clopidogrel should be replaced by ASA 5 days before surgery.
- At present carotid stenting has a slightly higher short-term complication rate and similar medium-term outcomes. The use of protection systems does not decrease the complication rate. The restenosis rate is higher after stenting. Whether this translates into higher long-term event rates is not yet known. The complication rate of carotid stenting is age dependent and increases beyond the age of 65–68 years.
- The combination of clopidogrel (75 mg) plus ASA (75–100 mg) is recommended in patients after carotid stenting for 1–3 months based on extrapolation from studies of coronary stents.

Two large randomized trials (NASCET and ESC) found a clear benefit of carotid surgery compared to medical treatment in patients with high-degree stenosis of the ICA [63–69]. Taken together the trials found an absolute risk reduction of 13.5% over 5 years for the combined endpoint of stroke and death in favor of carotid endarterectomy [69]. The risk reduction is even higher in stenosis >90%. In patients with 50–69% ICA stenosis the 5-year absolute RR for the endpoint ipsilateral stroke is 4.6%. This benefit is mainly seen in males. Patients with <50% ICA stenosis do not benefit from carotid endarterectomy. The short-term complication rates (stroke and death) were 6.2% for stenosis >70% and 8.4% for 50–69% stenosis. ASA should be given prior to, during and after carotid surgery [70].

Several studies randomized patients with significant ICA stenosis to carotid endarterectomy or balloon angioplasty with stenting. Surgeons and interventional neuroradiologists had to pass a quality control. SPACE randomized 1200 symptomatic patients with a >50% stenosis (NASCET criteria) or >70% (ESC criteria) within 6 months after TIA or minor stroke to carotid endarterectomy or stenting [71]. The primary endpoint, ipsilateral stroke or death within 30 days, was 6.84% in patients undergoing stenting and 6.34% in patients who were operated. A post hoc subgroup analysis identified age <68 years as a factor in a lower complication rate in patients treated with stenting. The complication rate of surgery was not age-dependent [72]. The use of a protection system did not influence the complication rate. The EVA3S study was terminated prematurely after 527 patients were randomized due to a significant difference in the 30-day complication rate favoring carotid surgery (9.6% vs. 3.9%; OR 2.5; 95% CI 1.25–4.93) [73]. Taken together the results of the two studies show a lower complication rate for endarterectomy [74]. The reported medium-term outcomes were comparable and the restenosis rate was higher after carotid stenting.

> Symptomatic patients with significant stenosis of the internal carotid artery (ICA) should undergo carotid endarterectomy. At present carotid stenting has a slightly higher short-term complication rate and similar medium-term outcomes.

Intracranial stenosis

- Symptomatic patients with intracranial stenosis or occlusions should be treated with antiplatelet therapy.
- In patients with recurrent events, stenting can be considered.

The WASID-II study recruited 569 patients with intracranial stenosis and randomized them to either oral anticoagulation (INR 2.0–3.0) or ASA (1300 mg/day). The study was terminated prematurely due to a higher rate of bleeding complications with warfarin [75]. Therefore ASA is recommended in these patients. Whether the high dose of ASA is needed is not known. Lower doses are better tolerated and appear to have equal efficacy in other ischemic stroke etiologies. Predictors for a recurrent ischemic event were the degree of stenosis, stenosis in the vertebrobasilar system and female sex [76]. In patients with recurrent ischemic events stenting might be considered [77, 78], although not based on the results of randomized trials.

Chapter Summary

- **Antihypertensive therapy** reduces the risk of stroke. Most likely all antihypertensive drugs are effective in secondary stroke prevention. More important than the choice of a class of antihypertensives is to achieve the systolic and diastolic blood pressure targets (<140/90 mmHg in non-diabetics and <130/80 in diabetics). In many cases this requires combination therapy and lifestyle modification.
- **Statin** therapy reduces the rate of recurrent stroke and vascular events. The target range of LDL is 70–100 mg/dl.
- Aggressive lowering of **blood glucose** does not reduce the risk of stroke and might even increase mortality.
- Treatment of increased plasma levels of **homocysteine** with vitamin B6, B12 and folic acid is not effective in secondary stroke prevention.
- **Hormone replacement** after menopause is not effective in the secondary prevention of stroke and may even increase the risk of fatal strokes.
- Patients with **TIA or ischemic stroke** should receive antiplatelet drugs. The choices are acetyl-salicylic acid (ASA 50–150 mg), the combination of ASA (2 × 25 mg) and extended-release dipyridamole (ER-DP 2 × 200 mg) or clopidogrel (75 mg).
- Patients with a **cardiac source** of embolism, in particular atrial fibrillation (AF), should be treated with oral anticoagulation (INR 2.0 to 3.0). Patients with contraindications or unwilling to use oral anticoagulation should receive ASA 100–300 mg/day. In cerebral ischemia of **non-cardiac** origin oral anticoagulation is not superior to ASA and is not recommended.
- Symptomatic patients with significant **stenosis** (degree of stenosis between 70% and 95%) of the **internal carotid artery** (ICA) should undergo carotid endarterectomy or carotid stenting. Patients should receive ASA prior to, during and after endarterectomy or the combination of clopidogrel (75 mg) plus ASA (75–100 mg) after carotid stenting for 1–3 months.
- Symptomatic patients with **intracranial stenosis** or occlusions should be treated with antiplatelet therapy. In patients with recurrent events, stenting can be considered.

References

1. Grau AJ, Weimar C, Buggle F, Heinrich A, Goertler M, Neumaier S, et al. Risk factors, outcome, and treatment in subtypes of ischemic stroke: the German stroke data bank. *Stroke* 2001; **32**:2559–66.

2. Wolf PA, Cobb JL, D'Agostino RB. Epidemiology of stroke. In Barnett HJM, Mohr JP, Stein BM, Yatsu FM, eds. *Stroke: Pathophysiology, Diagnosis and Management*. New York: Churchill Livingston; 1992: 3–27.

3. Hill MD, Yiannakoulias N, Jeerakathil T, Tu JV, Svenson LW, Schopflocher DP. The high risk of stroke immediately after transient ischemic attack: a population-based study. *Neurology* 2004; **62**:2015–20.

4. Lovett J, Coull A, Rothwell P. Early risk of recurrence by subtype of ischemic stroke in population-based incidence studies. *Neurology* 2004; **62**:569–73.

5. Weimar C, Roth MP, Zillessen G, Glahn J, Wimmer ML, Busse O, et al. Complications following acute ischemic stroke. *Eur Neurol* 2002; **48**:133–40.

6. Coutts SB, Eliasziw M, Hill MD, Scott JN, Subramaniam S, Buchan AM, et al. An improved scoring system for identifying patients at high early risk of stroke and functional impairment after an acute transient ischemic attack or minor stroke. *Int J Stroke* 2008; **3**(1):3–10.

7. Weimar C, Goertler M, Rother J, Ringelstein EB, Darius H, Nabavi DG, et al. Systemic Risk Score Evaluation in Ischemic Stroke Patients (SCALA): a prospective cross sectional study in 85 German stroke units. *J Neurol* 2007; **254**(11):1562–8.

8. Giles MF, Rothwell PM. Risk of stroke early after transient ischaemic attack: a systematic review and meta-analysis. *Lancet Neurol* 2007; **6**(12):1063–72.

9. Rothwell PM, Giles MF, Chandratheva A, Marquardt L, Geraghty O, Redgrave JN, et al. Effect of urgent treatment of transient ischaemic attack and minor stroke on early recurrent stroke (EXPRESS study): a prospective population-based sequential comparison. *Lancet* 2007; **370**(9596): 1432–42.

10. Yusuf S, Teo KK, Pogue J, Dyal L, Copland I, Schumacher H, et al. Telmisartan, ramipril, or both in patients at high risk for vascular events. *N Engl J Med* 2008; **358**(15):1547–59.

11. Rashid P, Leonardi-Bee J, Bath P. Blood pressure reduction and secondary prevention of stroke and other vascular events. A systematic review. *Stroke* 2003; **34**:2741–9.

12. Flather MD, Yusuf S, Kober L, Pfeffer M, Hall A, Murray G, et al. Long-term ACE-inhibitor therapy in

patients with heart failure or left-ventricular dysfunction: a systematic overview of data from individual patients. *Lancet* 2000; **355**:1575–81.

13. Progress Collaborative Group. Randomised trial of a perindopril-based blood-pressure lowering regimen among 6105 individuals with previous stroke or transient ischaemic attack. *Lancet* 2001; **358**:1033–41.

14. Schrader J, Lüders S, Kulschewski A, Berger J, Zidek W, Treib J, et al. The ACCESS Study: evaluation of acute candesartan cilexetil therapy in stroke survivors. *Stroke* 2003; **34**:1699–703.

15. Yusuf S, Diener HC, Sacco RL, Albers G, Bath P, Bornstein N, et al. Randomized trial of telmisartan therapy to prevent recurrent strokes and major vascular events among 20,332 individuals with recent stroke. *N Engl J Med* 2008; **359**:1225–37.

16. Paciaroni M, Hennerici M, Agnelli G, Bogousslavsky J. Statins and stroke prevention. *Cerebrovasc Dis* 2007; **24**(2–3):170–82.

17. Amarenco P, Labreuche J, Lavallee P, Touboul PJ. Statins in stroke prevention and carotid atherosclerosis: systematic review and up-to-date meta-analysis. *Stroke* 2004; **35**(12):2902–9.

18. Grundy SM, Cleeman JI, Merz CN, Brewer HB, Jr., Clark LT, Hunninghake DB, et al. Implications of recent clinical trials for the National Cholesterol Education Program Adult Treatment Panel III Guidelines. *J Am Coll Cardiol* 2004; **44**(3):720–32.

19. Heart Protection Study Collaborative Group. MRC/BHF Heart Protection Study of cholesterol lowering with simvastatin in 20,536 high-risk individuals: a randomised placebo-controlled trial. *Lancet* 2002; **360**:7–22.

20. Collins R, Armitage J, Parish S, Sleight P, Peto R. Heart Protection Study Collaborative Group. Effects of cholesterol-lowering with simvastatin on stroke and other major vascular events in 20536 people with cerebrovascular disease or other high-risk conditions. *Lancet* 2004; **363**:757–67.

21. The Stroke Prevention by Aggressive Reduction in Cholesterol Levels (SPARCL) Investigators. High-dose atorvastatin after stroke or transient ischemic attack. *N Engl J Med* 2006; **355**:549–59.

22. Endres M, Laufs U. Discontinuation of statin treatment in stroke patients. *Stroke* 2006; **37**(10):2640–3.

23. Blanco M, Nombela F, Castellanos M, Rodriguez-Yanez M, Garcia-Gil M, Leira R, et al. Statin treatment withdrawal in ischemic stroke: a controlled randomized study. *Neurology* 2007; **69**(9):904–10.

24. Wilcox R, Bousser MG, Betteridge DJ, Schernthaner G, Pirags V, Kupfer S, et al. Effects of pioglitazone in

patients with type 2 diabetes with or without previous stroke: results from PROactive (PROspective pioglitAzone Clinical Trial In macroVascular Events 04). *Stroke* 2007; **38**(3):865–73.

25. Gerstein HC, Miller ME, Byington RP, Goff DC, Jr., Bigger JT, Buse JB, et al. Effects of intensive glucose lowering in type 2 diabetes. *N Engl J Med* 2008; **358**(24):2545–59.

26. Patel A, MacMahon S, Chalmers J, Neal B, Billot L, Woodward M, et al. Intensive blood glucose control and vascular outcomes in patients with type 2 diabetes. *N Engl J Med* 2008; **358**(24):2560–72.

27. Toole JF, Malinow MR, Chambless LE, Spence JD, Pettigrew LC, Howard VJ, et al. Lowering homocysteine in patients with ischemic stroke to prevent recurrent stroke, myocardial infarction, and death: the Vitamin Intervention for Stroke Prevention (VISP) randomized controlled trial. *JAMA* 2004; **291**(5):565–75.

28. The Heart Outcomes Prevention Evaluation (HOPE) 2 Investigators Homocysteine lowering with folic acid and B vitamins in vascular disease. *N Engl J Med* 2006; **354**:1567–77.

29. Viscoli CM, Brass LM, Kernan WN, Sarrel PM, Suissa S, Horwitz RI. A clinical trial of estrogen-replacement therapy after ischemic stroke. *N Engl J Med* 2001; **345**:1243–9.

30. Antiplatelet Trialists Collaboration. Collaborative overview of randomised trials of antiplatelet therapy – I: prevention of death, myocardial infarction, and stroke by prolonged antiplatelet therapy in various categories of patients. *BMJ* 1994; **308**:81–106.

31. Antithrombotic Trialists' Collaboration. Collaborative meta-analysis of randomised trials of antiplatelet therapy for prevention of death, myocardial infarction, and stroke in high risk patients. *BMJ* 2002; **524**:71–86.

32. Born G, Patrono C. Antiplatelet drugs. *Br J Pharmacol* 2006; **147** Suppl 1:S241–51.

33. Algra A, van Gijn J. Cumulative meta-analysis of aspirin efficacy after cerebral ischaemia of arterial origin. *J Neurol Neurosurg Psychiatry* 1999; **65**:255.

34. Patrono C, Garcia Rodriguez LA, Landolfi R, Baigent C. Low-dose aspirin for the prevention of atherothrombosis. *N Engl J Med* 2005; **353**(22):2373–83.

35. Topol E, Easton D, Harrington R, Amarenco P, Califf R, Graffagnino C, et al. Randomized, double-blind, placebo-controlled, international trial of the oral IIb/IIIa antagonist lotrafiban in coronary and cerebrovascular disease. *Circulation* 2003; **108**:16–23.

36. Yusuf S, Zhao F, Mehta SR, Chrolavicius S, Tognoni G, Fox KK, et al. Effects of clopidogrel in addition to

aspirin in patients with acute coronary syndromes without ST-segment elevation. *N Engl J Med* 2001; **345**:494–502.

37. CAPRIE Steering Committee. A randomised, blinded, trial of clopidogrel versus aspirin in patients at risk of ischaemic events (CAPRIE). *Lancet* 1996; **348**:1329–39.

38. Diener H, Bogousslavsky J, Brass L, Cimminiello C, Csiba L, Kaste M, et al. Acetylsalicylic acid on a background of clopidogrel in high-risk patients randomised after recent ischaemic stroke or transient ischaemic attack: the MATCH trial results. *Lancet* 2004; **364**:331–334.

39. Bhatt DL, Fox KA, Hacke W, Berger PB, Black HR, Boden WE, et al. Clopidogrel and aspirin versus aspirin alone for the prevention of atherothrombotic events. *N Engl J Med* 2006; **354**(16):1706–17.

40. Bhatt DL, Flather MD, Hacke W, Berger PB, Black HR, Boden WE, et al. Patients with prior myocardial infarction, stroke, or symptomatic peripheral arterial disease in the CHARISMA trial. *J Am Coll Cardiol* 2007; **49**(19):1982–8.

41. Diener HC, Cuhna L, Forbes C, Sivenius J, Smets P, Lowenthal A. European Stroke Prevention Study 2. Dipyridamole and acetylsalicylic acid in the secondary prevention of stroke. *J Neurol Sci* 1996; **143**:1–13.

42. Diener HC, Darius H, Bertrand-Hardy JM, Humphreys M. Cardiac safety in the European stroke prevention study 2 (ESPS2). *Int J Clin Pract* 2001; **55**:162–3.

43. The ESPRIT Study Group. Aspirin plus dipyridamole versus aspirin alone after cerebral ischaemia of arterial origin (ESPRIT): randomised controlled trial. *Lancet* 2006; **367**:1665–73.

44. Diener HC, Sacco R, Yusuf S, for the Steering Committee and PRoFESS Study Group. Rationale, design and baseline data of a randomized, double-blind, controlled trial comparing two antithrombotic regimens and telmisartan vs. placebo in patients with strokes: the prevention regimen for effectively avoiding second strokes (PRoFESS) trial. *Cerebrovasc Dis* 2007; **23**:368–80.

45. Diener HC, Ringleb PA, Savi P. Clopidogrel for secondary prevention of stroke. *Expert Opin Pharmacother* 2005; **6**:755–64.

46. Diener HC. Modified-release dipyridamole combined with aspirin for secondary stroke prevention. *Aging Health* 2005; **1**:19–26.

47. Topol EJ, Byzova TV, Plow EF. Platelet GPIIb-IIIa blockers. *Lancet* 1999; **353**:227–31.

48. EAFT Group. Secondary prevention in non-rheumatic atrial fibrillation after transient ischaemic attack or minor stroke. *Lancet* 1993; **342**:1255–62.

49. Saxena R, Koudstaal PJ. Anticoagulants for preventing stroke in patients with nonrheumatic atrial fibrillation and a history of stroke or transient ischemic attack. *Stroke* 2004; **35**:1782–3.

50. Hart R, Pearce L, Miller V, Anderson D, Rothrock J, Albers G, et al. Cardioembolic vs. noncardioembolic strokes in atrial fibrillation: Frequency and effect of antithrombotic agents in the stroke prevention in atrial fibrillation studies. *Cerebrovasc Dis* 2000; **10**:39–43.

51. Nieuwlaat R, Capucci A, Camm AJ, Olsson SB, Andresen D, Davies DW, et al. Atrial fibrillation management: a prospective survey in ESC member countries: the Euro Heart Survey on Atrial Fibrillation. *Eur Heart J* 2005; **26**(22):2422–34.

52. Fuster V, Ryden LE, Cannom DS, Crijns HJ, Curtis AB, Ellenbogen KA, et al. ACC/AHA/ESC 2006 guidelines for the management of patients with atrial fibrillation: full text: a report of the American College of Cardiology/American Heart Association Task Force on practice guidelines and the European Society of Cardiology Committee for Practice Guidelines (Writing Committee to Revise the 2001 guidelines for the management of patients with atrial fibrillation) developed in collaboration with the European Heart Rhythm Association and the Heart Rhythm Society. *Europace* 2006; **8**(9):651–745.

53. Hylek EM, Evans-Molina C, Shea C, Henault LE, Regan S. Major hemorrhage and tolerability of warfarin in the first year of therapy among elderly patients with atrial fibrillation. *Circulation* 2007; **115**(21):2689–96.

54. ACTIVE Writing Group on behalf of the ACTIVE Investigators, Connolly S, Pogue J, Hart R, Pfeffer M, Hohnloser S, et al. Clopidogrel plus aspirin versus oral anticoagulation for atrial fibrillation in the Atrial fibrillation Clopidogrel Trial with Irbesartan for prevention of Vascular Events (ACTIVE W): a randomised controlled trial. *Lancet* 2006; **367**:1903–12.

55. The Stroke Prevention in Reversible Ischemia Trial (SPIRIT) Study Group. A randomized trial of anticoagulants versus aspirin after cerebral ischemia of presumed arterial origin. *Ann Neurol* 1997; **42**:857–65.

56. Mohr JP, Thompson JL, Lazar RM, Levin B, Sacco RL, Furie KL, et al. A comparison of warfarin and aspirin for the prevention of recurrent ischemic stroke. *N Engl J Med* 2001; **345**:1444–51.

57. The ESPRIT Study Group. Medium intensity oral anticoagulants versus aspirin after cerebral ischaemia of arterial origin (ESPRIT): a randomised controlled trial. *Lancet Neurol* 2007; **6**(2):115–24.

58. Algra A, De Schryver E, van Gijn J, Kappelle L, Koudstaal P. Oral anticoagulants versus antiplatelet therapy for preventing further vascular events after

transient ischaemic attack or minor stroke of presumed arterial origin. *Cochrane Database Syst Rev* 2006; 3:CD001342.

59. Levine SR, Brey RL, Tilley BC, Thompson JL, Sacco RL, Sciacca RR, et al. Antiphospholipid antibodies and subsequent thrombo-occlusive events in patients with ischemic stroke. *JAMA* 2004; **291**(5):576–84.

60. Beletsky V, Nadareishvili Z, Lynch J, Shuaib A, Woolfenden AR, Norris J, et al. Cervical arterial dissection. Time for a therapeutic trial? *Stroke* 2003; 34:2856–60.

61. Lyrer P, Engelter S. Antithrombotic drugs for carotid artery dissection. *Stroke* 2004; **35**(2):613–4.

62. Engelter ST, Brandt T, Debette S, Caso V, Lichy C, Pezzini A, et al. Antiplatelets versus anticoagulation in cervical artery dissection. *Stroke* 2007; **38**(9):2605–11.

63. Barnett HJ, Taylor DW, Eliasziw M, Fox AJ, Ferguson GG, Haynes RB, et al. Benefit of carotid endarterectomy in patients with symptomatic moderate or severe stenosis. *N Engl J Med* 1998; 339:1415–1425.

64. European Carotid Surgery Trialists' Collaborative Group. Randomised trial of endarterectomy for recently symptomatic carotid stenosis: final results of the MRC European Carotid Surgery Trial (ECST). *Lancet* 1998; 351:1379–87.

65. European Carotid Surgery Trialists' Collaborative Group. MRC European carotid surgery trial: interim results for symptomatic patients with severe carotid stenosis and with mild carotid stenosis. *Lancet* 1991; 337:1235–43.

66. Ferguson GG, Eliasziw M, Barr HWK, Clagett GP, Barnes RW, Wallace MC, et al. The North American symptomatic carotid endarterectomy trial: surgical result in 1415 patients. *Stroke* 1999; 30:1751–8.

67. Rothwell PM, Warlow CP, on behalf of the European Carotid Surgery Trialists' Collaborative Group. Prediction of benefit from carotid endarterectomy in individual patients: a risk-modelling study. *Lancet* 1999; 353:2105–10.

68. Rothwell PM, Eliasziv M, Gutnikov SA, Fox AJ, Taylor DW, Mayberg MR, et al. Analysis of pooled data from the randomized controlled trials of endarterectomy for symptomatic carotid stenosis. *Lancet* 2003; 361:107–16.

69. Rothwell P, Eliasziw M, Gutnikov S, Warlow C, Barnett H, Carotid Endarterectomy

Trialists Collaboration. Endarterectomy for symptomatic carotid stenosis in relation to clinical subgroups and timing of surgery. *Lancet* 2004; 363:915–24.

70. Chaturvedi S, Bruno A, Feasby T, Holloway R, Benavente O, Cohen SN, et al. Carotid endarterectomy – an evidence-based review: report of the Therapeutics and Technology Assessment Subcommittee of the American Academy of Neurology. *Neurology* 2005; **65**(6):794–801.

71. Ringleb PA, Allenberg J, Bruckmann H, Eckstein HH, Fraedrich G, Hartmann M, et al. 30 day results from the SPACE trial of stent-protected angioplasty versus carotid endarterectomy in symptomatic patients: a randomised non-inferiority trial. *Lancet* 2006; **368** (9543):1239–47.

72. Stingele R, Berger J, Alfke K, Eckstein HH, Fraedrich G, Allenberg J, et al. Clinical and angiographic risk factors for stroke and death within 30 days after carotid endarterectomy and stent-protected angioplasty: a subanalysis of the SPACE study. *Lancet Neurol* 2008; **7**(3):216–222.

73. Mas JL, et al, for the EVA-3S Investigators. Endarterectomy versus stenting in patients with symptomatic severe carotid stenosis. *N Engl J Med* 2006; **355**:1660–71.

74. Kern R, Ringleb PA, Hacke W, Mas JL, Hennerici MG. Stenting for carotid artery stenosis. *Nat Clin Pract Neurol* 2007; **3**(4):212–20.

75. Chimowitz MI, Lynn MJ, Howlett-Smith H, Stern BJ, Hertzberg VS, Frankel MR, et al. Comparison of warfarin and aspirin for symptomatic intracranial arterial stenosis. *N Engl J Med* 2005; **352**(13):1305–16.

76. Kasner SE, Chimowitz MI, Lynn MJ, Howlett-Smith H, Stern BJ, Hertzberg VS, et al. Predictors of ischemic stroke in the territory of a symptomatic intracranial arterial stenosis. *Circulation* 2006; **113**(4):555–63.

77. Zaidat OO, Klucznik R, Alexander MJ, Chaloupka J, Lutsep H, Barnwell S, et al. The NIH registry on use of the Wingspan stent for symptomatic 70–99% intracranial arterial stenosis. *Neurology* 2008; **70**(17):1518–24.

78. Jiang WJ, Xu XT, Du B, Dong KH, Jin M, Wang QH, et al. Comparison of elective stenting of severe vs moderate intracranial atherosclerotic stenosis. *Neurology* 2007; **68**(6):420–6.

Chapter 20

Neurorehabilitation

Sylvan J. Albert and Jürg Kesselring

Introduction and overview

Stroke is one of the most common causes of long-term disability in adults, especially in elderly people. Although progress in the acute treatment of stroke (e.g. thrombolysis, the concept of stroke units) has occurred over recent years, neurorehabilitation (mainly organized inpatient multidisciplinary rehabilitation) remains one of the cornerstones of stroke treatment. The overall benefit of stroke units results not only from thrombolysis – only a small proportion of all stroke patients (less than 10%) are treated with this regimen – but more generally from the multidisciplinary stroke unit management, including treatment optimization, minimization of complications, and elements of early neurorehabilitation [1, 2].

After the acute treatment, stroke patients with relevant neurological deficits should in general be treated by a specialized neurorehabilitation clinic or unit. The best timing for transferring a patient after initial treatment (e.g. on a stroke unit) to a specialized neurorehabilitation ward or clinic is still under discussion, but early initiation of rehabilitation is mandatory for outcome optimization (whereas ultra-early high-intensity training in the first hours to few days might be problematic).

Neurorehabilitation nowadays is considered as a multidisciplinary and multimodal concept to help neurological patients to improve physiological functioning, activity and participation by creating learning situations, inducing several means of recovery including restitution, functional remodeling, compensation and reconditioning [1]. A key point in successfully diminishing negative long-term effects after stroke and achieving recovery is the *work of a specialized multidisciplinary team* (physicians, nursing staff, therapists, others) with structured organization and processes and the stroke patient taking part in a multimodal, intense treatment program which is well adapted in detail to the individual goals of rehabilitation and deficits. The

WHO's ICF (The International Classification of Functioning, Disability and Health; 2001) is now widely accepted as a useful tool in goal-setting, making its way into clinical practice. It adds a social perspective with emphasis on participation.

There is growing evidence indicating a better outcome of neurorehabilitation in stroke with early initiation of treatment, high intensity, specifically aimed and active therapies and the coordinated work and multimodality of a specialized team [3].

Neuroplasticity
Mechanisms of neuroplasticity

While for many decades of the last century it was believed that, "once development is complete, the sources of growth and regeneration of axons and dendrites are irretrievably lost. In the adult brain the nerve paths are fixed and immutable: everything can die, nothing can be regenerated" [4], a paradigm shift has taken place. A few years later in 1936 it was reported that therapeutic exercises influence the course of spontaneous recovery of a brain affection [5]. It has been a long way, however, to what we now know, first by measurement of the effects of rehabilitation, that the central nervous system of the adult human being has an astounding potential for recovery and adaptability, which can be selectively promoted [6].

The extent of recovery in stroke is dependent on many factors, the initial size and location of the cerebral lesion being the predominant factor. Recovery (e.g. measured by motor scores) takes place more quickly and more effectively up to the first 8–12 weeks after a lesion and afterwards the recovery curve flattens. As an exception, in severe disorders recovery can vary and these patients may even show onset of functional recovery after a longer period [7].

Such recovery of the central nervous system over the course of time after the onset of stroke is possible due to a mechanism described as neuroplasticity, which can be observed and investigated by different approaches, e.g. from a clinical to a neurobiological and neuropathological point of view. Hebb first described neuroplasticity with regard to the function of synapses [8], and later this principle was also linked to the functioning of neurons in the wider context of neuronal networks.

Several (overlapping and interacting) mechanisms of neuronal plasticity can be identified [7, 9–11], which include:

- *Vicariation* (vice = instead of) describes the hypothesis that the functions of damaged areas can be taken over by different regions of the brain. In clinical practice this ability may vary widely and may be insufficient for a large group of patients with remaining difficulties after brain damage. With functional imaging, however, it could be demonstrated that vicariation takes place in cortical representation areas. Another clinical example is the change in lateralization of speech in some younger patients.
- *Plasticity of areas of cortical representation* was described in animal models in connection with the variable size of cortical representation "loco typico" of motor fields [12, 13]. Later such enlargement of cortical representations was also demonstrated in humans. By using transcranial magnetic stimulation (TMS) mapping in stroke patients, the area of cortical representation of the abductor minimi muscle (ADM) transiently increased even after a single training session. These findings suggest a very variable cortical representation [14]. Using functional positron emission tomography (PET) and functional magnetic resonance tomography (fMRI) different patterns of activation have been described (for a summary refer to Ward [11]). In an illustrative longitudinal study [15], a small group of stroke patients with comparable circumscribed M1 lesions (similar to experimental lesions in animal models) affecting the motor control of the contralateral hand were assessed over several months. In the first follow-up, ipsi- and contralateral activation patterns were noted. After several months, activation was again ipsilesional and closer to the former representation and more dorsal for the function of finger-extension as compared to controls, reflecting functional

reorganization in the motor cortex adjacent to the lesion. To summarize fMRI and PET studies after focal ischemic brain lesions resulting in motor deficits with damage to corticospinal tract, it is suggested that

- interruption of projections from the primary motor cortex (M1) leads to increased recruitment of secondary motor areas such as the dorsolateral premotor cortex and supplementary motor areas [16]. For this early *compensation* detailed longitudinal fMRI studies show initial upregulation in primary and secondary motor regions (ipsi- and/or contralateral) but also activity of other non-primary structures of the sensorimotor network [9], followed by
- more precise activation patterns with more focused and efficient brain activity in a later phase reflecting *reorganization* [17], and which are reminiscent of normal activation patterns. Enhanced activity of the ipsilesional primary motor cortex induced by motor training is paralleled by improved motor function [18].

For better understanding of these mechanisms a main strategy for recovery in such patients seems to be the goal of achieving the best results by recruitment and adaptation of surviving secondary motor areas in both hemispheres [16]: in addition to a static point-by-point view of the somatotopic organization of the motor homunculus recent studies also demonstrate the representation of movements within the primary sensorimotor cortex, and, on the other hand, second-ary motor areas have direct projections to spinal cord motor neurons, although they are less numerous than those from M1. A persistent activation, however, of many different areas may also indicate a less successful or failed reorganization in chronic stroke patients: the higher the involvement of the ipsilesional motor net-work, the better the recovery. In this respect *interaction between lesional and contralesional hemispheres* may also play an important role [19].

Basic underlying mechanisms of these findings include both different functional use of existing networks and synapses, but also to a certain extent structural changes. In the early course of ischemic stroke, pathophysiological mechanisms in the perilesional region are initiated, which include upregulation of plasticity-related proteins, brain-derived neurotrophic factor, synapsin I and certain neurotransmitters. These modifications probably lead to morphological changes, e.g. synaptic plasticity and sprouting as discussed below, especially on days 3–18 after stroke [19–23].

Sprouting of neurons after damage of the neuron itself is well known in the peripheral nervous system, where axons may re-grow after Wallerian degeneration. In the central nervous system of the adult, however, this mechanism is reduced (but not excluded) for several reasons, including the lack of Schwann cells (functioning as a leading structure for sprouting in the peripheral nerve system), barriers of gliosis produced by glia cells, incomplete remyelinization by oligodendrocytes, production of inhibitory factors by these cells and low production of growth factor GAP-43 in the adult central nervous system, which is available in the peripheral nerve system over the entire lifespan [7]. However, in animal models sprouting of neurons after lesions and also after interventions to reduce production of inhibitory factors has already been shown to lead to a better outcome. Sprouting of dendrites is much more common than the limited sprouting of axons.

Collateral sprouting can lead to a change of function in a damaged neuron by receiving new synaptic input from dendrites of non-lesioned sprouting neurons.

Synaptic plasticity refers to the altered synaptic function when cells are communicating, leading to plastic changes, stated as "cells that fire together, wire together" by Hebb [8]. Changes in synaptic activity can be measured by alterations in the number of NMDA receptors and are morphologically seen as "spines" between two neurons.

Diaschisis is a term used by von Monakow (1914) to describe the phenomenon that a focal lesion may also lead to changes in brain functioning of areas located far away. An example demonstrated by several recent neuroimaging studies is an enhanced contralesional cerebellar activity after cortical infarction.

Furthermore an *enriched environment* must also be mentioned in terms of neuroplasticity [7, 16], as has been demonstrated in animal models: rats with an ischemic lesion due to middle cerebral artery occlusion showed much better recovery when held in an enriched environment with free access to physical activity and social interactions [24].

Neuroplasticity is the dynamic potential of the brain to reorganize itself during ontogeny, learning, or following damage. In clinical neurorehabilitation this potential is utilized by creating a stimulating learning atmosphere and using stimulation techniques.

Inducing neuroplasticity

There are many parallels between postlesional neuroplasticity (re-learning) and normal learning in the development of human individuals leading to changes of *behavior* by repetitive interactions with the social environment. In clinical neurorehabilitation the main effect of the *multidisciplinary teamwork and applied therapies is to create a stimulating learning atmosphere* that matches the patient's individual needs and deficits. Such learning conditions also take place in the *therapeutic sessions* (see below) and in everyday life on the neurorehabilitation ward in interactions with physicians and the nursing team. A valuable principle to force the individual to learn is the use of *constraint-induced therapies (CIT)*, which however, cannot be used in the treatment of the majority of stroke patients (see below). In addition other *stimulation techniques* and *enhancement by use of medications* are under evaluation.

Supporting neuroplasticity by peripheral and brain stimulation techniques

Although not yet to be recommended for clinical routine, several trials have been undertaken and are currently ongoing to evaluate non-invasive cortical stimulation techniques with the purpose of enhancing neuroplasticity and recovery, using clinical outcome measures or fMRI. The main techniques are repetitive transcranial magnetic stimulation (rTMS) and transcranial direct current stimulation (TDCS), which can be used for both cortical enhancement and inhibition, depending on the set-up parameters. Furthermore epidural electrical stimulation (EES) is an invasive approach using a grid of electrodes implanted neurosurgically. Therefore its practical use in stroke patients is limited.

The main theory behind influencing cortical activity is the hypothesis of contralesional hemisphere overexcitability, but also involved are effects of locally disturbed function on other areas described as vicariation and changes of cortical representation (see above). The main approaches to brain stimulation are to increase the excitability of the cortex in the ipsilesional hemisphere and/or suppression of the contralesional hemisphere. This can be achieved noninvasively in conscious humans using repetitive transcranial magnetic stimulation (rTMS) and transcranial direct current stimulation (TDCS).

In rTMS an electric current is induced in the underlying cortex by a magnetic field which then activates the axons of cortical neurons. Low-frequency rTMS around 1 Hz results in decreased cortical excitability (which persists after the application of rTMS) and is therefore used on the contralesional hemisphere for downregulation. Higher frequencies of more than 5 Hz increase cortical excitability and can be applied to stimulate the cortex on the ipsilesional hemisphere. Special patterns of rTMS (theta bursts) have been used in humans, and are reported to have longer-lasting modulatory capacity [25].

In TDCS two electrodes (one active and one reference) are placed on the skin, delivering weak polarizing electrical current leading to different effects in the cortex, depending on the polarity: anodal TDCS has an excitatory effect, cathodal TDCS induces inhibition via presumed hyperpolarization. Usually 10–20 minutes of TDCS at 1–2 mA are regarded as safe and painless.

With the application of these newer treatment methods in stroke patients, recent findings suggest a 10–20% functional improvement in single sessions as well as in a small but increasing number of longer-term therapeutic trials. As far as is known now, cortical stimulation appears to be a safe and promising intervention for stroke patients; however, more trials are needed to assess the long-term benefit and to optimize protocols [16, 26, 27].

On the other hand peripheral techniques indirectly influencing cortical activity are under evaluation.

Reduction of sensori-motor input from the intact hand was shown to lead to improved performance of the paretic hand in stroke patients using cutaneous anesthesia [28]. This effect might – at least partially – also play a role in constraint-induced therapies (CIT).

Increasing input from the paretic hand using somatosensory stimulation may also improve motor function [29, 30], but only limited data are available now. Motor training of the paretic hand itself increases somatosensory input as well as constraint-induced therapies (CIT) (Figure 20.1).

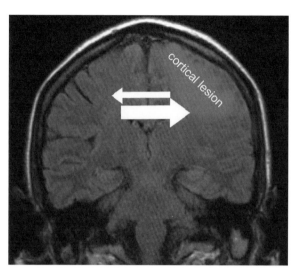

Figure 20.1. Non-invasive brain stimulation in stroke refers partly to the "contralesional hemisphere over-excitability hypothesis" – repetitive transcranial magnetic stimulation (rTMS) or transcranial direct current stimulation (TDCS) can be used for both cortical enhancement and inhibition, depending on the set-up parameters used.

Supporting neuroplasticity by pharmacological interventions

No single medication evaluated for its beneficial effect by modulating plasticity in the human motor cortex in stroke patients has reached class I evidence so far. Only a few preliminary studies using this approach have been conducted, and the results of some studies are contradictory. Levodopa, d-amphetamine, methylphenidate, donepezil and fluoxetine are found to be beneficial in trials evaluating motor recovery after stroke, but in one study d-amphetamine was found to have no effect. Negative effects on outcome were noted for benzodiazepines, haloperidol, prazosine and clonidine [31].

However, larger controlled trials are needed before such treatments can be generally recommended. Stroke patients presenting a reduced ability to take part in therapies due to diminished alertness and drive should be carefully evaluated for depression first. If treatment with stimulating antidepressants is not successful or not possible, the use of levodopa or a central stimulating agent may be an alternative treatment option (see Table 20.1).

Non-invasive cortical stimulation techniques (repetitive transcranial magnetic stimulation and direct current stimulation) are used in rehabilitation to

Table 20.1. Selected medications used in the course of neurorehabilitation.

Indication	Substance	Remarks
Post-stroke depression	venlafaxine	75–300(+) mg/day
	citalopram	20–40 mg/day; also useful in pathological crying
	mirtazapine	with sleep disorders; 15–45 mg/day (at bedtime); combination with venlafaxine and other possible
	trazodone	with agitation; 50–200 mg/day (main dosage at bedtime); can also be used in the elderly
Diminished drive	l-dopa/benserazide	evaluate 100/25–200/50 mg/day (studies for motor recovery undertaken with pulsed use in combination with physical therapies)
	methylphenidate	start with 10 mg/day, restricted substance, inpatient evaluation
Agitation, psychosis	quetiapine	25–300(+) mg/day; in elderly patients start with 12.5–25 mg
Agitation, sleep disorder	pipamperone	20–80(+) mg/day (at bedtime) for sleep disorder of the elderly
Post-stroke epilepsy	valproate	800–1800(+) mg/day; sometimes also used in central pain syndrome
	carbamazepine	600–1200(+) mg/day; sometimes also used in central pain syndrome and paroxysmal symptoms
	phenytoin	250–300(+) mg/day
	levetiracetame *and other antiepileptic drugs*	1000–3000 mg/day; 2000(+) mg/day in monotherapy (i.v. application possible: several benzodiazepines, valproate, phenytoin, levetiracetame)
	clonazepam, lorazepam *and other benzodiazepines*	i.v. application in status epilepticus; other indications include anxiety, sleep disorder, depression (temporarily) negative effect on cognition and learning; adverse drug reaction with agitation in the elderly
Pain/shoulder-arm pain	ibuprofen *and other NSAIDs*	combine with positioning and physical therapies
Shoulder-hand syndrome	prednisone	start trial with 50–70 mg/day
Central pain syndrome	amitryptiline	especially useful in constant burning pain; consider very slow initiation, e.g. 10 mg/day (50–75 mg/day) only 2nd line in depression
	pregabaline	slow elevation diminishes side-effects; 75–300(600) mg/day
	gabapentine	slow elevation diminishes side-effects; 900–3600 mg/day
	tramadole	combination with pregabaline or gabapentine; 50–150(+) mg/day
	oxycodone	in severe central pain syndrome; add-on; 5–50(+) mg/day

Table 20.1. (*cont.*)

Indication	Substance	Remarks
Bladder dysfunction	oxybutynin	detrusor spasticity; 7.5–15(20) mg/day
	alfuzosine *and other α-inhibitors*	increased urethral sphincter activity or detrusor sphincter dyssynergia
	desmopressin	in severe nycturia; 20 µg/day given intranasally at bedtime
Reflux, gastritis, ulcers (prevention)	omeprazole, pantoprazole *and other proton pump inhibitors*	consider administration twice daily in critically ill patients
Spasticity	botulinum toxin A	period of >3 months between intramuscular injections to diminish risk of antibodies
	baclofen	30–75(+) mg/day orally; intrathecal application in severe (spinal) spasticity
	tizanidine	4–24 mg/day (orally baclofen and tizanidine have very limited effects in cerebral spasticity)

Notes: Please note that (1) substances mentioned are examples of their group; (2) several of the indications are "off-label"; please verify with your national regulation standards; (3) there are not enough data for all of the mentioned substances to provide evidence-based recommendations (expert opinion or observational studies); (4) medications for secondary prophylaxis, dementia, cardiovascular diseases and infections are not included.

enhance neuroplasticity and recovery. In preliminary studies, some medications such as levodopa were found to be beneficial for motor recovery.

Structured multidisciplinary neurorehabilitation

Importance of multidisciplinary teamwork for stroke recovery

In addition to thrombolysis the multidisciplinary management in a stroke unit or by a stroke team has been shown to improve outcome significantly by reducing death rates and dependency (NNT 7 for thrombolysis versus NNT 9 for stroke unit treatment) [2]. The positive effect of stroke units is achieved by structural organization and interdisciplinary management, but also by the early use of elements of neurorehabilitation.

According to a large meta-analysis ($n = 1437$) the benefit of postacute treatment in *organized inpatient multidisciplinary rehabilitation* (as compared to treatment on a general ward and other nonspecific rehabilitation clinics) is associated with reduced odds of death, institutionalization and dependency. Of 100 patients treated by organized multidisciplinary neurorehabilitation as compared to general treatment, an extra five returned home in an independent state [32]. Therefore the beneficial elements of acute and postacute stroke treatment should be combined.

The amount of rehabilitation treatment in the acute phase may vary widely, as a multicenter study examining physical activity within the first 14 days of acute stroke unit care has shown: in the daytime patients spent more than 50% of the time resting in bed, 28% sitting out of bed, and only 13% engaged in activities with the potential to prevent complications and improve recovery of mobility. Furthermore patients were alone for 60% of their time [33]. The best timing for transferring a patient after initial treatment to a specialized neurorehabilitation ward or clinic is still under discussion, and concerns regarding optimal timing and intensity might also contribute to the problem (see below).

After acute stroke treatment medically stable patients with relevant neurological deficits should be treated in a specialized neurorehabilitation clinic or stroke unit in an in- or outpatient setting to take advantage of the impact of the work of a specialized multidisciplinary team with structured organization and processes: the patient takes part in a multimodal, intensive treatment program which must be adapted to the individual goals of rehabilitation with regular interdisciplinary re-evaluation.

A short and useful definition for an *organized inpatient multidisciplinary rehabilitation* includes: [33]

- interdisciplinary goal-setting;
- input from a multidisciplinary team of medical, nursing and therapy staff with an expertise in stroke and rehabilitation whose work is coordinated through regular weekly meetings;
- involvement of patients and family in the rehabilitation process;
- program of staff training.

This approach should be centered on the individual patient and family/caregivers, interacting closely with a multidisciplinary team consisting of physicians, nurses, physical and occupational therapists, kinesiotherapists, speech and language pathologists (SLP), psychologists, recreational therapists and social workers [3]. The required equipment in a neurorehabilitation department must be defined in detail to ensure structural quality. A description of medical and organizational processes using a quality-management system and "learning from mistakes", e.g. using a critical incidence reporting system (CIRS), is also important for rehabilitation centers.

At the onset of the rehabilitation process a multi-disciplinary assessment of deficits and resources is mandatory, including clinical neurological examination, assessment of functional performance, activities of daily living (ADL), social and personal background and coping strategies. To achieve recovery of physical and psychological functions and to reintegrate the patient into his/her social environment, therapies and other interventions must be adapted to the individual abilities and disabilities. In the course of rehabilitation the patients' progress and abilities are critically discussed and re-evaluated in the multidisciplinary team in at least weekly sessions with an adaptation and reconsideration of treatment strategies and goals (see below), if necessary [34–36].

Treatment in an organized inpatient multidisciplinary setting improves the outcome after stroke significantly. The positive effect of stroke units is gained by structural organization and interdisciplinary management, but also by the early use of elements of neurorehabilitation.

Timing and intensity

Clinical studies indicate that an early start and high intensity of therapies are decisive for a favorable long-term outcome. On the basis of pathophysiological data, the first 3 weeks after stroke are considered as a particularly promising period: in animal models active training leads to better functional recovery and sprouting, whereas inactivity results in additional loss of ability [12, 20, 23]. However, some experimental studies in rats show that very early (starting within 24 hours) and intense forced activity could lead to an enlargement of lesion areas. The occurrence of these negative consequences is explained by cytotoxic effects of glutamate, metabolic collapse of the penumbra region, inhibition of upregulation of signal proteins, focal hyperthermia and other factors [37–41]. Other recent animal studies, however, support the early initiation of appropriate activation. Early motor activation after focal ischemia starting at day 5 had a superior outcome (functional measures and more dendritic sprouting) as compared to a later beginning (at days 14 and 30) [20]. Furthermore in primates reorganization of cortical representation areas was found to be more effective after early activation (within 7 days) [12, 42]. Finally, in contrast to the above-mentioned studies, a better functional result without signs of enlargement of lesion areas was achieved by early motor training in rats beginning 24 hours after maturation of ischemic lesions [43].

Clinical data are consistent with these findings. In humans, however, other factors should be taken into account: immobilization increases the rate of complications after acute stroke, including thrombosis, infections, and ulcers. Early mobilization in the first days and structured training at an early stage on a stroke unit enhances the rate of discharges to the home with a lower degree of disabilities [44] as compared to later activation on a medical ward. Better long-term outcome is reported in stroke patients with early start of an organized inpatient multidisciplinary rehabilitation within 7 days in a multicenter study ($n = 1760$) with reduction of disability and better quality-of-life measures [45]. In another large study

($n = 969$) specifically examining the impact of the timing of the initiation of neurorehabilitation and functional recovery, a highly significant correlation of early treatment start and functional outcome was detected [46].

Not only early initiation of treatment but also the *intensity of rehabilitative therapies* is of significant importance, as shown in a meta-analysis [47] with higher mobility, autonomy, and improved executive functions when different therapeutic modalities are performed with increased intensity. Therapy intensity was also related to shorter lengths of stay and to improvements in patients' functional independence.

A higher intensity of therapies can also be achieved by the additional use of *rehabilitation robotics* in the multidisciplinary approach, as established for arm functioning and walking.

To summarize:

- immobilization after stroke is counterproductive (and should be reserved for specific rare situations, e.g. in the case of instable brain perfusion due to arterial stenosis) and
- an appropriate amount of activity should take place very early after the onset of stroke
- with the initiation of specific and intense individually adapted neurorehabilitation of the medically stable patient, ideally within the first days after stroke
- including in the course of treatment a high proportion of multimodal therapies.

Early mobilization and structured training at an early stage improves the outcome after stroke.

Goal-setting and assessment in stroke rehabilitation

Assessment outcome in stroke is directly linked to the model of illness and definition of treatment goals. Most widely accepted is the "The International Classification of Functioning, Disability and Health" (ICF) proposed by the WHO in 2001. In determining treatment goals the medical model is extended by adding a social perspective and defining "participation" as an important objective. Treatment goals measure the physical and psychological status, examining the impact of deficits on social aspects such as everyday life, social communication, or ability to work. Even if some somatic functions cannot be regained directly, higher social goals can be reached

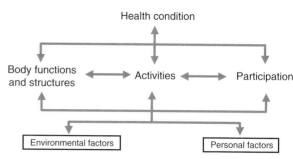

Figure 20.2. The ICF (The International Classification of Functioning, Disability and Health; WHO 2001) transforms the former WHO concept of "disability" into activity and stresses the interrelation of the several components: activity, body functions, body structures, participation, including two context factors: environmental and personal factors. (Figure adapted from "International Classification of Functioning, Disability and Health", World Health Organization, 2001.)

by establishing compensatory strategies. Interdisciplinary goal-setting is crucial for determining the exact treatment schedule, for estimating the duration of neurorehabilitation and for evaluating rehabilitative potential (Figure 20.2).

Assessment in stroke is crucial to demonstrate the course of recovery and benefit of neurorehabilitation and also to deliver instruments for research purposes. It adds *evaluation of quality of life* to *activity* as an outcome parameter. Activity can be assessed by *activity scales* and *scales of activities of daily living*.

Activity scales evaluate abilities and have their value in detailed measurement of aspects of specific therapies or in motor function research [48]. The most commonly used *activity scales* are:

- The Rivermead Mobility Index (RMI) [49]: a clinically relevant measure of disability which concentrates on body mobility. The RMI contains a series of 14 questions and one direct observation, and covers a range of activities from turning over in bed to running. Its validity as a measure of mobility after head injury and stroke was tested by concurrent measurement of mobility using gait speed and endurance, and by standing balance. The RMI forms a scale and can be used in hospital or at home. A modified version has been developed [50] in which the number of test items was reduced from 15 to eight items in order to measure mobility-related items that physical therapists consider essential for demonstrating treatment effects in patients following stroke, with the aim of better sensitivity.

- The Motor Assessment Scale (MAS) [51] is a brief assessment of eight areas of motor function and one item related to muscle tone. Each item is scored on a scale from 0 to 6. It is aimed at the functional capacities of stroke patients, and the items are: supine to side lying, supine to sitting over the edge of a bed, balanced sitting, sitting to standing, walking, upper-arm function, hand movements and advanced hand activities. Modified Motor Assessment Scale (MMAS): also included is a single item, general tonus, intended to provide an estimate of muscle tone on the affected side, which attracts criticism as being difficult to rate. In a special version [52] item descriptions were modified and the general tonus item was deleted.
- The Get-up and Go Test [53] requires patients to stand up from a chair, walk a short distance, turn around, return, and sit down again. Balance function is scored on a five-point scale. In the development the same patients undergo laboratory tests for gait and balance, showing good correlation with laboratory tests. The get-up and go test is regarded as a satisfactory clinical measure of balance in elderly people.
- The Action Research Arm Test (ARAT) [54] is an evaluative measure to assess specific changes in limb function among individuals who have sustained cortical damage resulting in hemiplegia. The ARAT consists of 19 items grouped into four subscales: grasp, grip, pinch, and gross movement. It assesses the ability to handle objects differing in size, weight and shape and therefore can be considered to be an arm-specific measure of activity limitation.
- The Nine Hole Peg Test (NHPT) [55] is composed of a square board with nine pegs and the patient is instructed to take pegs from a container, one by one, and place them into the holes on the board, as quickly as possible. It is aimed at measuring fine manual dexterity. The NHPT is easy to perform and estimates parts of the upper limb function.

Of the numerous scales to assess activities of daily living (ADL) the Barthel Index (BI) and the Functional Independence Measure (FIM), which includes additional items assessing the function of cognition, are most commonly used.

The Barthel Index (BI) [56] measures the extent to which somebody can function independently and has mobility in activities of daily living (ADL); i.e. feeding, bathing, grooming, dressing, bowel control, bladder control, toilet use, transfers (bed to chair and back), mobility (on level surfaces) and stair climbing, resulting in a cumulative score between 0 and 100 and also indicating the need for assistance in care. The Barthel Index (BI) is a widely used measure of functional disability but there are numerous extensions and modifications, e.g. the modified 10-item version by Collin et al. (1988), the extended BI (EBI) by Prosiegel et al. (1996) and the Early Rehabilitation Barthel Index (ERI) proposed by Schönle (1995).

The Functional Independence Measure (FIM) [57] was developed based on the Barthel Index and measures overall performance on ADL. It determines the need for assistance by another person (burden of care) and includes a cognitive domain score.

For assessing the ability of a person to live independently within a community an *instrumental activities of daily living* (IADL) is necessary, which includes several important and more complex functions that go beyond the items of basic self-care. It is debatable, however, which of the items, such as performing light housework, preparing a meal, taking medications, shopping for groceries or clothes, using the telephone and managing money, and many others, should be included.

For an overview on the scales used for *instrumental activities of daily living* and *measurements of quality of life* refer to Graham [48].

Stroke-specific instruments include the *Stroke Impact Scale* (SIS) [58], which is a self-report (patient and caregiver) health status measure to assess multidimensional stroke outcomes: in addition to functional status such as strength and hand function, activities of daily living and other dimensions of health-related quality of life, such as communication, memory and thinking, and social role function, are also considered. The SIS can show persisting difficulties in the physical domain of stroke patients who had been considered independent using ADL measures.

> Interdisciplinary goal-setting is crucial for determining the exact treatment schedule, for estimating duration as well as intensity of neurorehabilitation and for evaluating rehabilitative potential. Assessment is obligatory using validated scales.

Motor rehabilitation

Motor impairment is the most common deficit in stroke, often resulting in reduced independence and mobility. Beside the concepts of physical, occupational and other therapies (see below) the following methods are aimed especially at motor recovery.

Treadmill training

Walking is an important objective in stroke rehabilitation, conventional gait training programs on the floor being routine practice. With the aim of enhancing the efficacy of gait training and also of easing the burden on the therapists, three groups of treadmill training concepts have been developed and evaluated:

- body-weight supported treadmill training (BWSTT): partial body weight support can be used to gain better stepping kinematics in stroke patients unable to walk;
- treadmill training without body-weight support;
- gait machines, such as the Lokomat or Gait Trainer GTI, in addition to body-weight supported treadmill training, can provide a "gait pattern" even for seriously paretic limbs.

In rehabilitation practice these methods are used in addition to conventional modalities, leaving no doubt about the benefit in terms of easing the burden on the therapists and overall being regarded as useful for certain patients. In addition, measurement of gait indicators such as velocity and distance can be easily monitored. Several studies investigated the efficacy on different outcome parameters of gait [59–63]. Most of the studies can be criticized for low treatment contrast since control groups also received intense conventional training, and in addition different outcome parameters and intensities make a comparison of the results harder. However a meta-analysis [64] concludes that there is weak evidence for the overall effectiveness in improvement of gait endurance. The authors recommend that currently BWSTT should be reserved for patients whose physical condition is too weak to tolerate intense training.

Gait-training devices in stroke rehabilitation (their benefit having already been shown by Beer et al. [65] in neurorehabilitation of other diseases, e.g. multiple sclerosis) are currently being investigated as to the potential benefit for certain subgroups of stroke patients (with similar patient selection criteria) but the results are not available yet. It has been assumed that there might be an additional benefit for patients with neglect or pusher syndrome. As for treadmill training without body-weight support no evidence was found for better effectiveness compared to conventional gait training [66], at least for crucial parameters such as functional walking ability and walking speed by Laufer et al. [67]. However, benefits are seen when integrating treadmill training with structured speed dependence as a complementary tool in gait rehabilitation including physiotherapy, resulting in better gait speed and cadence after a 2-week training program for hemiparetic outpatients [68].

Gait training with rhythmical acoustical pacing

Auditory stimulation is useful combined with treadmill training [69], resulting in gait symmetry improved with acoustic pacing. Non-blinded studies illustrate the positive effect of conventional gait training with rhythmic cueing by a metronome or embedded in music, resulting in better stride length and walking speed [70, 71].

Constraint-induced therapy (CIT)

The principles of CIT and constraint-induced movement therapy (CIMT) were described by Taub in 1993 [72]; however, their relevance to practical neurorehabilitation and experimental neuroscience came later: at that time Taub argued that, after stroke, patients try unsuccessfully to use the affected side. Discouragement due to initial failure leads to "learned non-use". Later three principles for this kind of therapy were formulated, consisting of constraining the unaffected limb, forcing use of the affected limb, and intensive practice. Using this method motor rehabilitation of the upper limb is possible, if a selective function for the paretic wrist and fingers is present before initiation of treatment with CIMT. Therefore its use as a general treatment method in stroke is limited. A placebo-controlled study applying CIMT over a 2-week period in patients with stroke onset at 3–9 months before therapies showed highly significantly greater improvements than in the control group in motor and functional improvement [73], still detectable at 2-year follow-up (Figure 20.3) [74].

Repetitive training, aerobic exercises and specific muscle strength training

According to learning theories and knowledge derived from studies of neuronal plasticity, a repetition of tasks in rehabilitation in order to achieve better functional outcome is mandatory. A review of repetitive task training after stroke revealed modest

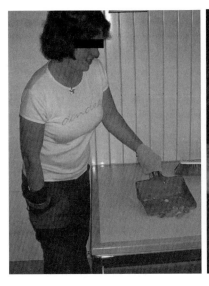 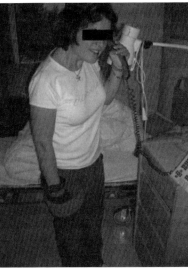

Figure 20.3. The principles of constraint-induced therapy (CIT) and constraint-induced movement therapy (CIMT) described by Taub are: constraining the unaffected limb, enforced use of the affected limb, and repetitive practice. The illustration shows a patient training the affected left arm in everyday life situations and therapeutic exercises.

improvement in lower limb function only, not in upper limb function [75].

Stroke patients suffer not only from neurological deficits but also to varying extents from physical deconditioning and sometimes also from cardiac co-morbidity [64]. Several studies address the possible benefit of general strengthening and aerobic exercises. In a retrospective analysis whole-body intensive rehabilitation was found to be feasible and effective in chronic stroke survivors [76]. In an observational study aerobic capacity and walking capacity were found to be decreased in hemiplegic stroke patients but were directly correlated with each other [77]. Adding physical fitness programs, e.g. by water-based exercise for cardiovascular fitness in stroke patients [78] or task-related circuit training [79, 80], was found to be useful, leading to better outcome not only in physical fitness but also in various secondary measures such as walking speed and endurance, muscle strength, maximal workload, and others [79, 80].

One concern in *specific muscle strength training* is increasing abnormal tone, leading to worsening of functional recovery. However, current opinions based on acquired data have changed; e.g. an observational study [81] showed that targeted strength training significantly increased muscle power in patients with muscle weakness of central origin without any negative effects on spasticity. Instead it was beneficial for functional outcome, showing that strength is related statistically to functional and walking performance.

Mirror therapy

In mirror therapy a mirror is placed at 90° close to the midline of the patient, positioning the affected limb behind the mirror. Using this arrangement the patient is instructed to watch the non-affected limb in the mirror with both eyes and perform excercises. Hereby he or she is getting the visual impression that the limb in the mirror – attributed as the affected limb – is now fully functioning. The role of mirror therapy in motor rehabilitation is not clear yet, but recently, after methodologically weak publications, a promising randomized controlled trial ($n = 40$) has been published for upper limb rehabilitation of subacute stroke patients with severe motor affection without aphasia or apraxia [82]: approximately 1 hour of mirror therapy daily in addition to a conventional rehabilitation program was more beneficial in terms of motor recovery and hand-related functioning than a similar treatment without mirroring. The beneficial effect on hand functioning started post-treatment and continued during the 6-month follow-up evaluation rated by Functional Independence Measure subscales. Several underlying mechanisms have been discussed, e.g. substitution of mirror illusions of a normal movement of the affected hand for decreased proprioceptive information, thereby helping to activate the premotor cortex and promoting rehabilitation by enhancing connections between visual input and premotor areas [83]. Contralateral activation of visual fields was also shown using fMRI [84], with the result that healthy subjects view their hand as their opposite hand by mirroring, activating the visual cortex opposite to the seen hand. Mirror therapy could be an additional option for the rehabilitation of severely paretic limbs, but more data need to be collected.

> Treadmill training, repetitive training, mirror therapy and constraint-induced therapy are newly investigated training principles and can be used especially for enhancing motor recovery.

Concepts of physiotherapy

The predominant common concepts of physiotherapy, the Bobath, Brunnstrom, proprioceptive neuromuscular facilitation (PNF) and Vojta methods, have in common that they claim to have a neurophysiological basis, in which facilitation and inhibition play a basic role. From an evidence-based point of view there is no doubt about the benefits of physiotherapy (see above) but there have not been sufficient data available to identify one of these special concepts as superior. The Bobath method is the leading approach in many central European countries, whereas in northern America and Scandinavia the Brunnstrom method is more common.

The Bobath concept was developed from the 1940s on by the physical therapist Berta Bobath and the physician Dr Karel Bobath, who also supplied the neurophysiological background to their concept. Basically the Bobath concept involves "24 h management" in which first of all the patient's basal and everyday needs are targets of the therapeutic and nursing management. The concept of neuronal reorganization aims at preventing the development of pathological movements by recognizing variations of "normal central postural control mechanism" regulations. The evaluation according to Bobath includes assessments of tonus, reciprocal inhibition and movement patterns. The treatment itself uses several stimuli, including positioning, tactile control, single movement elements and others. As knowledge of neurophysiology has changed, it is no surprise that some of the former explanations may sound outdated from a modern point of view. But several modern principles of plasticity and learning can be identified in the concept, e.g. repetition, task specificity, goal orientation, avoidance of "learned non-use" and forced-use therapy. In addition the concept has

developed, and changes in several aspects of its practical implementation have occurred.

The Brunnstrom approach is based on a concept developed by the Swedish physical therapist Signe Brunnstrom. It also uses facilitation techniques but, in contrast to the Bobath concept, in spastic hemiparesis synergetic patterns are regarded as early adaptations which are eventually transitioned by therapy into voluntary activation of movements.

> The Bobath concept includes assessments of tonus, reciprocal inhibition and movement patterns. The treatment itself uses several stimuli, including positioning, tactile control, single movement elements and others. In comparative studies, no advantage has been found for one technique over the other, including the Bobath, Brunnstrom and other techniques.

Rehabilitation of speech disorders

Aphasia with its affection of different modalities, including speech, comprehension, reading, and writing, is a common consequence of stroke, mainly of the left hemisphere. Because of its enormous impact on patients' lives rehabilitative therapy is mandatory and uses principles such as forced-use for treatment concepts [85]. Even more than in other therapeutic modalities, the importance of a high treatment intensity has been demonstrated: a meta-analysis [86] shows that studies which demonstrated a significant treatment effect of speech therapy on average provided 8.8 hours of therapy per week for about 11 weeks. In contrast, the negative studies only provided an average of 2 hours per week for about 23 weeks. Furthermore the total number of hours of aphasia therapy applied were directly linked to outcome, as measured by the Token Test, for example.

Rehabilitation of aphasia needs to be intense and newer studies correct the former uncertainty regarding the effectiveness of aphasia therapy. In the acute stage intense daily therapies are recommended. While spontaneous recovery can also be expected to some extent within the first year, only a minimal effect size is reported after 1 year post-onset [85]. Therefore there is a need for therapy in chronic aphasia and an appeal for episodic concentration of therapies has been made, as positive effects were found after intensive (3 hours/day) short-term (10 consecutive days) intervention using communication language games in a group-therapy setting [87]. These intensive therapies of several hours daily demand high cognitive functioning of treatable stroke patients [88]. For transfer of results from the therapeutic situation into the patients' environments there is also an indication for lower-frequency therapies of long duration.

The effect of aphasia therapy was also demonstrated using functional imaging such as PET [89]. From functional imaging it is known that clinical aphasia syndromes in practice are not strictly linked to anatomical regions and furthermore, with these methods, the courses of recovery and less successful progress can be revealed [90, 91], showing that successful regeneration from post-stroke aphasia depends more on the integration of available language-related brain regions than on recruiting new brain regions. Using PET and rTMS interference, restoration (for the right-handed patient) of the left hemisphere network seems to be more effective, although in some cases right hemisphere areas are integrated successfully.

Several studies examined the additional benefit from brain stimulation techniques [92] and medication on recovery from aphasia with positive results. However, it is premature to deduce a recommendation for clinical routine, as for aphasic patients there is currently no evidence that these task-specific improvements are persistent or have any impact on real-life communication abilities [93].

Dysarthria is an impairment of speech intelligibility, which in about half of cases is due to lacunar syndrome [94]. Extracerebellar infarcts causing dysarthria were located in all patients along the course of the pyramidal tract. At follow-up evaluation of 38 patients, 40% were judged to have normal speech, 23 patients had mild residual dysarthria, and only seven suffered from ongoing severe speech disturbances, underlining the rather good prognosis under standard rehabilitation.

> Rehabilitation of aphasia needs to be intense and newer studies support the efficacy of speech therapy.

Special topics
Dysphagia

Dysphagia is a potentially life-threatening complication of many neurological disorders, and stroke is the most common cause of neurogenic swallowing disorder.

The main dangers are:

- incidence of bolus, leading to acute blockage of airways;
- pneumonia due to aspiration;
- dysphagia can also lead to malnutrition.

On the other hand swallowing and food intake are important for the quality of life and autonomy of patients and will for many patients be considered an important goal of rehabilitation, according to the ICF (The International Classification of Functioning, Disability and Health; WHO 2001).

Dysphagia occurs in the acute state of stroke in more than 50% of patients, probably leading to aspiration in more than about 20% of them. In a meta-analysis of more than 15 studies using techniques such as fiberoptic endoscopic examination of swallowing (FEES) a wide variety of dysphagia rates between 30% and 78% [95, 96] was identified. The rate of pneumonia in stroke is at least twice as high in dysphagic patients: in a meta-analysis nine trials were identified with a rate of pneumonia in patients identified as dysphagic ranging from 7% to 68%, with the highest number reflecting patients with proven aspiration [97]. In a study focusing on cause-specific mortality after first cerebral infarction of more than 440 patients in the first month after stroke, mortality resulted predominantly from neurological complications. Afterwards mortality remained high because of respiratory and cardiovascular factors, but mainly because of pneumonia [98]. It is therefore encouraging that the detection of dysphagia was found to be highly associated with preventing pneumonia, when appropriate treatment by the clinician can be initiated, using, for example, variations in food consistency and fluid viscosity or implementation of swallowing techniques [99, 100]. The rate of detection, however, varies depending on the examination method and is highest for instrumental testing, which surpasses clinical testing protocols [96].

Neurogenic swallowing disorders are common in the course of stroke due to widespread involvement of different brain areas, including cortical (mainly sensory and motor cortex, premotor cortex) and brainstem areas, e.g. nuclei of caudal cranial nerves and "central pattern generators" within the medulla oblongata.

Evaluation of swallowing functions includes *clinical evaluation*, consisting of:

- *clinical neurological examination* with emphasis on bulbar symptoms, dysarthria, disturbed sensation and reflexes of the oropharynx;
- noting the most important *warning signs*: (a) gurgling voice, (b) bubbling respiration, (c) history of recurrent respiratory infections, (d) coughing, especially while/after eating or drinking;
- performing *clinical bedside tests:* various tests exist, such as the 50 ml water test with successive ingestion of 5 ml clear and clean water portions in ascending volume (which can be combined with oximetry) with monitoring of warning.

Particularly if technical evaluation is not performed, offering food should begin with simple consistencies. A more structured, elaborated and easy-to-use bedside test, the Gugging Swallowing Screen (GUSS) [100], allows a graded rating with separate evaluations for nonfluid and fluid nutrition, starting with nonfluids, and assesses the severity of aspiration risk and recommends a special diet accordingly.

If a stroke patient presents with warning signs and/or has failed a bedside test at least three main targets should be considered:

- *avoiding aspiration*: mandatorily discontinue oral food/fluid intake until a detailed treatment plan is set up;
- *nutrition*: choose an alternative pathway, e.g. nasogastric tube (up to 4 weeks) or in many cases percutaneous endoscopic gastrostomy;
- *quality of life, regaining autonomy*: continuing diagnosis and description of the swallowing problems *previous* to individual therapy, which in most cases will include technical evaluation (adapted from Prosiegel et al. [101]).

The rate of detection of dysphagia is higher with *technical evaluation*, which furthermore allows determination of the degree of swallowing disorder and checking of, for example, the appropriateness of compensatory maneuvers and adaptation of food/fluid consistency. The methods predominantly used are:

- *Fiberoptic endoscopic examination of swallowing (FEES)* [102]: the value of laryngoscopy has become appreciated for its direct view of the larynx, its ability to identify salient findings, and its value in guiding treatment, and therefore FEES has

become a standard procedure. At the onset of the swallow the pharyngeal air space is obliterated by tissue contacting other tissue and the bolus passing through, resulting in a so-called "swallow whiteout" without direct vision. However, when the swallow is over, its success or failure can be judged by the residue of colored test food and fluids [103]. FEES has only limited ability to assess the upper esophageal sphincter (UES) and its dysfunctioning.

- *Videofluoroscopic swallowing study (VFSS):* the stroke patient must be able to sit in front of a fluoroscope. First anatomical structures and landmarks are identified at rest without contrast. Then radiopaque material (usually barium) mixed with liquid and food of varying consistencies is administered [104].

The main *pathological findings* of the technical examinations include:

- leaking/pooling: fluids/food reach the pharynx in an uncontrolled way;
- penetration: fluids/food are reaching the aditus laryngis prematurely, above the vocal cords;
- retention: fluids/food remain in the hypopharynx after swallowing, e.g. in the sinus piriformis (carrying the risk of later aspiration);
- aspiration, including silent aspiration: fluids/food pass the vocal cords. It is especially dangerous if coughing or other cleaning procedures are not promptly initiated. To rate the findings of such examinations the Rosenbek penetration–aspiration scale is established (Figure 20.4) [105].

After defining the individual problems of swallowing dysfunction, an adequate treatment schedule can be set up, including several *therapeutic compensatory interventions*, for example:

- modify bolus volume, consistency, viscosity;
- change method of food/liquid delivery;
- modify sequence of delivery;
- change rate of food/liquid delivery;
- alter behavior (e.g. dry/clearing swallows, postural changes);

and *rehabilitative* techniques which include:

- swallow maneuvers (supraglottic swallow, effortful swallow);
- exercises (to increase strength of muscle groups);
- sensory stimulation techniques (thermal-tactile stimulation and others) [103].

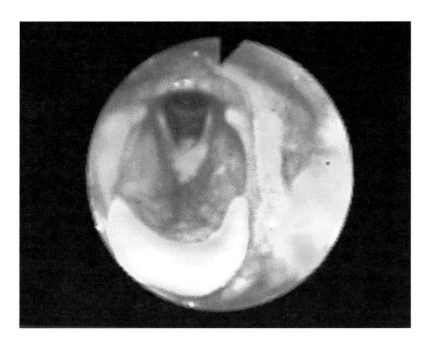

Figure 20.4. Fiberoptic endoscopic examination of swallowing (FEES). Findings from an 18-year-old female (cerebral venous sinus thrombosis) with tracheostomy showing severe dysphagia with penetration, residuals, and "silent" aspiration (patient shows no coughing at any time). Later withdrawal of the cannula after laryngopharyngeal sensory training (aeration with fenestrated cannula and a valve) was successful.

Dysphagia is a common and dangerous problem after stroke and can be detected by clinical assessment and technical evaluation (fiberoptic endoscopy or videofluoroscopy). It must be treated by modification of the ingested substances and rehabilitative techniques.

Tracheostomy

Patients admitted with tracheostomy often also need intense dysphagia management. Endoscopic evaluation of the cannula should be performed, looking for the correct distal position (to avoid lesions of the trachea by chronic pressure) and, if a model with fenestration is used, checking the fenestration (which is often closed by material or granuloma, or the fenestration of the cannula might not be suitable anatomically for the individual patient). Basically when withdrawal from the cannula is formulated as a goal because a patient with tracheostomy improves as regards dysphagia, level of consciousness and/or pulmonary function, one should try to increase the duration of episodes with aeration of the larynx and pharynx in order to diminish sensory loss of the mucosa and to increase swallowing function. This can be achieved by using a cannula with fenestration and/or deblockage of the cannula and a valve. Respiration and swallowing function must be controlled

carefully. If long-term tracheostomy is needed, percutaneous tracheotomy should be avoided because of the high rate of long-term complications, with high rates of bleeding, granulomas, pain and other problems such as the often difficult exchange by caregivers [101, 106].

Treatment of spasticity

The treatment of spasticity requires mainly physiotherapy, nursing care, occupational therapy and in many cases orthotic management. Whereas spasticity as a consequence of a stroke might in many cases also have a certain beneficial compensatory aspect, it can also lead to increased disability, loss of function, pain, and hindered care, and also carries the risk of secondary complications. If physical treatment reaches a limit, in generalized symptoms of spasticity one might want to consider the option of oral agents and intrathecal baclofen, but orally given medication such as baclofen in cortical or subcortical stroke has a disappointing effect vs. side-effect ratio in most cases. In focal or sometimes multifocal spasticity, *botulinum toxin* as a part of a longer-term strategy is an often successful treatment option in many cases, requiring patient assessment and definition of the goals of treatment [107]. Botulinum toxin (which exists in seven different serotypes, proteins A–G) acts on

297

cholinergic neuromuscular junctions to block transmitter release. Type A was the first botulinum toxin for medical use. Applied into the muscles by injection, a positive effect can be expected after between several days and 1 week, lasting for 3–6 months. Often one or two treatment sessions with botulinum toxin are helpful to regain therapeutic benefit from intense physical therapies. In general, botulinum toxin is considered a safe therapeutic agent [108]; however, there have been safety warnings regarding the adherence to the maximum dosage per session and time interval between injections because of case reports about exacerbation of preexisting swallowing disorders and neurological deterioration in higher-dosage applications.

Practically, the use of electromyography for application helps to improve the cost-effectiveness and the use of lower dosages. As several products of botulinum toxin A and B with different rates of effectiveness per unit are available, documentation of the product used is indispensable.

If multimodal treatment of spasticity (maybe also considering serial casting) fails, surgical therapy in some cases may finally be a therapeutic option.

In the event of an increase in spasticity in the course of treatment, symptomatic factors such as infections, bladder dysfunctioning, fractures, thrombosis and many others should be considered.

> Spasticity can be treated with physiotherapy, nursing care and occupational therapy. If physical treatment comes to a limit, oral agents, intrathecal baclofen and botulinum toxin are treatment options.

Cognitive recovery after stroke

Besides defined neuropsychological syndromes, cognitive impairment after a stroke is very common and may persist in the postacute and also the chronic phase. Individual assessment includes evaluation of several aspects of attention, intelligence, memory, executive functions and personality prior to devising an individual treatment schedule, which can be neuropsychologically specific but should also be interdisciplinary, as the impairment usually has an impact on several aspects of the rehabilitation progress and the ability to cope with the activities of daily living. Depending on treatment goals, a more practical evaluation including out-of-hospital observations can also be useful. For detailed guidelines on cognitive rehabilitation refer to Cappa et al. [109].

Restoration or preservation of cognition is an important and increasingly recognized field in stroke rehabilitation. Impairment of attention, memory, and other domains has to be considered when setting up treatment goals.

Spatial neglect

Spatial neglect is a common syndrome following stroke, most frequently of the right hemisphere, predominantly but not exclusively of the parietal lobe. It is a complex deficit in attention and awareness which can affect extrapersonal space and/or personal perception. Elements of spatial neglect may also be seen with infarctions of the left hemisphere; however, symptoms are clinically less consistent than in right hemispheric neglect [110].

The therapeutic process is often prolonged. In multidisciplinary neurorehabilitation, perception via the affected side is enforced as much as possible, and additional alertness training as well as visual, proprioceptive and vestibular stimulation techniques are used [111, 112]. In addition to focal disturbances, in this condition a hemispheric imbalance may be of clinical relevance. Only a few pilot studies have been published to evaluate the benefit of cortical stimulation techniques, e.g. Shindo et al. [113] used inhibitory low-frequency rTMS over the unaffected posterior parietal cortex for six sessions over 2 weeks in a small pilot study, resulting in decreased unilateral spatial neglect for at least 6 weeks. Several rTMS-workgroups, however, have already reported successfully provoking a "model neglect" in healthy subjects [114], which might be useful in further research.

> Spatial neglect is a frequent syndrome of right hemispheric stroke and needs active and prolonged attention in the rehabilitation process.

Other neuropsychological syndromes

Hemianopia has a large impact on daily activities which appears in problems in reading, orientation and safety in traffic. Basic rehabilitative management includes stimulation from the hemianopic side (e.g. positioning of the bed, talking). While spontaneous recovery might occur at least up to several months, treatment options such as visual field training are controversial. Using compensatory visual field training compared to a control group no formal change of visual defect was reported by Nelles et al.

[115], although the training improved detection of and reaction to visual stimuli. Other groups recently reported an improvement of the visual field of up to 5° for ischemic lesions and up to 10° benefit for stroke after a hemorrhage, using reaction perimetry treatment [116].

Space perception disorders can lead to spatial disorientation (affecting a person's topographical orientation), well known in right-hemisphere infarction. A misperception of the body's orientation in the coronal plane is seen in stroke patients with a "pusher syndrome". They experience their body as oriented upright when it is in fact tilted to one side, and therefore use the unaffected arm or leg to actively push away from the unparalyzed side and typically try to resist any attempt to passively correct their body posture. The syndrome is a distinctive clinical disorder after unilateral left or right brain lesions in the posterior thalamus or in the insula and postcentral gyrus [117]. The recovery under physical therapy, by trying to enhance sensorimotor input from the contralateral side, is often prolonged.

Apraxia is a syndrome of left-hemisphere infarction. It often severely hinders ADL independence (apart from contributing to speech disorders as speech apraxia) and treatment of apraxia should definitely be part of the overall neurorehabilitation program [109]. Although the literature on recovery and treatment is limited, apraxia has been shown to be improved by occupational therapy. For a review of apraxia treatment and also on other aspects of occupational therapy refer to Steultjens et al. [118].

> Hemianopia, visual perception deficits, and apraxia are frequent and disabling. They deserve active screening and should be considered in goal-setting.

Rehabilitation of brainstem syndromes

The locked-in syndrome (LiS) typically originates from a ventro-pontine lesion, resulting in a complete quadriplegia and anarthria without coma (in stroke caused by basilar artery occlusion or brainstem hemorrhage). In most cases communication remains possible (by simple or elaborate speech coding), using spared vertical eye movements or blinking. For the clinician it is important to know this syndrome and to make an early diagnosis. The levels of cognitive function in cases of pure brainstem lesions are normal in many cases, while additional brain injuries are most likely responsible for associated cognitive deficits in LiS [119]. Patients should receive early and intensive multidisciplinary rehabilitation with the goal of establishing communication, with evaluation of the use of patient–computer interfaces such as infrared eye-movement detectors and others. In the first treatment episode the prognosis is undetermined, as a small proportion of patients to some extent develop motor recovery [120]. According to the authors, in spite of severe disability most of these patients do not want to die.

> The locked-in syndrome – quadriplegia and anarthria without coma – is usually caused by basilar artery occlusion and represents a challenge to rehabilitation teams.

Like in other brainstem syndromes, pathological crying can also occur in locked-in syndrome (SSRI medication should be evaluated; see Table 20.1).

Brainstem lesions should be carefully evaluated for dysphagia. Individual assessment is necessary in severe brainstem syndromes with vegetative state or minimally conscious state.

Other common problems

Bladder dysfunction: urine incontinence occurs frequently in the acute state of stroke and after 1 year 20% of survivors suffer from it. The patient should be investigated for residual urine by ultrasound or intermittent catheterization, and infection should be ruled out. Disorders of storage can be treated by bladder retraining and pelvic floor exercises. In storage problems provoked by detrusor spasticity, which can occur with or without urethral sphincter dysfunction, treatment with anticholinergic drugs such as oxybutynin should be evaluated (see Table 20.1).

Pain in the post-stroke episode may be due to different causes, e.g. associated with spasticity (see above) or related to a central post-stroke syndrome. Mostly affections of the brainstem, thalamic structures or spinal stroke contribute to this problem. This specific pain can be episodic but more often is constant. Treatment options include physiotherapy, and medication (see Table 20.1) such as antidepressants, anticonvulsants and opioid analgetics. Because of the chronic course, psychological support to improve coping may be necessary.

Hemiplegic shoulder (arm) pain has multiple causes. The shoulder joint in hemiplegia is sensitive to traumatization of various structures and inferior subluxation can lead to injuries, including tendons, capsule or peripheral nerves and plexus. It is important to keep the shoulder correctly positioned to prevent subluxation by orthotic management. Hemiplegic shoulder pain in stroke may be due to adhesive capsulitis (50%), shoulder subluxation (44%), rotator cuff tears (22%), and shoulder-hand syndrome (16%) [121]. The etiology of shoulder-hand syndrome with pain of the shoulder or arm and edema of the hand and arm is controversial; many authors consider it a form of reflex sympathetic dystrophy/complex regional pain syndrome, probably initiated by mechanisms mentioned above. Management includes positioning, orthotic management, physical therapy including steps for reduction of edema, and analgetics. In more severe cases intermediate dosage treatment with oral prednisone is effective [122].

Depression: post-stroke depression (PDS) occurs in at least one-third of patients in the first year after onset, although estimates differ widely between studies due to varying definitions, populations, exclusion criteria and the timing of assessments [123]. PDS often hinders the course of rehabilitation and influences recovery and outcome following stroke. It is often underdiagnosed because of overlapping symptoms with the stroke itself. It manifests itself in subtle signs, such as refusal to participate in treatments. Antidepressive treatment with SSRI and related substances (see Table 20.1) is the first treatment choice; in addition studies suggest adaptations of cognitive-behavioral therapy techniques and brief supportive therapy to be beneficial [3]. In a Cochrane review, however, there was no evidence for improvements of PDS by medication. The authors [123] indicate that the heterogeneity of the studies and problematic patient selection, with exclusion of certain neurological deficits such as aphasia, might have led to the result.

Driving after stroke: in a study investigating relative crash risk associated with medical conditions ($n = 4448$) the diagnosis "previous stroke" was only a nearly significant risk [124]. There is no doubt that driving ability in the post-stroke period needs assessment, and a study [125] shows that patients are in danger of making inappropriate decisions about their driving capabilities without professional advice and/or evaluation. As a first step there are certain medical and neurological conditions where clinical judgement will confirm stroke patients as being incapable of driving, e.g. persistent complete hemianopia, neglect and relevant cognitive impairment, whereas pure motor deficits can often be solved by car adaptation.

The extent of further evaluation ranges from screening tests, specific neuropsychological assessments and simulator tests to full road tests. If a post-stroke patient is evaluated as not capable of driving, a reassessment in the further course of rehabilitation with appropriate therapies can be a goal. It has also been shown that simulator-based driving training improved driving ability, especially for well-educated and less disabled stroke patients [126].

Partnership and sexual functioning: partnership is in many cases affected by the post-stroke condition, owing to altered physical and psychological conditions with their implications for everyday life and communication. Couple psychotherapy can be initiated and also improvements to assistance in the various fields can indirectly help relieve the often serious problems. Summarized in a review [127], observational studies suggest that the frequency and range of sexual disorders after stroke are high and a noticeable decline in sexuality occurs in both genders after stroke; furthermore partner dissatisfaction is high. In addition to the direct consequences of stroke, psychosocial issues and depression are likely to contribute to the problem. Pre-existing vascular disorders may also cause erectile difficulties as well as antihypertensive agents and other drugs. As the problems are often complex, treatment suggestions have to be comprehensive. Erectile dysfunctioning can be treated with phosphodiesterase type 5 inhibitors or intracavernosal prostaglandin E-1 injections.

Hypersexuality rarely occurs, and is treatable with behavioral therapy, SSRI and antiandrogens.

Social problems after stroke can severely affect various aspects of patients' lives, such as unemployment, invalidity, financial problems, problems with health insurance, difficulties with housing, family issues, social contacts and other factors. Social counseling is therefore mandatory in the course of stroke rehabilitation, which includes, for example, information about social security systems, social services, self-help and stroke groups.

Acknowledgement

The authors would like to thank Serafin Beer for helpful discussion and comments on the manuscript.

Chapter Summary

Neuroplasticity is the dynamic potential of the brain to reorganize itself during ontogeny and learning, or following damage. The central nervous system of the adult human being has an astounding potential for regeneration and adaptability, which can be selectively supported and used for rehabilitation.

Several mechanisms of neuronal plasticity can be identified:

- *Vicariation* describes the hypothesis that functions of damaged areas can be taken over by different regions of the brain.
- *Plasticity of areas of cortical representation*: damage to the brain leads to an increased recruitment of secondary areas of representation as early compensation, followed by a later phase of reorganization.
- *Sprouting of neurons* as in the peripheral nervous system. In the central nervous system of the adult, however, this mechanism is reduced, but not absent.
- *Diaschisis* describes the phenomenon that a focal lesion may also lead to changes in brain functioning of areas located far away.

Neuroplasticity can be supported by:

- A multidisciplinary team in a structured setting. Treatment in a stroke unit has been shown to improve the outcome significantly (number needed to treat 7 for thrombolysis versus 9 for stroke unit treatment). In this setting input from a team of medical, nursing and therapy staff, optimal timing and early initiation (i.e. within 7 days) of intensive rehabilitation, and the definition of treatment goals following physical and psychological status evaluation, are beneficial.
- Special training, such as treadmill training, constraint-induced therapy (CIT: the unaffected limb is constrained to enforce the use of the affected limb under intensive practice), repetitive training or mirror therapy.
- Peripheral and brain stimulation techniques: repetitive transcranial magnetic stimulation (rTMS) leads to decreased or increased cortical excitability, depending on the frequency. It can be used for downregulation of the contralesional or stimulation of the ipsilesional hemisphere. With transcranial direct current stimulation (TDCS), a weak polarizing electrical current is delivered to the cortex.
- Pharmacological interventions: in preliminary studies, some medications such as levodopa and others were found to be beneficial for motor recovery, while others, e.g. benzodiazepines, had a negative effect on outcome.

Speech disorders need intense training because of their enormous impact on the patient's life. Newer studies with therapies taking place daily for several hours correct the former uncertainty regarding the effectiveness of aphasia therapy. Brain stimulation techniques and medication might add additional benefit.

Dysphagia occurs in the acute state of stroke in more than 50% of patients, probably leading to aspiration in more than about 20% of them. To detect dysphagia, clinical evaluation can be combined with technical tests such as fiberoptic endoscopic examination of swallowing (FEES) and videofluoroscopic swallowing studies (VFSS). After defining the individual problems in swallowing dysfunction, adequate therapeutic compensatory interventions, for example modification of bolus volume and viscosity, and rehabilitative techniques, such as exercise or sensory stimulation, can be set up. Patients admitted with tracheostomy often also need intense dysphagia management.

Spasticity can be treated with physiotherapy, nursing care and occupational therapy. If physical treatment reaches a limit, oral agents, intrathecal baclofen and botulinum toxin are treatment options.

For the treatment of **spatial neglect**, perception via the affected side is enforced as much as possible and additional alertness training as well as visual and proprioceptive stimulation techniques are used. Only a few pilot studies have been published to evaluate the benefit of cortical stimulation techniques (e.g. inhibitory low-frequency rTMS).

References

1. Beer S, Clarke S, Diserens K, Engelter S, Müri R, Schnider A, et al. Neurorehabilitation nach Hirnschlag. *Schweiz Med Forum* 2007; **7**:294–7.

2. Warlow C, Sudlow C, Dennis M, Wardlaw J, Sandercock P. Stroke. *Lancet* 2003; **362**(9391):1211–24.

3. Duncan PW, Zorowitz R, Bates B, Choi JY, Glasberg JJ, Graham GD, et al. Management of Adult Stroke Rehabilitation Care: a clinical practice guideline. *Stroke* 2005; **36**(9):e100–43.

4. Cajal R. *Degeneration and Regeneration of The Nervous System*. London: Oxford University Press; 1928.

5. Foerster O. Übungstherapie In *Handbuch der Neurologie*, Vol. 8. Berlin: Julius Springer; 1936.

6. Kesselring J. Neurorehabilitation: a bridge between basic science and clinical practice. *Eur J Neurol* 2001; **8**(3):221–5.

7. Nelles G. Neuronale Plastizität. In Nelles G, ed. *Neurologische Rehabilitation*. Stuttgart: Thieme; 2004:1–13.

8. Hebb DO. *The Organisation of Behavior: a neuropsychological approach*. New York: Wiley; 1949.

9. Duffau H. Brain plasticity: from pathophysiological mechanisms to therapeutic applications. *J Clin Neurosci* 2006; **13**(9):885–97.

10. Nudo RJ. Mechanisms for recovery of motor function following cortical damage. *Curr Opin Neurobiol* 2006; **16**(6):638–44.

11. Ward NS. Future perspectives in functional neuroimaging in stroke recovery. *Eura Medicophys* 2007; **43**(2):285–94.

12. Nudo RJ, Milliken GW. Reorganization of movement representations in primary motor cortex following focal ischemic infarcts in adult squirrel monkeys. *J Neurophysiol* 1996; **75**(5):2144–9.

13. Nudo RJ, Milliken GW, Jenkins WM, Merzenich MM. Use-dependent alterations of movement representations in primary motor cortex of adult squirrel monkeys. *J Neurosci* 1996; **16**(2):785–807.

14. Liepert J, Graef S, Uhde I, Leidner O, Weiller C. Training-induced changes of motor cortex representations in stroke patients. *Acta Neurol Scand* 2000; **101**(5):321–6.

15. Jaillard A, Martin CD, Garambois K, Lebas JF, Hommel M. Vicarious function within the human primary motor cortex? A longitudinal fMRI stroke study. *Brain* 2005; **128**(Pt 5):1122–38.

16. Ward NS, Cohen LG. Mechanisms underlying recovery of motor function after stroke. *Arch Neurol* 2004; **61**(12):1844–8.

17. Ward NS, Brown MM, Thompson AJ, Frackowiak RS. Neural correlates of motor recovery after stroke: a longitudinal fMRI study. *Brain* 2003; **126**(Pt 11):2476–96.

18. Calautti C, Baron JC. Functional neuroimaging studies of motor recovery after stroke in adults: a review. *Stroke* 2003; **34**(6):1553–66.

19. Ward NS, Brown MM, Thompson AJ, Frackowiak RS. Neural correlates of outcome after stroke: a cross-sectional fMRI study. *Brain* 2003; **126**(Pt 6):1430–48.

20. Biernaskie J, Chernenko G, Corbett D. Efficacy of rehabilitative experience declines with time after focal ischemic brain injury. *J Neurosci* 2004; **24**(5):1245–54.

21. Griesbach GS, Hovda DA, Molteni R, Wu A, Gomez-Pinilla F. Voluntary exercise following traumatic brain injury: brain-derived neurotrophic factor upregulation and recovery of function. *Neuroscience* 2004; **125**(1):129–39.

22. Wall PD, Egger MD. Formation of new connexions in adult rat brains after partial deafferentation. *Nature* 1971; **232**(5312):542–5.

23. Witte OW. Lesion-induced plasticity as a potential mechanism for recovery and rehabilitative training. *Curr Opin Neurol* 1998; **11**(6):655–62.

24. Johansson BB, Ohlsson AL. Environment, social interaction, and physical activity as determinants of functional outcome after cerebral infarction in the rat. *Exp Neurol* 1996; **139**(2):322–7.

25. Huang YZ, Edwards MJ, Rounis E, Bhatia KP, Rothwell JC. Theta burst stimulation of the human motor cortex. *Neuron* 2005; **45**(2):201–6.

26. Harris-Love ML, Cohen LG. Noninvasive cortical stimulation in neurorehabilitation: a review. *Arch Phys Med Rehabil* 2006; **87**(12 Suppl 2):S84–93.

27. Talelli P, Cheeran BJ, Teo JT, Rothwell JC. Pattern-specific role of the current orientation used to deliver theta burst stimulation. *Clin Neurophysiol* 2007; **118**(8):1815–23.

28. Floel A, Nagorsen U, Werhahn KJ, Ravindran S, Birbaumer N, Knecht S, et al. Influence of somatosensory input on motor function in patients with chronic stroke. *Ann Neurol* 2004; **56**(2):206–12.

29. Alon G, Levitt AF, McCarthy PA. Functional electrical stimulation (FES) may modify the poor prognosis of stroke survivors with severe motor loss of the upper extremity: a preliminary study. *Am J Phys Med Rehabil* 2008; **87**(8):627–36.

30. Alon G, Levitt AF, McCarthy PA. Functional electrical stimulation enhancement of upper extremity functional recovery during stroke rehabilitation: a pilot study. *Neurorehabil Neural Repair* 2007; **21**(3):207–15.

31. Ziemann U, Meintzschel F, Korchounov A, Ilic TV. Pharmacological modulation of plasticity in the human motor cortex. *Neurorehabil Neural Repair* 2006; **20**(2):243–51.

32. Langhorne P, Duncan P. Does the organization of postacute stroke care really matter? *Stroke* 2001; **32**(1):268–74.

33. Bernhardt J, Dewey H, Thrift A, Donnan G. Inactive and alone: physical activity within the first 14 days of acute stroke unit care. *Stroke* 2004; **35**(4):1005–9.

34. Kesselring J. Neuroscience and clinical practice: a personal postscript. *Brain Res Brain Res Rev* 2001; **36**(2–3):285–6.

35. Kesselring J, Coenen M, Cieza A, Thompson A, Kostanjsek N, Stucki G. Developing the ICF Core Sets for multiple sclerosis to specify functioning. *Mult Scler* 2008; **14**(2):252–4.

36. Mauritz KH. Rehabilitation von neurologischen Erkrankungen: Schlaganfall. In Nelles G, ed. *Neurologische Rehabilitation*. Stuttgart: Thieme; 2004: 204–17.

37. DeBow SB, McKenna JE, Kolb B, Colbourne F. Immediate constraint-induced movement therapy causes local hyperthermia that exacerbates cerebral cortical injury in rats. *Can J Physiol Pharmacol* 2004; **82**(4):231–7.

38. Humm JL, Kozlowski DA, James DC, Gotts JE, Schallert T. Use-dependent exacerbation of brain damage occurs during an early post-lesion vulnerable period. *Brain Res* 1998; **783**(2):286–92.

39. Kozlowski DA, James DC, Schallert T. Use-dependent exaggeration of neuronal injury after unilateral sensorimotor cortex lesions. *J Neurosci* 1996; **16**(15):4776–86.

40. Risedal A, Zeng J, Johansson BB. Early training may exacerbate brain damage after focal brain ischemia in the rat. *J Cereb Blood Flow Metab* 1999; **19**(9):997–1003.

41. Schallert T, Fleming SM, Leasure JL, Tillerson JL, Bland ST. CNS plasticity and assessment of forelimb sensorimotor outcome in unilateral rat models of stroke, cortical ablation, parkinsonism and spinal cord injury. *Neuropharmacology* 2000; **39**(5):777–87.

42. Barbay S, Plautz EJ, Friel KM, Frost SB, Dancause N, Stowe AM, et al. Behavioral and neurophysiological effects of delayed training following a small ischemic infarct in primary motor cortex of squirrel monkeys. *Exp Brain Res* 2006; **169**:106–16.

43. Marin R, Williams A, Hale S, Burge B, Mense M, Bauman R, et al. The effect of voluntary exercise exposure on histological and neurobehavioral outcomes after ischemic brain injury in the rat. *Physiol Behav* 2003; **80**(2–3):167–75.

44. Indredavik B, Bakke F, Slordahl SA, Rokseth R, Haheim LL. Treatment in a combined acute and rehabilitation stroke unit: which aspects are most important? *Stroke* 1999; **30**(5):917–23.

45. Musicco M, Emberti L, Nappi G, Caltagirone C. Early and long-term outcome of rehabilitation in stroke patients: the role of patient characteristics, time of initiation, and duration of interventions. *Arch Phys Med Rehabil* 2003; **84**(4):551–8.

46. Maulden SA, Gassaway J, Horn SD, Smout RJ, DeJong G. Timing of initiation of rehabilitation after stroke. *Arch Phys Med Rehabil* 2005; **86**(12 Suppl 2): S34–S40.

47. Jette DU, Warren RL, Wirtalla C. The relation between therapy intensity and outcomes of rehabilitation in skilled nursing facilities. *Arch Phys Med Rehabil* 2005; **86**(3):373–9.

48. Graham A. Measurement in stroke: activity and quality of life. In Barnes M, Dobkin B, Bougousslavsky J, eds. *Recovery after Stroke*. Cambridge University Press; 2005: 135–60.

49. Collen FM, Wade DT, Robb GF, Bradshaw CM. The Rivermead Mobility Index: a further development of the Rivermead Motor Assessment. *Int Disabil Stud* 1991; **13**(2):50–4.

50. Lennon S, Johnson L. The modified Rivermead mobility index: validity and reliability. *Disabil Rehabil* 2000; **22**(18):833–9.

51. Carr JH, Shepherd RB, Nordholm L, Lynne D. Investigation of a new motor assessment scale for stroke patients. *Phys Ther* 1985; **65**(2):175–80.

52. Loewen SC, Anderson BA. Reliability of the Modified Motor Assessment Scale and the Barthel Index. *Phys Ther* 1988; **68**(7):1077–81.

53. Mathias S, Nayak US, Isaacs B. Balance in elderly patients: the "get-up and go" test. *Arch Phys Med Rehabil* 1986; **67**(6):387–89.

54. Lyle RC. A performance test for assessment of upper limb function in physical rehabilitation treatment and research. *Int J Rehabil Res* 1981; **4**(4):483–92.

55. Mathiowetz V, Kashman N, Volland G, Weber K, Dowe M, Rogers S. Grip and pinch strength: normative data for adults. *Arch Phys Med Rehabil* 1985; **66**(2):69–74.

56. Mahoney FI, Barthel DW. Functional evaluation: the Barthel Index. *Md State Med J* 1965; **14**:61–5.

57. McDowell I, Newell C. *Measuring Health: A Guide to Rating Scales and Questionnaires*. Oxford University Press; 1996.

58. Duncan PW, Wallace D, Lai SM, Johnson D, Embretson S, Laster LJ. The stroke impact scale version 2.0. Evaluation of reliability, validity, and sensitivity to change. *Stroke* 1999; **30**(10):2131–40.

59. da Cunha IT Jr, Lim PA, Qureshy H, Henson H, Monga T, Protas EJ. Gait outcomes after acute stroke rehabilitation with supported treadmill ambulation training: a randomized controlled pilot study. *Arch Phys Med Rehabil* 2002; **83**(9):1258–65.

60. Kosak MC, Reding MJ. Comparison of partial body weight-supported treadmill gait training versus aggressive bracing assisted walking post stroke. *Neurorehabil Neural Repair* 2000; **14**(1):13–19.

61. Nilsson L, Carlsson J, Danielsson A, Fugl-Meyer A, Hellstrom K, Kristensen L, et al. Walking training of

patients with hemiparesis at an early stage after stroke: a comparison of walking training on a treadmill with body weight support and walking training on the ground. *Clin Rehabil* 2001; **15**(5):515–27.

62. Sullivan KJ, Knowlton BJ, Dobkin BH. Step training with body weight support: effect of treadmill speed and practice paradigms on poststroke locomotor recovery. *Arch Phys Med Rehabil* 2002; **83**(5):683–91.

63. Visintin M, Barbeau H, Korner-Bitensky N, Mayo NE. A new approach to retrain gait in stroke patients through body weight support and treadmill stimulation. *Stroke* 1998; **29**(6):1122–8.

64. Wood-Dauphinee S, Kwakkel G. The impact of rehabilitation on stroke outcomes: what is the evidence. In Barnes M, Dobkin B, Bougousslavsky J, eds. *Recovery after Stroke*. Cambridge University Press; 2005:162–88.

65. Beer S, Aschbacher B, Manoglou D, Gamper E, Kool J, Kesselring J. Robot-assisted gait training in multiple sclerosis: a pilot randomized trial. *Mult Scler* 2008; **14**(2):231–6.

66. Liston R, Mickelborough J, Harris B, Hann AW, Tallis RC. Conventional physiotherapy and treadmill re-training for higher-level gait disorders in cerebrovascular disease. *Age Ageing* 2000; **29**(4):311–18.

67. Laufer Y, Dickstein R, Chefez Y, Marcovitz E. The effect of treadmill training on the ambulation of stroke survivors in the early stages of rehabilitation: a randomized study. *J Rehabil Res Dev* 2001; **38**(1):69–78.

68. Pohl M, Mehrholz J, Ritschel C, Ruckriem S. Speed-dependent treadmill training in ambulatory hemiparetic stroke patients: a randomized controlled trial. *Stroke* 2002; **33**(2):553–8.

69. Roerdink M, Lamoth CJ, Kwakkel G, van Wieringen PC, Beek PJ. Gait coordination after stroke: benefits of acoustically paced treadmill walking. *Phys Ther* 2007; **87**(8):1009–22.

70. Mandel AR, Nymark JR, Balmer SJ, Grinnell DM, O'Riain MD. Electromyographic versus rhythmic positional biofeedback in computerized gait retraining with stroke patients. *Arch Phys Med Rehabil* 1990; **71**(9):649–54.

71. Thaut MH, McIntosh GC, Rice RR. Rhythmic facilitation of gait training in hemiparetic stroke rehabilitation. *J Neurol Sci* 1997; **151**(2):207–12.

72. Taub E, Miller NE, Novack TA, Cook EW 3rd, Fleming WC, Nepomuceno CS, et al. Technique to improve chronic motor deficit after stroke. *Arch Phys Med Rehabil* 1993; **74**(4):347–54.

73. Wolf SL, Winstein CJ, Miller JP, Taub E, Uswatte G, Morris D, et al. Effect of constraint-induced movement therapy on upper extremity function 3 to 9 months after stroke: the EXCITE randomized clinical trial. *JAMA* 2006; **296**(17):2095–104.

74. Wolf SL, Winstein CJ, Miller JP, Thompson PA, Taub E, Uswatte G, et al. Retention of upper limb function in stroke survivors who have received constraint-induced movement therapy: the EXCITE randomised trial. *Lancet Neurol* 2008; **7**(1):33–40.

75. French B, Thomas LH, Leathley MJ, Sutton CJ, McAdam J, Forster A, et al. Repetitive task training for improving functional ability after stroke. *Cochrane Database Syst Rev* 2007;(4):CD006073.

76. Wing K, Lynskey JV, Bosch PR. Whole-body intensive rehabilitation is feasible and effective in chronic stroke survivors: a retrospective data analysis. *Top Stroke Rehabil* 2008; **15**(3):247–55.

77. Courbon A, Calmels P, Roche F, Ramas J, Rimaud D, Fayolle-Minon I. Relationship between maximal exercise capacity and walking capacity in adult hemiplegic stroke patients. *Am J Phys Med Rehabil* 2006; **85**(5):436–42.

78. Chu KS, Eng JJ, Dawson AS, Harris JE, Ozkaplan A, Gylfadottir S. Water-based exercise for cardiovascular fitness in people with chronic stroke: a randomized controlled trial. *Arch Phys Med Rehabil* 2004; **85**(6):870–4.

79. Dean CM, Richards CL, Malouin F. Task-related circuit training improves performance of locomotor tasks in chronic stroke: a randomized, controlled pilot trial. *Arch Phys Med Rehabil* 2000; **81**(4):409–17.

80. Rimmer JH, Riley B, Creviston T, Nicola T. Exercise training in a predominantly African-American group of stroke survivors. *Med Sci Sports Exerc* 2000; **32**(12):1990–6.

81. Badics E, Wittmann A, Rupp M, Stabauer B, Zifko UA. Systematic muscle building exercises in the rehabilitation of stroke patients. *NeuroRehabilitation* 2002; **17**(3):211–14.

82. Yavuzer G, Selles R, Sezer N, Sutbeyaz S, Bussmann JB, Koseoglu F, et al. Mirror therapy improves hand function in subacute stroke: a randomized controlled trial. *Arch Phys Med Rehabil* 2008; **89**(3):393–8.

83. Altschuler EL, Wisdom SB, Stone L, Foster C, Galasko D, Llewellyn DM, et al. Rehabilitation of hemiparesis after stroke with a mirror. *Lancet* 1999; **353**(9169):2035–6.

84. Dohle C, Kleiser R, Seitz RJ, Freund HJ. Body scheme gates visual processing. *J Neurophysiol* 2004; **91**(5):2376–9.

85. Barthel G, Meinzer M, Djundja D, Rockstroh B. Intensive language therapy in chronic aphasia: which

aspects contribute most? *Aphasiology* 2008;
22(4):408–21.

86. Bhogal SK, Teasell R, Speechley M. Intensity of aphasia therapy, impact on recovery. *Stroke* 2003; **34**(4):987–93.

87. Meinzer M, Djundja D, Barthel G, Elbert T, Rockstroh B. Long-term stability of improved language functions in chronic aphasia after constraint-induced aphasia therapy. *Stroke* 2005; **36**(7):1462–6.

88. Breitenstein C, Kramer K, Meinzer M, Baumgartner A, Floel A, Knecht S. Intense language training for aphasia: contribution of cognitive factors. *Nervenarzt* 2009; **80**(2):149–50, 152–4.

89. Musso M, Weiller C, Kiebel S, Muller SP, Bulau P, Rijntjes M. Training-induced brain plasticity in aphasia. *Brain* 1999; **122** (Pt 9):1781–90.

90. Heiss WD, Thiel A, Kessler J, Herholz K. Disturbance and recovery of language function: correlates in PET activation studies. *Neuroimage* 2003; **20** Suppl 1:S42–9.

91. Winhuisen L, Thiel A, Schumacher B, Kessler J, Rudolf J, Haupt WF, et al. The right inferior frontal gyrus and poststroke aphasia: a follow-up investigation. *Stroke* 2007; **38**(4):1286–92.

92. Monti A, Cogiamanian F, Marceglia S, Ferrucci R, Mameli F, Mrakic-Sposta S, et al. Improved naming after transcranial direct current stimulation in aphasia. *J Neurol Neurosurg Psychiatry* 2008; **79**(4):451–3.

93. Cappa SF. Current to the brain improves word-finding difficulties in aphasic patients. *J Neurol Neurosurg Psychiatry* 2008; **79**(4):364.

94. Urban PP, Wicht S, Vukurevic G, Fitzek C, Fitzek S, Stoeter P, et al. Dysarthria in acute ischemic stroke: lesion topography, clinicoradiologic correlation, and etiology. *Neurology* 2001; **56**(8):1021–7.

95. Mann G, Hankey GJ, Cameron D. Swallowing disorders following acute stroke: prevalence and diagnostic accuracy. *Cerebrovasc Dis* 2000; **10**(5):380–6.

96. Martino R, Foley N, Bhogal S, Diamant N, Speechley M, Teasell R. Dysphagia after stroke: incidence, diagnosis, and pulmonary complications. *Stroke* 2005; **36**(12):2756–63.

97. Smithard DG, O'Neill PA, Parks C, Morris J. Complications and outcome after acute stroke. Does dysphagia matter? Stroke 1996; **27**(7):1200–4.

98. Vernino S, Brown RD, Jr., Sejvar JJ, Sicks JD, Petty GW, O'Fallon WM. Cause-specific mortality after first cerebral infarction: a population-based study. *Stroke* 2003; **34**(8):1828–32.

99. Hinchey JA, Shephard T, Furie K, Smith D, Wang D, Tonn S. Formal dysphagia screening protocols prevent pneumonia. *Stroke* 2005; **36**(9):1972–6.

100. Trapl M, Enderle P, Nowotny M, Teuschl Y, Matz K, Dachenhausen A, Brainin M. Dysphagia bedside screening for acute-stroke patients: the Gugging Swallowing Screen. *Stroke* 2007; **38**(11):2948–52.

101. Prosiegel M, Aigner F, Diesener P, Gass C, George S, Hanning C, et al. Qualitätskriterien und Standards für die Diagnostik und Therapie von Patienten mit neurologischen Schluckstörungen. Neurogene Dysphagien – Leitlinien der DGNKN. *Neurol Rehabil* 2003; **9**(3–4):157–81.

102. Langmore SE, Schatz K, Olsen N. Fiberoptic endoscopic examination of swallowing safety: a new procedure. *Dysphagia* 1988; **2**(4):216–19.

103. Langmore SE. Endoscopic evaluation of oral and pharyngeal phases of swallowing. *GI Motility online* (2006), doi:10.1038/gimo28, nature.com 2006.

104. Gramigna GD. How to perform video-fluoroscopic swallowing studies. GI Motility online (2006), doi:10.1038/gimo95, nature.com 2006.

105. Rosenbek JC, Robbins JA, Roecker EB, Coyle JL, Wood JL. A penetration-aspiration scale. *Dysphagia* 1996; **11**(2):93–8.

106. Hess DR. Tracheostomy tubes and related appliances. *Respir Care* 2005; **50**(4):497–510.

107. Ward AB. Spasticity treatment with botulinum toxins. *J Neural Transm* 2008; **115**(4):607–16.

108. Rosales RL, Chua-Yap AS. Evidence-based systematic review on the efficacy and safety of botulinum toxin-A therapy in post-stroke spasticity. *J Neural Transm* 2008; **115**(4):617–23.

109. Cappa SF, Benke T, Clarke S, Rossi B, Stemmer B, van Heugten CM. EFNS guidelines on cognitive rehabilitation: report of an EFNS task force. *Eur J Neurol* 2005; **12**(9):665–80.

110. Beis JM, Keller C, Morin N, Bartolomeo P, Bernati T, Chokron S, et al. Right spatial neglect after left hemisphere stroke: qualitative and quantitative study. *Neurology* 2004; **63**(9):1600–5.

111. Karnath HO, Christ K, Hartje W. Decrease of contralateral neglect by neck muscle vibration and spatial orientation of trunk midline. *Brain* 1993; **116** (Pt 2):383–96.

112. Thimm M, Fink GR, Kust J, Karbe H, Sturm W. Impact of alertness training on spatial neglect: a behavioural and fMRI study. *Neuropsychologia* 2006; **44**(7):1230–46.

113. Shindo K, Sugiyama K, Huabao L, Nishijima K, Kondo T, Izumi S. Long-term effect of low-frequency repetitive transcranial magnetic stimulation over the unaffected posterior parietal cortex in patients with unilateral spatial neglect. *J Rehabil Med* 2006; **38**(1):65–7.

114. Nyffeler T, Cazzoli D, Wurtz P, Luthi M, von Wartburg R, Chaves S, et al. Neglect-like visual exploration behaviour after theta burst transcranial magnetic stimulation of the right posterior parietal cortex. *Eur J Neurosci* 2008; **27**(7):1809–13.

115. Nelles G, Esser J, Eckstein A, Tiede A, Gerhard H, Diener HC. Compensatory visual field training for patients with hemianopia after stroke. *Neurosci Lett* 2001; **306**(3):189–92.

116. Schmielau F, Wong EK Jr. Recovery of visual fields in brain-lesioned patients by reaction perimetry treatment. *J Neuroeng Rehabil* 2007; **4**:31.

117. Karnath HO. Pusher syndrome – a frequent but little-known disturbance of body orientation perception. *J Neurol* 2007; **254**(4): 415–24.

118. Steultjens EM, Dekker J, Bouter LM, Leemrijse CJ, van den Ende CH. Evidence of the efficacy of occupational therapy in different conditions: an overview of systematic reviews. *Clin Rehabil* 2005; **19**(3):247–54.

119. Schnakers C, Majerus S, Goldman S, Boly M, Van Eeckhout P, Gay S, et al. Cognitive function in the locked-in syndrome. *J Neurol* 2008; **255**(3):323–30.

120. Smith E, Delargy M. Locked-in syndrome. *BMJ* 2005; **330**(7488):406–9.

121. Lo SF, Chen SY, Lin HC, Jim YF, Meng NH, Kao MJ. Arthrographic and clinical findings in patients with hemiplegic shoulder pain. *Arch Phys Med Rehabil* 2003; **84**(12):1786–91.

122. Braus DF, Krauss JK, Strobel J. The shoulder-hand syndrome after stroke: a prospective clinical trial. *Ann Neurol* 1994; **36**(5):728–733.

123. Hackett ML, Anderson CS, House A, Halteh C. Interventions for preventing depression after stroke. *Cochrane Database Syst Rev* 2008(3):CD003689.

124. Sagberg F. Driver health and crash involvement: a case-control study. *Accid Anal Prev* 2006; **38**(1):28–34.

125. Fisk GD, Owsley C, Pulley LV. Driving after stroke: driving exposure, advice, and evaluations. *Arch Phys Med Rehabil* 1997; **78**(12):1338–45.

126. Akinwuntan AE, De Weerdt W, Feys H, Pauwels J, Baten G, Arno P, et al. Effect of simulator training on driving after stroke: a randomized controlled trial. *Neurology* 2005; **65**(6):843–50.

127. Rees PM, Fowler CJ, Maas CP. Sexual function in men and women with neurological disorders. *Lancet* 2007; **369**(9560):512–25.

Index